Microbiology in Clinical Practice

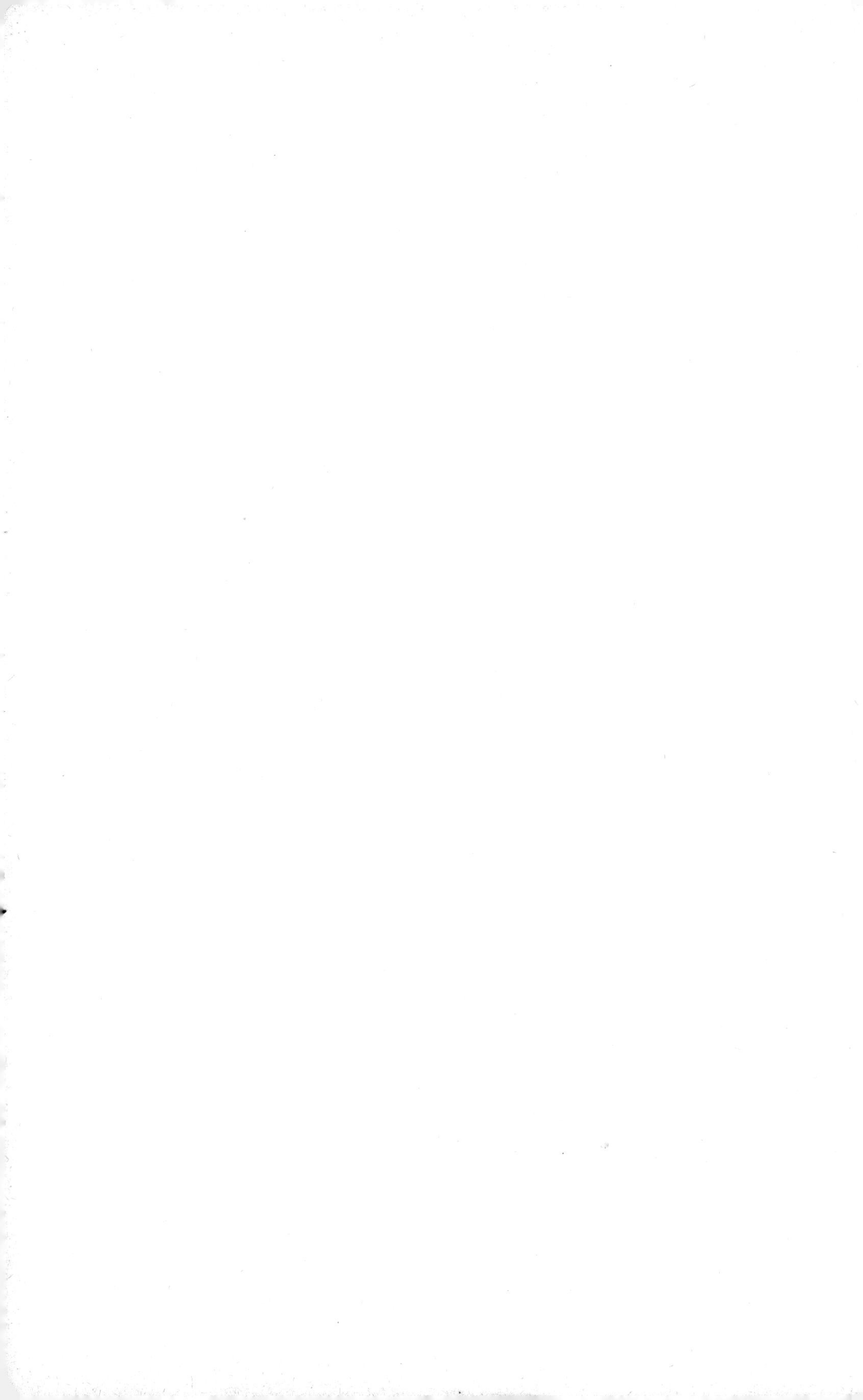

Microbiology in Clinical Practice

D. C. Shanson MB, MRCPath

Consultant Clinical Microbiologist,
St Stephen's Hospital, London SW 10

Senior Lecturer in Medical Microbiology,
Westminster Medical School, London

WRIGHT · PSG

Bristol London Boston
1982

Department of Clinical Microbiology,
St Stephen's Hospital,
London SW10 9TH. 1982

Published by:
John Wright & Sons Ltd, 42–44 Triangle West, Bristol BS8 1EX, England.
John Wright PSG Inc., 545 Great Road, Littleton, Massachusetts 01460, U.S.A.

British Library Cataloguing in Publication Data
Shanson, D. C.
Microbiology in clinical practice.
1. Medical microbiology
I. Title
616′.01′024616 QR46

ISBN 0 7236 0577 7

Library of Congress Catalog Card Number: 81-71446

Typeset and printed in Great Britain by
John Wright & Sons (Printing) Ltd. at the Stonebridge Press, Bristol BS4 5NU

Dedicated to

ELIZABETH, ESTHER and SARAH

Preface

This book is primarily intended for junior hospital doctors and senior medical students as a comprehensive guide in applying microbiological knowledge to the clinical management of infection. Microbiological and relevant clinical information are integrated as far as possible throughout the book. Some elementary knowledge of the subject is assumed but the first three chapters on general principles of microbiology and chemotherapy should assist quick revision. Although longer than some of the books on bacteriology that medical students are advised to read, the presentation of facts in an easily understood form, and their relationship to clinical problems, should fill a 'vacuum'. Medical students should particularly learn the main causative organisms, the principal diagnostic investigations and recommended drugs for each type of infection.

The book should be of particular value to clinical doctors sitting the first part of the MRCP examination, the Diploma in Child Health, or the primary FRCS examination, to medical students taking the Final MB examinations, and to pathology or microbiology trainees studying for the examinations of the Royal College of Pathologists. Science graduates and senior MLSO staff should also find the book useful for referring to microbiological facts in a clinical context. Further reading sections are included at the end of each chapter and an up-to-date brief survey of antimicrobial drugs is included in the appendix at the end of the book.

I am especially grateful to Professor D. C. E. Speller, of the Department of Clinical Microbiology at the Bristol Royal Infirmary, for valuable comments on early drafts and for encouraging me to write in the first place. I wish to particularly thank Dr Elizabeth Price, Senior Lecturer in Medical Microbiology at the Institute of Child Health, London, for reading the entire book and making many helpful criticisms during its preparation. Thanks are also due to many other colleagues and I would like to mention Dr T. Rogers, Senior Lecturer in Medical Microbiology at Westminster Medical School, Dr A. Pallett and Dr S. Namnyak, Senior House Officers in Pathology at St Stephen's Hospital, and Miss Teresa Johnson, medical student, for reading individual chapters and for helpful comments. There were several secretaries who typed the manuscript, but I would particularly like to thank Miss Lesley Heape and Miss Carolyn Fuller for patiently unravelling most of my hieroglyphics. I am grateful to Dr S. Crook, Senior Registrar in Medical Microbiology, at St Stephen's Hospital, for help with reading the proofs. Finally I am grateful to the publishers, John Wright and Sons Ltd, and to Mr Roy Baker, in particular, for their understanding and co-operation during the preparation of the book.

D. C. Shanson

Acknowledgements for Illustrations

I am grateful to the owners of the copyright for permission to use the following illustrations.

Professor S. Selwyn, Department of Medical Microbiology, Westminster Medical School and the Department of Medical Illustration, Westminster Hospital, London, for:

Fig. 3.3: Antibiotic synergy plate. Reproduced from *The Beta-Lactam Antibiotics* (fig. 6, p. 143), Hodder & Stoughton Educational.
Fig. 8.1: Elek plate for *C. diphtheriae.*
Fig. 9.2: Gas–liquid chromatography tracing.
Fig. 10.1: Rash of meningococcal septicaemia.
Fig. 21.2: Reduviid cone-nosed triatomid bug.
Fig. 22.2: *Plasmodium falciparum* in a blood film.
Fig. 23.1: *Ascaris lumbricoides.*
Fig. 23.2: Threadworm ova.
Fig. 23.3: *Schistosoma haematobium* ovum.

Professor A. J. Dudgeon and the Board of Governors of the Hospital for Sick Children, London, for:

Fig. 7.1: Congenital rubella: unilateral cataract

Professor A. J. Dudgeon and the Medical Department, The British Council, for:

Fig. 7.2.: Pathogenesis of congenital rubella. Reproduced from Dudgeon J. (1969), *British Medical Bulletin*, vol. 25, no. 2, p. 160, Fig. 1.

Mr S. Brown and the Department of Medical Photography, Kensington and Chelsea Group of Hospitals, London, for:

Fig. 3.2: Stokes antibiotic sensitivity plate.
Fig. 18.2: '3 tube' antibiotic combination test.

Dr Y. Clayton, and the Institute of Dermatology, London, for:

Fig. 13.1: Forearm of a patient with tuberculoid leprosy.
Fig. 16.1: Tinea capitis.
Fig. 16.2: Tinea corporis.
Fig. 16.3: *Microsporum canis* macroconidia.
Fig. 16.4: *Malassezia furfur* in skin scraping.

Mr S. Rice and Dr E. Price, Department of Medical Microbiology, Queen Elizabeth Hospital for Children, London, for:

Fig. 12.1: Electron micrograph of Influenza A virus.
Fig. 14.2: Electron micrograph of *Campylobacter jejuni.*
Fig. 14.3: Electron micrograph of Rota virus.

Dr June D. Almeida, and the Wellcome Research Laboratories, Beckenham, Kent, for:

Fig. 15.2: Electron micrograph of hepatitis B antigen
Medical Education (International). Ltd., for:
Fig. 12.2: Gram-stained smear of sputum from a patient with pneumococcal pneumonia. Reproduced from Shanson D. C. (1979), *Medicine*, 3rd Series, vol. 23, p. 1183.

International Medicine and Franklin Scientific Publications for:
Fig. 12.3: Chest X-ray of a patient with Legionnaires' disease
Reproduced from Shanson D. C. (1980), *International Medicine*, vol. 1, no. 3, 2–5, Fig. 3.

Professor C. L. Berry, Department of Morbid Anatomy, The London Hospital Medical College, London, for:
Fig. 18.1: Chapter 18, *Staph. aureus* endocarditis vegetation on triscupid heart valve.

We acknowledge the kind help of the Pharmaceuticals Division, ICI.

ERRATA

On the Contents page —
Abbreviations are on page xxi
The Foreword is on page xxiii

On page 40 (*Table 3.5*) —
Candida and *Histoplasma*
should come under Ketoconazole,
not under Griseofulvin

Contents

'Priority' Reading in this Book for Medical Students

Information which is especially relevant for undergraduate study is included in the following parts of the book:

Chapter		Recommended 'priority' reading
1	Use of the laboratory	*Reading of the whole of these three chapters suggested*
2	Classification and pathogenicity of microbes	
3	Chemotherapy—general principles	
4	Pyrexia of unknown origin	*Most of each of these chapters, but details of treatment, e.g. doses of drugs, not necessary*
5	Septicaemia	
6	Opportunistic infections	
7	Obstetric and neonatal infections	
8	Infections of children	*Respiratory infections, rubella and immunization*
9	Anaerobic infections	*Reading of the entire chapter*
10	Infections of central nervous system	*Reading of the entire chapter, especially meningitis due to the three primary pathogens*
11	ENT and eye infections	*Most of this chapter*
12	Infections of the lower respiratory tract	*Most of this chapter*
13	Mycobacterial and actinomycete infections	*TB, leprosy and actinomycosis*
14	Infections of the gastro-intestinal tract	*Enteric fever, gastro-enteritis, food poisoning, dysentery and giardiasis*
15	Hepatic infections	*Mainly viral hepatitis*

16	Skin infections	*Boils, carbuncles, erysipelas and cellulitis, impetigo, ringworm (dermatophytes), burns*
17	Bone and joint infections	*Acute osteomyelitis, septic and 'reactive' arthritis*
18	Infections of the heart	*Reading of the entire chapter*
19	Infections of the urinary tract	*Definitions, 'significant bacteriuria', predisposing factors, main causative organisms, screening, infection of children, the main investigations (but excluding localization tests)*
20	Sexually transmitted diseases	*Syphilis, gonorrhoea, chlamydial infections, genital herpes, candida/trichomonas vaginitis, scabies and pediculosis pubis*
21	Zoonoses	*Introductory section and a few main examples of bacterial, protozoal, viral zoonoses, etc.*
22	Arthropod-borne infections and viral haemorrhagic fevers	*Tables mainly included for reference and quick revision; malaria, visceral leishmaniasis and yellow fever*
23	Worms	*Main tapeworms, roundworms, flukes; schistosomiasis, hydatid and filarial worms are particularly important*

24	Hospital infection	*General considerations at beginning of chapter and staphylococcal wound sepsis*
25	Disinfection and sterilization	*Most of this chapter*

Appendix 1 Basic characteristics of some important bacterial pathogens

At the end of each chapter references that are particularly recommended for further study by undergraduates are indicated.

Abbreviations

AFB	Acid-fast bacilli
AHG	Anti-human immunoglobulin
ALLO	Atypical *Legionella*-like organism
ASO	Anti-streptolysin O titre
BFP	Biological false positive reaction
CAT	Computerized axial tomography
CAP	Cellulose acetate precipitin amoebic antibody test
CFT	Complement fixation test
CIE	Counter-current immunoelectrophoresis
CLED	Cysteine lactose electrolyte-deficient medium
CMV	Cytomegalovirus
CNS	Central nervous system
CSF	Cerebrospinal fluid
CSSD	Central sterile supply department
CVP	Central venous pressure
DCA	Desoxycholate citrate agar
DGI	Dark-ground illumination
DIC	Disseminated intravascular coagulation
ECHO	Enteric cytopathogenic human orphan
ELISA	Enzyme-linked immunosorbent assay
EMSU	Early morning specimen of urine
ENL	Erythema nodosum leprosum
FTA	Fluorescent treponemal antibody test
GCFT	Gonococcal complement fixation test
GLC	Gas–liquid chromatography
HAV	Hepatitis A virus
HBcAg	Hepatitis B core antigen
HBsAg	Hepatitis B surface antigen
HDCSV	Human diploid cell strain vaccine
HPLC	High pressure liquid chromatography
HVS	High vaginal swab
Ig	Immunoglobulin
IPPR	Intermittent positive pressure respiration
IVP	Intravenous pyelogram
LGV	Lymphogranuloma venereum
LPS	Lipopolysaccharide
MBC	Minimum bactericidal concentration
MCU	Micturating cysto-urethrography
MIC	Minimal inhibitory concentration
MIF	Macrophage inhibition factor
MOEH	Medical Officer for Environmental Health
MSU	Mid-stream sample of urine
NBT	Nitroblue tetrazolium dye test
NSA	Non-sporing anaerobic
NSU	Non-specific urethritis
PPD	Purified protein derivative
PUO	Pyrexia of unknown origin

QAC	Quaternary ammonium compound
RES	Reticulo-endothelial system
RPCFT	Reiter protein complement fixation test
RSV	Respiratory syncytial virus
RTD	Routine test dilution
Rubella HAI	Rubella haemagglutination antibody inhibition test
SLE	Systemic lupus erythematosus
SSPE	Sub-acute sclerosing panencephalitis
TAB	Typhoid and parathyphoid A and B vaccine
TCBS	Thiosulphate-citrate-bile salt-sucrose agar
TPHA	*Treponema pallidum* haemagglutination antibody test
TPI	*Treponema pallidum* immobilization antibody test
TRIC	Trachoma inclusion conjunctivitis agent
TSSU	Theatre sterile supply unit
VCT	Vancomycin, colistin and trimethoprim medium
VDRL	Venereal disease reference laboratory antibody test
WBC	White blood cell count
WR	Wassermann reaction

Foreword

D. C. E. Speller MA, BM, BCh(Oxon), FRCP, MRCPath

Professor of Clinical Bacteriology,
University of Bristol

Honorary Consultant Microbiologist,
Bristol Royal Infirmary

Those of us who teach clinical microbiology, and who ourselves recognize the particular interest of the specialty, are often at a loss to recommend a general book on the subject. Microbiology textbooks, arranged according to genera and species of micro-organisms, do not commend themselves to those whose interests are the diagnosis and practical management of infection. Too often virology, mycology and parasitology are separately dealt with as advanced secondary specialties. Which book can be recommended to a clinical medical student who wishes to read more deeply of medical microbiology than he can in textbooks of medicine or infectious diseases? Which book for the young surgeon or physician approaching his professional examinations? Which for the trainee pathologist, to complement books of more laboratory-directed information?

This need for clinically based books has been recognized recently, and I have watched the development of Dr Shanson's extensive clinical microbiology with interest. I warmly welcome the finished book. Infections caused by all types of micro-organism, including recently recognized syndromes, are included, and they are presented in practically useful sections—mainly by body systems, but also by aetiological agent, age group or epidemiological pattern, when these are more relevant. With the practical advice on the use of the laboratory and on therapy, this book should make an important contribution to the knowledge and management of infective disease.

SECTION A

General Principles

Chapter 1

Classification and pathogenicity of microbes

So, naturalists observe, a flea
Hath smaller fleas that on him prey;
And these have smaller fleas to bite 'em,
And so proceed ad infinitum.

Jonathan Swift, *On Poetry*

The microbial causes of human disease include viruses, chlamydiae, rickettsiae, mycoplasmas, bacteria, fungi and protozoa. Basic features of these are included in *Table 1.1*. Arthropods and worms are discussed in later chapters.

Viruses differ greatly from all the other microbes as they consist essentially of only nucleic acid surrounded by a protein coat (capsid) and contain only one instead of two types of nucleic acid. Once inside human cells, the viruses remove the normal nuclear control of the cells to take over cellular metabolism for the synthesis of new virions. Chlamydiae and rickettsiae are also obligate intra-cellular parasites, have both DNA and RNA, and multiply by binary fission. Mycoplasmas, bacteria and fungi can be cultured in cell-free media unlike the above intra-cellular microbes.

Bacterial causes of disease are mainly 'lower' bacteria which are unicellular. Multiplication is predominantly by asexual binary fission although biological variation is facilitated in some species by 'sex', especially with Gram-negative species such as *Escherichia coli*. Only a few 'higher' bacteria cause disease in man, such as *Actinomycetes israelii* which are filamentous Gram-positive bacilli.

Protozoa pathogenic to man are divided into three main groups:

i. Sarcodina (amoebae), e.g. *Entamoeba histolytica*
ii. Sporozoa, e.g. *Plasmodium falciparum, Toxoplasma gondii*
iii. Mastigophora (flagellates), e.g. *Trichomonas vaginalis, Giardia lamblia, Leishmania* and *Trypanosoma* species

CLASSIFICATION OF BACTERIA

There are three main groups of bacteria:

i. Bacteria that are readily Gram-stained
ii. Acid-fast bacilli
iii. Spirochaetes

Table 1.1. Classification of microbes

Type of microbe	*Nucleic acids*	*Multiplication*		*Approx. size, μm*	*Seen by light microscope*	*Cell wall*	*Cyto-plasmic membrane*	*Sensitive to 'antibiotics'*	*Other features*
		Intracellular	*Extracellular*						
Viruses	DNA or RNA	+ (Virus takes over control of cell to synthesize new virions)	–	0·01–0·3	No	No	No	No	Host cell may show inclusions
Chlamydiae e.g. *C. trachomatis*, *C. psittaci*)	DNA +RNA	+ (Multiplication by binary fission)	–	0·3	No	No	Yes	Yes (e.g. tetra-cyclines)	Host cell shows character-istic inclusions
Rickettsiae *Coxiella* (e.g. *R. prow-azeki*)	DNA +RNA	+ (Multiplication by binary fission)	– (Occasional exceptions)	0·3	Sometimes just visible by special stains	Rudimentary cell wall	Yes	Yes (e.g. tetra-cyclines)	'Typhus' trans-mitted by arthropods
Mycoplasmas (e.g. *M. pneu-moniae*, *M. hominis*)	DNA +RNA	+ (Multiplication involves 'ele-mentary bodies	+	0·12–0·3	Sometimes just visible by special stains	No	Yes	Yes (e.g. tetra-cyclines)	Pleomorphic cells
Bacteria	DNA +RNA	±	+ (Multiplication by binary fission)	0·5–0·8 long	Yes	Yes (Muramic acid usually present)	Yes	Yes	Rigid cell wall
Fungi	DNA +RNA	+	+	Larger than bacteria (>5 long, >0·5 wide)	Yes	Yes Thicker than bacterial wall + con-tains sterol	Yes	No sensitive to anti-fungal drugs	Members of plant kingdom but no chlorophyll
Protozoa	DNA +RNA	± (Depends on particular species)	±	Larger than fungi	Yes	Yes	Yes	Not usually	

Bacteria that are Readily Gram-stained

These are classified into Gram-positive (blue-purple) or Gram-negative (pink-red) cocci or bacilli (*Table 1.2*).

Practical details of the Gram-stain are given in the Appendix to Chapter 2, p. 28. After the application of the methyl violet dye, Gram-positive bacteria stain blue and this colour is retained in spite of decolorization with acetone (or alcohol). Gram-negative bacteria initially stain blue after the methyl violet is applied, but the colour is lost after the application of acetone (or alcohol). They then take up the pink counterstain (saffronin, methyl red or carbol fuchsin).

The reason for the difference in colour after Gram-staining is not fully understood, but it is probably related to the large amount of mucopeptide and teichoic acid in the cell walls of Gram-positive bacteria. The fact that Gram-positive bacteria are more acidic than Gram-negative bacteria may account for their greater affinity for a basic dye. Even more important may be the greater permeability of Gram-negative cell walls which allow the methyl violet–iodine dye complex to diffuse out after treatment with acetone more readily than the cell walls of Gram-positive bacteria.

Within each subgroup, there are aerobic or anaerobic examples. The majority of bacterial pathogens can grow either aerobically or anaerobically, i.e. they are 'facultative anaerobes' such as *Staphylococcus aureus* or *Escherichia coli*; in *Table 1.2* these have been included as 'aerobes'. There are a few bacterial species which are strict aerobes, such as *Pseudomonas aeruginosa*, which will not grow at all anaerobically. Some bacterial species are strict anaerobes, such as *Clostridium tetani* or *Bacteroides fragilis*, which will not grow at all aerobically.

Exceptional Gram-stainable bacteria include *Legionella pneumophila* and *Borrelia vincenti*. *Legionella pneumophila* requires prolonged staining with the counterstain to be seen in tissues, although it appears readily as Gram-negative bacilli in smears made from colonies on agar media. *Borrelia vincenti* is the only spirochaetal pathogen that is easily seen by a Gram-stain.

Acid-fast Bacilli

Mycobacterial species are not readily seen by a Gram-stain, although they are weakly Gram-positive bacilli. Ziehl-Neelsen or other acid-fast stains are required for staining these organisms which have cell walls containing abundant lipids. Examples include *Mycobacterium tuberculosis* and *Mycobacterium leprae*.

Spirochaetes

Spirochaetes are thin-walled spiralled flexible organisms which are motile by means of an axial filament. They are not seen in a Gram-stain (except *B. vincenti*), but may be seen either by dark-ground illumination microscopy, or in a silver stain under the light microscope. Borrelia spirochaetes in the blood may also be seen in a Giemsa stain.

The three groups of spirochaetes include:

i. *Treponema*
   Spirochaetes with regular spirals, approximately 1 μm apart from each other, 5–15 μm long and about 0·2 μm wide, e.g. *Treponema pallidum* (cause of syphilis)

Table 1.2. Simple classification of Gram-stainable bacterial pathogens

Bacteria					*Genus*	*Species examples*
Gram-positive Bacteria	*Cocci*	Aerobic	(Clusters)		*Staphylococcus*	*S. aureus*
						S. albus (*S. epidermidis*)
			(Chains/pairs)		*Streptococcus*	*S. pneumoniae*, *S. pyogenes*
						S. viridans, *S. faecalis*
		Anaerobic			*Streptococcus*	*S. putridus*
	Bacilli	Aerobic	(Sporing)		*Bacillus*	*B. anthracis*
			(Non-sporing)		*Corynebacterium*	*C. diphtheriae*
					Listeria	*L. monocytogenes*
					Nocardia	*N. asteroides*
		Anaerobic	(Sporing)		*Clostridium*	*C. tetani*
						C. welchii (*perfringens*)
			(Non-sporing)		*Propionibacterium*	*P. acnes*
					Actinomycetes	*A. israelii*
Gram-negative Bacteria	*Cocci*	Aerobic	(Pairs)		*Neisseria*	*N. meningitidis*
						N. gonorrhoeae
		Anaerobic			*Veillonella*	
	Bacilli	Aerobic	*a.* Enterobacteria	e.g.	*Escherichia*	*E. coli*
					Klebsiella	*K. aerogenes*
					Proteus	*P. mirabilis*
					Serratia	*S. marcescens*
					Salmonella	*S. typhi*
					Shigella	*Sh. sonnei*
			b. Pseudomonas		*Pseudomonas*	*P. aeruginosa*
			c. Vibrios		*Vibrio*	*V. cholerae*
					Campylobacter	*C. jejuni*
			d. Parvobacteria		*Haemophilus*	*H. influenzae*
					Brucella	*B. abortus*
					Bordetella	*B. pertussis*
					Pasteurella, *Yersinia*	*P. multocida*, *Y. pestis*
			e. Legionella		*Legionella*	*L. pneumophila*
			f. Spirillum		*Spirillum*	*S. minus*
		Anaerobic			*Bacteroides*	*B. fragilis*

ii. *Leptospira*
Spirochaetes which have tightly coiled spirals, 5–15 μm long and about 0·1 μm wide. Characteristically, there is often a 'hooked' end, e.g. *Leptospira icterohaemorrhagiae* (cause of Weil's disease).

iii. *Borrelia*
Large spirochaetes, 10–30 μm long and about 0·3 μm wide, with irregular spirals 2–4 μm apart from each other, e.g. *Borrelia recurrentis* (a cause of relapsing fever).

CLASSIFICATION OF VIRUSES

The classification of viruses depends on several factors including the type of nucleic acid present, the arrangement of the capsids into a cubical (icosahedral), helical or complex symmetry, the number of capsomeres, the size of the virus particle and whether the virion is naked or enveloped (often indicated by ether resistance or sensitivity, respectively, as well as by electron microscopic appearance). The main viruses causing disease in man are classified in *Table 1.3*.

One way of memorizing which viruses contain DNA is to remember that 'PHA*D*' is for *D*NA viruses, with *P* for Pox and Papova, *H* for herpes, *AD* for Adenoviruses. Virtually all the remaining pathogenic human viruses are RNA viruses including the self-explanatory pico*rna* viruses ('PicoRNA' viruses).

Some DNA viruses may cause tumours in man. These include papilloma virus causing warts, Epstein-Barr virus causing Burkitt's lymphoma and associated with naso-pharyngeal carcinoma, and herpes simplex virus which is associated with carcinoma of the cervix (*see* Jawetz et al., 1980).

CLASSIFICATION OF FUNGI

The fungi causing diseases in man belong to the class 'fungi imperfecti'. There are four main groups of pathogenic fungi: moulds (filamentous fungi), true yeasts, yeast-like fungi and dimorphic fungi.

i. *Filamentous fungi*
These grow as long filaments called 'hyphae' and the branched hyphae intertwine to form a 'mycelium'. Reproduction is by spores including sexual spores which are used for identification. Culture in vitro of these fungi on Sabouraud's medium often shows 'powdery' colonies due to the presence of abundant spores, e.g. *Trichophyton mentagrophytes*.

ii. *True yeasts*
These are unicellular round or oval fungi. Reproduction is by budding from the parent cell. Cultures in vitro characteristically show 'creamy' colonies, e.g. *Cryptococcus neoformans*.

iii. *Yeast-like fungi*
These are like yeasts since they may appear as round or oval cells and grow by budding. They may also form long non-branching filaments known as 'pseudohyphae', e.g. *Candida albicans*.

iv. *Dimorphic fungi*
These grow as yeast forms in the body and at 37 °C on culture media. They also form mycelia in the environment and on culture media at 22 °C. Several examples of this group of fungi grow intra-cellularly in reticulo-endothelial cells in infected patients, e.g. *Histoplasma capsulatum*.

Table 1.3. Classification of viruses

Nucleic acid	*Capsid arrangement*	*Naked or enveloped*	*Size of virus particle*, nm	*Number of capsomers*	*Virus family*	*Virus examples*	*Diseases*
DNA	Cubical (icosahedral)	Enveloped	100–200	162	Herpes viruses	Herpes simplex, I and II	Mucocutaneous herpetic lesions
						Varicella-zoster	Chickenpox and 'shingles'
						Cytomegalovirus	Cytomegalovirus inclusion disease
						Epstein-Barr virus	Glandular fever and Burkitt's lymphoma
DNA	Cubical	Naked	70–90	252	Adeno-viruses	Over 30 serological types of adenoviruses	Pharyngo-conjunctivitis Lower respiratory infections in infants
						Adenovirus type 8	Epidemic kerato-conjuncti-vitis ('shipyards eye')
DNA	Cubical	Naked	45–55	72	Papova-viruses	Papilloma virus	Warts
						SV 40 type viruses	Progressive multifocal leucoencephalopathy
DNA	Complex	Complex coat	Approx. 200 × 400		Pox viruses	Variola	Smallpox (now extinct)
						Monkeypox	Monkeypox (rarely affects man)
						Vaccinia	Vaccinial skin lesions after vaccination
						Orf	Contagious pustular dermatitis—orf
						Molluscum contagiosum	Molluscum contagiosum

Table 1.3 (cont.)

Nucleic acid	Capsid arrangement	Naked or enveloped	Size of virus particle, nm	Number of capsomers	Virus family	Virus examples	Diseases
RNA	Cubical	Enveloped	30–90		Toga viruses	Alpha and flavi viruses	Arthropod borne fevers, e.g. equine encephalitis, yellow fever
RNA	Cubical	Naked	20–30	32	Picorna-viruses	Enteroviruses—polio	Poliomyelitis
						—echo	Respiratory and CNS infections
						—coxsackie A/B	Respiratory, CNS and heart infections
						Rhinoviruses	Colds
RNA	Cubical	Naked	60–80		Reo-viruses	Rotavirus (wheel-like shape)	Gastro-enteritis
RNA	Helical	Enveloped	80–120		Ortho-myxo-viruses	Influenza A/B viruses	Influenza
					Paramyxo-viruses	Para-influenza viruses	Para-influenza
						Respiratory syncytial virus	Bronchiolitis, 'croup' and colds
						Mumps	Mumps
						Measles	Measles
RNA	Helical	Enveloped	Approx. 70 × 170		Rhabdo-viruses ('bullet' shaped)	Rabies virus	Rabies
RNA	Helical	Enveloped	90–100		Bunya-viruses	California arborviruses	Arthropod-borne fevers
RNA	Unknown	Enveloped	50–300		Arena-viruses	Lassa fever virus	Lassa fever
						Lymphocytic chorio-meningitis	Aseptic meningitis
RNA	Complex	Enveloped	80–130		Corona-viruses	Coronaviruses	Upper respiratory infections

Fungi can also be classified according to whether they cause superficial or deep mycoses in infected patients and some examples are included in *Table 1.4*. The deep mycoses most frequently occur in immunocompromised patients. Disease might also arise from the ingestion of mycotoxins in food: aflatoxins may be produced by *Aspergillus flavus* in cereals in underdeveloped countries and ingestion of these toxins may cause liver damage possibly also predisposing to the development of hepatoma.

Table 1.4 Classification of fungi

Fungi	*Type of fungus*	*Disease examples*	*Geographical distribution*
Fungi causing superficial mycoses			
Dermatophytes including *Microsporum*, *Trichophyton* and *Epidermophyton* species	Filamentous	Tinea (ringworm) of skin, nails or hair	Worldwide
Aspergillus niger	Filamentous	Otitis externa	Worldwide
Candida albicans	Yeast-like	Oral thrush, monilial vaginitis Intertrigo, nappy rash Paronychia, granulomas in chronic mutocutaneous candidiasis	Worldwide
Malassezia furfur	Yeast-like	Pityriasis versicolor	Worldwide
Fungi causing deep mycoses			
Aspergillus fumigatus	Filamentous	Pulmonary or disseminated aspergillosis	Worldwide
Mucor	Filamentous	*Mucor mycosis*	Worldwide
Allescheria boydii } *Madurella* species }	Filamentous	Madura mycosis ('Madura foot')	Tropics and subtropics
Candida albicans	Yeast-like	Septicaemia, endocarditis, bronchial and renal infections	Worldwide
Cryptococcus neoformans	True yeast	Cryptococcal meningitis or pulmonary infection (Torulosis)	Worldwide
Histoplasma capsulatum	Dimorphic	Pulmonary or disseminated histoplasmosis	U.S.A. mainly
Blastomyces dermatidis	Dimorphic	North American blasto-mycosis	North America
Sporotrichum schenkii	Dimorphic	Sporotrichosis	U.S.A. and France mainly
Coccidioides immitis	Dimorphic (closest)*	Coccidioidomycosis (San Joaquin Valley fever)	U.S.A.—South Western

* 'Sporangia' in tissues, filamentous at 22 °C.

PATHOGENESIS: FACTORS AFFECTING THE 'VIRULENCE' AND SPREAD OF MICROBES

Pathogenicity

Microbes can be classified into 'pathogens', 'commensals' which are found in the normal body flora and 'saprophytes' which are found in environmental sites such as soil or plants. However, such a classification is of limited value since there are many examples of 'commensals', such as *Escherichia coli, Staph. saprophyticus* or *Streptococcus viridans* or saprophytes, such as *Mycobacterium kansasii* or *Legionella pneumophila* which may cause disease in patients under certain circumstances. The 'pathogenicity' of a microbe depends on host as well as on microbial factors and microbes can be usefully classified into 'conventional pathogens', 'conditional pathogens' and 'opportunist pathogens' (*see* p. 466, Chapter 24). Host factors include the age of the patient, genetic factors, general host defences and local host defences against infection (*see* Chapter 6 and Immunodeficiency, in Chapter 8).

'Koch's postulates' have sometimes been useful for establishing the pathogenic relationship between a microbe and a disease. These postulates include the following: (1) the particular microbe is always associated with a given disease (this microbe may be either the cause or an incidental result of the disease); (2) the microbe may be isolated in the laboratory from specimens from a patient with the disease; (3) it is possible to produce a similar disease in animals by inoculation of the microbe into animals. *Mycobacterium tuberculosis* causing tuberculosis may be taken as an example where these three postulates may be fulfilled, but there are many other examples where complete fulfilment of these postulates does not occur, as with *Treponema pallidum* and syphilis, Epstein-Barr virus and glandular fever, *Chlamydia trachomatis* and non-specific urethritis.

Factors Affecting 'Virulence'

There is a lot of variation between strains of the same microbial species or between different species, in the 'virulence' of the microbe when considering the likelihood of disease being produced in a given 'host'. An experimental measure of the 'virulence' can sometimes be obtained by estimating the LD_{50} (lethal dose) which is the dose of organisms required to kill 50% of the animal population inoculated with the particular microbe. The more virulent the strain the lower is the LD_{50}.

The main known factors that affect virulence are concerned with pathogenicity, such as toxins and capsules in bacteria, examples of which are included in *Table 1.5*. In recent years, there has been an increased interest in bacterial adhesiveness factors, such as the pili of gonococci or of *E. coli* strains that cause urinary tract infections (*see* Chapter 19). It has also become apparent that the 'virulence' of bacterial strains may also depend on the presence of transmissible genes contained in plasmids or mediated by bacteriophage. The adhesiveness to the ileal mucosa of an *E. coli* strain that produces enteritis in pigs is dependent on the presence of the K88 capsular antigen, a factor which is plasmid mediated. Enterotoxin production by this *E. coli* strain is also dependent on the presence of the appropriate plasmid. In man, the toxins produced by *Corynebacterium diphtheriae* and the erythrogenic toxin produced by *Strep. pyogenes* strains in

Table 1.5. Factors affecting 'virulence' of bacteria—some examples

Virulence factor	*Bacterial examples*	*Comment*
I. *Toxins*		
i. 'Classical exotoxins'	Gram-positive bacteria mainly, e.g. *Clostridium tetani* toxin; *Clostridium welchii* toxin; *Clostridium botulinum* toxin; *Corynebacterium diphtheriae* toxin	i. Exotoxins are highly toxic polypeptides excreted by living bacteria (micrograms kill animals). They act at specific target sites, e.g. CNS, heart ii. They are highly antigenic (exception is *C. tetani* toxin) iii. Converted to antigenic non-toxic toxoids by formalin iv. The toxin is neutralized by anti-toxin v. The toxins are often destroyed by heat
ii. Other exotoxins	Streptococcal erythrogenic toxin	Produced by *Strep. pyogenes* strains causing scarlet fever
	Staph. aureus enterotoxin:	Heat stable
	Bacillus anthracis toxic complex:	Consists of three factors which combined in a complex cause oedema, haemorrhage and collapse
	Vibrio cholerae enterotoxin; *Escherichia coli* enterotoxin; *Shigella dysenteriae* entero/neurotoxins	These enterotoxins may produce diarrhoea after stimulating epithelial adenylate cyclase
iii. 'Classical endotoxins'	Gram-negative bacteria mainly, e.g. *Salmonella typhi*; *Neisseria meningitidis*; *Escherichia coli*; *Pseudomonas aeruginosa*	i. Endotoxins are lipopolysaccharide (LPS) molecules in the outer layer of Gram-negative cell walls (released when organisms disintegrate). Lipid A is the main toxic component (hundreds of micrograms kill animals). They act non-specifically on RES cells stimulating release of mediators affecting vascular permeability and release of prostaglandins that may cause fever ii. The sugar chains present in the polysaccharide core of LPS confer 'O' antigen specificity and also affect virulence ('rough' strains instead of 'smooth' strains when the projecting sugar chains are shortened and the Gram-negative bacteria become less virulent) iii. Not converted to toxoids by formalin

Table 1.5 (cont.)

Virulence factor	*Bacterial examples*	*Comment*
		iv. Toxins do not naturally stimulate neutralizing anti-toxin although antibodies to polysaccharide 'O' antigens result v. Endotoxins are relatively heat stable vi. May be detected by the Limulus test vii. Severe endotoxaemia in patients may cause disseminated intravascular coagulation or/and fatal cardiovascular collapse
iv. Enzymes	e.g. *Staph. aureus* coagulase	Role of enzymes in man often unclear Coagulase may contribute to 'walling off' of staphylococcal lesions
	Strep. pyogenes streptolysins	Streptolysins can induce lysosomal discharge and kill polymorphs and inhibit chemotaxis
II. *Capsules and other surface antiphagocytic factors*	e.g. Capsule of *Haemophilus influenzae* Pittman type b (polysaccharide) Capsule of *Strep. pneumoniae* (polysaccharide) Capsule of *Bacillus anthracis* (polyglutamic acid) K antigen of *Escherichia coli* (polysaccharide) Vi antigen of *Sal. typhi* 'M protein' of *Strep. pyogenes*	These factors may contribute to the 'invasiveness' of some virulent bacteria by rendering the bacteria relatively resistant to either phagocytosis or killing within polymorphs or macrophages. Certain capsulated bacteria may multiply in macrophages and be disseminated throughout the body as a result, e.g. *Sal. typhi* bacilli with Vi antigen If specific antibody (opsonins) has developed to the capsule or surface component the anti-phagocytic effect may be reduced
	Protein A of *Staph. aureus*	Blocks phagocytosis of opsonised pathogenic strains of *Staph. aureus* possibly by interfering with attachment of Fc portions of IgG opsonins to surface of polymorphs

scarlet fever patients are dependent on genes mediated by temperate phages. The fact that particular microbes appear to be more or less virulent at different times, might be due in part to the presence or absence of these types of transmissible genes. Scarlet fever is much less frequent than 50 years ago although streptococcal sore throats are still common. Skin sepsis due to *Staph. aureus* strains in hospital maternity units appears to be much less serious than in the 1950s. The microbial and the other factors that affect the virulence, and the spread of pathogens are often unclear (*see* Williams, 1976).

Factors affecting Spread

Epidemiological factors affecting the 'host' are relevant to the spread of microbes including the numbers of susceptible individuals in a geographically defined area, the proximity of the individuals to each other and to the source of infection, and the presence of other factors necessary for the transmission of infection, such as the correct climate or season, the presence of an essential arthropod vector, etc. These and other factors are discussed where relevant in the subsequent chapters where sporadic, endemic or epidemic infections are described.

Microbial factors that affect the spread depend partly on the 'virulence' of the microbe and partly on the ability of the microbe to survive or multiply in a given inanimate environment ('fomites' such as bedclothes, 'vehicles' such as milk or water) or on the hands of patients or hospital staff or in animals/arthropods. Above all, the microbe must have the ability to initiate an infection in a patient in as low a dose as possible, have an effective portal of entry for establishing infection, as well as a method of exit from the body where it can be shed in large numbers for as long as possible. 'Carrier' states clearly aid the transmission of bacteria. Gram-positive bacteria survive reasonably well in 'dry' environments while Gram-negative bacteria and some spirochaetes survive best in moist situations.

Microbes are either transmitted horizontally, i.e. between individuals of the same generation (such as the plague bacillus) or vertically, i.e. between individuals of different generations (such as congenital rubella from mother to infant). Hepatitis B is one example of an infection that is vertically transmitted between many millions of people in the underdeveloped world.

Infection is either endogenous, from the patient's own flora, or exogenous, from a source outside such as another patient or person, an animal, a 'vehicle' or 'fomite'. Modes of transmission of microbes include: (1) direct contact, such as with *Neisseria gonorrhoeae*; (2) ingestion, such as with *Vibrio cholerae*; (3) inoculation, such as with a 'sharps' injury transmitting hepatitis B, mosquito bite transmitting malaria or dog bite transmitting rabies; (4) inhalation, such as with measles virus, rhinoviruses or *Mycobacterium tuberculosis*. Numerous diseases are transmitted by the airborne route either by sprays of infected droplets or secretions (by coughing, sneezing or spitting) which contaminate clothing, hands, handkerchiefs (such as with rhinoviruses causing common colds) or by respiratory droplet nuclei (such as with measles virus). The droplet nuclei (1–10 μm in diameter) result from the evaporation of large droplets and may travel long distances as they become suspended in the air.

SYNOPSIS OF MEDICALLY IMPORTANT BACTERIA

See section on basic characteristics of bacteria that can be Gram-stained, p. 516.

Further Reading

Christie A. B. (1980) *Infectious Diseases: Epidemiology and Clinical Practice*, 3rd ed. Edinburgh, Churchill Livingstone.

*Cruickshank R., Duguid J. P., Marmion B. P. et al. (1975) *Medical Microbiology*. Edinburgh, Churchill Livingstone.

Emond R. T. D. (1974) *A Colour Atlas of Infectious Diseases*. London, Wolfe Medical Books.

Jawetz E., Melnick J. C. and Adelberg E. A. (1980) *Review of Medical Microbiology*, 14th ed. Los Altos, California, Lange Medical Publications, pp. 506–535.

Lambert H. P. (1979) The pathogenesis of diarrhoea of bacterial origin. In: Reeves D. and Geddes A. (ed.) *Recent Advances in Infection*. Edinburgh, Churchill Livingstone.

Mandell G. L., Douglas R. G. and Bennett J. E. (1979) *Principles of Infectious Diseases*, 2 vols. Chichester, John Wiley.

*Mims C. (1976) *The Pathogenesis of Infectious Disease*. London, Academic Press.

Olds R. J. (1975) *A Colour Atlas of Microbiology*. London, Wolfe Medical Books.

Stokes E. J. and Ridgway G. L. (1980) *Clinical Bacteriology*, 5th ed. London, Edward Arnold.

*Stratford B. C. (1977) *An Atlas of Medical Microbiology: Common Human Pathogens*. Oxford, Blackwell Scientific Publications.

*Timbury M. (1978) *Notes on Medical Virology*, 6th ed. Edinburgh, Churchill Livingstone.

Williams R. E. O. (1976) The flux of infection. *Proc. R. Soc. Med.* **69**, 797–803.

Wilson G. J. and Miles A. A. (1975) *Topley and Wilson's Principles and Practice of Bacteriology, Virology and Immunity*, 6th ed. London, Edward Arnold.

Youmans G. P., Paterson P. Y. and Sommers H. M. (1980) *The Biological and Clinical Basis of Infectious Diseases*, 2nd ed. Philadelphia, Saunders.

* This reference is particularly recommended for further reading by undergraduates.

Chapter 2

Use of the microbiology laboratory—general principles

This chapter is mainly concerned with the general principles involved in making the best use of the laboratory. The principles of the diagnosis of microbial disease are also discussed in relation to the examination of the specimens and interpretation of the results from the laboratory. The use of the laboratory should not be confined to the sending of specimens. Hospital doctors and medical practitioners in the community should be aware of the other work of the laboratory and the role of the consultant clinical microbiologist (*Table 2.1*).

COLLECTION OF CLINICALLY RELEVANT SPECIMENS

Unfortunately, microbiology as well as other pathology laboratories receive thousands of requests that cannot reasonably be expected to influence the management of the patient. The best use of the laboratory involves sending only relevant specimens so that the highest quality work can be done on a reasonable number of specimens. This is especially important when the economic situation of a country greatly limits the laboratory resources. Screening investigations of large numbers of patients are rarely justified—exceptions include routine antenatal screening tests (*see* p. 366). Examples of unnecessary investigations include 'routine' microscopy and culture of urine specimens from all non-catheterized adult patients in hospital, including those without symptoms suggestive of urinary tract infection. However, patients who are about to have a cystoscopy or urological surgery should normally have screening tests for urinary tract infection before such procedures (*see* p. 92). Sputum microbiology is not usually helpful in patients with chronic bronchitis who have infective exacerbations, since the presence of the two main bacterial pathogens, *Haemophilus influenzae* and *Strep. pneumoniae*, can easily be predicted (*see* p. 216).

While patients in hospital are often over investigated or inappropriately investigated, those in general practice are not investigated as often as is necessary. For example, the general practitioner could probably use the laboratory more often, with benefit to the individual patient or community, for investigating the frequency and dysuria syndrome, genital tract infection including sexually transmitted diseases, diarrhoea in children, febrile or abdominal symptoms after recent travel abroad and the justified screening of women for immunity to rubella.

Table 2.1. Work of the microbiology laboratory and role of the consultant clinical microbiologist

Type of work	*Role of the consultant clinical microbiologist*
A. Microbiological examination of specimens	1. To have regular contact with clinical colleagues to help ensure that the investigations are most appropriate for the clinical conditions suspected and that good quality specimens are sent 2. To organize the laboratory, with the assistance of senior non-medical staff, so that clinically relevant investigations are carried out reliably, safely and economically. Important results are promptly communicated to colleagues and discussed
B. Consultations on the investigation and management of patients with infection problems	1. Seeing patients on the wards, their temperature charts and drug sheets, etc., together with clinical colleagues, and helping with rational decisions about the optimal use of the laboratory, anti-microbial drugs and other aspects of management 2. Discussing 'difficult' clinical problems and management of outbreaks of infectious disease in the general population with general practitioners, community health physicians, medical officers for environmental health and public health authorities
C. Control of hospital infection	The consultant microbiologist is usually ultimately responsible for advice on a day-to-day basis for the prevention and control of hospital infection. He/She also helps to design and implement policies on the use of antibiotics, isolation procedures, sterilization and disinfection, etc. Cross-infection incidents are investigated and controlled.
D. Teaching and research	Education of medical, nursing, pharmacy and other staff about infections, the use of antibiotics, disinfectants, etc. Research on epidemiology, diagnosis, treatment or prevention of infections

The need to consider investigations for parasitic diseases is increasing because of the current widespread opportunities for travel to 'exotic' places; malaria is now commonly imported into Britain and should be urgently diagnosed by the examination of suitable blood films (*see* p. 431).

Detailed examples of relevant specimens from patients in both hospital and general practice are discussed in subsequent chapters.

PROVISION OF ESSENTIAL CLINICAL INFORMATION

The laboratory needs to select appropriate tests on each specimen according to the clinical information given which is usually only immediately available on the accompanying request form. Examples of the information routinely required include age, brief relevant details of the main clinical condition, the date of onset of the illness, information about recent/current/imminent antibiotic therapy, details of known antibiotic allergies, history of recent travel abroad, and, for serological tests, the dates of past immunizations or suspected contact with a source of infection.

PRIOR DISCUSSION WITH THE MICROBIOLOGIST

Certain types of investigation need to be adequately discussed with the microbiologist beforehand so that the best use of the laboratory is achieved. These include assays of antibiotics, the isolation of viruses, animal inoculation tests and the investigation of possible cross-infection incidents. Patients who may have serious infection can often be discussed with the clinical microbiologist at the bedside; the microbiologist may then help to suggest the most appropriate investigations and also advise on the subsequent management of the patient.

COLLECTION OF GOOD QUALITY SPECIMENS

When many poor quality specimens are sent, the laboratory produces many useless results! The collection of good quality microbiology specimens is dependent on:

a. The optimal time of specimen collection
b. The correct types of specimen
c. Well-collected specimens with minimum contamination from the normal flora of the patient or the person collecting the specimens
d. Adequate quantities of each specimen and an appropriate number of specimens.
e. Clearly labelled and 'safe' specimens

Optimal Time of Collection of Specimens

Specimens for the culture of bacteria must be collected before the start of antibiotics if a good quality specimen is to be sent to the laboratory. Small doses of antibiotic may damage organisms so that they may not multiply in culture media even though the antibiotic might not necessarily have had any useful clinical effect.

Blood cultures and blood films for malarial parasites are usually best collected just as the patient's temperature starts to rise (*see* Chapters 4 and 5). However, when infective endocarditis is suspected, three blood culture sets can be collected within a 24-hour period irrespective of the temperature of the patient (*see* Chapter 18).

Specimens for electron microscopy or isolation of viruses are most likely to give positive results when collected during the most acute stages of the disease. Rotaviruses may be seen by electron microscopic examination of faeces from an infant with acute gastro-enteritis and coxsackie B virus may be isolated from the throat swab or faeces of a patient with acute myocarditis/pericarditis.

Serology is usually most satisfactory when a four-fold or greater rising antibody titre to a pathogen can be demonstrated in paired sera. This is most likely to be achieved by collecting the first serum sample as early on in the disease as possible. Patients with pyrexia of unknown origin (PUO) should have the first serum collected and saved when they first attend (*see* p. 78).

Correct Types of Specimen

Specimens which are the most appropriate for the clinical condition are required. For example, patients with possible bacterial meningitis should have blood cultures as well as cerebrospinal fluid collected. Cervical, urethral and preferably rectal swabs should be collected rather than high vaginal swabs from female patients with suspected gonorrhoea. Per-nasal swabs should always be collected from children who may have pertussis rather than a throat or ordinary nose swab, although the ideal is to collect both per- and post-nasal swabs. Pus is always preferable to swabs but is essential for the isolation of mycobacteria. There are numerous other examples of 'correct' and 'wrong' types of specimens which are discussed in the subsequent chapters on infections (*see also* Appendix p. 28).

Well-collected Specimens with Minimum Contamination from the Normal Flora

In practice, nursing staff are often asked to collect specimens for microbiology investigations by medical staff; all staff should become aware of the importance of minimizing the contamination of specimens. Examples of poor quality specimens include saliva instead of sputum or a salivary-mucoid sputum sample instead of a mucopurulent specimen from a patient with pneumonia.

Mid-stream specimens of urine need careful collection to avoid excessive contamination by normal perineal or genital flora (*see* p. 362). A throat swab collected from a patient with a sore throat should not touch the buccal mucosa or tongue, which should be depressed by a spatula, but should sample the site of the inflamed posterior pharynx or tonsils. A high vaginal swab should be collected using a vaginal speculum with care not to touch the lower vagina or perineum. Blood or cerebrospinal fluid (CSF) cultures can be ruined by contamination from the skin flora of the patient or from the doctor collecting the specimens unless scrupulous aseptic and antiseptic techniques are used to avoid contamination.

In certain situations, it may be impractical to obtain a truly representative sample of the site of infection. A patient may have chronic osteomyelitis of the tibia with sinuses discharging through the skin and a superficial swab of the skin around the sinus opening may yield growth of various bacteria which need not necessarily reflect the pattern of pathogens present in the deep infected bone site. The limitations of microbiological investigations under these circumstances needs to be clearly understood. More invasive procedures, such as open bone biopsy and culture may be indicated in selected patients. In some patients with suspected opportunistic lung infections, techniques such as trans-tracheal aspiration, bronchial washing and trans-bronchial biopsy, percutaneous needle lung biopsy or open lung biopsy may be justified. Tuberculous peritonitis might not become diagnosed until laparotomy is carried out and peritoneal biopsies examined.

Adequate Quantity and Appropriate Number of Specimens

The volume of blood for culture from an adult should be at least 10 ml per blood culture set and at least two blood culture sets should be collected from patients with suspected bacteraemia. The collection of adequate quantities of early morning sputum or the whole of the early morning specimen of urine, on three successive days, is required for the isolation of *Mycobacterium tuberculosis* (*see* p. 244).

At least two samples of faeces on different days are desirable from patients with diarrhoea for the culture of salmonellae or shigellae. When the convalescent carriage of *Salmonella typhi* is investigated in a food handler, ten samples of faeces should be cultured (*see* p. 263). Serological investigations usually require paired sera. However, in some instances, further serum samples should also be collected: in Legionnaires' disease, for example, the antibody titres may occasionally not be raised in the first two serum samples, but may be raised in a third sample collected 1–6 weeks after the second sample. Other examples of the importance of collecting the correct quantity or number of specimens are included in later chapters.

Clearly Labelled and 'Safe' Specimens

The 'Howie code of practice' gives guidelines on the safe collection, transport and examination of specimens for pathology. Samples for microbiological investigations should be placed in leak-proof containers. (In practice, these containers are often not perfectly leak proof and each container should be enclosed in a plastic bag preferably in a separate pocket from the accompanying request form.) Examples of microbiological hazards to staff handling leaking containers include acquiring enteric infections from faeces, tuberculosis from sputum from an open case of pulmonary TB, and hepatitis from leaking blood. Any specimen from a patient with suspected hepatitis needs to have a 'hepatitis risk' label clearly attached and the accompanying request form should also be similarly labelled (*see also* Chapter 24, p. 492).

TRANSPORT OF SPECIMENS TO THE LABORATORY

Specimens should be as fresh as possible for the optimal isolation of microbes. Many pathogenic organisms do not survive for long in clinical specimens kept at room temperature including gonococci, *Haemophilus*, *Bacteroides*, anaerobic cocci and most viruses. On the other hand, some organisms contaminating specimens from the normal flora, such as coliforms or coagulase-negative staphylococci, may rapidly grow in specimens kept at room temperature. Urine or sputum samples should reach the laboratory within 2 hours of collection whenever possible (*see* p. 363 and p. 226). If delays are expected, urine samples should either be refrigerated or dip slides immediately inoculated.

Various transport media, such as Stuart's transport medium, should be used for the transport of pus or swabs for bacterial culture when delays in transport of more than half an hour are anticipated, or when neisseria infections are suspected. However, the inoculated transport media should be sent to the laboratory as soon as possible and, in any case, not later than 4 hours after their inoculation. It is possible for coliforms to multiply even in transport media after a few hours at room temperature, causing a significant change in the results of culture.

The investigation of eye, genital tract or suspected pertussis infections is best carried out at the bedside where suitable culture media are directly inoculated (and direct smears made when relevant). If this is not possible, Stuart's transport medium may be used for eye or genital tract swabs and Lacey's pertussis transport medium for the per-nasal swabs (*see* p. 137).

A few specimens need to be fresh enough to still be warm when they arrive in the laboratory! Examples include cerebrospinal fluid from a patient with suspected meningitis, since otherwise meningococci may rapidly die, and faeces from a patient with possible acute amoebic dysentery so that a search can be made for motile trophozoites of *Entamoeba histolytica*.

Viral transport medium, containing a balanced amino-acid salt solution at an appropriate pH with added antibiotics, is necessary for transporting swabs for viral culture to the laboratory (*see* Appendix 2) but a similar medium *NOT* containing antibiotics should be used for the transport of specimens when chlamydia isolation is required. CSF for virological investigation should be examined within a couple of hours of collection or else kept at −70 °C (e.g. overnight).

There are many other potential problems with the transport of specimens to the laboratory and these are discussed in subsequent chapters.

PROCEDURES IN THE LABORATORY FOR MICROBIOLOGICAL DIAGNOSIS

The following section is a summary of some basic procedures and principles used for the laboratory diagnosis of microbial disease.

Naked Eye Examination of Specimens

This helps to determine whether a specimen is suitable and may also give some immediate clues about the presence of an infection. A saliva sample instead of an expectorated sputum sample should be discarded and a request made to send a sputum sample. If the specimen is a sample of pus, or a purulent sputum or a turbid CSF, there is immediate evidence of infection. A foul-smelling sample of pus may suggest the presence of anaerobes.

Occasionally naked eye examinations alone allow a diagnosis to be made, for example a tapeworm segment or roundworm may be apparent in a specimen of faeces. A 'rice water' stool sample may indicate infection by *Vibrio cholerae*, an 'anchovy sauce' sputum sample would suggest invasive amoebiasis affecting the lungs, sulphur granules in pus would indicate the presence of actinomycosis, and blood and mucus in a liquid specimen of faeces would suggest the possibility of dysentery.

Microscopy

'Wet' preparations for ordinary light microscopy are useful for the examination of CSF, urine or body fluid specimens to look for evidence of pus cells and organisms, faeces for trophozoites, ova and cysts, vaginal secretions for *Trichomonas* and *Candida*, and skin, nails and hair, after clearing in warm potassium hydroxide, for evidence of fungal infection.

Dark-ground illumination (DGI) microscopy is mainly used today to look for the spirochaete, *Treponema pallidum*, in suspected primary or secondary syphilitic lesions in male homosexual patients.

Gram-stained smears are probably more widely used than any other type of microscopic investigation to help determine the predominant types of bacterial pathogens present in pus, sputum, tissue, CSF or specimens from other sites. Rapid and valuable information is often obtained about the likelihood of the presence of infection and the type of infection when pus cells and numerous Gram-stainable organisms are seen in fresh well-collected specimens. Unfortunately, the quality of the smears is frequently reduced by sending swabs in Stuart's transport medium, since the material is diluted out although the culture results may be improved; ideally pus or a swab not sent in Stuart's medium would be sent in addition for the purpose of making a smear. There are numerous examples of the value of Gram-stains of clinical specimens included in the following chapters. A few examples where the Gram-stains may be of life-saving importance include the rapid diagnosis of bacterial meningitis on examination of a Gram-stain deposit of CSF, and the diagnosis of staphylococcal pneumonia by looking at a Gram-stain smear of sputum. Gram-stains are also performed on suspect positive blood cultures to give valuable rapid diagnosis of serious infections. In the identification of colonies appearing on culture media the Gram-stain is an essential first step. In some instances, the Gram-stain may give positive results although the cultures are subsequently negative, because antibiotics have been given. Very occasionally, the Gram-stained smear may be the only means of making the diagnosis, such as when a throat swab taken from a painful pharyngeal ulcer is examined and large numbers of fusiforms and spirochaetes are seen indicating that the diagnosis is Vincent's angina.

Microscopy for acid-fast bacilli in specimens is usually carried using either the Ziehl-Neelsen acid alcohol stain or fluorescent auramine-phenol techniques. Acid-fast stains of sputum allow a rapid presumptive diagnosis of open pulmonary tuberculosis to be made and, in suspected tuberculous meningitis, the finding of acid fast bacilli in the CSF deposit or spider web clot is of enormous importance. Leprosy bacilli still cannot be cultured in vitro, but the diagnosis may sometimes be confirmed when acid fast stains show the presence of the bacilli using a modified Ziehl-Neelsen technique. These investigations are discussed in detail in Chapter 13.

'Negative' staining with Indian ink might be occasionally useful to demonstrate thick capsules, such as those seen in cryptococci in a CSF deposit from a patient with cryptococcal meningitis.

Romanowsky stains such as Leishman or Giemsa stains of blood films, bone marrow aspirate or other specimens may immediately confirm the diagnosis of malaria, leishmaniasis, trypanosomiasis, babesiosis or other parasitic diseases. With most of these diseases, direct microscopic investigations are the main way in which the diagnosis is confirmed. Cultures are usually not applicable and serological investigations do not necessarily give evidence of current disease.

Immunofluorescent microscopy is increasingly important for the rapid diagnosis of viral respiratory and other infections. These techniques allow microbial antigens to be seen as well as the whole organisms. Rapid immunofluorescent techniques are particularly useful for the early recognition of respiratory syncytial virus infections in infants. Other examples, where rapid immunofluorescent techniques may be useful, include the detection of herpes simplex or rabies viruses in brain biopsy specimens, *Chlamydia trachomatis* in conjunctival scrapings, and treponemes in a smear from a suspected syphilitic genital lesion. Immunofluorescent microscopy is widely used to help in the identification of organisms on culture plates, such as *Neisseria gonorrhoeae*, and also in serological antibody investigations, such as fluorescent treponema antibody or fluorescent amoebic antibody tests. These techniques are usually very sensitive and may be highly specific in certain situations, but positive and negative controls have to be carefully examined in each batch of tests.

Histological haematoxylin and eosin microscopy of fixed sections of specimens may often reveal evidence of infection. Examples where an infective diagnosis may be suggested include a lymph gland biopsy showing evidence of either toxoplasmosis, tuberculosis or pyogenic infection or lung biopsy showing cytomegalovirus inclusion cells. Histological Gram or Ziehl-Neelsen stains are also frequently useful for finding evidence of pyogenic or mycobacterial infections of tissues and PAS or silver stains may be useful to find evidence of fungal sections. Silver stains may be necessary to see *Pneumocystis* or *Legionella* in lung specimens from patients with unusual types of pneumonitis. Sometimes these specimens are obtained from post-mortem material.

Electron microscopy is mainly used for the rapid diagnosis of rotavirus or herpes infections. In the past, this type of microscopy was important for the rapid differentiation of smallpox from typical chickenpox or other skin infections. Smallpox is now officially an extinct disease but this technique may be useful for confirming that certain skin lesions are due to ectopic vaccinial infection. Electron microscopy can also be used to confirm the diagnosis of other infections including Orf.

Detection of Microbial Antigens

In addition to the immunofluorescent techniques referred to above, microbial antigens may be often detected in specimens by immunoelectrophoretic methods. Pneumococcal polysaccharide antigen may often be detected in sputum, serum or urine of patients with pneumococcal pneumonia. Immunoelectrophoresis is a valuable rapid diagnostic method in this situation, when patients have already been given an antibiotic and conventional sputum or blood cultures are negative but, even in the absence of antibiotic therapy, this test is often positive when the cultures are negative. As with all immunological methods the use of the correct buffers and care with other technical details plus the use of adequate controls is necessary for the best results. The detection of pneumococcal, haemophilus or meningococcal antigens in a CSF specimen by immunoelectrophoresis is also valuable but good antisera must be used and may have to be imported from Scandinavia. Hepatitis B antigens such as HBsAg and hepatitis e antigens may be detected using gel immuno-precipitation techniques, but a wide range of other serological techniques are available for investigation of hepatitis including radio-immunoassay techniques (*see* p. 297). The demonstration of e antigen in serum may correlate with infectivity. Cryptococcal antigen can sometimes be detected in the CSF of patients with cryptococcal meningitis using a latex agglutination technique (*see* p. 188). It is likely that the detection of microbial antigens in specimens will become increasingly important in the future.

Gas–Liquid Chromatographic Techniques

Gas–liquid chromatographic (GLC) techniques have become increasingly useful for the rapid detection of anaerobic infections. Specimens of pus from abdominal, gynaecological or brain abscesses may be shown to have multiple volatile fatty acids present which indicate anaerobic infection within a few hours of collection of the specimen of pus and this may affect decisions about the chemotherapy of infection. Positive blood culture broths can also similarly be looked at by GLC techniques for evidence of anaerobic septicaemia. These techniques are also useful for the species identification of anaerobes. They have also been used to identify *Legionella pneumophila* which has a unique fatty acid structure in the cell wall including long-chain fatty acids such as iso-16-O fatty acid.

Isolation of Microbes

The importance of collecting good quality relevant specimens before the start of antimicrobial chemotherapy, and the direct inoculation of prompt transportation of specimens, has already been stressed. In general, the isolation of the causative microbes of infectious diseases is the most reliable way in which a diagnosis can be confirmed. Examples include the isolation of *Salmonella typhi* from the blood cultures of a patient with suspected typhoid fever, or *Mycobacterium tuberculosis* from the cervical lymph gland of a patient with suspected tuberculous lymphadenitis.

Isolation of bacteria or fungi from specimens collected from sites normally sterile, such as blood or CSF, is usually easy to interpret but, when the clinical significance is in doubt, discussions between the clinician and microbiologist about the patient are always necessary. An *E. coli* isolated from one out of three blood culture bottles only and not from any bottle of two subsequent blood cultures, sets in a patient not receiving any antibiotic is usually not clinically significant. However, any organism that is isolated from the blood cultures on two or more different occasions is significant until 'proved otherwise', even 'skin contaminants' such as diphtheroids or *Staph. albus* may, for example, occasionally cause infective endocarditis. A diphtheroid-like organism isolated from a CSF sample might eventually be identified as *Listeria monocytogenes*.

Even using the best isolation techniques, results of culture may be negative in patients with tuberculosis, meningococcal meningitis, infective endocarditis, deep mycoses and many viral infections. When interpretation of an isolate from a blood culture is uncertain, antibody studies using the patient's serum against the patient's isolate may be helpful. For example, fluorescent streptococcal antibody titres may be performed against a streptococcus isolated from one bottle only from a patient with a possible endocarditis (*see* p. 344).

Bacterial or fungal isolations from specimens collected from sites with normal flora, such as sputum, are often difficult to interpret. Factors that need to be considered in interpretation of the results include knowledge of the likely quality of the specimens at the time of the collection, the history of its transport to the laboratory, the microscopy results, the number of times the organism has been isolated from such specimens, and the numbers of organisms present in each specimen. A sputum specimen may yield growth of large numbers of an organism such as *Pseudomonas*, which is not relevant to the infection in that patient; for example a sputum from a child with cystic fibrosis may not yield growth of the *Staph. aureus* or *Haemophilus influenzae* which is actually causing clinical infection, because it is obscured by the *Pseudomonas* which has multiplied in the sputum at room temperature during delayed transport in the hospital. The problems of interpretation of specimen results are discussed in subsequent chapters (*see*, for example, Chapter 9, p. 158, Chapter 12, p. 227, Chapter 13, p. 245, Chapter 6, p. 104 and Chapter 19, p. 365).

Virological or chlamydia isolation methods may yield positive results within a few days when good specimens are collected in the early stages of the disease. Notes on virological investigations are included in Appendix 2, p. 30.

Serology

Indirect evidence of infection obtained only by serological methods is much less satisfactory than the isolation of the causative organism and, in many instances, 10 days or longer has to pass before a rising antibody titre can be demonstrated. Nonetheless, in sub-acute or chronic infections such as Q fever or brucellosis, the diagnostic information obtained by serology is often valuable. Some other examples of infections where serology is often relied on to confirm the diagnosis are psittacosis, *Mycoplasma* pneumonia, Legionnaires' disease, amoebic liver abscess, syphilis and pulmonary aspergilloma. The importance of collecting an acute serum as early as possible in the illness has been mentioned. A rise in antibody titre between two serum samples collected 10–14 days apart is best demonstrated by simultaneous testing of the two sera against the appropriate microbial antigens. At least a four-fold rise in titre or a single very high titre of antibody, possibly with specific IgM antibody present, may indicate recent infection (for example in rubella, *see* p. 132). The precise details of the date of onset of the illness and the dates on which the serum samples were collected are essential information. Past immunizations may also be taken into account in some infections, e.g. typhoid.

Certain serological tests are of very limited value and are only rarely indicated. Examples include the Widal test (*see* p. 263) and the gonococcal complement fixation test (*see* p. 387).

Animal Inoculation Tests

Animal houses have been closed in many hospitals during the last 15 years because of the improved alternative methods of diagnosis that have become available. Nevertheless, there are still a few possible indications for inoculation of specimens into animals. These include the use of guinea-pigs for the isolation of *Mycobacterium tuberculosis* from certain very important surgical specimens that cannot be repeated (*see* p. 247), inoculation of mice or guinea-pigs, or the isolation of *Leptospira* from patients with suspected acute leptospirosis (*see* p. 407), and the isolation of coxsackie A viruses from specimens from patients with respiratory or central nervous system infections by the intracerebral inoculation of suckling mice (hardly ever used routinely). Arbovirus, rickettsia and toxoplasma organisms can also sometimes be isolated by injecting specimens into rodents but this is not routinely indicated in Britain. Guinea-pigs are essential for the isolation of *Legionella pneumophila* from environmental samples, such as water, during the investigation of outbreaks of Legionnaires' disease.

The 10-day-old chick embryo may be used to isolate or differentiate herpes simplex viruses types I and II (on the chorioallantoic membrane), pox viruses such as vaccinia (on the chorioallantoic membrane), influenza viruses (allantoic and amniotic cavities), chlamydiae and rickettsiae (yolk sac).

Skin Tests

Skin tests with microbial antigens are of limited value for the diagnosis of infection. These tests may give indirect evidence of past or current contact with a pathogen and the Mantoux skin test is probably the commonest example (*see* p. 248). Antigens extracted from opportunist *Mycobacterium* species may be useful for obtaining indirect evidence of infection due to these species (*see* p. 254). Conversion of a skin test from negative to positive, in an individual patient, may provide more valuable evidence of current infection. In the U.S.A., the histoplasmin skin test is frequently used in a similar way to the Mantoux skin test. However, negative skin mantoux and histoplasmin reactions do not exclude the possibility of current infection. A positive skin test may be due to past immunization, for example a positive Mantoux test may follow BCG immunization. The Frei skin test may help to diagnose lymphogranuloma venereum infection and the Casoni skin test has been used to investigate patients with suspected hydatid disease. Serum should be collected for antibody tests before the histoplasmin, Frei or Casoni skin tests are performed. If the serum complement fixation tests for lymphogranuloma venereum (psittacosis antigen group) or hydatid are positive to a significant titre it may not be necessary to perform the skin tests. In the case of the Casoni test, this may be of particular advantage since the test performed in an individual with hydatid disease can become complicated by marked local inflammatory reactions.

The main use of microbial skin tests is to detect infection or the development of immunity to microbes. They may also be used to test for allergy to microbial antigens, for example in patients with asthma due to allergy to *Aspergillus* (*see* p. 237).

Quality Control

Most microbiology laboratories in Britain participate in quality control programmes to check that the laboratory can reliably undertake various microbiological procedures. The reference laboratory sends simulated specimens to the diagnostic laboratories and reports are returned to the reference laboratory in a stated time. External quality control programmes have helped to improve the performance of some laboratories in relation to the isolation and identification of organisms as well as the issuing of relevant and accurate antibiotic sensitivity reports.

Internal quality control is also useful within each laboratory where occasional simulated samples, containing known organisms or known concentrations of antibiotics for assay, are put through the laboratory by the consultant as simulated specimens. When the results obtained by the laboratory are not satisfactory an analysis of the methods used is made and repeat samples are put through the laboratory until a satisfactory result is obtained.

The usefulness of the results obtained by even the most reliable laboratory is dependent upon the factors that have been discussed in this chapter, including the relevance, quality and transportation of the specimens. The satisfactory interpretation of the results depends on a good level of communication between the clinicians and microbiologists.

ANTIBIOTIC SENSITIVITY TESTS

These tests which are frequently carried out routinely during the examination of microbiological specimens are discussed in Chapter 3.

Further Reading

Baker F. J. and Breach M. R. (1980) *Medical Microbiological Techniques*. London, Butterworths.

*Cruickshank R., Duguid J. P., Marmion B. P. et al. (1975) *Medical Microbiology*, 12th ed., Vols. 1 and 2. Edinburgh, Churchill Livingstone.

Evans E. G. V. (1979) Diagnosis of systemic fungal infections. In: Reeves D. and Geddes A. (ed.) *Recent Advances in Infection*. Edinburgh, Churchill Livingstone.

Garrod L. P. (1961) *Clinical Bacteriology, St Bartholomew's Hospital Journal*, October 1961, pp. 223–227.

*Howie Sir James (1979) Clinicians and microbiologists should get together. *Journal of Infection* **1**, 19–22.

Lipsky B. A. and Plorde J. J. (1978) Bacterial culture specimens, categories, collection and interpretation. *Postgraduate Medicine* **64**, 80–92.

Newsom S. W. B. (1979) Automated and rapid methods for the diagnosis of infectious diseases. In: Reeves D. and Geddes A. (ed.) *Recent Advances in Infection*. Edinburgh, Churchill Livingstone.

Shanson D. C. (1976) How not to do it: clinical microbiology investigations. *Hospital Update* **2**, 589–598.

Spencely M., Parker M. J., Dewar R. A. D. et al. (1979) The clinical value of microbiological laboratory investigations. *Journal of Infection* **1**, 23–36.

Stokes E. J. (1979) Quality control in microbiology. In: Reeves D. and Geddes A. (ed.) *Recent Advances in Infection*. Edinburgh, Churchill Livingstone.

Stokes E. J. and Ridgway G. L. (1980) *Clinical Bacteriology*, 5th ed. London, Edward Arnold.

*Timbury M. G. (1978) *Notes on Medical Virology*, 6th ed. Edinburgh, Churchill Livingstone.

Tyrell D. A. J., Phillips I., Goodwin C. J. et al. (1979) *Microbial Disease: The use of the Laboratory in Diagnosis, Therapy and Control*. London, Edward Arnold.

* This reference is particularly recommended for further study by undergraduates.

Appendix to Chapter 2

1. Some microbiological methods

Basic methods for the isolation and identification of bacterial pathogens are referred to in Chapters 1, 9 (Anaerobic infections), 13 (Mycobacterial infections) and *see* section on p. 516. The detailed investigations required for each type of infection are discussed in subsequent chapters.

MAKING SMEARS: THE GRAM-STAIN AND ACID-FAST STAINS

Making Smears

Ideally swabs collected from septic wounds should be smeared directly onto sterile glass slides at the bedside. If Stuart's transport medium is used for transporting the swab, the smear obtained in the laboratory from this medium is often not satisfactory since material has been diluted out in the transport medium. Ideally, if Stuart's transport medium is used then an additional swab should be transported specifically for the purpose of making a smear. Good swabs received in the laboratory and those from Stuart's transport medium do not require any further moistening before the smear is made. However if a dry swab is received in the laboratory some prior moistening may be necessary:

A loopful of sterile water or saline should be transferred to the centre of a labelled glass slide. This swab should be rubbed over the centre of the slide to make a thin smear.

Smears from pus and from centrifuged deposits, urine, CSF or other fluids are made by spreading a loopful of pus or deposit over the centre of the slide. Larger quantities of deposit may be necessary when smears are examined for acid-fast bacilli and then a sterile pasteur pipette may be used for transferring the deposit to the slide. Work on sputum specimens should always be carried out in an approved B_1 safety cabinet in case acid fast bacilli are present in the specimens.

Gram-stain

After the smear is made, it is allowed to dry at room temperature and then fixed by gentle heat in a bunsen flame. The Gram-stain steps are:

1. *Methyl violet*
   Flood the slide with methyl violet for about 1 minute
   Wash with tap water
2. *Lugol's iodine*
   Flood the slide with Lugol's iodine for about 1 minute
   Then wash with tap water
3. *Acetone*
   Add acetone to the slide for only 1–3 seconds or until such time as no more blue colour runs out of the smear
   This time of decolorization is critical since, if the acetone is left on the

slide for an excessive period, Gram-positive organisms may appear to be Gram-negative
As soon as decolorization is complete, wash the acetone off with tap water

4. *Dilute carbol fuchsin*
   Flood the slide with dilute carbol fuchsin as the counterstain and leave for about 1 minute. Then wash the stain off with tap water. (Alternatives to carbol fuchsin are saffronin or neutral red.)
5. Wipe the undersurface of the slide with blotting paper and allow the slide to dry at an angle at room temperature

Gram-positive organisms stain blue or purple or black
Gram-negative organisms stain pink or red
(*See also* Gram-stain, Chapter 1, p. 5)

ZIEHL-NEELSEN STAIN FOR ACID-FAST BACILLI

1. Flood the slide with strong carbol fuchsin and apply heat gently under the slide with a lighted taper so that steam rises for about 5 minutes
2. Wash in running tap water, and then in 3% acid alcohol for 1–3 minutes
3. Flood the slide with Loeffler's methylene blue and leave for about 30 seconds
4. Wash in tap water
5. Examine the acid alcohol fast stain with the oil immersion lens of the light microscope for at least 10 minutes

2. *Basic virological investigations*

The collection of specimens for virology investigations should preferably be discussed with the laboratory beforehand.

Specimens Collected for Electron Microscopy or Fluorescence Microscopy

Some frequent examples include:

1. Faeces from patients with suspected rotavirus gastro-enteritis should be sent in the same type of container as used for samples for bacteriological examination
2. Naso-pharyngeal secretions: these are best collected by aspirating secretions through a disposable catheter into a trap which is connected at the other end to a suitable mechanical sucker that applies a gentle suction (no more than 26 pounds negative pressure). These specimens are collected from children with suspected viral respiratory tract infections. The open ends of the trap are heat-sealed before it is sent to the laboratory. It is important that the specimen is transported without delay since it is also

used for isolation of viruses. The secretions are used to make smears for rapid immunofluorescent microscopy using antisera to respiratory syncytial virus, para-influenza viruses, etc.

3. Vesicular fluid from possible herpetic lesions can be collected into capillary tubes. The base of the vesicle can be gently scraped with a sterile disposable needle (as used for venepuncture) and the needle used to make a smear on the centre of a glass slide. The slide is dried at room temperature and

Table 2.2. Virological investigations

Clinical condition	*Specimens*	*Viruses suspected include*	*Usual investigations*		
			Microscopy	*Isolation*	*Serology*
Skin or mucosal vesicles	Vesicle fluid scrapings (swab of lesion for culture only)	Herpes simplex	+	+	
		Varicella-zoster	+		
		Vaccinia	+	+	
Respiratory infection	Throat swab Naso-pharyngeal aspirate or washings Paired sera (faeces)	Influenza Para-influenza Respiratory syncytial virus	+	+	+
		Rhinoviruses		+	
		Adenoviruses (enteroviruses)		+	+
Rubella or measles	Paired sera	Rubella or measles			+
Aseptic meningitis	CSF Faeces Throat swab Paired sera	Enteroviruses		+	(+)
		Mumps		+	+
Encephalitis	As for aseptic meningitis plus brain biopsy	Enteroviruses Mumps Herpes simplex Measles	+	+	+
Pericarditis, myocarditis	Throat swab Faeces Paired sera	Coxsackie B (Influenza)		+	+
Gastro-enteritis	Faeces	Rotaviruses	+		
Hepatitis	Serum	Hepatitis B Hepatitis A			+
Eye infection	Conjunctival scrapings	Herpes simplex		+	
		Adenoviruses		+	
		*Chlamydia trachomatis**	+	+	
Congenital infections	Throat swab Urine Paired sera, mother and baby	Cytomegalovirus		+	+
		Rubella			+

* Chlamydia is not a virus—microscopy for inclusions in epithelial cells by iodine or immunofluorescent stains.
—culture requires special transport medium without antibiotics for culture.

another dry slide is taped to it. Electron microscopy can be performed on material that is washed off the slide as well as from the vesicular fluid in the capillary tube. Herpes simplex virus looks identical to varicella-zoster virus since both are herpes viruses

Table 2.3. Isolation of viruses

Viruses	Methods of isolation		
	Tissue culture	*Other*	*Method of detection*
Myxoviruses and paramyxoviruses			
Influenza	Monkey kidney cells[a]	Amniotic cavity fertile egg	Haemadsorption of erythrocytes on tissue cultures
Para-influenza	Monkey kidney cells		
Mumps	Monkey kidney cells		
Measles	Human amnion cells		CPE and neutralization
Respiratory syncytial virus	Human epithelium cells (Hep_2/or HeLa cells)		CPE and immunofluorescence
Rhinoviruses			
Rhinovirus M	Monkey kidney cells		CPE and neutralization
Rhinovirus H	Human embryo lung[b]		
Herpes viruses			
Herpes simplex	HeLa or Hep_2 cells[c]	CAM of egg	CPE and neutralization
Varicella-zoster	Human embryo lung and human amnion cells		
Cytomegalovirus	Human embryo lung		
Enteroviruses			
Polio	Monkey kidney and HeLa cells		CPE and neutralization
Coxsackie A	(Monkey kidney)	Suckling mice	
Coxsackie B	Monkey kidney and HeLa cells		CPE and neutralization
Echo	Monkey kidney cells		
Adenoviruses	HeLa or Hep_2 cells		CPE, Complement fixation and neutralization
Poxviruses			
Vaccinia		CAM of egg	Characteristic pocks
Rubella	Rabbit kidney 13 cells		Interference

[a] Monkey kidney and human amnion cells, examples of primary tissue cultures.
[b] Human embryo (diploid) lung is an example of a semi-continuous cell line.
[c] HeLa and Hep_2 cells, examples of continuous cell lines.
CPE, cytopathogenic effect.
CAM, chorioallantoic membrane of fertile hen's egg.

Specimens for Virus Isolation

Virus transport medium is necessary for throat swabs or swabs of skin sites but is not necessary for faeces, CSF or pharyngeal secretions sent immediately to the laboratory in a trap. When vesicle fluid or scrapings are collected from skin or mucosa, some of this material should be put directly into viral transport medium for virus isolation. A morning specimen of urine may be collected for the isolation of cytomegalovirus when this condition is suspected and sent promptly to the laboratory. If a short delay is anticipated, the urine sample may be mixed with a suitable sorbitol-containing viral transport medium.

If delays in transport of specimens for virology are unavoidable, refrigeration at 4 °C in a Thermos flask is necessary. CSF may be stored overnight at −70 °C, but no specimens for virology should be put into the deep freeze section of an ordinary fridge which may be at around −20 °C, since viruses may die rapidly at this temperature.

Respiratory syncytial virus is particularly labile and is relatively sensitive to cold; specimens should not be refrigerated but inoculated into tissue cultures as soon as possible, in the laboratory if not on the ward.

Suitable specimens and some virological investigations are summarized in *Tables 2.2* and *2.3*. Specimens for virus isolation are collected as early on in the acute stage of the disease as possible, and usually not later than 7 days after the onset of symptoms. Serum is also collected in the acute stage and a second specimen taken after an interval of about 2 weeks. When enteroviruses are isolated, paired sera are used to carry out neutralization tests against the isolated virus. Serological investigations for respiratory tract infections include complement fixation tests for influenza, para influenza, respiratory syncytial virus as well as non-viral causes of atypical pneumonia, including *Mycoplasma pneumoniae, Coxiella burnetii* and *Chlamydia psittaci*.

Chapter 3

Antimicrobial chemotherapy—general principles

Antimicrobial agents include antibiotics, anti-viral drugs, anti-fungal agents and anti-protozoal drugs. They demonstrate 'selective toxicity', i.e. the drugs can be administered to man with reasonable safety while having marked toxic effects on certain microbes.

Host defence mechanisms are usually necessary for the final elimination of microbial pathogens and it is not essential to use 'bactericidal' drugs to treat most infections. Important exceptions where 'bactericidal' agents are indicated include the chemotherapy of infective endocarditis or of opportunistic infections in immunocompromised patients.

The most important information about a drug concerns its clinical efficacy in the treatment of infections and this can be best assessed by well-conducted clinical trials.

MODE OF ACTION OF ANTIMICROBIAL DRUGS

The bacterial cell wall is very different from the mammalian cell wall. Certain antibiotics, such as penicillin, act by interrupting the synthesis of the cell wall during the process of division. They will be ineffective against organisms, such as *Mycoplasma*, which do not have a cell wall. Other antibiotics, such as sulphonamides, act by inhibiting folic acid synthesis. Man can utilize dietary folic acid to synthesize purines and pyrimidines which are necessary for nucleic acid synthesis but bacteria cannot. Many bacteria must synthesize their own folic acid by metabolizing para-aminobenzoic acid to dihydrofolic acid and then to tetrahydrofolic acid. Sulphonamides have a similar chemical structure to *p*-aminobenzoic acid and, when present in excess, the sulphonamides are taken up by a process of 'competitive inhibition' in preference to the *p*-aminobenzoic acid, thus blocking folic acid synthesis. In the next stage of purine synthesis, the enzyme dihydrofolate reductase may be inhibited by trimethoprim. A similar enzyme is also present in man but trimethoprim has a much greater affinity for the bacterial enzyme.

The specific 'target sites' where antimicrobial agents act are summarized in *Table 3.1*. An indication of whether an antibiotic is usually bactericidal or basteriostatic is also included in the table, but in practice this is dependent on the concentration of the drug present. Certain drugs such as erythromycin may be bacteriostatic at low concentrations, but bactericidal at high concentrations.

Table 3.1. Mode of action of antimicrobial drugs

Target site	*Drug*	*Comment*	*Cidal Static*
Cell wall	Vancomycin Bacitracin	Inhibit peptidoglycan formation	Cidal
	Beta-lactams: e.g. penicillin ampicillin cloxacillin cephalosporins	Interfere with cross-linkages of peptidoglycan molecules—in low concentrations septum formation is inhibited	Cidal (osmotic lysis of bacteria with defective cell walls when high concentrations of drug present)
Cytoplasmic membrane	Polymyxins	Affinity for membrane in Gram-negative bacilli	Cidal
	Amphotericin B Nystatin	Affinity for 'sterol' in fungal membranes	Static
Ribosomes	Tetracyclines	Interfere with transfer RNA—amino acid attachment—protein synthesis inhibited	Static
	Chloramphenicol	Interfere with translocation	Static
	Erythromycin Lincomycin Fusidic acid	Interfere with translocation—protein synthesis inhibited	Static with low concentrations, cidal with high concentrations
	Aminoglycosides	Interfere with mRNA attachment to ribosome	Cidal
Nucleic acid replication	Rifampicin	RNA replication interfered with	Cidal
	Nalidixic acid	DNA replication interfered with	Cidal
	Metronidazole	DNA replication interfered with	Cidal
	5-Fluorocytosine Griseofulvin	Nucleic acid synthesis inhibited of some fungi	
	Idoxuridine Cytarabine	DNA synthesis in DNA viruses interfered with	

SPECTRUM OF ACTIVITY OF ANTIMICROBIAL AGENTS

Narrow Spectrum Drugs

Penicillin is a good example of a 'narrow spectrum' antibiotic with activity mainly against the Gram-positive bacteria. Streptomycin, gentamicin and other aminoglycosides are examples of 'narrow spectrum' antibiotics with activity mainly against Gram-negative bacteria. Metronidazole is a recent example of a 'narrow spectrum' antibiotic with activity almost entirely against strictly anaerobic bacteria and some protozoa. 'Narrow spectrum' antibiotics are included in *Tables 3.2* and *3.3*. These tables also indicate a few important activities of these drugs outside of the main narrow spectrum, such as penicillin activity against Gram-negative cocci and erythromycin activity against *Legionella* species.

Broad Spectrum Drugs

Broad spectrum antibiotics are active against many Gram-positive and Gram-negative bacteria and examples include tetracyclines, ampicillin and cephalosporins (*see Table 3.4*). They are often used for the 'blind' treatment of infections when the likely causative pathogen is 'unknown'. Unfortunately, there is much 'abuse' of broad spectrum antibiotics in clinical practice (*see below*).

Table 3.2. Narrow spectrum antibiotics mainly active against Gram-positive bacteria: examples of susceptible microbes*

Antibiotic example	*Gram-positive cocci*	*Gram-positive bacilli*	*Gram-negative cocci*	*Gram-negative bacilli*	*Other*
Penicillin	*Strep. pyogenes* *Strep. pneumoniae* '*Strep. viridans*' *Staph. aureus* (a few strains only) Anaerobic cocci	*C. diphtheriae* *L. monocytogenes* *Clostridium* spp.	*N. meningitidis* *N. gonorrhoeae*	*P. multocida* Vincent's fusiforms *B. necrophorus*	Treponemes *Leptospira* spp.
Cloxacillin	*Staph. aureus* (*Strep. pyogenes*)				
Fusidic acid	*Staph. aureus*				
Erythromycin	*Staph. aureus* *Strep. pyogenes* *Strep. pneumoniae* '*Strep. viridans*'	*C. diphtheriae* *Propionibacterium acnes*		*Campylobacter* spp. *Legionella* spp.	*Mycoplasma pneumoniae*
Clindamycin and Lincomycin	*Staph. aureus* *Strep. pyogenes*			*Bacteroides fragilis*	
Novobiocin	*Staph. aureus* Streptococci				
Vancomycin	*Staph. aureus* '*Strep. viridans*'	*Clostridium difficile*			

* The majority of strains of the species mentioned are susceptible unless otherwise stated.

Table 3.3. Narrow spectrum antibiotics mainly active against Gram-negative bacilli: examples of susceptible microbes

Antibiotic example	*Gram-positive cocci*	*Gram-positive bacilli*	*Gram-negative cocci*	*Gram-negative bacilli*	*Other*
Aminoglycosides: Streptomycin Kanamycin Gentamicin Tobramycin Amikacin	*Staph. aureus* (especially gentamicin)			*E. coli* *Klebsiella* spp. *Proteus* spp. Other 'coliforms'* *Pseudomonas aeruginosa* —gentamicin, tobramycin and amikacin only	*M. tuberculosis* (streptomycin mainly and to lesser extent kanamycin)
Polymyxins				*Pseudomonas aeruginosa* and 'coliforms'	
Nalidixic acid (urinary anti-bacterial)				*E. coli* and other 'coliforms'	
Mecillinam				*E. coli* and other 'coliforms' *Salmonella* spp.	
Metronidazole (active only against anaerobic bacteria and protozoa)	Anaerobic cocci	*Clostridium* spp.		*Bacteroides fragilis* *Bacteroides necrophorus* *Bacteroides melaninogenicum* Fusiforms	

* 'Coliforms' does not include *Pseudomonas*.

Antituberculous drugs are mentioned in the chapter on mycobacterial infections. Antimicrobial drugs which are active against viruses, fungi and protozoa are included in *Tables 3.5* and *3.6*.

GENERAL PRINCIPLES OF USE OF ANTIMICROBIAL DRUGS

There are five main questions that should be considered before antibiotics are prescribed (*Fig. 3.1*).

Evidence of Infection?

When there is no good clinical evidence of infection, antibiotics are rarely necessary, the main exception being prophylaxis which is discussed below.

Infections Unlikely/Likely to Respond to Treatment?

Antibiotics usually cannot be expected to hasten the patient's recovery from a mild attack of gastro-enteritis or influenza and few doctors would prescribe antibiotics for the common cold. However, if salmonella gastro-enteritis leading to septicaemia is suspected in an infant or elderly person, urgent investigations and prompt antibiotic treatment is essential.

Relevant Specimens Before Treatment?

The great importance of collecting blood and other specimens for culture from patients with suspected serious infections before the start of antimicrobial therapy, has already been stressed in the previous chapter. The main possible exception is suspected bacterial meningitis in a patient seen in general practice (*see* p. 172). The results of antibiotic sensitivity tests are of critical importance for the subsequent rational chemotherapy of many serious infections.

Timing the Start of Treatment?

In patients with life-threatening infections in hospital, antimicrobial treatment is indicated as soon as the specimens have been collected for microbiology. During the first 24 hours of treatment, it is often possible to have useful guidance for the optimal choice of agent from the result of a Gram-stain of sputum, CSF, pus or blood culture.

Which Drug?

Ideally a narrow spectrum antibiotic should be selected for treating specific infections rather than a broad spectrum antibiotic, since narrow spectrum drugs are less likely to disturb the patient's normal flora and cause superinfection or spread of antibiotic-resistant strains. Examples include benzylpenicillin treatment for a patient with streptococcal cellulitis or pneumococcal pneumonia, oral penicillin V for a patient with a streptococcal sore throat, flucloxacillin for treating a *Staph. aureus* wound infection, erythromycin for treating infected eczema where the patient has a mixture of *Staph. aureus* and *Strep. pyogenes*, and

Table 3.4. Broad spectrum antibiotics: examples of susceptible microbes

Antibiotic example	*Gram-positive cocci*	*Gram-positive bacilli*	*Gram-negative cocci*	*Gram-negative bacilli*	*Other*
Tetracyclines	*Strep. pneumoniae* *Strep. pyogenes* *Staph. aureus*	*Clostridium* spp. *P. acnes*	*N. gonorrhoeae*	*Haemophilus influenzae* 'Coliforms' *Brucella* spp. *Yersinia* spp. *V. cholerae* (El Tor)	*Mycoplasma pneumoniae* *Coxiella buretii* *Chlamydia trachomatis* *Chlamydia psittaci*
Chloramphenicol	*Staph. aureus* *Strep. pneumoniae*		*N. meningitidis*	*Haemophilus influenzae* *Salmonella typhi* *E. coli* and other 'coliforms' *Bacteroides fragilis*	Rickettsiae
Ampicillin	*Strep. pneumoniae* *Strep. pyogenes* *Strep. faecalis* *Staph. aureus* (a few strains only)	*L. monocytogenes* *C. diphtheriae* *Clostridium* spp.	*N. gonorrhoeae* *N. meningitidis*	*Haemophilus influenzae* *E. coli* and other 'coliforms' (— not *Klebsiella*)	
Carbenicillin	(Streptococci)			*Pseudomonas aeruginosa* (some strains) *Proteus* species (indole positive)	
Cephalosporins (*see* p. 541)	*Strep. pyogenes* *Strep. pneumoniae* *Strep. aureus*	*Clostridium* spp.	*N. gonorrhoeae*	*E. coli* and other 'coliforms' including *Klebsiella*	
Trimethoprim (often given with sulphonamides as cotrimoxazole)	*Staph. aureus* *Streptococci*		*Neisseria* spp.	*Haemophilus influenzae* *E. coli* and other 'coliforms' including *Klebsiella* spp. *Salmonella typhi*	

Table 3.4. (cont.)

Antibiotic example	*Gram-positive cocci*	*Gram-positive bacilli*	*Gram-negative cocci*	*Gram-negative bacilli*	*Other*
Sulphonamides (often given with trimethoprim as cotrimoxazole)	*Staph. aureus* Streptococci		*N. meningitidis*	*E. coli* and other 'coliforms' (many strains resistant)	
Nitrofurantoin	*Staph. saprophyticus*			*E. coli* and other 'coliforms' (not reliable for *Proteus*)	
Rifampicin	Staphylococci Streptococci		*N. meningitidis*	*E. coli* and other 'coliforms'; *S. typhi*	*M. tuberculosis*

Table 3.5. Drugs active against viruses and fungi: examples of susceptible microbes

Drug	*Usage*	
Antiviral		
Idoxuridine	Topical	Herpes simplex virus
Cytarabine	Systemic	Herpes simplex virus
Vidarabine	Systemic	Herpes simplex virus
Acycloguanosine	Systemic (topical)	Herpes simplex virus Varicella-zoster virus
Amantadine	Systemic	Influenza A viruses
Methisazone	Systemic	Vaccinia and variola viruses
Interferon (species specific)	Systemic and topical	'Broad spectrum' anti-viral agent ('theoretical' at present)
Antifungal		
Polyenes:		
Amphotericin B	Systemic or topical	*Candida albicans*; *Cryptococcus*; *Aspergillus; Histoplasma*
Nystatin	Topical (including gut)	*Candida albicans*
Natamycin	Topical	*Candida albicans*
Imidazoles:		
Clotrimazole	Topical	*Candida albicans*; dermatophytes
Miconazole	Topical (and systemic)	*Candida albicans*; dermatophytes
Econazole	Topical	*Candida albicans*; dermatophytes
Ketoconazole	Systemic	South American *Coccidiomyces*; dermatophytes
Griseofulvin	Systemic	*Candida*; *Histoplasma*; dermatophytes
5-fluorocytosine	Systemic	*Candida albicans* (some strains); *Cryptococcus* (some strains)

Table 3.6. Anti-protozoal drugs

Drug example	*Some susceptible protozoa examples*	
Metronidazole	*Trichomonas vaginalis*	*Entaemoeba histolytica, Giardia lamblia*
Emetine		*Entaemoeba histolytica*
Pyrimethamine, Sulphadiazine	*Toxoplasma gondii*	Some *Plasmodium* strains (prophylaxis)
Spiramycin	*Toxoplasma gondii*	
Chloroquine, Quinine		*Plasmodium* (malaria) strains (treatment)
Primaquine		*Plasmodium vivax* (treatment liver cycle)
Pentamidine, Cotrimoxazole (high dosage)	*Pneumocystis carinii*	

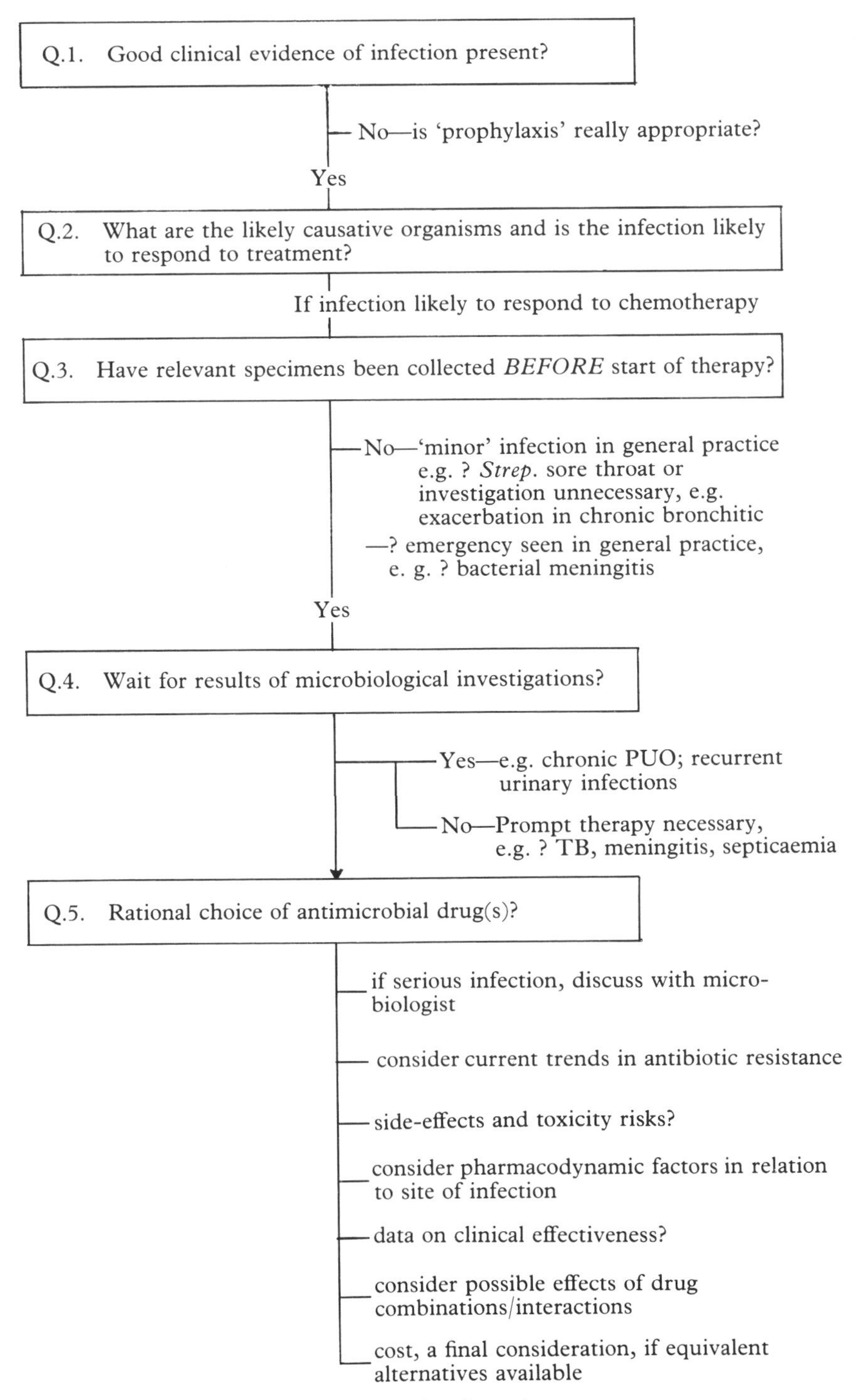

Fig. 3.1. Main questions to consider before starting chemotherapy.

procaine penicillin for treating gonorrhoea. However, 'narrow spectrum' treatment of many infections due to coliforms is not feasible since the agents available, such as aminoglycosides or polymyxins, are usually too potentially toxic. These narrow spectrum agents need to be restricted for the treatment of serious infections. In practice, broad spectrum antibiotics such as ampicillin, cotrimoxazole or a cephalosporin are used to treat many infections due to Gram-negative bacilli.

If the patient has recently received antibiotics, such as ampicillin, this should be taken into account when choosing an antibiotic, since the infecting organism might be resistant to the recently prescribed antibiotic.

Knowledge of the likely site of infection and of the pharmacodynamic characteristics of antimicrobial drugs is also important in the selection of the suitable agent. If, for example, there is a soft tissue infection or abscess due to *Staph. aureus*, a drug that penetrates well such as fusidic acid may be considered in combination with another anti-staphylococcal drug (surgical drainage may also be considered necessary). Chloramphenicol is suitable for treating some central nervous system bacterial infections since high concentrations are obtained in the CSF and the drug penetrates the brain barrier well.

Patient factors influence the selection of an antibiotic. If the patient has a suspected streptococcal sore throat and is allergic to penicillin, erythromycin may be used instead. Tetracycline should not be given to children or pregnant mothers because of the possible discolouration of teeth and the potential harmful effects on bones. Sulphonamides are best avoided in pregnancy and during the neonatal period as their use may be associated with the development of neonatal kernicterus.

Combinations of Antibiotics

Disadvantages of giving combinations of antibiotics include increasing the likelihood of the development of side effects or toxicity, superinfection and hospital cross-infection with antibiotic-resistant bacterial strains, the possibility of antagonism between the drugs against the infecting organism and increased costs. Examples of increased side effects or toxicity include the higher incidence of skin rashes or blood dyscrasias with trimethoprim and sulphonamides combined than with each agent alone and the increased incidence of nephrotoxicity when cephalosporins and gentamicin are combined. Superinfection and hospital cross-infection with multiple antibiotic-resistant strains of *Klebsiella* have especially occurred in patients receiving combinations of ampicillin plus cloxacillin, or cotrimoxazole and other antibiotic combinations. The more 'broad spectrum' the combined cover, the more likely that fungi, such as *Candida albicans*, will cause superinfections in hospital patients.

A good example of antagonism is the combination of penicillin and tetracycline; if these drugs are combined in a patient with pneumococcal infection the tetracycline, acting as a bacteriostatic drug, inhibits the division of pneumococci and antagonizes the action of penicillin which, as a bactericidal agent, acts mainly on dividing pneumococcal cells.

In practice, there are certain situations where combinations of antibiotics are valuable. These include:

1. *Mixed or 'unknown' infections*
   When each antibiotic alone cannot treat all of the main infecting organisms that are present in a mixed infection. An example of a justified combination in this situation includes the use of gentamicin and metronidazole together in a patient with serious abdominal sepsis where gentamicin is used mainly against coliforms and metronidazole mainly against *Bacteroides*.
2. *Synergistic combinations*
   Bactericidal synergistic antibiotic combinations are often necessary for treating patients with infective endocarditis, such as penicillin plus gentamicin for a patient with *Strep. faecalis* endocarditis. Bactericidal synergistic combinations may also be necessary for treating septicaemia due to Gram-negative bacilli in a severely neutropenic patient.
3. *Prevention or delay of development of drug resistance*
   When antituberculous drugs such as isoniazid, streptomycin or rifampicin are used alone resistant mutants may readily emerge during the course of treatment. This risk is greatly reduced by the use of combinations of antituberculous drugs (*see* p. 249). Other examples include the combination of fusidic acid with erythromycin or other anti-staphylococcal antibiotics for the treatment of *Staph. aureus* infections, and the combination of gentamicin and carbenicillin for the treatment of pseudomonas infections.

   Jawetz has suggested that the effects of antibiotic combinations may be predictable in general terms:
   a. A bactericidal drug combined with another bactericidal drug may produce a synergistic combination.
   b. A bacteriostatic drug combined with a bactericidal drug is likely to be antagonistic.
   c. A bacteriostatic drug combined with another bacteriostatic drug is usually merely additive.

However, there are so many species and strain variations and so many different antibiotics with different antimicrobial properties that it is often impossible to predict accurately the effect of a particular combination of drugs against a particular isolate. The laboratory can perform antibiotic combination tests on an isolate from a patient with a serious infection to determine whether synergy, antagonism, addition or indifference occurs in vitro. These tests are mainly carried out when managing difficult cases of endocarditis.

For a full account of antibiotic combinations the reader is referred to Simmons (1980).

PHARMACODYNAMIC FACTORS

Knowledge of the basic pharmacology of antimicrobial agents is important both for choosing an agent and for using the selected drug optimally. Pharmacodynamic factors determine whether a drug is likely to reach the site of infection in adequate concentration. Knowledge of the potential side effects and toxicity gives an indication of the extent to which such therapeutic concentrations can be safely achieved (i.e. the therapeutic index is assessed). Factors concerning the patient's age and weight, renal and hepatic function, and dialysis procedures may need careful consideration. In pregnancy, drugs that could damage the foetus must be avoided.

Administration by the Oral Route

Drugs can be either not absorbed, only partially absorbed or well absorbed after oral administration:

1. *Non-absorbable drugs*

   Non-absorbable antimicrobial drugs which are active topically against the normal flora or pathogens in the alimentary tract include neomycin, vancomycin, polymyxin and nystatin. However, if there is extensive disease affecting the gut, it is possible that some of these drugs could be exceptionally absorbed to cause toxic effects, such as neomycin in patients with ulcerative colitis or hepatic failure.

2. *Partially absorbed drugs*

   There are numerous drugs which are incompletely absorbed including penicillins, ampicillin, cloxacillin, tetracyclines and erythromycin. Gastric acid partially destroys some penicillins, such as penicillin G, but penicillin V (phenoxymethylpenicillin), ampicillin and cloxacillin are relatively acid resistant. Absorption of some drugs is delayed or reduced by giving them after eating a meal and this especially applies to ampicillin, tetracycline and cloxacillin. Milk and other substances containing divalent cations, such as calcium ions, can chelate tetracyclines so that they remain in the bowel. The disturbance to the normal bowel flora and the incidence of alimentary tract side effects such as diarrhoea is generally greatest with drugs that are only partially absorbed, especially if they are 'broad spectrum', such as ampicillin or tetracycline. It is best to administer many oral antimicrobial agents before meals. Nausea and vomiting, as well as bowel disease or recent surgery, may also reduce the absorption of some drugs.

   The parenteral rather than the oral route should be used to initially administer drugs to most patients who have acute serious infections because of the many variables affecting absorption.

3. *Well-absorbed drugs*

   In recent years, there have been successful attempts to improve the absorption of many types of antibiotics. Examples include the introduction of esters of ampicillin such as talampicillin and pivampicillin, of mecillinam such as pimecillinam, and of carbenicillin such as carfecillin, and the introduction of a modified isoxazolyl penicillin (flucloxacillin) which is slightly better absorbed than cloxacillin. The non-active esters of the beta-lactam drugs mentioned above protect the drugs from the gastric acid and, after passing through the stomach, enzymes release the active beta-lactam drug which is absorbed to give much higher serum levels than those achieved by administering the original beta-lactam drug. However in the case of carfecillin, the serum carbenicillin levels obtained are still too low to be useful therapeutically and adequate concentrations of carbenicillin may only be achieved in the urine.

   Amoxycillin is a similar but different drug to ampicillin which is absorbed twice as well as ampicillin. It also has a longer half-life in the serum than ampicillin. Oral amoxycillin should probably be used in preference to oral ampicillin for treating infections, although, at present, ampicillin costs less. Cephalexin and cephradine are two similar oral cephalosporins which are extremely well absorbed. Paradoxically, the serum levels of cephradine after oral administration are much higher than when the same drug is administered by the intra-muscular route. This phenomenon also occurs with chloramphenicol which is well absorbed after oral administration.

Parenteral Administration of Antimicrobial Agents

Rapid serum therapeutic concentrations of antibiotics are achieved by administering the drugs by the intravenous route which is important when treating patients with life-threatening infections such as septicaemia.

Erythromycin, tetracycline and chloramphenicol are more reliably administered by the intravenous than the intra-muscular routes when parenteral administration is indicated, but the potential hepatotoxicity of intravenous tetracycline needs to be remembered. Certain systemic acting drugs can only be administered intravenously, such as vancomycin or amphotericin B, and these may occasionally cause phlebitis. Some drugs, such as cephalothin, polymyxins or cefoxitin, particularly painful when administered by the intra-muscular route, are preferably administered intravenously.

When drugs are administered intravenously, there are dangers of introducing superinfections at the drip site or from the infusion bottle or cannula, and these risks should be avoided (*see* p. 489). In general, bolus administration through the drip tubing is probably preferable to continuous infusions of drug, but care is often necessary to administer the drug slowly by the bolus route as recommended by the manufacturer. Carbenicillin and some other drugs have to be administered by slow intermittent intravenous infusions and there are also incidental risks of electrolyte imbalance that must be taken into account. Less sodium ions may be administered when an alternative drug such as ticarcillin or azlocillin is used, for example, instead of carbenicillin. Drug interactions may also occur in infusion bottles if, for example, gentamicin is added to a bottle containing carbenicillin. Penicillin drugs, if administered by the continuous intravenous infusion method (perhaps, for example, when treating streptococcal endocarditis), might be partially inactivated by dextrose solutions.

Distribution and Bioavailability

After administration the antimicrobial agent should be distributed in the body to reach the site of infection. The exact pattern of distribution largely depends on physico-chemical and other properties of the drug including its lipid solubility, protein-binding and tissue-binding affinities, ability to cross cell membranes and penetrate into cells, and ability to cross the blood brain barrier. In general, very lipid soluble drugs, such as chloramphenicol, are widely distributed. Drugs which are water soluble and poorly soluble in lipids, such as gentamicin may be mainly distributed in the plasma and extracellular fluid. Certain antibiotics may achieve high concentrations in particular sites of body fluids in relation to the serum concentrations. Examples include fusidic acid and lincomycin which may penetrate bone well. About 30% of the serum levels of chloramphenicol are obtained in the CSF, whereas only low relative concentrations of aminoglycosides are obtained in this fluid. Penicillins and cephalosporins do not significantly penetrate into the CSF except when there is meningeal inflammation present or when toxic doses are given.

The role of protein binding is debatable when compared with other factors. When a drug is very highly protein bound, there may be little unbound drug available to be in a biologically active free form, but the strength of the binding may also vary between different drugs. Cloxacillin and fusidic acid are highly protein-bound drugs, whereas cephradine is poorly protein bound and erythromycin is moderately protein bound; in clinical practice, all of these drugs may be effective for treating *Staph. aureus* infections. Other pharmacodynamic factors, such as serum levels, the half-life of the drug, the concentrations at the site of infection, and the degrees of tissue binding, may sometimes be more important than the degree of binding to plasma proteins.

Renal Excretion

Many antimicrobial drugs including nalidixic acid, nitrofurantoin, penicillins, cloxacillin, cephalosporins, mecillinam, trimethoprim, sulphonamides, polymyxin, aminoglycosides and amphotericin B are mainly excreted by the renal route. The maintenance doses of these drugs may have to be reduced or the interval between the doses increased when there is impaired renal function to avoid toxicity, and assays of serum antibiotic levels are often necessary for the more toxic drugs. The aminoglycosides are mainly excreted by glomerular filtration, but penicillins and some cephalosporins are excreted by the tubular route which may sometimes be delayed by simultaneously administering probenecid.

Biliary and Faecal Excretion

Some drugs are mainly excreted in the bile, such as rifampicin, erythromycin and novobiocin. The drug may then be excreted in the faeces. Other drugs which are mainly excreted by the renal route may also be partly excreted in the bile, such as ampicillin, and this may have a practical application, such as in the treatment of typhoid carriers. However, when there is biliary tract obstruction, the concentrations of ampicillin in the bile may be much less than in a normal biliary tract and this may be relevant for the treatment of cholangitis or the typhoid carrier state.

Metabolism

Many antimicrobial drugs are partially or completely metabolized to microbiologically inactive compounds which are subsequently excreted. The liver is the main site of inactivation for chloramphenicol, metronidazole and fusidic acid, and to some extent lincomycin. Rifampicin and isoniazid are deacetylated in the liver. The rate of acetylation of isoniazid is genetically determined and there is a bimodal distribution of the population into rapid acetylators and slow acetylators of isoniazid. When there is hepatic damage, the doses of drugs metabolized by the liver may need adjustment.

Drug Interactions

When more than one antimicrobial agent or other drugs are administered simultaneously, there may be an interaction with the antibiotic which is pharmacological or microbiological. A good example of this is the interaction between diuretics, such as fusemide, and cephalosporins which increase the potential nephrotoxicity of the cephalosporins. The risk of nephrotoxicity is also increased when gentamicin is given at the same time as cephalosporins. Microbiological effects of antibiotic combinations have already been mentioned above, but, when the pH of the urine is altered, the activity of certain drugs such as nitrofurantoin or gentamicin may be affected.

Certain drugs, such as aminoglycosides including gentamicin, may interfere with normal neuromuscular transmission and the anaesthetist needs to take this into account when using muscle relaxants in surgical patients. Antimicrobial agents that are bound to plasma might displace other drugs and cause unwanted effects such as griseofulvin interacting with warfarin which may result in haemorrhages. Some antimicrobial drugs may induce increased hepatic enzyme function and bring about undesirable effects with other drugs; rifampicin or doxycycline may, for example, cause oral contraceptives to be more rapidly metabolized.

Duration of Therapy

The factors that influence the required duration of therapy include the choice of drug, the clinical evidence of relapse rates with different durations of therapy (if known), the degree of antimicrobial sensitivity of the pathogen, the dose, the route of administration, as well as the site of infection and the host defence mechanisms.

A week is usually recommended for a course of antibiotic for treating many bacterial infections. However, some infections can be effectively treated with less than 3 days' treatment or, in a few instances, after only one dose of drug, while other infections require longer than a week's therapy (*Table 3.7*). Unnecessary long treatment increases the chances of side effects or toxicity as well as causing increased costs. In hospital practice, there is a further important reason for checking that patients are not given antibiotic therapy longer than is strictly necessary and this is the increased risks of acquiring hospital infections caused by antibiotic-resistant organisms.

USE OF MICROBIOLOGICAL INVESTIGATIONS IN THE MANAGEMENT OF THERAPY

The use of the laboratory for obtaining a rapid presumptive microbiological diagnosis has already been mentioned above. Once certain organisms have been identified, the antimicrobial sensitivity can usually be predicted; examples include *Strep. pyogenes* which is always sensitive to penicillin, *Candida albicans* which is always sensitive to nystatin or amphotericin B and *Strep. pneumoniae* which is nearly always sensitive to penicillin. In many hospitals, the antimicrobial sensitivities of other common pathogens can also be predicted, for example *Staph. aureus* strains are usually sensitive to cloxacillin. For the treatment of severe infections and of most bacterial infections in hospital, it is essential to base subsequent rational therapy on the results of the laboratory antibiotic tests.

Table 3.7. Duration of therapy

Example	*Traditional duration of treatment recommended*	*Comments*
Penicillin treatment for gonorrhoea	Single dose (procaine penicillin)	Repeat doses necessary for 'complicated' gonorrhoea
Penicillin treatment for streptococcal sore throat	5- or 10-day course	Lower relapse rate after 10-day course
Ampicillin/amoxycillin for 'simple' urinary tract infection	1 week	3-day course, as effective as 1 week course,—2 doses possibly may suffice*
Penicillin/chloramphenicol for confirmed meningococcal meningitis	1–2 weeks	Required duration not known
Chloramphenicol treatment for typhoid fever	At least 2 weeks	Shorter courses associated with higher relapse rates
Penicillin treatment of streptococcal endocarditis	At least 6 weeks	For endocarditis due to penicillin sensitive *Strep. viridans* treatment for 3–4 weeks may be adequate as long as aminoglycosides are added during the first 2 weeks (Streptococcal prosthetic valve endocarditis requires at least 8 weeks' treatment even if aminoglycosides are used in combination)
Chemotherapy for pulmonary tuberculosis	*In 1960s: 1·5–2 years* *In 1980: 9 months*	6-month courses might prove effective if pyrazinamide is included in the combined therapy*
Erythromycin treatment for Legionnaires' disease	*3 weeks*	Shorter courses can become complicated by a fatal relapse

* Further evaluations of these short courses are being carried out.

Antibiotic Disc Diffusion Sensitivity Tests

These tests predict the usefulness of different antimicrobial agents when used at the usual therapeutic doses. They give a very approximate measure of the degree of sensitivity and there are occasions when the sensitivity tests in vitro do not correlate with the clinical results of treatment either for technical or for other reasons. Good host defences might occasionally help to give the impression of 'successful' antibiotic therapy, even when the infecting organism was apparently resistant to the drug selected. In general, when there is a serious infection due to a bacterial strain which is resistant to an antibiotic on controlled disc tests, it is unlikely that the patient will respond clinically to treatment with that antibiotic (*see also* Failure of antibiotic therapy *below*).

Organisms likely to be causing infection rather than colonization are selected for disc tests. However, in practice, this distinction between infecting and colonizing organisms is sometimes difficult.

The secondary (indirect) antibiotic sensitivity test results on pure cultures of the isolates are usually available two days after the receipt of the clinical specimen. Primary (direct) antibiotic sensitivity tests can be carried out by placing antibiotic discs directly on agar plates that have been inoculated with the clinical sample, such as urine or pus; the results of antibiotic sensitivity tests may then be available after only overnight culture. In practice, primary antibiotic sensitivity disc tests are carried out on samples from patients with serious infections, such as a CSF from a patient with purulent meningitis, pus from an abdominal abscess, and infected urine from a patient with suspected pyelonephritis. The antibiotic discs are often selected according to the results of a Gram-stain of the specimen.

There are many potential technical problems involved with 'routine' antibiotic disc tests. A standardized method is necessary where—

1. The inoculum is adjusted to give a uniform, dense but not quite confluent growth (especially important for sulphonamides and cephalosporins).
2. A standard sensitivity medium is used, which also preferably has inhibitors of sulphonamides (*p*-aminobenzoic acid) or trimethoprim (thymidine) removed.
3. Discs, strips or rings containing antibiotics have to contain suitable known amounts of drug and the discs should be stable on storage and reproducible results obtained between batches.
4. The conditions of incubation and other factors also must be standardized as well as the method of interpreting the inhibition zones around discs. Most laboratories report an organism as either 'sensitive', 'moderately sensitive' or 'resistant' to the antibiotic. When 'moderately sensitive' is reported, it is usually meant that the infection due to the organism might respond to larger than usual doses of the antibiotic.

The use of good controls with each batch of tests is essential. A rotary 'Stokes Method' is often used today in Britain to help to control the results (*see Fig. 3.2* and Stokes and Ridgway, 1980). In this system, control organisms with known full sensitivity, such as the 'Oxford' strain of *Staph. aureus* or known strains of *E. coli* or *Pseudomonas aeruginosa*, are compared with the appropriate test strains on the same plate. When the inhibition zone of the test organism is similar to that of the control sensitive strain, the test is reported as 'sensitive'. When the test strain

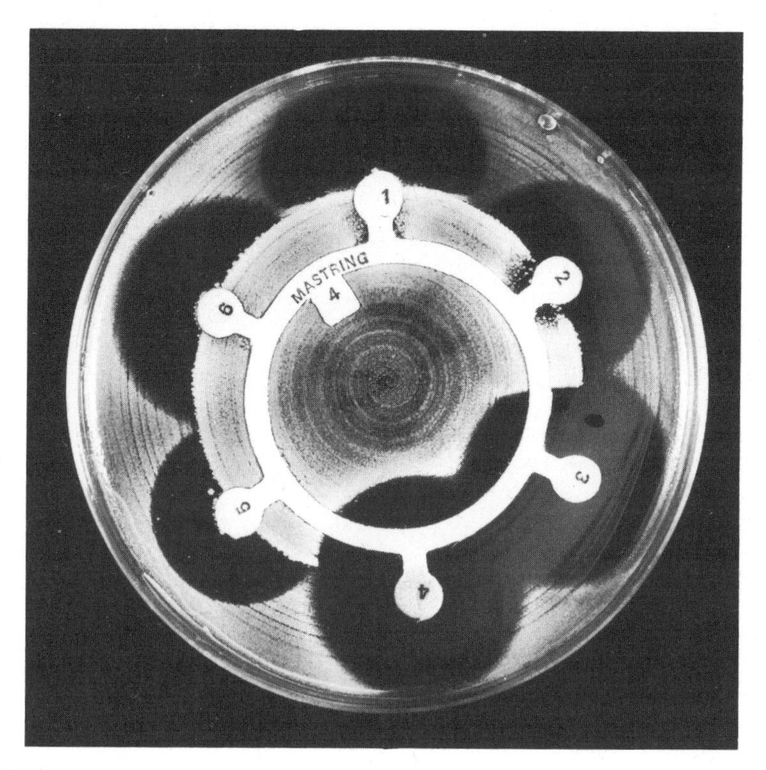

Fig. 3.2. Stokes antibiotic sensitivity test plate showing *Staph. aureus* strain with a multiple antibiotic resistance pattern in the centre.

grows within 3 mm of the disc and the control strain shows a large zone of inhibition, the test organism is reported as 'resistant'.

Participation by the laboratory in quality control programmes helps the laboratory to ensure that the results of antibiotic sensitivity test methods are reliable.

Slow-growing organisms, such as mycobacteria, require special methods of sensitivity tests (*see* p. 247).

Minimal Inhibitory Concentration (MIC)

A range of concentrations of an antibiotic can be incorporated into a suitable broth in a series of tubes, known as the 'tube dilution technique', or into solid medium in a series of plates ('agar MIC'). The broth or agar is inoculated with a standardized inoculum of the test organism. A control organism with a known MIC is also tested simultaneously. After incubation, the minimal inhibitory concentration of the drug is the concentration required to inhibit the organism (the relevant tube is often apparent on inspection for turbidity or change of colour of a pH indicator).

The MIC is only routinely determined for a few clinical isolates from patients with serious infections where optimal antimicrobial therapy is essential.

Examples include streptococci from blood cultures from patients with infective endocarditis and some bacterial strains causing septicaemia in immunosuppressed patients.

Minimum Bactericidal Concentration (MBC)

When the MIC determination mentioned above has been carried out on a bacterial isolate in broth, the tubes may be subcultured onto blood agar to determine the minimum concentration of drug required to kill the organism (MBC). This test is only occasionally necessary in a 'routine' laboratory but is indicated on streptococci and some other organisms causing infective endocarditis (*see* Chapter 18).

Antibiotic Combinations

Sometimes synergy (*Fig. 3.3*) is suggested by disc test results when the zones near the junction of the drugs are larger than around each drug alone. When the zone around one drug is reduced in the presence of the other drug antagonism is suggested. Accurate determination can only be determined by quantitative studies using a 'chessboard' or 'cellophane transfer techniques', where a range of concentrations of each drug alone and in combination is tested. These tests are mainly necessary in patients with endocarditis when a bactericidal synergic drug combination has to be selected. The classical example is the use of a penicillin with an aminoglycoside for treating *Strep. faecalis* endocarditis.

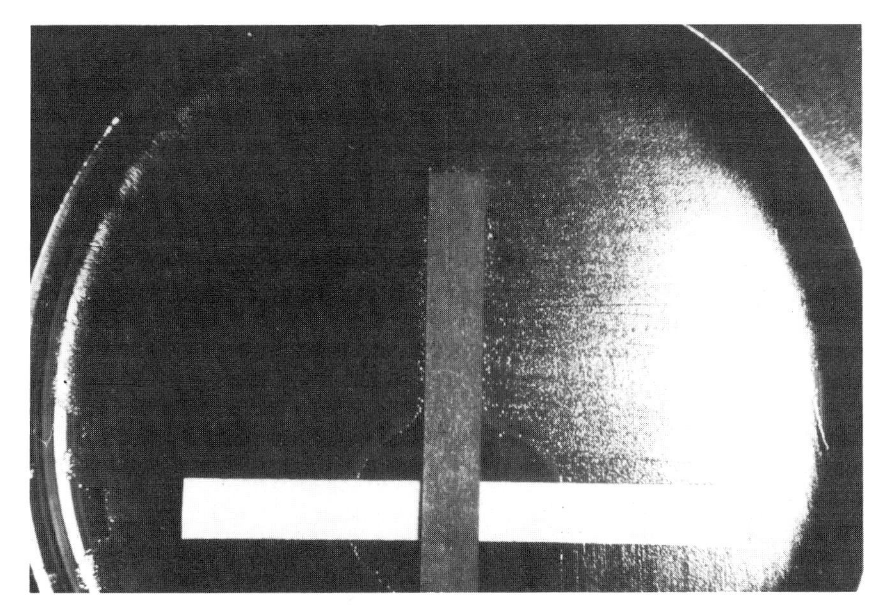

Fig. 3.3. Antibiotic synergy plate showing synergy between penicillin (vertical strip) and streptomycin (horizontal strip) against a strain of *Enterococcus*.

Serum Bactericidal Assay Test

This type of assay is a simple method to assess antibiotic treatment in a patient with serious infection. Fresh serum is collected from the patient just before and shortly after a dose of antibiotic (such as 1 hour after i.m. penicillin) and is double diluted in broth to which a standard inoculum of the bacterial isolate is added. After incubation the tubes showing no growth are subcultured onto blood agar (as this 'no growth' might be due to a static action only) and the serum bactericidal titre against the patient's own infecting organism is then determined. Ideally a greater than one-in-eight post dose bacterial titre should be aimed at during the treatment of infective endocarditis (*see* p. 349).

This test can also be carried out in patients with septicaemia or deep sepsis, especially when the patient is severely neutropenic or has immunodeficiency. Optimal bactericidal therapy is then necessary and the dose can be adjusted according to the results of the serum bactericidal assay. If the patient's organism is not killed by even a one in two dilution of the patient's serum collected 1 hour after a 'large' dose of the antibiotic, a change of drug or the use of a synergistic bactericidal combination of drugs may need further urgent consideration.

ANTIBIOTIC ASSAYS

Assays of antibiotics in serum, CSF, pus or sputum may occasionally be necessary to determine whether adequate concentrations of antimicrobial agents are obtained at the likely sites of infection, or to see if an accumulation of the drug is occurring in the serum which might lead to potentially toxic concentrations. Antibiotic assays should always be discussed between the clinician and microbiologist before samples are collected. Great care is necessary to collect serum or other fluids for assay at the most appropriate times in relation to the times of administration of the doses and all these times should be accurately recorded. Serum samples collected around the expected peak times should be able to give an indication of the likely effectiveness of the treatment (and, for gentamicin, this usually means 1 hour after an intramuscular dose of gentamicin or half an hour after an intravenous dose of gentamicin; another example is the collection of a peak serum $1\frac{1}{2}$ hours after an oral dose of amoxycillin). When toxicity tests need to be assessed, serum samples are generally best collected just before the next dose of drug and these are known as 'trough' or 'pre-dose' serum samples.

Examples of special situations where antibiotic assays should be considered are included in *Table 3.8*. Aminoglycoside serum assays are probably the most frequently performed antibiotic assays. The main aminoglycoside drugs assayed are gentamicin, tobramycin, amikacin and streptomycin and this is necessary to avoid ototoxicity and, to a lesser extent, nephrotoxicity, and also to check that adequate doses are given to patients with serious infections. Serum samples are usually collected after at least two doses of drug have been given, as repeated dosage is necessary before an 'equilibrated' (or steady state) pattern of serum levels is established in a patient. Rapid assay results are often available within 3–5 hours of collection of the sample using microbiological methods. In some recent immunoassay tests the results may be available within 30 minutes. Rapid assay results are particularly valuable during the first 1 or 2 days of treatment of

Table 3.8. Indications for antibiotic assays

Example	*Specimens for antibiotic assay*	*Type of assay*
Gram-negative septicaemia, peritonitis, or other serious infections treated with aminoglycosides	Serum 'pre-' and 'post-dose' samples	Serum aminoglycoside assays, e.g. gentamicin assays
Infective endocarditis, when treated with oral amoxycillin	Serum samples	Serum amoxycillin assays (*see* Chapter 18)
Infective endocardits or serious staphylococcal infections treated with vancomycin	Serum 'pre'- and 'post-dose' samples	Serum vancomycin assays
Meningitis treated with chloramphenicol (neonates)	Serum and CSF samples	Serum and CSF chloramphenicol assays
Renal tuberculosis treated with streptomycin	Serum samples	Serum streptomycin assays

patients with acute life-threatening Gram-negative septicaemias. Gentamicin is the most frequently assayed drug in the serum.

Serum Gentamicin Assay

Purpose: Safe and effective gentamicin therapy
Indications:
1. Impaired renal function
2. Elderly patients
3. When gentamicin is to be given for more than 1 week even though renal function is apparently normal initially
4. Poor clinical improvement (?) as inadequate dosage—discuss with clinical microbiologist

Information required for laboratory:
1. Approximate age (and ideally weight)
2. State of renal function (serum urea/creatinine levels)
3. Time of last dose of gentamicin
4. Times of taking blood for assay
   (trough and peak levels usually desirable)
5. Dose regime
6. Length of time the patient has been on gentamicin
7. Other antibiotics, current or recent (for example, beta-lactams, such as cephalosporins)

Interpretation of gentamicin assay results:
Close collaboration between clinician and microbiologist is essential for interpretation of the results in each patient.
1. *Ototoxicity*
   Toxic effects are most likely to occur during long durations of therapy and when there are high serum trough levels (greater than 2 mg per litre). For example: the patient with a serum trough level of 4 mg/l, gentamicin daily for 10 days or longer, has a relatively high risk of developing vestibular VIII cranial nerve side effects such as giddiness, nausea and vomiting.
   Repeated serum gentamicin levels are often necessary in patients requiring prolonged therapy and daily levels are indicated in patients with severe impairment of renal function.
   Comparison of the results from one day to the next will help to show evidence of drug accumulation (increasing trough levels) and then the doses of gentamicin should be reduced if ototoxicity is to be avoided.
2. *Effectiveness of therapy*
   The initial therapy should not depend on the results of antibiotic assay. It is important to give sufficiently large doses to patients with life-threatening infections during the first 24 hours of therapy. The initial doses can be determined by reference to a dosage table or to a Mawer's nomogram (in an adult patient of approx. 70 kg weight with normal renal function, the total dose of gentamicin usually recommended is at least 6 mg per kg per day). When the renal function is impaired, a full 'loading' dose is still indicated although the 'maintenance' doses may need reduction. Rapid gentamicin assay results can be available to help monitor therapy from the second day of treatment and at repeated intervals depending on the clinical situation.

The MICs of most coliforms to gentamicin are less than 5 mg/l and minimal serum gentamicin levels of 5 mg/l should be achieved 1 hour after an intramuscular (half an hour after an intravenous) dose of gentamicin, in patients with Gram-negative septicaemia. The peak gentamicin levels should preferably be greater than 8 mg/l for treating Gram-negative septicaemia in severely neutropenic patients or for the treatment of serious *Pseudomonas aeruginosa* infections. The microbiologist might arrange for an MIC to gentamicin of an organism from a blood culture or CSF from 'difficult' infections so that a more exact idea of the desirable post-dose gentamicin levels can be ascertained. Ideally, the serum peak gentamicin levels should exceed the MIC by a factor of at least two. However to help avoid toxicity, the peak serum gentamicin levels should probably not exceed 15 mg/l although trough levels are mainly used to help in the determination of the risks of toxicity.

Methods of Antibiotic Assay

Most antibiotic assays in Britain are at present carried out by microbiological assay methods. These methods are time consuming, and involve skilled techniques and the use of adequate internal quality control serum samples. Information about other antibiotics given to a patient at the same time as the antibiotic for assay is essential so that the most appropriate assay method can be selected. A suitable drug-inactivating enzyme can sometimes be added to the serum (for example beta-lactamase to destroy cephalosporins). The assays are usually carried out by plate diffusion methods. With serum gentamicin assays a standard klebsiella assay organism is used to inoculate the surface of an agar plate, holes are cut and serum standards containing known concentrations of gentamicin and test sera are used to fill the holes in the same plate. After either overnight incubation at 35 °C or rapid incubation (such as after 3 hours at 40 °C), the inhibition zones are measured on an optical zone reader. The zone diameters of the standards are plotted on a graph against log gentamicin concentration. The test concentrations can be calculated by marking the test zone diameters on the standard curve and reading off the corresponding test concentrations. There are many potential pitfalls with these techniques. Most British laboratories participate in national quality control programmes in order to help check the reliability of the assays.

Other methods of antibiotic assays include immunoassay methods such as fluorimetric assay or radio-immunoassay techniques, and radio-active enzyme methods such as a gentamicin acetyl transferase method which requires a liquid scintillation counter. In the last few years, high pressure liquid chromatography (HPLC) techniques have been used to assay many antimicrobial drugs including cephalosporins and chloramphenicol. The assay of chloramphenicol is particularly important in neonates to help avoid 'grey syndrome' while still achieving effective chloramphenicol concentrations.

CAUSES OF FAILURE OF ANTIMICROBIAL CHEMOTHERAPY

The causes for the apparent failure of a course of chemotherapy include failures to apply the principles discussed above and are summarized below.

1. *Clinical Condition not Susceptible to Antimicrobial Treatment*

A frequent cause of apparently failed antibiotic treatment is the hidden collection of a substantial quantity of pus which needs to be located and surgically drained. Alternatively, the patient may have a reticulosis, a drug reaction or other non-microbial cause of fever which could not be expected to respond to antimicrobial chemotherapy. In some cases, an infection may be present which will not respond to antibiotic treatment, such as glandular fever. Even when 'pathogens' have been isolated, it is possible that there is a mixed infection. Superinfection with antibiotic-resistant organisms may also occur during treatment.

2. *Failure to use the Laboratory Properly*

Specimens may not have been collected before the start of antibiotic therapy and this is especially serious if there is a life-threatening infection present, such as infective endocarditis. Inappropriate poorly collected or improperly transported specimens may have been received by the laboratory (*see* Chapter 2).

3. *Limitations of Laboratory Methods and Laboratory Errors*

The laboratory may fail to recognize the causative organism of infection in good quality specimens, either because of the lack of sensitivity of the diagnostic methods or because of technical errors. Errors in the laboratory identification and antibiotic sensitivity tests may occasionally occur.

4. *Wrong Choice of Antibiotics*

The choice of drugs has been discussed above. An obvious example of a wrong choice of drug is ampicillin for treating oestomyelitis which is due to a penicillinase-producing *Staph. aureus* strain.

5. *Wrong Doses*

Inadequate doses may have been given. This is particularly important in a patient with a serious infection such as Gram-negative septicaemia; dosage of gentamicin, for example, may not have been monitored by antibiotic assays. Drugs should be given sufficiently frequently, taking into account the expected half-life of the drug in a particular patient.

6. *Inadequate Duration*

Relapses of infection may occur if drugs are not given for long enough.

7. *Wrong Route of Administration*

The unreliable absorption of certain drugs, e.g. after oral administration, or occasionally after an intramuscular injection, becomes especially important when serious infections are treated.

8. *Use of Antagonistic Antibiotic Combinations*

This is most likely to occur when a bacteriostatic agent, such as tetracycline, is used at the same time as a bactericidal agent, such as penicillin (*see* p. 43).

9. *Development of Antimicrobial Resistance*

There are many examples of the possible development of resistance to the antimicrobial agent given during a course of therapy. Examples include the development of resistance by staphylococci to rifampicin or fusidic acid, or of tubercle bacilli to streptomycin when these drugs are used alone. Resistance transfer mediated by plasmids, sometimes to several antibiotics at once, may occur between gut organisms during treatment. This transfer of resistance may sometimes occur between an organism which is non-pathogenic in a particular patient, to a pathogen. For example, a strain of *Salmonella* may become resistant to ampicillin or trimethoprim by acquiring a plasmid for resistance to these antibiotics from an antibiotic-resistant strain of *E. coli* in the bowel of the patient.

RESISTANCE TO ANTIMICROBIAL DRUGS

There are many different mechanisms for antimicrobial drug resistance and knowledge of the genetic basis for these has increased greatly in recent years. Drug resistance trends are often unpredicted. For example, the sudden emergence in 1976–1977 of gentamicin resistance in *Staph. aureus* strains occurred in many countries, although no resistance of this type had been reported during the previous ten years. Another example was the appearance for the first time of penicillinase-producing *Neisseria gonorrhoeae* strains in different parts of the world including the U.S.A., Britain, the Far East and Africa in 1976–1977. A brief account of antibiotic drug resistance is included in this section.

Natural Drug Resistance

An entire bacterial species may be resistant to an antibiotic before the introduction of the drug. Examples include *Strep. pyogenes* resistant to gentamicin, *Staph. aureus* resistant to polymyxins, *Proteus mirabilis* resistant to polymyxins, *Pseudomonas aeruginosa* resistant to cloxacillin, *Mycoplasma pneumoniae* resistant to penicillin and *Candida albicans* resistant to griseofulvin. Of course, there are many other examples. Reasons for innate drug resistance include lack of penetration of the drug through the cell wall, lack of a suitable cell wall target site or other target receptors in the cell, and susceptibility to naturally produced drug-destroying enzymes that may have existed before the introduction of the drug commercially.

Acquired Drug Resistance and 'Cross Resistance'

The two main groups of antimicrobial drug resistance mechanisms are mechanisms involving drug-destroying enzymes or intrinsic type resistance mechanisms.

Drug-destroying Enzymes

Penicillinases and cephalosporinases are beta-lactamases which hydrolyse the beta-lactam ring of various penicillin and cephalosporin drugs. The beta-lactamases that are produced by some *Staph. aureus* strains, *E. coli*, *Klebsiella*, *Proteus*, *Pseudomonas*, *Haemophilus influenzae*, *Neisseria gonorrhoeae* and other bacterial strains may differ in their ability to destroy particular beta-lactam antibiotics and to cause 'cross-resistance'. For example, the penicillinase which is produced characteristically by hospital *Staph. aureus* strains is responsible for cross-resistance in these strains between penicillin and ampicillin, amoxycillin, carbenicillin, ticarcillin and azlocillin, but there is no significant cross-resistance between penicillin and cloxacillin or cephradine as these latter semi-synthetic beta-lactam drugs are relatively insusceptible to this penicillinase.

Drug-destroying enzymes are responsible for high level antibiotic resistance in some Gram-negative bacilli including resistance to many aminoglycosides. Examples include aminoglycoside phosphotransferases, acetyltransferases and adenyltransferases and, depending on the particular enzymes present in a strain, an organism may be resistant to several different aminoglycosides. Some *E. coli* or *Klebsiella* strains may be resistant to streptomycin and kanamycin but sensitive to gentamicin and tobramycin, while other strains for example may be cross-resistant to streptomycin, kanamycin, gentamicin and tobramycin but sensitive to amikacin.

Intrinsic-Type Resistance Mechanisms

Permeability barriers to drugs can be developed as an intrinsic resistance mechanism. This occurs with tetracycline resistance in some *Staph. aureus* strains and amikacin resistance in some Gram-negative bacilli.

Development of an altered metabolic pathway can allow bacterial strains to be no longer inhibited by a drug, for example sulphonamide resistance in *E. coli* strains can be due to these strains requiring less extracellular *p*-aminobenzoic acid for folic acid synthesis.

Alteration of a target site in the cell is a frequent mechanism of drug resistance. Examples include alteration of the ribosome binding sites for some aminoglycosides, e.g. in some streptomycin-resistant *Staph. aureus* or *E. coli* strains.

Methicillin resistance in *Staph. aureus* strains is due to an unknown type of intrinsic resistance mechanism. There is some cross-resistance in these strains between methicillin and cloxacillin, flucloxacillin and cephalosporins.

Adaptation (Tolerance)

There are many examples of laboratory 'training' of organisms to become gradually adapted to grow in the presence of increasing concentrations of a drug and such an adaptive process is often not important clinically. However, there are some instances of the gradual development of low levels of drug resistance in clinical isolates. For example, the MIC of penicillin for gonococcal strains gradually increased from 0·007 mg/l in the early 1950s up to about 10 to 30 times this level for some strains during the 1960s. These latter relatively penicillin-resistant gonococcal strains can still be effectively treated by using high doses of parenteral penicillin with probenecid. By the early 1970s, there were occasional infections due to gonococcal strains with MICs of about 1·0 mg/l and these infections were difficult to treat unless penicillin was given in enormous doses.

'Single Step' Chromosomal Mutation and the Selection of Drug-Resistant Mutants

The rapid development of a high level of antimicrobial drug resistance in an infecting strain may occur during a course of treatment when the drug is used alone. This particularly applies in staphylococci to streptomycin, rifampicin, novobiocin and, to a lesser extent, fusidic acid and erythromycin. The frequency of spontaneous mutation of chromosomal genes that control the susceptibility to a drug can be between 10^{-6} and 10^{-12} per generation. For the above drugs, the development of drug-resistant mutants can occur at a relatively high frequency and, once resistant mutants appear, they may become selected out in the presence of the drug so that after a short time only drug-resistant mutants are isolated from the patient. When, for example, streptomycin is used alone to treat an *E. coli* urinary infection, a few mutants may appear rapidly resistant to streptomycin and within a few days the whole population of *E. coli* appears resistant to streptomycin. A high degree of resistance can appear due to a single base change in the DNA of *E. coli* so that the ribosome is altered and is no longer susceptible to the action of streptomycin. Chromosomal resistance is also important in the treatment of tuberculosis; the chances of acquired resistance occurring due to the selection of chromosomal-resistant mutants of tubercle bacilli is much less if at least two effective anti-tuberculous drugs are used together rather than separately (for example streptomycin plus isoniazid or rifampicin plus isoniazid).

Infectious Drug Resistance (Transmissible Drug Resistance)

It is now realized that most of the clinically important acquired drug resistance in antibiotic resistant strains of *Staph. aureus* and many antibiotic-resistant strains of Gram-negative bacilli are 'R' factor (plasmid) mediated. Plasmids are extra-chromosomal packets of DNA which may code for antibiotic resistance and be transferred from an antibiotic-resistant strain to a sensitive strain, thereby causing the sensitive strain to become antibiotic resistant. The Japanese workers who first described plasmids in the early 1960s in strains of *Shigella*, coding for simultaneous multiple antibiotic resistance to tetracycline, streptomycin, sulphonamide and chloramphenicol, suggested that the plasmids could have originated in antibiotic-resistant *E. coli* strains and that the transfer of plasmids from *E. coli* to *Shigella* strains was possible by a conjugation mechanism, involving the sex pilus of donor bacterial cells. Since then many different plasmids have been described in Gram-negative bacteria which may transfer 'en bloc' multiple antibiotic resistance between different strains of the same species, between strains of different species, and between strains of different genera.

Plasmids mediating antibiotic resistance in *Staph. aureus* strains differ in two main ways from those that mediate antibiotic resistance in strains of Gram-negative bacteria. Firstly, the plasmid transfer from an antibiotic-resistant donor strain of *Staph. aureus* to an initially sensitive recipient strain is by means of transducing bacteriophages, during close intercell contact, instead of the conjugation method associated with Gram-negative bacilli. Secondly, the plasmids in *Staph. aureus* strains usually code genetically for only one or two different antibiotic resistances at a time, such as penicillin or/and tetracycline resistance, whereas one plasmid in a Gram-negative bacillus often simultaneously codes for resistance to several different antibiotics. A multiple antibiotic-resistant strain of *Staph. aureus* may contain two or more different antibiotic-resistance plasmids.

Plasmids naturally occur in strains of *E. coli* and other species in the normal human flora, but the incidence of plasmids is probably higher in countries where antibiotics are directly available to the general population such as in Mexico, Greece and some Asian countries. In the absence of any antibiotic prescribing, many of the bacterial strains spontaneously lose the plasmids. In the countries mentioned above, it is particularly possible for plasmids in the normal human bowel flora to be transferred to certain strains of intestinal pathogens, such as *Salmonella* and *Shigella*. In this way it is likely that a plasmid for chloramphenicol resistance, for example, became transferred to different strains of *Salmonella typhi*. Chloramphenicol-resistant typhoid bacilli have caused recent outbreaks of typhoid fever in Mexico and the Far East. Transfer of plasmid-carrying bacteria can occur between the flora of man and animals. The best example was the spread of multiple antibiotic-resistant strains of *Salmonella typhimurium*, phage type 29, resistant to streptomycin, ampicillin, tetracycline and furazolidine from cattle to man in the late 1960s.

Plasmids may evolve to gain more antibiotic-resistant determinants and sometimes to lose them. 'Transposons' are small pieces of DNA which, unlike plasmids, cannot replicate themselves but which may 'jump' between different plasmids and between plasmids and chromosomes and these DNA pieces are long enough to carry recognizable genes. One example of an important gene carried by an antibiotic-resistant transposon is known as 'TEM1'. The TEM gene on the transposon controls the production of beta-lactamase and this transposon is incorporated into plasmids which then mediate resistance to beta-lactam antibiotics, such as ampicillin, in some strains of *E. coli*, *Klebsiella*, and other coliforms, *Haemophilus influenzae*, Pittman capsulated type b and *Neisseria gonorrhoeae*. The transfer of the TEM-containing transposon from a beta-lactamase-producing *E. coli* strain to an initially beta-lactam-sensitive strain of *Haemophilus* or a gonococcal organism is probably a very rare event. However, once this event has occurred, the new strain may itself spread to cause infections and the plasmid containing the TEM transposon may also spread between different *Haemophilus* or gonococcal strains relatively easily so that a great increase in the distribution of this plasmid occurs. This spread of the plasmid is particularly likely when there is widespread use of ampicillin or other beta-lactam drugs. At the present time, the TEM gene for beta-lactamase production is distributed in 17 different bacterial genera in many countries of the world.

Other examples of plasmid-mediated enzymes include the aminoglycoside-inactivating enzymes and chloramphenicol acetyltransferase. Intrinsic resistance mechanisms can also be mediated by plasmids and an example is tetracycline resistance in *Staph. aureus* strains.

Epidemiology of Antibiotic Resistance

The incidence of antibiotic resistance in strains of different bacterial species depends on three main groups of factors including:

1. The occurrence of plasmids or transposons which mediate drug resistance in bacteria.
2. The patterns of use of antimicrobial drugs in hospitals or in the general population or in animals.

   The greater the quantities of drugs used and the longer the drugs have been in use, the more likely it is that strains resistant to the antibiotics will develop and spread. Certain types of usage are strongly associated with the development of resistance, such as topical use of gentamicin, fusidic acid or neomycin which may result in the development and spread of bacterial strains resistant to these antibiotics.
3. The degree of cross-infection with antibiotic-resistant strains of bacteria. This is particularly relevant in hospitals.

Multiple antibiotic resistance in *Staph. aureus* strains in the general wards of many hospitals has declined during the 1970s so that the majority of strains are only penicillin resistant, whereas, in the 1950s and early 1960s, multiple antibiotic resistance in *Staph. aureus* was a serious problem. Today occasional problems with outbreaks due to multiple antibiotic-resistant strains may still occur. Methicillin and gentamicin-resistant *Staph. aureus* strains are now causing increasing cross-infection problems in many major hospitals in different parts of the world.

Gram-negative multiple antibiotic resistance is prevalent but in the majority of hospitals the incidence of resistance to gentamicin or modern cephalosporins, such as cefuroxime or cefoxitin, is low, usually less than 5% of *E. coli* strains being resistant to these antibiotics. The situation in relation to individual antibiotics will vary, from year to year, between different hospital units as well as between different hospitals in various parts of a country and between different countries. The incidence of antibiotic resistance in Gram-negative bacilli in the general population is greatest in undeveloped countries where incorrect use and overuse of antibiotics is common.

ANTIBIOTIC PROPHYLAXIS

Antibiotics are probably overused for prophylactic purposes and this has contributed to the development and spread of antibiotic resistance in bacterial strains, as well as to cross-infection incidents with antibiotic-resistant strains of bacteria. A serious outbreak of *Klebsiella* infections in a neurosurgical unit was only brought under control when 'prophylactic' ampicillin, which was routinely given to surgical patients, was stopped (*see* Price and Sleigh, 1970). Cephalosporins are frequently used for 'prophylaxis' in surgical patients and it is likely that one of the consequences of this is an increased incidence of superinfections due to *Pseudomonas aeruginosa* strains.

In each instance where antibiotic prophylaxis is considered, the risks to the patient from no prophylaxis and the risks from side effects or toxic effects of the antimicrobial drugs selected should be assessed. Also the evidence that prophylaxis with particular drugs will be effective in preventing infection due to the particular likely causative organisms should be considered. Whenever possible narrow spectrum drugs rather than broad spectrum drugs should be used against a specific microbe to minimize the disturbance to the normal flora and the risks of superinfection; this is particularly important in hospital in-patients. A clear differentiation of prophylaxis as opposed to 'early treatment' is desirable but not always possible.

Medical Indications for Prophylaxis

There are only a few main examples of justified medical prophylaxis. These include:

a. *Rheumatic fever*
Long term prophylaxis with oral penicillin V is indicated in children who have had rheumatic fever to prevent a further *Strep. pyogenes* infection which could otherwise lead to another attack of rheumatic fever.

b. Meningococcal meningitis
Immediate prophylaxis for close contacts in the family (or institution) of a case of meningococcal meningitis is necessary with either sulphonamides or rifampicin depending on the local prevalence of sulphonamide-resistant meningococci (*see* Chapter 10, 173). The use of penicillin in this situation would be a good example of inappropriate prophylaxis since penicillin does not eliminate naso-pharyngeal carriage of meningococci.

Recurrent urinary tract infections

Low dose long term cotrimoxazole (or trimethoprim alone) prophylaxis may be indicated in selected patients, especially children, to prevent recurrent urinary tract infections (*see* Chapter 19, 374).

Surgical Indications for Prophylaxis

Lower limb amputation

Gas gangrene post-operatively may occur unless specific prophylaxis is given to cover amputations, major hip surgery or other surgery on the lower limbs of a patient, especially when ischaemic arterial disease is present. Benzylpenicillin is indicated with the first dose given shortly before the start of the operation, so that penicillin is present throughout the operation, and in the immediate post-operative period to prevent germination of spores of *Cl. welchii*. Povidone iodine pre-operative compresses may also be used at the site of the operation.

Prevention of endocarditis in dental patients

The possibly fatal consequences of endocarditis developing, following bacteraemia, with organisms known to cause endocarditis in patients with known susceptible heart lesions, justifies the use of prophylactic antibiotics even though the chances of endocarditis occurring without any prophylaxis are small. For susceptible patients undergoing dental extractions or other 'at risk' dental procedures, a parenteral administration of a mixture of short- and long-acting penicillins is given 20 minutes before the procedure, or, alternatively, supervised high dose oral amoxycillin is given 1 hour before the procedure. Patients with prosthetic heart valves require parenteral prophylaxis using a combination of penicillin and gentamicin. If previous antibiotics have been given to the patient, or, if the patient is allergic to penicillin, other prophylactic regimes may be indicated (*see* Chapter 18).

Prevention of endocarditis in other surgical patients

Appropriate prophylaxis is required for susceptible patients undergoing genito-urinary instrumentation or surgery, as well as for those requiring heart surgery (*see* Chapter 18).

Prevention of wound and other surgical sepsis in patients requiring colorectal surgery

Antibiotic prophylaxis as well as an adequate mechanical pre-op. bowel preparation is desirable to reduce the chances of post-op. sepsis complications. Potentially serious complications may occur such as subphrenic or pelvic abscess, peritonitis or Gram-negative bacteraemia, as well as local wound infection.

Metronidazole, started immediately pre-operatively, given during the operation and for a short period post-operatively, is a useful prophylactic agent which reduces the surgical sepsis associated with *Bacteroides*. An aminoglycoside (or possibly a cephalosporin) may be given peri-operatively also to reduce aerobic sepsis due to *E. coli* and other coliforms.

Some authorities recommended the local instillation of an antibiotic into a wound, such as cephaloridine, but although this may reduce wound sepsis rate it does not necessarily reduce the incidence of serious deep surgical sepsis or bacteraemia.

Prevention of sepsis following other types of surgery

Examples include:

a. Orthopaedic surgery

Apart from the prevention of post-operative gas gangrene, antibiotic prophylaxis is probably justified for hip replacement operations. The consequences of sepsis following the insertion of a prosthetic hip joint are so great that antibiotic prophylaxis is fully justified using systemic peri-operative cloxacillin active against staphylococcal organisms and continued for two days post-operatively. An alternative is the use of gentamicin in bone cement to be locally active against some *Staph. epidermidis* (albus) strains as well as *Staph. aureus* and some Gram-negative bacilli. Alternatively, a systemic cephalosporin can be given but this has the disadvantage of broad spectrum activity with the increased risk of *Pseudomonas* or cephalosporin-resistant coliform infections of the wound (and urinary tract in elderly patients).

b. Gynaecological surgery

A short peri-operative prophylactic course of metronidazole plus a cephalosporin may reduce sepsis rates following vaginal and abdominal hysterectomy.

c. Biliary tract surgery

Cephazolin given peri-operatively may reduce sepsis rates in selected patients undergoing biliary tract surgery. Patients who have stones or 'sludge' in the bile duct, those with recent cholecystitis, and patients who are over 70 years old may benefit from this type of prophylaxis.

d. Urological surgery
Prevention of Gram-negative bacteraemia during instrumentation of surgery on an infected urinary tract (*see* p. 92).

e. Vascular surgery involving the insertion of a prosthesis
If a Dacron aortic graft or other vascular prosthesis becomes infected the results may be catastrophic. The prophylactic use of a modern cephalosporin such as cefuroxime, to be active against staphylococci and Gram-negative bacilli, may be justified during the operation and for a period of up to 48 hours post-operatively.

In all of the above situations, prophylaxis is not required before the 'at risk' period begins and the first dose is usually necessary just before the start of surgery. The duration of the 'at risk' period is usually short and prophylaxis is rarely necessary for more than 48 hours post-operatively.

ANTIBIOTIC POLICIES

In recent years, the need to encourage the discriminate use of antibiotics in hospital, and to limit the development and spread of antibiotic-resistant bacterial strains, has been increasingly recognized. Some hospitals have produced antibiotic policies to limit the development of antibiotic resistance, to encourage rational use of established drugs and to limit the use of 'new' drugs, and also partly to reduce costs.

Restriction of the use of certain antibiotics, such as erythromycin and tetracycline, and the use of some antibiotics only in combination, such as rifampicin and fusidic acid, have sometimes helped to delay the development and limit the spread of antibiotic-resistant strains of *Staph. aureus* or of Gram-negative bacilli. In particular, the avoidance of valuable antibiotics for topical use is a common feature of many antibiotic policies. Each hospital needs its own policy since the prevalence of resistant strains, plasmids, etc. will vary to some extent from hospital to hospital and the consultant microbiologist has a particularly important role in this respect. In most hospitals today, the greatest antibiotic-resistance properties are encountered in strains of Gram-negative bacilli and restriction of the use of gentamicin and new cephalosporin drugs, such as cefuroxime, may be particularly advisable.

An effective means of isolating patients and other methods limiting cross-infection with antibiotic-resistant strains is also essential at the same time as an antibiotic policy. This subject is discussed more fully in Chapter 24 and references on antibiotic policies are included in the further reading list.

Further Reading

*Ayliffe G. A. J. (1979) Trends in resistance and their significance in primary pathogenic bacteria. In: Reeves D. and Geddes A. (ed.) *Recent Advances in Infection*. Edinburgh, Churchill Livingstone.

Ball P. (1981) Toxicity of antibacterial agents. *Medicine International* **1**, 102–105.

Cartwright R. Y. (1981) Antifungal agents. *Medicine International* **1**, 173–177.

Collier L. H. and Oxford J. (ed.) (1980) *Developments in Antiviral Therapy*. London, Academic Press.

Falkow S. (1975) *Infectious Multiple-Drug Resistance*. London, Pion.

*Garrod L. P. (1972) Causes of failure in antibiotic treatment. *Br. Med. J.* **4**, 473–476.

Garrod L. P., Lambert H. P. and O'Grady F. (1981) *Antibiotic and Chemotherapy* 5th ed. Edinburgh, Churchill Livingston.
Grüneberg R. N. (ed.) (1980) *Antibiotics and Chemotherapy: Current Topics*. Lancaster, U.K., MTP Press. (NB Includes chapters on antibiotic policies, antibiotic combination and prophylaxis.)
Hirsch M. S. and Swartz M. N. (1980) Antiviral agents. *N. Engl. J. Med.* **302**, 903–909; 949–953.
Kucers A. and Bennett N. M. (1979) *The Use of Antibiotics,* 3rd ed. London, Heinemann.
Mawer G. E., Ahmed R., Dobbs S. M. et al. (1974) Prescribing aids for gentamicin. *Br. J. Clin. Pharm.* **1**, 45.
Mouton R. P., Brumfitt W. and Hamilton-Miller J. M. T. (ed.) (1977) *The Rational Choice of Antibacterial Agents*. Middlesex, Kluwer-Harrap Handbooks.
Noone P. (1979) *A Clinician's Guide to Antibiotic Therapy,* 2nd ed. London, Blackwell Scientific Publications.
Phillips I. (1979) Antibiotic policies. In: Reeves A. and Geddes A. (ed.) *Recent Advances in Infection*. Edinburgh, Churchill Livingstone.
Price D. J. E. and Sleigh J. D. (1970) Control of infection due to *Klebsiella aerogenes* in a neurosurgical unit by withdrawal of all antibiotics. *Lancet* **2**, 1213.
Reeves D. S., Bint A. J. and Bullock D. W. (1978) Use of antibiotics: sulphonamides, co-trimoxazole and tetracyclines. *Br. Med. J.* **2**, 410–413.
Richards H. and Datta N. (1981) Transposons and trimethoprim resistance. *Br. Med. J.* **282**, 1118–1119.
Shanson D. C. and Hince C. J. (1977) Serum gentamicin assays of 100 clinical serum samples by a rapid 40 °C klebsiella method compared with overnight plate diffusion and acetyltransferase assays. *J. Clin. Pathol.* **30**, 521–525.
Simmons N. A. (1980) Combinations of antibacterial drugs. In: Grüneberg R. N. (ed.) *Antibiotics and Chemotherpay: Current Topics*. Lancaster, U.K., MTP Press.
Speller D. C. E. (ed.) (1980) *Antifungal Chemotherapy*. Chichester, John Wiley.
Stokes E. J. and Ridgway G. (1980) *Clinical Bacteriology*, 5th ed. London, Edward Arnold.
Williams R. J. and Williams J. D. (1980) The cephalosporin group of antibiotics. In: Grüneberg R. N. (ed.) *Antibiotics and Chemotherapy: Current Topics*. Lancaster, U.K., MTP Press.
Wise R. (1978) Use of antibiotics: penicillins. *Br. Med. J.* **1**, 1679–1681.

* Particularly recommended for further study by undergraduates.

SECTION B

Specific Clinical Topics

Chapter 4

Pyrexia of unknown origin (PUO)

DEFINITION OF PUO

A patient, who presents with pyrexia as a predominant clinical feature that has lasted for 10 days or longer without an obvious cause, is customarily considered as a case of PUO. However, in practice, even when the pyrexia has been present for only a few days, the clinical problem may be considered as one of 'acute' PUO. If the PUO persists for three weeks or longer, the patient's problem becomes one of 'chronic' PUO.

MAJOR CAUSES OF PUO

Infective causes are responsible for about three-quarters of cases of 'acute' PUO, but for only about one-third of cases of 'chronic' PUO (*Table 4.1*).

Viruses, such as enteroviruses, adenoviruses or myxoviruses, cause the majority of infections associated with 'acute' PUO whereas the infective problems causing 'chronic' PUO mainly include the causes of chronic pyogenic sepsis and tuberculosis (*Table 4.2*).

Table 4.1. Major causes of PUO

Causes	*Acute** *PUO, %*	*Chronic†* *PUO, %*
1. Infections	69	36
2. Neoplasms	6	19
3. Collagen diseases	3	13
4. Other causes include:		
a. Granulomas		
b. Endocrine		
c. Drug reactions		
d. CNS abnormalities		
e. Malingering		

* Data from a study of PUO cases by Effersoe, 1960–63.
† Data from a study of 100 cases of PUO by Petersdorf and Beeson, (1961).

Neoplasms are important causes of 'chronic' PUO (*Table 4.1*). Pyrexia may particularly be the main clinical feature associated with certain malignant neoplasms such as lymphomas, leukaemia, hepatoma or hypernephroma.

Table 4.2. Infective causes of chronic PUO

*Cause**	*No. of cases*
Tuberculosis	11
Hepato-biliary tract sepsis	8
Adbominal cryptic abscesses	4
Endocarditis	5
Pyelonephritis	3
Psittacosis	2
Brucellosis	1
Gonorrhoea	1
Malaria	1

*Data from a study of 36 infected cases out of a total of 100 cases with chronic PUO (Petersdorf and Beeson, 1961).

Collagen diseases such as Systemic Lupus Erythematosus (SLE), Polyarteritis nodosa, or dermatomyositis are sometimes the cause of 'chronic' PUO (*Table 4.1*).

Granulomas such as sarcoidosis or Crohn's disease are often associated with pyrexia.

Endocrine or metabolic diseases are rarely the cause of PUO since there are usually other prominent clinical features present, which help to suggest the diagnosis. Thyrotoxicosis may occasionally present with pyrexia as a main feature. Familial Mediterranean Fever, associated with raised aetiocholone hormones, is a very rare disease in Britain.

Alcoholic patients with liver disease sometimes present with pyrexial illness which is due to alcoholic hepatitis or other non-infective causes; however, since these patients are predisposed to many different infections, including pneumococcal and Gram-negative infections, they may sometimes have to be investigated for the infective causes of PUO.

Drug reactions are sometimes the cause of PUO.

Central nervous system abnormalities are very rarely the cause of PUO. Disturbances of the temperature regulating centre around the hypothalamus may cause PUO and rarely occurs following infiltration of this region of the brain by a neoplasm or granuloma.

Malingering should be particularly considered in a patient who has had many previous hospital admissions and who shows no pyrexia when the taking of the temperature has been carefully supervised.

INFECTIVE CAUSES OF PUO

Classification

A clinically useful method of classifying the infective causes of PUO depends on whether the PUO arises because of *non-specific infection*, at an inaccessible site, or *specific infection* due to a particular pathogen (*Table 4.3*).

Non-specific Causes

Cryptic abscesses ('hidden' abscesses) are common causes of PUO which are frequently found at abdominal or pelvic sites. Important examples of abdominal

Table 4.3. Classification of infective causes of PUO

A. Non-specific causes		
Site of infection important—infection may be caused by many different (non-specific) organisms		
Examples:		
1. Cryptic abscesses in—	liver abdomen pelvis retroperitoneal or mediastinal sites	
2. Infective endocarditis		
3. Urinary tract infections		
4. Ear, sinus or dental infections		
B. Specific causes		
Specific diseases, each caused by specific pathogens		
Examples:		
1. Bacterial diseases	Tuberculosis Typhoid Brucellosis	Leptospirosis Relapsing fever Nocardiosis
2. Viral diseases	Glandular fever Cytomegalovirus disease Hepatitis A or B	Sandfly fever Yellow fever Lassa fever
3. Rickettsial, coxiella diseases	Typhus Q fever	
4. Chlamydial diseases	Psittacosis Cat Scratch Fever	
5. Protozoal diseases	Malaria Amoebiasis Kala-azar	Toxoplasmosis Trypanosomiasis Pneumocystis
6. Fungal diseases	Cryptococcosis Candidiasis	Histoplasmosis Aspergillosis
7. Helminth diseases	Toxocariasis Filarial	Fasciola

cryptic abscesses include para-colic abscess, sometimes associated with neoplasia or diverticular disease, liver abscess, subphrenic abscess, frequently post-operative, and perinephric abscess. Many different bacterial species, often mixed together, can cause collections of pus at these sites including those found in the faecal flora: *E. coli*, other coliforms and *Bacteroides fragilis, Staph. aureus, Streptococcus milleri* and other streptococci.

Infective endocarditis frequently presents clinically as PUO and must particularly be assumed to be the diagnosis in any patient who has both a pyrexia and heart murmur until proved otherwise. The range of organisms that may cause infection of a heart valve is very wide (*see* Chapter 18).

Urinary tract infection may occur without obvious symptoms such as dysuria or frequency of micturition and cause PUO. Pyelonephritis is particularly liable to occur when there is an abnormality of the urinary tract present, such as a calculus. Occasionally the first urine sample collected fails to reveal a urinary tract infection bacteriologically when an obstruction is present. Gram-negative bacilli, staphylococci or enterococci are the usual causes of urinary tract infections (*see* Chapter 19).

Ear infection is a frequent cause of PUO in children, due to *Strep. pneumoniae, Strep. pyogenes, Staph. aureus* or *Haemophilus influenzae* (*see* Chapter 11).

Dental sepsis has recently become increasingly recognized as an important cause of PUO. Abscesses in the gums may not always be accompanied by an obvious toothache.

Specific Causes

Scores of different diseases may cause the patient to present clinically with PUO and some examples are mentioned below or are included in *Table 4.3*.

Tuberculosis, due to *Mycobacterium tuberculosis*, is a very important specific cause of PUO in many countries. In Britain, tuberculosis is still a frequently encountered disease and most often occurs amongst immigrants and elderly white males (*see* Chapter 13).

Glandular fever (Infectious Mononucleosis) due to the Epstein-Barr virus, is a common cause of PUO in young adults.

Toxoplasmosis, due to the protozoon *Toxoplasma gondii*, is frequently associated with pyrexia and lymphadenopathy in children and adults.

Typhoid fever, due to *Salmonella typhi*, or paratyphoid fever due to *Salmonella paratyphi A, B* or *C*, clinically presents with PUO as the characteristic main feature during the early stages of the illness. Enteric fever is one of the most important causes of PUO in patients who have recently travelled abroad but some patients acquire their infections in Britain (*see* Chapter 14).

Malaria, malignant tertian due to *Plasmodium falciparum*, or benign tertian to *Plasmodium vivax* or *ovale*, or quartan due to *Plasmodium malariae*, is an increasingly frequent cause of PUO in patients returning to Britain after a recent visit abroad. Malignant tertian malaria especially needs to be rapidly diagnosed if unnecessary fatalities are to be avoided.

Brucellosis, due to *Brucella abortus* or *melitensis*, often presents as PUO either 'acute' or 'chronic' and is endemic in many parts of Southern Europe, Africa and the Middle East and in a few regions of Britain.

Kala-azar (Visceral leishmaniasis) due to *Leishmania donovani*, commonly presents as PUO and is particularly seen in patients who have recently travelled to Britain from countries bordering on the Mediterranean or the Middle East.

Amoebiasis, especially hepatic amoebiasis, due to *Entamoeba histolytica* frequently presents as PUO in Britain amongst immigrant patients who have previously lived in the Indian subcontinent.

Leptospirosis, *Legionnaires' disease* and *secondary syphilis* are a few examples of diseases which may occasionally cause a patient to present with an acute PUO problem.

Opportunistic infections due to cytomegalovirus, *Pneumocystis carinii*, *Babesia*, aspergilli, *Candida*, *Cryptococcus neoformans*, in immunodeficient or immunosuppressed patients are discussed separately (*see* Chapter 6).

INVESTIGATION OF PUO

The main investigation steps required to diagnose the cause of PUO are summarized in *Table 4.4*. The first, and the most important single step, is the taking of a good clinical history from the patient.

Table 4.4. Main steps for diagnosing the cause of PUO

Step 1.	History of patient:	Age, immigrant? Recent travel abroad? Occupation? Contact with cases of infectious diseases or animals? Unpasteurized milk products? Taking drugs?
Step 2.	Physical examination:	On admission and repeated frequently
Step 3.	Temperature chart:	Pattern of pyrexia (*see Fig. 4.1*)
Step 4.	Special investigations:	i. Basic routine investigations ii. Further special investigations selected for each patient
Step 5.	Laparotomy	Considered for undiagnosed chronic PUO cases with 'clues' of hepatic, abdominal or pelvic disease
Step 6.	Therapeutic trials	Therapy for a specific disease, for an adequate duration

History of the Patient

Points in the history taking that need special attention include the following.

1. Age and whether the patient is an immigrant in Britain

A young adult is more likely to have glandular fever than a person in middle age. A child is particularly likely to have infection as the cause of PUO. A middle-aged or elderly adult with PUO has a greater chance of collagen disease or neoplasia as the cause than a child. If the patient is a young adult immigrant with PUO, the chances that tuberculosis is the cause must be high.

2. Duration of the pyrexia

The duration of the illness needs to be known so that the patient can be provisionally categorized as an 'acute' or 'chronic' PUO case. The causes of 'chronic' PUO tend to be different from those of 'acute' PUO (*see* Causes of PUO *above*).

3. Recent travel abroad

Increasing numbers of tourists and immigrants enter Britain after a recent visit abroad to a country where malaria, typhoid, visceral leishmaniasis, amoebiasis, brucellosis or tick typhus is endemic because of easier air travel to 'exotic' places. Malaria and typhoid are the two most common imported infections which may prove fatal unless rapidly diagnosed. These two infections require immediate consideration in any patient with fever who has recently travelled abroad. Most patients with imported infections have been abroad during the previous 6 months. Although viral haemorrhagic fevers must also be considered in patients returning from Africa, the chances of a PUO being due to malaria or typhoid fever are enormously higher than Lassa fever. An enquiry should be included about what prophylaxis had been taken against malaria in those who passed through malarial areas; often it is inadequate. In a small number of patients an attack of PUO, due to *P. vivax* malaria, may occur a few years after having returned from a malarial area, sometimes associated with a precipitating factor, such as an operation.

Tuberculosis and hepatic amoebiasis are frequently the cause of chronic PUO in immigrants from Asia or Africa and the travel abroad may not have been very recent in these cases. These infections may become apparent several months or years after the patient arrived in Britain.

4. Occupation and place of residence

Veterinary surgeons, farmers and their families and others who may live or work on agricultural land are at greater risk of acquiring brucellosis or Q fever (from cattle or sheep) or leptospirosis (from rats, cattle, pigs), than city dwellers. Rat catchers, sewer workers and laboratory personnel working in animal houses are exposed to the risk of acquiring leptospirosis. Pathology laboratory staff are at particular risk of acquiring TB, although this risk has probably decreased in the last few years. There have been a few recent cases of laboratory-acquired typhoid.

5. Contact with pets or animals

The patient may have acquired a zoonosis from contact with an animal that has been kept as a pet: toxoplasmosis from cats, psittacosis from parrots, toxocariasis or leptospirosis from puppies, are some examples. Contact with an infected farm animal may have occurred during a holiday.

6. Contact with cases of infectious diseases

Patients may have a history of contact with a known case of tuberculosis, enteric fever or hepatitis, as examples, and this might be relevant.

7. Drinking unpasteurized milk or eating goat's cheeses or unpasteurized cream

Brucellosis, Q fever and bovine tuberculosis and *Salmonella dublin* infections are examples of zoonoses that may cause PUO after drinking unpasteurized milk. In Britain today, significant quantities of unpasteurized milk or cream are consumed in some regions including parts of the West Country, Cumbria and Scotland.

Brucella melitensis can survive for many days in goat's cheeses prepared from infected milk in some Mediterranean, African or Middle Eastern countries and a history of eating one of these recently prepared cheeses indicates the need to particularly consider brucellosis.

8. Taking of drugs

Any drugs the patient is on or has recently taken should be noted since one of these may have caused a febrile drug reaction. If the drug is an antibiotic or steroid the clinical or laboratory features of the disease causing the PUO may become modified.

Heroin drug addicts are at particular risk of developing endocarditis, staphylococcal cryptic abscesses or hepatitis B.

Physical Examination

In many patients with PUO there are few, if any, physical signs apparent to help make the correct diagnosis. However, occasionally important signs are observed such as splenomegaly, the development of a rash or lymphadenopathy. The ear drums need examination particularly in infants and children for signs of otitis media. A rectal examination, always needs to be included, and in women a pervaginal examination and visualization of the cervix is usually desirable also, to find any evidence of pelvic infection or masses. The gums and teeth need careful examination for any evidence of dental sepsis.

The physical examination needs to be repeated regularly since a transient rash, such as the abdominal rose spots of typhoid fever or splenomegaly associated with Kala-azar and other conditions may become evident although the spleen was not enlarged on admission of the patient to hospital.

Temperature Chart

The pattern of pyrexia is often of enormous diagnostic importance (*Fig. 4.1*). However, in patients receiving steroids or in elderly patients, the pyrexia may become less typical or even non-existent.

Intermittent fever, where the temperature rises and returns to normal between each pyrexia, characteristically occurs at regular intervals, sometimes with rigors, in malaria (*Fig. 4.1*), and irregularly in conditions such as cholangitis. In malaria, the temperature pattern may occasionally become less regular especially in the early stages of the disease or when there are mixed plasmodia infections. In Kala-azar, 'notched' peaks are sometimes observed. (Malaria and leishmaniasis are discussed in Chapter 22.) An undulating fever with drenching sweats is sometimes seen in brucellosis.

Remittent fever, where the temperature does not usually return to normal between each peak of pyrexia, is characteristically seen in patients with collections of pus who usually develop a high swinging fever (*Fig. 4.1*). A 'step ladder' pyrexia may typically occur in early typhoid fever which is also associated with a relative bradycardia.

No specific pattern of pyrexia usually occurs in patients with infective endocarditis and in many patients with brucellosis or tuberculosis.

SPECIAL INVESTIGATIONS

Special investigations include laboratory, radiological, radioisotope scanning and ultrasound investigations.

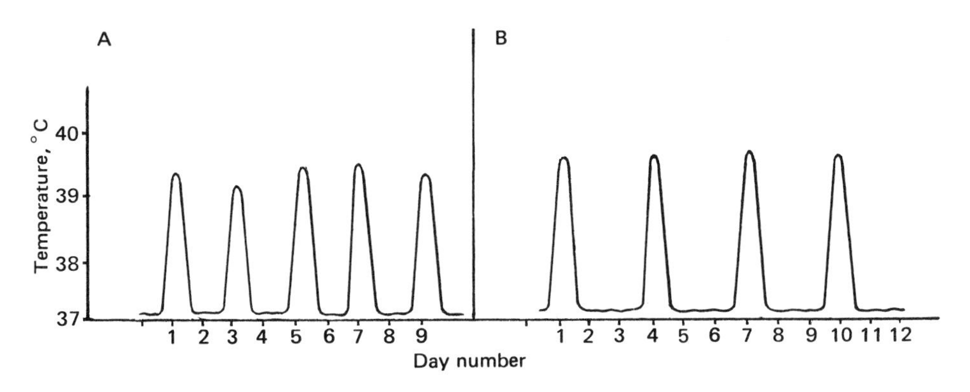

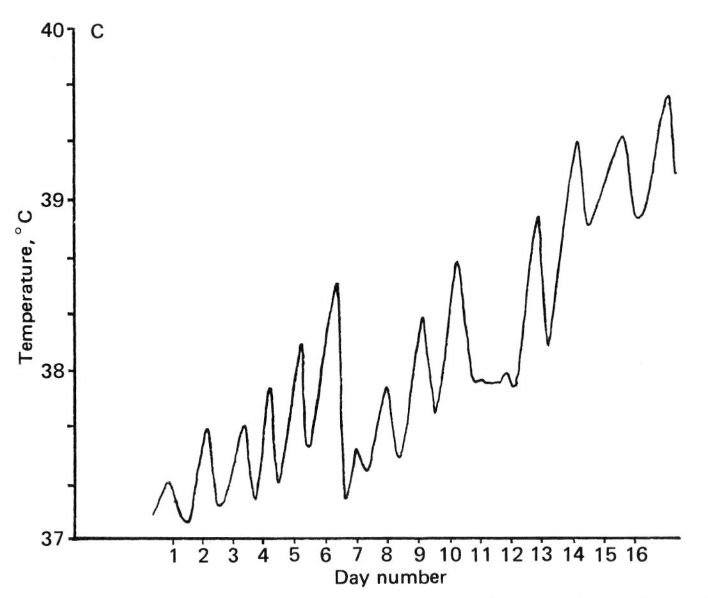

Fig. 4.1. Temperature charts. (A) and (B) are for intermittent fever; (C) is for a remittent fever. (A) Case of tertian malaria due to *P. vivax* infection; (B) case of quartan malaria due to *P. malariae* infection; (C) patient with subphrenic abscess.

Initial Special Investigations

A routine set of basic special investigations is necessary in nearly all patients with PUO (*Table 4.5*).

The basic investigations often reveal the diagnosis or give helpful clues. A high white blood cell count (WBC), such as 30 000 per mm^3 with a polymorph leucocytosis, together with a high swinging remittent pyrexia would be very suggestive of a cryptic abscess. Glandular fever is often diagnosed on the basis of atypical mononuclear cells in the blood film and may be confirmed subsequently by a positive Paul-Bunnell serological test. Malaria is usually rapidly diagnosed by the examination of the Giemsa/Leishman stained thick or thin blood films which should be collected while the temperature is rising. Severe neutropenia is

Table 4.5. Initial special investigations

Type of investigations	*Examples of usefulness*
A. Haematological:	
1. Haemaglobin	Anaemia a feature of Kala-azar, endocarditis, etc.
2. White blood count and differential film	Polymorph leucocytosis—pyogenic infection? Neutropenia—typhoid, malaria, leishmaniasis, SLE, severe drug reaction? Atypical mononuclear cells—glandular fever? Eosinophilia—helminths, drug reaction, polyarteritis
3. Thick and thin blood films when recent travel abroad	Malaria, trypanosome, filarial parasites or *Borrelia*?
4. Erythrocyte sedimentation rate	>100 mm/h-TB, collagen diseases, neoplasm?
B. Microbiological:	
1. *a.* Blood cultures	Specific pathogens isolated such as *Salmonella typhi*. Non-specific organisms isolated may indicate site of infection, e.g. *E. coli* mixed with *Bacteroides fragilis* may suggest abdominal, hepatic or pelvic cryptic abscess
b. Blood smears for parasites *see A.*3 above)	
2. Urine and faeces microscopy and cultures	Diagnosis of urinary and gastro-intestinal tract infections Sterile pyuria—TB of genito-urinary tract? —EMSU × 3 for AFB indicated
3. Throat swab culture	*Strep. pyogenes*—recent streptococcal infection and rheumatic fever?
4. Serology	Routinely collect and store an 'acute' serum on admission Paired sera to look for *RISING* antibody titre, (>4-fold) for evidence of infection with specific pathogens Occasionally a high single antibody titre is significant (*see also Table 4.6*)
C. Radiological	
Chest X-ray	Consolidation, empyema, lung abscess? TB—primary, secondary, miliary? Hilar lymphadenopathy—TB or sarcoidosis

EMSU × 3, early morning specimen of urine collected on three consecutive occasions.
SLE, systemic lupus erythematosus.

frequently observed in patients with leishmaniasis, malaria, enteric fever or overwhelming pyogenic infection.

Blood cultures are best collected in practice as soon as the temperature starts to rise, although in endocarditis it does not matter when the blood cultures are collected in relation to the pyrexia. Theoretically, the optimal time for collecting blood cultures in pyaemic conditions is during the hour before pyrexia occurs which is rarely of practical relevance. As long as the blood culture sets are collected before the start of any antibiotics, there is little benefit in collecting more than three sets of cultures. Each set of blood culture bottles should include anaerobic as well as aerobic media and the broths may need to be incubated for up to six weeks.

An 'acute' serum sample should always be collected at the start of the patient's investigations and stored so that it can be referred to subsequently at the same time as a later serum sample for serological tests if necessary.

Further Special Investigations

The basic investigations referred to above may need repetition at appropriate intervals. In addition further special investigations are selected which are relevant for each individual patient with PUO (*Table 4.6*).

Serological tests

In most instances, serological tests are performed simultaneously on the paired sera ('acute' and 'convalescent') which are collected with an interval of 10–14 days between them. Occasionally, a single high titre of a specific antibody may be suggestive of recent infection, especially when the IgM antibody is also positive, as with an IgM-positive fluorescent toxoplasma antibody test suggesting recent or current toxoplasmosis.

A Widal test is often of limited value (*see* Chapter 14), but should be included when the cultures are negative on a patient with an 'acute' PUO, especially if he has recently travelled abroad.

Brucella agglutinins and brucella complement fixation test (brucella CFT) and Q fever CFT are required on most PUO cases where the basic investigations have been unhelpful. These tests are especially indicated when the patient has drunk unpasteurized milk, is a vet or has another occupational reason for exposure to *Brucella* and fever, or has recently stayed in a brucellosis endemic area.

An ASO titre is essential when there is a clinical possibility of rheumatic fever.

Patients who have had malaise, sore throat or lymphadenopathy and who show a lymphocytosis or an 'infectious mononucleosis' picture in the blood film, need a Paul-Bunnell test (often performed initially as a 'monospot' test) and a toxoplasma dye test. The Paul-Bunnell may take up to 3 months to become positive and may need to be repeated a few times if initially negative. For Paul-Bunnell negative glandular fever patients, a cytomegalovirus CFT should be performed. Psittacosis, mycoplasma, Q fever, influenza complement fixation tests and legionella fluorescent antibody tests should be undertaken, particularly if there are respiratory symptoms.

Immigrant patients with a raised white blood count and swinging pyrexia may have an amoebic liver abscess and a serum fluorescent amoebic antibody test is especially useful in these patients.

Other examples of serological tests are included in *Table 4.6*.

Serum biochemical tests

Liver function tests are frequently abnormal when an infective process involves the liver. The aminotransferases are usually markedly elevated (in the thousands) when a patient presents with a pyrexial illness due to hepatitis A or B. The amino transferases are only moderately raised in Legionnaires' disease. The alkaline phosphatase is sometimes raised in patients with brucellosis or liver

Table 4.6. Further special investigations
Select further investigations appropriate to each patient

A. *Serological tests (usually paired sera required)—examples*:
Widal test
Brucella agglutinins and complement fixation test (CFT)
ASO titre
Q fever CFT
Leptospira CFT
Fluorescent amoebic antibody test
Fluorescent leishmanial antibody test
Toxoplasma dye test (and IgM)
Paul-Bunnell test for infectious mononucleosis
Cytomegalovirus CFT
HBsAg for Hepatitis B
Filarial CFT and fluorescent antibody tests
VDRL and TPHA for syphilis
Psittacosis, mycoplasma, influenza CFT's
Weil-Felix test (*Proteus* organisms agglutinins) for typhus
Legionella pneumophila fluorescent antibody test
Aspergillus, histoplasma, and other fungal precipitins and CFT
Anti-nuclear factor, DNA, smooth muscle, mitochondrial autoantibodies

B. *Special further cultures—examples*:
EMSU, gastric washings for tubercle bacilli
Urine and blood cultures for *Leptospira* using guinea-pig inoculations
Bone marrow culture for *Salmonella typhi* and tubercle bacilli

C. *Biopsies for microbiology and histology—examples*:
Bone marrow for leishmania, leukaemia
Lymph nodes for tubercle bacilli, toxoplasma, reticulosis, sarcoidosis
Liver biopsy for tubercles, sarcoidosis, cytomegalovirus
and for leishmania in certain marrow negative cases
Temporal arteries for temporal arteritis

D. *Biochemical tests—examples*:
Liver function tests—aminotransferases (viral hepatitis)
—alkaline phosphatase (*brucella*, cholangitis)
Electrophoresis —high IgM in leishmaniasis
α-Foeto protein —hepatoma

E. *Radiological—examples*:
Intravenous pyelogram —pyelonephritis, carbuncle on kidney, perinephric abscess, hypernephroma
Dental and sinus X-rays—sinusitis, dental sepsis
Spinal X-rays —TB or osteomyelitis of spine

F. *Skin tests—examples*:
Mantoux test—intradermal tuberculin delayed hypersensitivity test
Kveim test for sarcoidosis
Histoplasmin for histoplasmosis

G. *Ultrasound and echocardiography*
Abdominal or pelvic masses—abscesses, neoplasms—ultrasound
Regurgitation of blood across cardiac lesion, vegetations—echocardiography

H. *Scans*
Liver scans—liver abscesses, hepatoma
Whole body CAT scans—cryptic abscesses, neoplasms
Radioactive gallium or indium scans to locate pyogenic lesion

I. *Laparotomy—examples of findings at*:
Neoplasms—abdominal lymphomas,
—carcinoma, hepatoma
Tuberculous peritonitis
Cryptic abscesses in liver, abdomen or pelvis

VDRL, venereal disease reference laboratory antibody test.
TPHA, *Treponema pallidum* haemagglutination test.

abscess. These enzyme tests may of course be abnormal when there is significant non-infective hepatocellular damage or biliary tract disease.

The α-foetoprotein is often detected in the serum of patients with a PUO due to hepatoma.

Biopsies

Lymph nodes recently enlarged in the neck or other sites are frequently features of tuberculous glands or glands enlarged due to toxoplasmosis. Excision of the enlarged gland is often indicated and part of the gland should be sent in a sterile container, *without formalin*, for microbiology while another piece is also sent in formalin for histology.

A liver biopsy is often invaluable for the laboratory diagnosis of miliary tuberculosis and pieces of the biopsy should be sent for both histology and microbiology, as described for the lymph node biopsy.

Bone marrow biopsy is frequently positive for Leishman Donovan bodies in patients with PUO due to visceral leishmaniasis. Occasionally, the marrow biopsy is negative in this condition, in which case serum fluorescent leishmania antibody tests should be performed when the diagnosis is strongly suspected. The isolation of typhoid bacilli or tubercle bacilli from cultures of the bone marrow, when other cultures are negative, is exceedingly rare.

Scans and ultrasound

In practice isotopic scans of the liver and ultrasound of the abdomen, liver and pelvis are of enormous help in detecting cryptic abscesses. In the liver, the abscess may be pyogenic or amoebic; the serum fluorescent amoebic antibody test is useful for differentiating between these.

Neoplasms, such as hepatoma, abdominal lymphoma, may also sometimes be revealed by these techniques.

Whole body computerized axial tomography (CAT) scans can also be arranged in some centres to reveal cryptic abscesses or tumours in non-abdominal sites.

Labelling of the patients own white blood cells with radioactive gallium or indium, and injecting these back into the patient, may help to reveal cryptic collections of pus during subsequent scanning.

Radiology

A chest X-ray was included in the basic set of routine investigations. When non-pulmonary tuberculosis is suspected, especially in immigrants, X-rays of the spine and other bony sites are often required.

A plain X-ray of the abdomen can show calcified hydatid cysts in the liver (which may become secondarily infected), or schistosome infiltrated urinary bladder or occasionally a soft tissue mass that could be hypernephroma.

An intravenous pyelogram (IVP) will help show abnormalities of the urinary tract which may be infected, and occasionally reveals a perinephric abscess or carbuncle on the kidney or hypernephroma.

A 'skeletal survey' may also reveal osteomyelitis or metastatic carcinoma as the cause of a PUO—but there are usually clinical features apart from pyrexia which would suggest the need for this type of radiology. Lymphangiography may help to reveal a lymphoma as the cause of a PUO.

Skin tests

The Mantoux test is nearly always indicated in cases of 'chronic' PUO. If strongly positive in a young child, incubating tuberculosis must be suspected but positive reactions in immigrant adults are often due to previous tubercle infection. A persistently negative reaction in a PUO patient who is not overwhelmingly ill, and who is not on steroids, makes the diagnosis of tuberculosis unlikely. However, it is rarely possible for a Mantoux test to be negative in a patient with tuberculosis, especially abdominal tuberculosis. Conversion from a positive test to a negative test may be observed in some patients with sarcoidosis.

A wide range of fungal antigens are available including histoplasmin, coccidioidin and sporotrichin for injecting into the skin of patients with mycoses especially if they have recently visited an endemic area.

Laparotomy

The confirmation of the diagnosis of a cryptic abscess in the abdomen, pelvis or liver may only come at laparotomy which in any case is usually required to treat the condition by draining the collection of pus. At the same time, the cause of the hidden abscess, such as diverticular or neoplastic disease of the colon, may become apparent.

Laparotomy is also often the only way in which tuberculous peritonitis or other forms of abdominal TB can be diagnosed; suspicious lesions are biopsied for histology and microbiology.

Therapeutic Trials

Sometimes an infection such as typhoid, tuberculosis, malaria or leishmaniasis is clinically suspected as the cause of PUO, but the special investigations have so far failed to confirm the diagnosis. In this situation, a specific therapeutic trial is frequently justified, provided all the relevant microbiological tests have been undertaken first, and a few comments on these trials follow.

1. *?TB*: *p*-aminosalicylic acid and isoniazid or ethambutol and isoniazid are useful combinations since these agents do not have significant antimicrobial effects against organisms other than mycobacteria. The duration of the antituberculous trial is important; at least 3 or 4 weeks before a reduction in the pyrexia can be reasonably confidently expected; 2 weeks is inadequate for some cases.

2. *?Malaria*: a short course of chloroquine usually causes the pyrexia, due to chloroquine-sensitive strains of *Plasmodium*, to become reduced within a couple of days. Quinine may be necessary for treating malaria due to the relatively rare strains of chloroquine-resistant *Plasmodia* encountered in patients returning to Britain from the Far East and certain parts of S. America.

3. *? Enteric fever*: chloramphenicol usually causes a clinical response to treatment and a diminution of the pyrexia within 2 or 3 days of treatment when

the salmonellae are sensitive to chloramphenicol, which is the usual situation in patients diagnosed in Britain (*see* Chapter 14). Chloramphenicol is active against many different organisms, however, so this would not be a truly specific therapeutic trial.

4. ? *Visceral leishmaniasis*: parenteral administration of Pentostam (sodium stibogluconate) usually causes a marked clinical improvement within 1–2 days of starting treatment.

5. ? *Streptococcal endocarditis*: patients started on 'blind' combination of benzylpenicillin plus gentamicin often show a marked improvement in their general well being within 24 hours of starting treatment (*see* Chapter 18). These antibiotics are active against many different organisms and the therapeutic trial is not specific for either streptococci or endocarditis.

Steroids are sometimes used empirically to treat undiagnosed PUO cases and as these drugs can both clinically mask and worsen tuberculosis they should probably only be used in conjunction with antituberculous drugs.

Drug reactions can sometimes be diagnosed by stopping all the drugs the patient is on and then restarting them carefully, one drug at a time. The pyrexial reaction disappears on stopping the drugs and may reappear when the offending drug is reintroduced.

Further Reading

Bell Dion R. (1978) Diseases of immigrants. *Prescriber's Journal* **18**, 100–111.

Daggett P. (1978) A system for the investigation of pyrexia of uncertain origin. *Br. J. Hosp. Med.* **16**, 357.

Effersoe P. (1968) Patients with continuous fever at the Department of Contagious Diseases, Blegdamshospital, Copenhagen 1960–63. *Danish Med. Bull.* **15**, 231–239.

Geddes A. M. (1974) Unexplained fever. *Br. Med. J.* **4**, 397.

Geddes A. M. (1974) Undiagnosed fever—Rickettsial, viral and helminth infections. *Br. Med. J.* **4**, 454.

Munro J. F. (1978) Pyrexia of uncertain origin. *Medicine*, 3rd series, 7, 327–332.

Petersdorf R. G. and Beeson P. B. (1961) Fever of unexplained origin—report on 100 cases. *Medicine (Baltimore)* **40**, 1.

Chapter 5
Septicaemia

CLINICAL FEATURES

Characteristic clinical features of septicaemia include fever, rigors, mental confusion, tachycardia and hypotension. In the early stages, the clinical features may be very varied, especially in infants (*see* Chapter 7). Prompt recognition of septicaemia and immediate treatment based on the knowledge of the likely causative organisms is essential. Complications include septic shock, disseminated intravascular coagulation (DIC) and acute renal failure. The mortality rate depends on the age, the underlying condition and the treatment given; in many series the mortality rate varies between 15 and 35%. (*See also* Meningococcal meningitis in Chapter 10.)

CAUSATIVE ORGANISMS

During the past 40 years, the incidence of septicaemia due to streptococci and staphylococci has declined. Gram-negative septicaemia has become more frequent and septicaemia due to non-sporing anaerobes has become increasingly recognized. The relative incidence of the different causative organisms varies between hospitals according to the specialities practised, the incidence of hospital infection and the kind of community served by each hospital. The relative incidence of causative organisms in a typical district general hospital in Britain is as follows:

Type of causative organisms	*Approx. percentage of patients with septicaemia*
Gram-negative	49
Gram-positive	40
Anaerobic	10
Non-bacterial	1

The three most common organisms isolated from blood cultures are *E. coli*, *Staph. aureus* and *Strep. pneumoniae*. In about 94% of patients with positive blood cultures only one type of organism is isolated. However, drug addicts especially may have polymicrobial septicaemias (e.g. *Staph. aureus* plus *Pseudomonas aeruginosa*). Scores of different bacterial species may cause septicaemia and only some of the more important examples are mentioned below.

Gram-negative Septicaemia

E. coli is by far the most frequent cause of this condition. The release of endotoxins from Gram-negative organisms may result in septic shock. Many factors predispose to Gram-negative septicaemia including the increase in instrumentation and surgery performed in recent years (*Fig. 5.1*, *Tables 5.1* and *5.2*). The incidence of Gram-negative sepsis in hospital and also the effects of

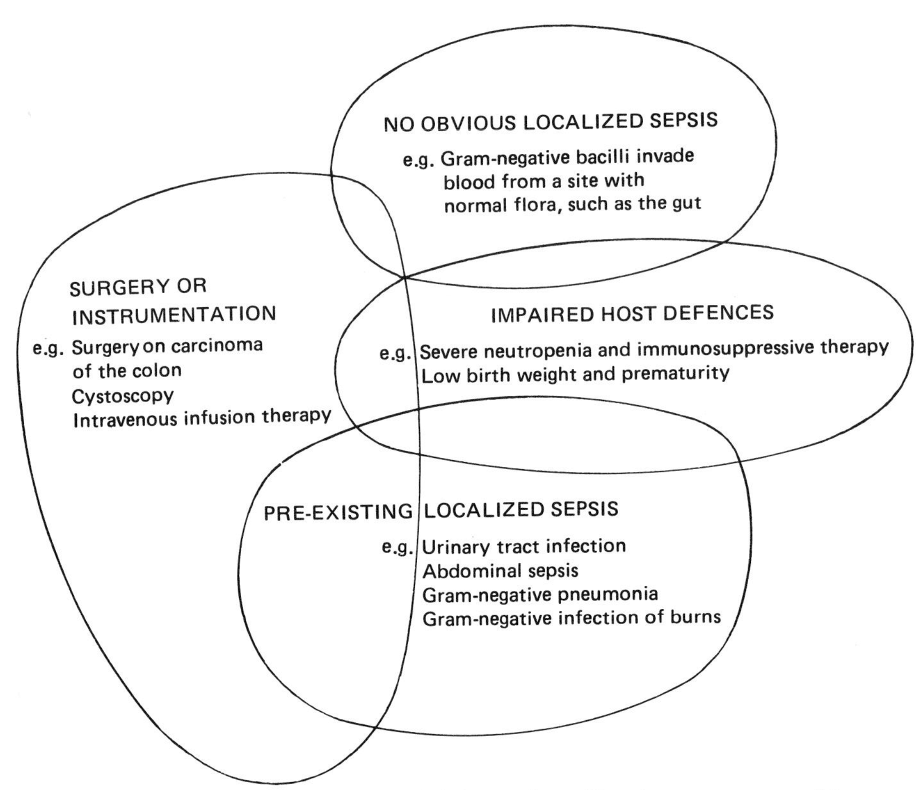

Fig. 5.1. Venn diagram showing the possible interactions of four important groups of factors predisposing to Gram-negative septicaemia.

Table 5.1. Gram-negative septicaemia—bacterial causes and underlying conditions

Blood culture isolates	*Approx. percentage of septicaemic cases in a typical British District Hospital %*	*Underlying conditions*
E. coli	22	Urinary tract infections
Klebsiella species	7	Abdominal sepsis
Proteus species	5	Hepato-biliary tract infection
Enterobacter species	1	Leukaemia
Salmonella species	4	Enteric fever Gastro-enteritis in the elderly and infants
Haemophilus influenzae	4	Respiratory and CNS infections in infants
Neisseria meningitidis	1	
Pseudomonas aeruginosa	3	Leukaemia
Serratia marcescens	less than 1	Respiratory and urinary tract infections Burns
Neisseria gonorrhoeae	less than 1	Female pelvic infection

Table 5.2. Pre-disposing factors for Gram-negative septicaemia

1. *Impairment of general host defences*	
i. *Examples by disease*	ii. *Examples by treatment*
Diabetes mellitus	Immunosuppression
Age extremes	—steroids
—premature babies	—radiotherapy
—very elderly	—cytotoxic drugs
Debilitation	Severe neutropenia
—malignancy	—cytotoxic drugs
—uraemia	
—hepatic failure	
Leukaemia, reticulosis	
Aplastic anaemia	
Myeloma	
Malabsorption	
Nephrotic syndrome	
Congenital immunodeficiency	
2. *Instrumentation and surgery* *Examples*:	
Surgery on the urinary tract or large bowel	
Intravenous therapy—central venous pressure lines	
Urinary catheterization, cystoscopy; trans-rectal prostatic biopsy	
Tracheostomy plus intermittent positive pressure ventilation and humidification	
Baby incubator and resuscitation equipment	
Radiological invasive techniques	
3. *Factors that may encourage spread of Gram-negative bacteria in hospital* These include:	
i. Poor hospital hygiene with numerous contaminated moist sites	
ii. Aseptic technique lapses	
iii. Disinfectant policy not followed	
iv. Antibiotic overusage	
v. Isolation policy not practised	

widespread use of broad spectrum antibiotics, such as ampicillin, in promoting infections due to antibiotic-resistant strains, are discussed in Chapters 6 and 24.

Gram-positive Septicaemia

Staph. aureus and streptococci cause the majority of Gram-positive septicaemias which usually complicate infections of the skin, soft tissues, lungs, bones and joints (*Table 5.3*). Some of the *Strep. pneumoniae* isolations from blood cultures may be associated with pneumonia without obvious clinical signs of septicaemia. Lancefield group B haemolytic streptococci are important causes of septicaemia in neonates (*see* Chapter 7).

The clinical features and complications of septicaemia due to *Staph. aureus* or other Gram-positive organisms may be indistinguishable from that due to Gram-negative bacteria. The septic shock and disseminated intravascular coagulation that can complicate staphylococcal septicaemia may posssibly be due to the effects of protein A of *Staph. aureus*. Metastatic abscesses and acute infective

Table 5.3. Gram-positive septicaemia—bacterial causes and underlying conditions

Blood culture isolates	*Approx. percentage of septicaemia cases in a district hospital, %*	*Underlying conditions*
1. *Streptococci*:		
Streptococcus pneumoniae	17	Respiratory tract infections—particularly pneumonia Meningitis; splenectomy
Streptococcus pyogenes	4	Cellulitis
Group B haemolytic streptococci	2	Obstetric and neonatal infections
Other haemolytic streptococci	<1	Skin infections
Streptococcus faecalis	<1	Urinary tract infection; endocarditis
Streptococcus milleri	2	Collections of pus in abdomen, liver, chest
'*Streptococcus viridans*'	1	Endocarditis
Microaerophilic streptococci	<1	Endocarditis
2. *Staphylococci*:		
Staphylococcus aureus	14	Skin, wound, bone and joint infections Drug addiction Pneumonia and lung abscess Endocarditis and infected pacemakers
Staphylococcus epidermidis	<1	Prosthesis in joint, CNS or heart infected; infected i.v. line
3. *Listeria monocytogenes*	<1	Reticulosis, splenectomy, immunosuppression

endocarditis affecting a previously healthy aortic valve can also complicate *Staph. aureus* septicaemia.

Anaerobic Septicaemia

Bacteroides fragilis and other *Bacteroides* species are the main causes of anaerobic septicaemia. These species can clinically cause a septicaemia that is indistinguishable from that produced by aerobic causes of Gram-negative septicaemia. Abdominal or gynaecological sepsis, is usually present and *Bacteroides* may be mixed with *E. coli* or other coliforms in the blood (*see* Chapter 9).

Anaerobic streptococci may occasionally invade the blood from an infected female genital tract or from oral sepsis.

Clostridial septicaemia due mainly to *Clostridium welchii* is rare today in Britain. These septicaemias are associated with severe toxaemia: haemolysis, shock, jaundice and acute renal failure often leading rapidly to death (*see* Gas gangrene and Septic abortion in Chapter 9).

Organisms Other than Bacteria occasionally Isolated from the Blood

These include:

Fungi:

Candida albicans—the most frequently isolated fungus from blood cultures (vented broths containing glucose are desirable for the isolation of fungi)

Other *Candida* species

Cryptococcus neoformans, *Histoplasma capsulatum*, *Aspergillus* species — rarely isolated from blood cultures

Rickettsiae and 'Coxiella':

Rickettsia species (causing typhus fevers), *Coxiella burnetii* — rarely isolated from blood; animal inoculation techniques necessary

Viruses:

Arboviruses and viral causes of haemorrhagic fevers such as Lassa fever virus; animal inoculation techniques or suitable tissue cultures in designated reference laboratories required.

MICROBIOLOGICAL INVESTIGATIONS OF SEPTICAEMIA

The main microbiological investigations available are:

1. *Blood cultures*
2. *Cultures of other infected sites*
   Swabs of infected burns, wounds, umbilicus, etc.
   Urine and sputum
   Faeces when alimentary tract infection suspected
3. *Detection of microbial products in serum*
   Counter-current immunoelectrophoresis (CIE) detection of pneumococcal, *Klebsiella* and other microbial antigens
   Limulus lysate test for detection of endotoxin of Gram-negative bacteria
   Gas–Liquid chromatography (GLC) to detect volatile fatty acids produced by anaerobes in blood cultures
4. *Blood cultures—new approaches*
   Radiometric, filtration, electrical impedance methods. These methods are still being developed and require further evaluation before they can become widely used (Washington, 1978)
5. *Animal inoculation*
   Isolation of rare fastidious pathogens from blood including *Legionella*, *Leptospira*, rickettsiae and viruses

For the vast majority of clinical situations, conventional cultures of blood and other possibly infected sites remains the main laboratory diagnostic approach. Occasionally when antibiotics have already been given, the CIE method may be useful during the first few days of antibiotic therapy. Gas-liquid chromatography techniques are sometimes useful for the rapid detection of anaerobes in positive blood cultures.

Conventional Blood Culture Techniques

At least two blood samples, preferably three, should be collected from a seriously ill patient with suspected septicaemia during a 1–3 hour period. Blind antibiotic therapy is indicated as soon as these and other appropriate cultures have been collected.

When the patient is less acutely ill there may be time to collect at least one of the blood samples just as the temperature is beginning to rise (the number of bacteria in the blood usually is greater at this time than when the temperature has reached its peak or is on the decline). In practice, if pathogenic bacteria are isolated from blood cultures at all, they are usually isolated from the first couple of sets collected.

Every blood culture set should routinely include aerobic and anerobic broths for inoculation at the bedside. Occasionally additional media may be recommended by the microbiologist.

The prevention of contamination of the blood cultures is of vital importance and an example of instructions for the collection of blood cultures is included in the appendix. Most bacteria that are isolated from blood cultures are either seen in Gram-stains of turbid blood culture broths or as colonies on blood agar subculture plates between 1 and 3 days after the collection of blood cultures. Only a few further bacterial strains are isolated after 5 days' incubation of the blood culture broths.

Interpretation of Blood Culture Isolates

Some isolates are likely to be clinically significant even if only isolated from one bottle of a blood culture set that includes three bottles of broth, for example an isolate of *Neisseria meningitidis* or *Salmonella typhi*. Other isolates are likely to be 'contaminants' from the skin of the patient or from a person collecting or examining the blood cultures, such as *Staph. epidermidis*, micrococci, diphtheroids and aerobic spore-bearing bacilli (which can sometimes be confused with Gram-negative bacilli such as coliforms), and frequently more than one type of 'contaminant' organism may be present in a blood culture set. However, any organism may be clinically significant (including *Staph. epidermidis* or other skin 'commensals') and the main microbiological requirement is to have isolated the same organism from at least two separate blood samples. If only one sample is obtained, then it is usually desirable to have demonstrated the organisms in more than one bottle of that blood culture set. In each patient the exact clinical circumstances, including whether or not the patient has received any recent antibiotic therapy, must be taken into account (*see also* Blood cultures, in Chapter 18).

ANTIBIOTIC TREATMENT OF SEPTICAEMIA

Immediate parenteral antibiotic treatment is necessary as soon as cultures have been taken but, when a collection of pus is suspected, this usually also requires urgent surgical drainage. When antibiotics are given by the intravenous route, they are preferably administered by bolus injections rather than by continuous infusions.

1. *'Blind' Antibiotic Treatment at the Start of Therapy*

The clinical evidence and knowledge of the underlying condition often suggests the type of likely causative organism but sometimes there are no obvious clinical clues present. Examples of *combinations* of antibiotics that are suitable for different situations as 'blind' initial parenteral treatment are:

a. *When there are 'no relevant clinical clues'*:

i. *Gentamicin*	Usually effective against *E. coli*, *Pseudomonas*, and other Gram-negative bacilli (and *Staph. aureus* partially) gentamicin dosage 6 mg/kg/day in three divided doses; maintenance doses depend on state of renal function
plus	
ii. *Cloxacillin*	Usually effective against *Staph. aureus* (and some streptococci) Cloxacillin dosage 1·5 g, 6-hourly (in an adult with normal renal function)
plus	
iii. *Benzylpenicillin*	Effect against *Strep. pneumoniae*, *Strep. pyogenes* and other streptococci (penicillin is the drug of choice for nearly all streptococcal infections) Benzylpenicillin dosage 1·5 Mu, 6-hourly (in an adult with normal renal function)

In penicillin-allergic patients, erythromycin lactobionate 1 g, intravenously and 6-hourly, can be used instead of penicillin and cloxacillin in an adult.

The above combination of gentamicin, cloxacillin and benzylpenicillin covers over 80% of the bacteria that are likely to cause septicaemia. However, *Bacteroides fragilis*, which may be associated with between 5 and 10% of septicaemias is not covered by this combination. In practice, there are usually clinical clues present to suggest the possibility of bacteroides infection (*see below*).

b. *Abdominal or pelvic sepsis when Gram-negative septicaemia is suspected*:

i. *Metronidazole*	Effective against *Bacteroides fragilis* and many other anaerobes. Metronidazole dosage 500 mg, 8-hourly, in an adult
plus	
ii. *Gentamicin*	Usually effective against *E. coli* and other Gram-negative bacilli (*see (a) above*)

c. *Severe neutropenia or immunosuppression*:

High initial doses of an aminoglycoside in combination with a beta-lactam antibiotic active against many *Pseudomonas aeruginosa* strains, are indicated in severely immunocompromised patients including some patients with acute leukaemia, e.g.

i. *Gentamicin* — Usually effective against *Pseudomonas aeruginosa, Klebsiella aerogenes, E. coli* and other Gram-negative bacilli (and *Staph. aureus* partially)
Gentamicin dosage 7·5 mg/kg/day in three divided doses (maintenance doses depend on state of renal function)

plus

ii. *Carbenicillin* — Effective against some *Pseudomonas aeruginosa* and other Gram-negative bacteria (as well as some streptococci)
Carbenicillin dosage 5 g, 6-hourly, slow intravenous administration

However, alternative combinations such as *tobramycin* plus *ticarcillin* may be preferred (*see also* Chapter 6).

d. Gram-negative septicaemia suspected in association with urinary tract infection

i. *Gentamicin* — Especially effective against *E. coli, Klebsiella* and other bacterial strains which may be resistant to ampicillin
Dosage (as in (*a*) *above*)

plus (optional)

ii. *Ampicillin* — Only effective against some *E. coli* and other Gram-negative strains which are sensitive to ampicillin
Ampicillin dosage 1 g, 6-hourly, in an adult with normal renal function

e. Gram-negative septicaemia suspected in association with meningococcal infection

A patient with a purpuric rash due to probable meningococcal septicaemia should be treated with benzylpenicillin (*see* Chapter 10).

f. Suspected Gram-positive septicaemia

Clinical evidence of septicaemia together with skin sepsis, acute osteomyelitis or other conditions associated with *Staph. aureus* or streptococcal infection indicates the need for initial suitable high dose anti-Gram-positive antibiotics in a non-penicillin-allergic patient.

i. *Cloxacillin* — Effective against penicillinase-producing strains of *Staph. aureus*
Cloxacillin dosage 2 g, 6-hourly, in an adult with normal renal function

plus

ii. *Benzylpenicillin* — Drug of choice for penicillin-sensitive strains of *Staph. aureus* (a few strains only) and also for *Strep. pyogenes* and other haemolytic streptococci
Benzylpenicillin dosage 3 Mu, 6-hourly in an adult with normal renal function

When *Staph. aureus* is strongly suspected, the addition of fusidic acid or gentamicin is often desirable, especially if there is associated infection in the lungs, e.g.

i. *Cloxacillin* — *As above*
plus
ii. *Gentamicin* — As a synergistic antistaphylococcal agent to combine with the cloxacillin
Dosage as in (*a*) above

If penicillin allergy is present the following combination is suggested:

i. *Erythromycin* — Usually effective against *Staph. aureus* and streptococci
Erythromycin lactobionate dosage 1 g, 6-hourly intravenously, in an adult
plus
ii. *Fusidic acid* — Usually effective against *Staph. aureus* (possibly in synergistic combination with erythromycin)
Fusidic acid dosage 500 mg, 8-hourly, orally or intravenously, in an adult.

g. Suspected clostridial septicaemia
A combination of benzylpenicillin, metronidazole and gentamicin will treat a mixed infection due to *Clostridium welchii*, other anaerobes and Gram-negative organisms (plus also to some extent *Staph. aureus*), but other aspects of management including hyperbaric oxygen and surgery may also be important (*see* Chapter 9).

h. Neonatal septicaemia
See Chapter 7, p. 117 and Chapter 10, p. 181.

2. *Subsequent Antibiotic Treatment*

Once the blood cultures are seen to be positive (e.g. turbidity, haemolysis or routine subculture positive) the antibiotic treatment can be appropriately modified. In the early stages a Gram stain of the blood culture broth may be valuable. Antibiotic sensitivity results are usually available within 1–3 days and will guide optimal chemotherapy. Benzylpenicillin is always indicated for non-penicillin-allergic patients whenever *Strep. pyogenes* or *Strep. pneumoniae* is isolated from the blood cultures.

Monitoring of treatment

Antibiotic assays are essential when aminoglycosides are given to patients with impaired renal function and also when a patient is not responding rapidly to treatment (*see* Serum gentamicin assays in Chapter 3). The doses of aminoglycoside or their frequency (or both) may be adjusted according to the results of repeated aminoglycoside assays.

The maintenance doses of gentamicin or tobramycin in an adult with normal renal function after the first 24 hours of therapy is usually in the range 80–160 mg. The frequency of maintenance doses given, until the results of gentamicin assay are available, can be adjusted according to the following rough guide of renal function and dosage:

Blood urea,		*Frequency of gentamicin*
mmol/l	*(mg%)*	*or tobramycin doses*
7	35	8-hourly
7–18	35–100	12-hourly
18–36	100–200	Daily
36	200	48-hourly or less frequently

The duration of antibiotic treatment required is usually at least 1 week, but this will greatly depend on the patient's clinical progress and the underlying clinical condition.

Causes of persistent septicaemia

Causes of persistent septicaemia in spite of appropriate antibiotic therapy include:

1. Presence of a collection of pus that needs surgical drainage
2. Infection of a prosthesis, e.g. an infected prosthetic heart valve
3. Mechanical obstruction associated with back pressure in a heavily infected site, e.g. calculus in an infected renal pelvis or bile duct
4. Impaired host defences such as severe neutropenia (*see* Chapter 6)
5. Development of antibiotic resistance in the original infecting strain

PREVENTION OF SEPTICAEMIA

Measures to prevent septicaemia include:

1. *Minimizing cross-infection and self-infection (autogenous infection) in hospital*
   By good hand washing and drying techniques, and the use of hand antiseptics where necessary, especially in high risk units.
   Isolation of patients with multiple antibiotic-resistant strains of Gram-negative bacilli or *Staph. aureus*.
   Adequate aseptic and disinfectant policies.
2. *Discriminate use of broad spectrum antibiotics*
   Sometimes a drastic reduction of antibiotic prescribing may be followed by a reduction in the incidence of septicaemia and wound infection (*see* Price and Sleigh, 1970).
3. *'Localized sepsis' recognized and appropriate antibiotic prophylaxis given for surgery or instrumentation on an infected site*
   Examples of 'localized sepsis' include urinary tract infection, biliary tract infection and abdominal abscesses. Prophylaxis should be started just before instrumentation or surgery is performed (*see also* Antibiotic prophylaxis, in Chapter 3).
   The control of hospital infection and Gram-negative sepsis is discussed in greater detail in Chapters 6 and 24.

Further Reading

A. C. P. Symposium (1980) Septic shock. *J. Clin. Pathol.* **33**, 888–896.
*Geddes A. M. (1978) Today's treatment, use of antibiotics: septicaemia. *Br. Med. J.* **2**, 181–184.

*Leading Article (1979) Meningococcal septicaemia. *Br. Med. J.* **2**, 953.
McHenry M. C. (1974) Bacteraemia caused by Gram-negative bacilli. *Med. Clin. North Am.* **58**, 623.
Price D. J. E. and Sleigh J. D. (1970) Control of infection due to *Klebsiella aerogenes* in a neurosurgical unit by withdrawal of antibiotics. *Lancet* **2**, 1213.
Shanson D. C. (1978) Blood culture techniques. In: Williams J. D. (ed.), *Modern Topics of Infection*. London, Heinemann.
Shanson D. C. and Singh J. (1981) The effect of adding cysteine to brain heart infusion broth on the isolation of *Bacteroides fragilis* from experimental blood cultures. *J. Clin. Pathol.* **34**, 221–223.
Simpson R. A. and Speller D. C. E. (1979) Detection of bacteraemia by countercurrent immuno-electrophoresis. *Lancet* **1**, 206.
Stokes E. J. (1974) *Blood Culture Technique*. Association of Clinical Pathology Broadsheet no. 81.
Stumacher R. J., Kovnat M. J. and McCabe W. R. (1973) Limitations of the usefulness of the Limulus assay for endotoxin. *N. Engl. J. Med.* **288**, 1261–1264.
Washington J. A. (1978) *The Detection of Septicaemia*. Florida, CRC Press.
Winslow E. J., Loeb H. S., Rahimtoola S. H. et al. (1973) Haemodynamic studies and results of therapy in 50 patients with bacteraemic shock. *Am. J. Med.* **54**, 421–432.

*Particularly recommended for further study by undergraduates.

Appendix to Chapter 5

Instructions for the collection of blood cultures (example at St Stephen's Hospital, London SW10, 1981)

Whenever possible at least two separate blood culture sets are collected before the start of antibiotic therapy.

The routine blood culture set consists of three bottles:

1. *Nutrient broth*, 10 ml, containing 0·05% 'Liquoid' (aerobic CO_2 bottle)
   5.0 ml blood is added to Bottle 1.
2. *Brain heart infusion broth, containing 0·05% cysteine*
   75 ml (anaerobic bottle)
   5·0 ml blood is added to Bottle 2
3. *Glucose broth* (0·1% glucose), 50 ml, containing 0·05% 'Liquoid'
   Between 5·0–10·0 ml blood are added to Bottle 3

Instructions for collection of blood cultures:

a. Wash and dry hands thoroughly
b. Inspect the venepuncture site (antecubital fossa usually)
c. Clean patient's skin thoroughly for 1–2 minutes with chlorhexidine in spirit. Allow the skin to dry before taking blood
d. Remove the Viscap covers of blood culture bottles with scissors avoiding contamination of the bottle tops

e. Wipe the penetrable part of the rubber on the bottle tops with separate swabs containing chlorhexidine in spirit. The rubber should be dry before puncturing with a needle

f. Withdraw 20 ml of blood into the syringe. Remove the needle and replace with a sterile needle, taking care not to touch the end of the syringe

g. Inoculate the blood into each bottle through the penetrable rubber. Mix gently by swirling

Where only a small volume of blood is obtained, as for example from a child, it is preferable to inoculate only bottles 1 and 2

h. Place the labelled bottles in an incubator as soon as possible (Bottle 1 is transferred to a CO_2 incubator in the laboratory)

i. Please write brief details of patient's relevant history on request form, including any recent antibiotic therapy

Chapter 6

Opportunistic infections

Many opportunistic infections are acquired in hospital and some are discussed in Chapters 5 and 24. Opportunistic infections are a major cause of illness and death in oncology patients and the leading cause of death in recipients of renal transplants. Severely immunocompromised patients may develop simultaneous infections with several different types of 'opportunist' organisms.

'OPPORTUNIST' ORGANISMS

The term 'opportunist' is not an exact one. 'Opportunist' organisms have three main characteristics:

1. They are usually organisms of low pathogenicity, e.g.
   Pseudomonas aeruginosa
   Staph. epidermidis
   Candida albicans
   Cytomegalovirus
   Babesia
2. They cause serious infections mainly when the host's defence mechanisms against infection are impaired, e.g.
   in patients receiving treatment for acute leukaemia or lymphoma, and recipients of renal or other transplants who are immunosuppressed
3. They can behave as 'conventional pathogens' but under opportunistic conditions may cause atypical clinical presentations or disseminated lesions, e.g.
   Mycobacterium tuberculosis causing a PUO illness in immunosuppressed patients due to miliary TB or
   Strongyloides stercoralis causing overwhelming life-threatening infection in a persistently immunosuppressed patient

Examples of opportunist organisms are included in *Table 6.1* together with brief notes on their associated infections and the specimens required for microbiological diagnosis.

'Opportunist' Bacteria

a. Gram-negative bacilli

Gram-negative bacilli are the most common 'opportunist' pathogens and their sources are either

Table 6.1. Some opportunistic infections and specimens needed for diagnosis

Organism	*Opportunistic infection*	*Specimens for diagnosis*
Bacterial:		
Pseudomonas aeruginosa *Klebsiella aerogenes* *Serratia marcescens* Other 'coliforms' and *Pseudomonas* species	*a.* Gram-negative pneumonia *b.* Gram-negative septicaemia (following invasion of blood by organisms, after localized infections, or from normal gut flora)	Blood cultures and sputum Blood cultures and specimens from infected sites including urine and sputum
Legionella pneumophila	Legionnaires' disease	Bronchial washings, sputum and blood cultures for culture for *Legionella*; paired sera for legionella fluorescent antibodies
Staph. aureus	Severe staphylococcal pneumonia, septicaemia or persistent abscesses	Blood cultures, sputum and pus for culture
Nocardia asteroides	Nocardiosis, especially involving lungs, subcutaneous tissues or kidneys	Sputum, pus from empyema or skin abscess, urine for microscopy and culture
Listeria monocytogenes	Listeriosis, involving lungs, blood or CNS	Blood cultures and CSF
Mycobacterium tuberculosis and BCG	Miliary tuberculosis. Disseminated and pulmonary BCG	Sputum, EMSUs, bone marrow and liver biopsy for microscopy and culture of acid-fast bacilli
Viral:		
Herpesviruses		
1. Herpes simplex	*a.* Severe or generalized herpetic infection of skin and mucous membranes *b.* Herpetic eye infection—danger of corneal dendritic ulcers *c.* Herpes simplex pneumonitis, hepatitis or encephalitis	Vesicular fluid and swabs of lesions into viral transport medium for culture; rapid examination of fluid or tissue by electron microscopy or fluorescent antibody method
2. Cytomegalovirus (CMV)	*a.* Disseminated cytomegalovirus inclusion disease and PUO *b.* CMV pneumonia *c.* CMV hepatitis	Throat swab and urine into CMV viral transport medium for prompt viral culture; liver biopsy and other tissue for microscopic examination for cytomegalovirus inclusions; paired sera for CMV, CFTs
3. Varicella-zoster virus (VZ)	*a.* Severe or disseminated zoster ('shingles') infection—may be rapidly fatal	Vesicle fluid for electron microscopy (culture not usually feasible)
	b. Varicella pneumonitis	Paired sera for VZ CFTs

Table 6.1 (continued)

Organism	*Opportunistic infection*	*Specimens for diagnosis*
Measles virus	Giant cell pneumonia, especially in children who have not previously had measles or who were not previously immunized when their host defences were apparently normal—carries high mortality rate. Especially dangerous in leukaemic children	Throat swab for virus culture; paired sera for measles CFTs
Hepatitis B virus, and non-A, non-B hepatitis virus	Symptomless carriage frequent in immunosuppressed and uraemic patients—high titres of hepatitis virus may be present—risks to attendant staff as well as other patients	Serum for HBsAg and other hepatitis serological tests (*see* Chapter 15)
Vaccinia virus	Vaccinia gangrenosum, disseminated vaccinial lesions and other vaccinial complications which may be fatal; smallpox vaccination is not indicated today and is especially contraindicated in immunocompromised patients	Vesicular material for electron microscopy and viral culture
Fungal:		
Yeasts:		
Candida albicans and other *Candida* spp.	Systemic candidiasis—bronchopulmonary oesophageal, peritoneal or renal lesions; septicaemia and endocarditis	Blood culture and culture and microscopy on specimens from relevant sites
Cryptococcus neoformans	Cryptococcosis—chronic granuloma in lungs or CNS	Sputum, CSF for microscopy and culture; blood cultures; tests for cryptococcal antigen in CSF
Filamentous fungi:		
Aspergillus fumigatus and other *Aspergillus* spp.	Pulmonary or disseminated *Aspergillus*. In the latter form lesions may occur in lungs, brain and liver. Rarely aspergillus endocarditis may be the main lesion	Sputum for microscopy and culture; blood cultures; biopsy material for microscopy and culture; serology—aspergillus precipitins (may be negative)
Mucor	Mucormycosis	Biopsy material for microscopy and culture

Table 6.1 (continued)

Organism	*Opportunistic infection*	*Specimens for diagnosis*
Dimorphic fungi:		
Histoplasma capsulatum	Histoplasmosis—pulmonary and disseminated histoplasmosis—mainly affecting patients who have stayed in N. America or W. Indies	Sputum, bone marrow aspirate, liver biopsy for microscopy and culture; blood cultures; serum for histoplasma CFT (may be negative)
Protozoal:		
Pneumocystis carinii	Pneumocystis interstitial pneumonia	Sputum, lung biopsy—silver stain microscopy
Toxoplasma gondii	Toxoplasmosis—severe and disseminated lesions may occur affecting brain and myocardium	Biopsy material of lymph nodes or other tissues for histology and paired sera for toxoplasma dye or fluorescent antibody tests
Babesia spp.	Babesiosis—fever, anaemia and myalgia in splenectomized patient (possibly following tick bite)	Thick and thin blood films for Giemsa staining—parasite seen in red cells
Worms:		
Strongyloides stercoralis	Disseminated strongyloidiasis—affecting many organs following invasion of blood from gut—may be fatal and occur many years after the original infestation (eosinophilia may be absent)	Faeces, jejunal biopsy, sputum or gastric aspirate for microscopy for the larvae

i. Endogenous — from the patient's alimentary tract flora, the most frequent source, causing 'autogenous' infections ('self-infections')

or

ii. Exogenous — from infected or colonized lesions from other patients or from moist contaminated sites in the hospital environment
Cross-infection may be associated with the spread of Gram-negative bacilli by the hands of hospital staff

Examples include *E. coli*, *Klebsiella aerogenes*, *Proteus mirabilis*, *Pseudomonas aeruginosa*, *Pseudomonas cepacia* and other *Pseudomonas* species, *Enterobacter*, *Acinetobacter*, and non-pigmented strains of *Serratia marcescens*. All of these organisms have been increasingly isolated from blood cultures during the last 30 years and this is largely due to the increased incidence of 'opportunistic' conditions (*see below* and Chapter 5).

There is a high incidence of opportunistic Gram-negative infections in special units such as oncology units, intensive care and special care baby units, neurosurgical units, liver units, renal units and burns units. Factors that predispose to Gram-negative infections in these units include instrumentation and the frequent administration of antibiotics. Many of the Gram-negative bacilli are multiple antibiotic resistant and this resistance is often R factor (plasmid) mediated; there may also be 'cross-infection' with plasmids mediating 'en bloc' multiple antibiotic resistance between different strains of the same species or between strains of different Gram-negative bacterial species. The epidemiology of infections occurring in intensive care units is typical of that seen in special units and this is discussed in Chapter 24.

Legionella pneumophila is a rare cause of opportunistic Gram-negative infection which may also cause serious or fatal lung infection and septicaemia in immunocompromised patients. Outbreaks of Legionnaires' disease, due to this organism, have recently occurred amongst oncology and transplant patients in North America and Britain.

b. Gram-positive bacteria

These are important causes of opportunistic infections although less frequent causes than Gram-negative bacilli. Examples include *Strep. pneumoniae* in splenectomized children (sometimes causing serious and recurrent infections), *Listeria monocytogenes* in lymphoma patients, *Staph. aureus* in neutropenic patients (causing pneumonia and septicaemia) and *Staph. aureus* or *Nocardia asteroides* in children with chronic granulomatous disease. *Strep. agalactiae* (Lancefield group B haemolytic streptococcus) may cause serious infections in low birth weight neonates (*see* Chapter 7) and may also rarely cause endocarditis in elderly debilitated patients. *Staph. epidermidis* is an increasingly frequent opportunist organism in immunocompromised or debilitated patients who have either an intravenous infusion or a catheterized urinary tract. This staphylococcus is also an important cause of infection in patients with a Spitz-Holter valve, a prosthetic heart valve or a hip joint prosthesis.

c. Anaerobic bacteria

Anaerobes are only infrequently the cause of opportunistic infections compared with the above aerobic bacteria. However, serious and persistent infection due to some non-sporing anaerobes is sometimes associated with an 'opportunistic' condition, e.g. empyema and septicaemia due to *Bacteroides* species in a patient with rheumatoid arthritis receiving steroids.

d. Acid-fast bacilli

Mycobacterium tuberculosis is an important 'opportunist' causing disseminated lesions in renal transplant and other patients receiving prolonged immunosuppressive drugs and in patients with lymphoma. BCG and some 'opportunist' ('anonymous') mycobacteria have also caused infections in immunocompromised patients although these are very rare compared with *M. tuberculosis*, for example disseminated life-threatening infection due to BCG in a child with chronic granulomatous disease.

Mycobacterium leprae can behave as an 'opportunist'; the types of lesion associated with infection are closely related to the immune response of the patient (*see* Chapter 13).

Opportunist Fungi

Fungal causes of opportunistic infection are rare compared to bacterial causes, but are important causes of life-threatening infections in persistently immunocompromised patients. Examples include *Candida albicans* and other *Candida* species, *Aspergillus fumigatus* and other *Aspergillus* species, *Cryptococcus neoformans*, mucor, *Histoplasma capsulatum* and *Coccidioides immitis*. The latter two fungi are mainly relevant in patients who have, at some time, stayed in the endemic regions of North America. *Candida* and *Aspergillus* species cause the majority of opportunistic fungal infections in Britain, followed by cryptococci. These infections particularly affect patients with decreased cellular immunity, including those with lymphomas or sarcoidosis and recipients of renal transplants after several months of immunosuppressive treatment. Previous broad spectrum antibiotic therapy is an important predisposing factor, especially for candida and aspergillus infections. Serious candida lesions may develop in pharyngeal-oesophageal, bronchial, renal and endocardial sites, sometimes in association with candidaemia. Patients who are having peritoneal dialysis can occasionally develop a candida peritonitis. Aspergillus infection mainly involves the lungs but subsequent dissemination can involve one or more other sites including the brain, pituitary, kidneys and heart. Not only may multiple sites become infected by one fungus, but simultaneous infection due to more than one type of fungus may also occur. The mortality rate of opportunistic fungal infections is high, especially in aspergillus infections in immunosuppressed patients.

Viral, Protozoal and Helminth Opportunist Organisms

Viruses, protozoa and helminths may cause life-threatening infections in patients with impaired cellular immunity (*see Tables 6.1–6.3*). The most frequent viral opportunist organisms belong to the herpes group: cytomegalovirus, varicella-zoster and herpes simplex. Varicella-zoster and herpes simplex can cause acute pneumonitis, severe muco-cutaneous infections and life-threatening disseminated lesions. Cytomegalovirus frequently causes subacute pulmonary infection as well as disseminated lesions (this virus may incidentally also contribute to the rejection of a transplanted kidney when the virus is originally present in the donor tissue). *Toxoplasma gondii* and *Babesia* species may cause life-threatening protozoal infections in immunodeficient patients. Babesia organisms usually cause infections in cattle. Humans may rarely be infected following a splenectomy. *Stongyloides stercoralis* may cause overwhelming infection in immunosuppressed patients who have contracted intestinal strongyloides many years previously in an endemic region such as Guyana.

Table 6.2. Impaired host defences and associated opportunistic infections

	Bacterial			Viral	Fungal			Protozoal
	Gram-negative bacilli, e.g. E. coli, Klebsiella, Pseudomonas Serratia	*Gram-positive cocci, e.g. Staph. aureus, Strep. pneumoniae*	*'Intracellular', e.g. Listeria, Legionella, M. tuberculosis*	*Herpes simplex, CMV, varicella-zoster, measles*	*Candida albicans*	*Cryptococcus neoformans*	*Aspergillus fumigatus*	*Pneumocystis carinii*
Granulocytopenia e.g. during treatment of acute leukaemia	+++	+++	+	+	++	+	+	+
Cellular immunity deficient e.g. in patients with lymphomas, acute lymphoblastic leukaemia, sarcoidosis, or recipients of transplants treated with prolonged immunosuppression	+	+	+++	+++	++	+++	+++	+++
Humoral immunity deficient e.g. post-splenectomy congenital immunoglobulin deficiency	+	+++	+	+	+	–	–	+

+++ Strong association.
++ Moderate association.
+ Weak association.
– No obvious association.

Table 6.3. Some opportunistic lung infections not responding to initial 'blind' antibiotic therapy

Causative organism	*Usual sources*	*Means of spread to other patients include*
Bacterial examples		
Mycobacterium tuberculosis	Usually reactivation of past tuberculous focus; occasionally follows contact	Inhalation of acid-fast bacilli from contact with open pulmonary TB
Legionella pneumophila	Contaminated water in air conditioning plants, humidifiers, shower equipment	Inhalation of aerosols containing *Legionella* from an environmental source (no case-to-case spread)
Nocardia asteroides	Contaminated air and dust; sputum from infected patient	Air and dust (*see* outbreak in renal transplant unit article by Houang et al. 1980)
Viral examples		
Cytomegalovirus Herpes simplex Varicella-zoster (VZ) virus	Usually reactivation of latent infection; VZ infection occasionally follows contact with a case of shingles or chickenpox	Spread of herpes simplex or cytomegalovirus possible by hands of hospital staff—probably unusual; spread of varicella-zoster by contact via infected respiratory droplets or vesicle material is likely to susceptible staff or patients (strict isolation and contact only with VZ-immune staff is necessary)
Measles virus	Respiratory droplets from another case	Inhalation of infected respiratory droplets
Fungal examples		
Aspergillus fumigatus *Cryptococcus neoformans*	Contaminated air and dust	Air and dust (case-to-case spread is probably rare)
Protozoal example		
Pneumocystis carinii	Unknown	Outbreaks may occur—epidemiology not known
Helminth example		
Strongyloides stercoralis	Dissemination to lungs and other sites from previous intestinal strongyloidiasis	(No case-to-case spread in hospital)

OPPORTUNISTIC CONDITIONS

The 'opportunistic conditions' present in an individual patient greatly influence the type of infections that the patient may develop. These conditions include:

1. *Impaired Host Defences*

This is the most important group of 'opportunistic conditions'. The three main types of impaired general host defences include severe neutropenia (granulocytopenia), impaired cellular immunity and impaired humoral immunity (*Table 6.2*).

Severe neutropenia is probably the most frequent type of impaired host defence mechanism encountered and it may result in serious infections. Infections in neutropenic patients are most often bacterial and death often results from either pneumonia or septicaemia (*see* Chapter 5). The chances of serious bacterial infections occurring is inversely related to the granulocyte count, when the granulocyte counts are less than 500–1000 per mm^3. The risk of infection is also closely related to the duration of severe neutropenia. Virtually all patients tend to develop serious bacterial infections when the blood granulocyte count has remained less than 300 per mm^3 for more than 2 or 3 weeks.

Patients with impaired cellular immunity may suffer from 'intracellular' (*Table 6.2.*), bacterial, viral, fungal, protozoal or helminth infections and simultaneous infection with different organisms is frequent. An impaired humoral immune response is particularly associated with serious bacterial infections. Severe impairment of an immunoglobulin response to infection is less frequent in adults than an impaired cellular immune response.

Impaired immunity and disorders affecting phagocytes may be due either to primary (congenital) or secondary (acquired) causes. Congenital immunodeficiency is discussed in Chapter 7 and is much less frequent than impaired host defences due to acquired causes. Secondary causes include:

a. Extremes of age
  e.g. low birth weight neonates and the elderly
b. Acquired diseases including
  i. *Diseases of the reticuloendothelial system*
    e.g. leukaemia, lymphoma, myeloma
  ii. *Immunoglobulin deficiency associated with disease*
    e.g. nephrotic syndrome, protein-losing enteropathy, severe malabsorption syndrome
  iii. *Metabolic disease*
    e.g. diabetes mellitus, uraemia, liver failure
  iv. *Sarcoidosis*
c. Treatment
  i. *Cytotoxic and immunosuppressive drugs*
    e.g. steroids, azathioprine, vincristine and other drugs used in the treatment of cancer and for recipients of transplants
    These drugs frequently cause neutropenia and severe immunodeficiency
  ii. *Radiotherapy*
    (e.g. whole-body irradiation for patients receiving bone marrow transplants is an extreme example)

2. *Instrumentation and Surgery*

These manipulations impair local mechanical barriers to infection and facilitate the invasion of organisms into the body, e.g. intravenous infusions and CVP lines, indwelling urinary catheters, tracheostomies and IPPR with use of ventilators and humidifiers.

Endogenous infection is most frequent with these invasive procedures but cross-infection is also common. The causative organisms often include multiple antibiotic-resistant strains of bacteria (*see* Intensive care units and hospital infection, in Chapter 24).

3. *Administration of Broad Spectrum Antibiotics*

The giving of broad spectrum antibiotics to patients with impaired host defences and/or recent instrumentation predisposes to superinfection by antibiotic-resistant strains of opportunist bacteria, such as *Klebsiella, Pseudomonas* or *Serratia,* or fungi, such as *Candida.*

N.B. Immunosuppressed patient + ampicillin = klebsiella infection
(in many patients)

4. *Structural Damage to an Organ or System*

For example, a kidney damaged by calculi or a lung damaged by previous infection provides a nidus for bacteria and other organisms.

5. *Foreign Bodies*

Implantation of foreign materials also provides a nidus for infection, often by organisms of low pathogenicity. For example, *Staph. epidermidis* and candida infections of arterio-venous shunts in renal dialysis patients, aortic dacron grafts, intravenous catheters, prosthetic heart valves, etc.

DIAGNOSIS OF OPPORTUNISTIC INFECTIONS

Clinical features are often lacking in immunocompromised patients with infection. Fever is frequently the only obvious feature. However, fever may also be due to non-infective causes including malignancy or drug reactions. Patients who have infection are generally more unwell than patients with fever due to non-infective causes, but the distinction is often difficult. In all febrile patients blood cultures, preferably two or three sets, should be collected before the start of prompt 'blind' chemotherapy. If possible, a urine sample should also be collected for culture before treatment starts. A clear bacteriological diagnosis, achieved in only 20–40% of patients, is valuable for subsequent optimal therapy. Knowledge of the patient's clinical state, chest X-ray findings, the types of 'opportunistic conditions' present, and the local prevalence of 'opportunist' organisms may cause certain infections to be suspected. The specimens required for each main type of infection are included in *Table 6.1.*

Diagnosis of the exact site of infection is frequently difficult in severely neutropenic patients. Signs of infection may be lacking due to deficiency in 'pus' cells and impaired inflammatory response. Common sites of infection that need to be considered include the lungs, pharynx and oesophagus, and peri-anal region. In some patients, bacteria from the faecal flora enter the blood from the normal gastro-intestinal tract. Although symptoms or signs at a localized site, such as the peri-anal region, may be minimal, appropriate swabs should be collected in addition to blood and urine cultures. Physical examination of the chest and chest radiograph may also show only minimal abnormalities when the patient presents with fever, and sputum may not be produced. When sputum is produced, the results of microscopy and culture are sometimes unhelpful but an immunoelectrophoresis of the sputum for pneumococcal antigen may help to indicate *Strep. pneumoniae* as one of the causative organisms. Trans-tracheal aspiration has proved increasingly useful in recent years for the investigation of lower respiratory tract infection in immunocompromised patients, as the aspirate is uncontaminated by saliva. The isolation of *Klebsiella aerogenes* and other Gram-negative bacilli, *Nocardia* and other organisms from the aspirate is likely to be clinically significant. In selected patients culture of bronchial washings can also provide useful microbiological results and *Legionella pneumophila* has been successfully isolated from this type of specimen. Bacteriological diagnosis is most frequently made by positive blood cultures irrespective of whether a site of infection has been located. *E. coli* strains are the most frequent Gram-negative bacilli isolated and, together with other Gram-negative bacilli, such as *Klebsiella*, account for about two-thirds of the blood culture isolates. *Staph. aureus, Strep. pneumoniae* or haemolytic streptococci are isolated from about one-third of the positive blood cultures.

A few days after cultures have been collected, and 'blind' antibiotic treatment started, there may be little evidence of any clinical response in some patients who have diffuse shadows apparent on a chest radiograph. Unusual opportunist organisms (*Tables 6.1–6.3*) need serious consideration in these circumstances. *Mycoplasma pneumoniae* and *Coxiella burnettii* may cause severe atypical pneumonia in a few patients and paired serology for the appropriate complement fixation tests should be arranged. In practice 'antibiotic-resistant' infections of the lungs in persistently immunocompromised patients are frequently due to *Mycobacterium tuberculosis*, fungi such as *Aspergillus*, and viruses such as cytomegalovirus. *Pneumocystis carinii* pneumonitis is an important but rare infection in patients with impaired cellular immunity and needs to be especially considered in children with diffuse bilateral shadowing on the chest radiograph. Diagnosis of *Pneumocystis* and other unusual opportunistic lung infections by open lung biopsy is probably the method of choice since adequate samples of tissue can then be examined by silver stains (such as Grocott's and other stains) to see the characteristic pneumocystis cysts or fungi. Histology may also reveal infection by *M. tuberculosis* or cytomegalovirus. However, open lung biopsy is not practical in many patients and less invasive procedures such as fibre-optic bronchoscopy with the collection of bronchial washings or biopsy material may be considered. 'Ordinary' sputum and trans-tracheal aspirates should be examined by microscopy and culture for fungi and acid-fast bacilli. A Grocott's silver stain of the sputum only rarely reveals pneumocystis infection in patients with pneumocystis pneumonitis.

Serological investigations for evidence of infection by *Candida albicans* (candida precipitins), *Aspergillus fumigatus* (aspergillus precipitins), cytomegalovirus (CMV, CFT), *Legionella pneumophila* (fluorescent legionella antibodies), and other opportunist organisms are useful when paired sera show a rising 'specific' antibody titre of four-fold or greater, or a single high titre. A positive specific IgM result is particularly helpful if cytomegalovirus or legionella infection is suspected. However, these antibody tests are frequently unhelpful since 'false negative' or only low serum antibody titres result in some patients with established infections, because the immune response is too poor to generate significant antibody titres. The detection of serum circulating antigens might prove more useful in the future than the detection of antibodies.

TREATMENT OF OPPORTUNISTIC INFECTIONS

Initial Treatment

The majority of infected compromised patients have bacterial infections which require prompt 'blind' treatment as soon as the cultures have been collected. Bactericidal antibiotic combinations using two drugs generally give the best results as the causative bacterial strains are likely to be sensitive to at least one of the antibiotics in the combination and, if sensitive to both the antibiotics, a synergic antibacterial effect may sometimes by achieved. The particular selection of 'blind' drugs depends on knowledge of the local prevalence of pathogens and their antibiotic sensitivity characteristics. *Pseudomonas aeruginosa* is an example of one organism which may frequently cause serious infections in neutropenic patients in one hospital centre, but not in another. (Consideration of recent positive cultures, such as a urine yielding growth of a *Klebsiella* strain resistant to a cephalosporin, and of any recent antibiotics given should also be included when selecting 'blind' antibiotics for treating a febrile illness.)

Selection of antibacterial agents from the following three groups has been recommended (to be given as combinations) for 'blind' therapy in the initial treatment of infections in neutropenic patients with leukaemia:

i. Aminoglycosides, such as gentamicin, tobramycin or amikacin—active against Gram-negative bacilli (and staphylococci)
ii. Cephalosporins, such as cephalothin, cephazolin, cefuroxime or cefoxitin—active against Gram-negative bacilli and Gram-positive cocci
iii. 'Anti-pseudomonas' penicillins, such as carbenicillin, ticarcillin, mezlocillin or azlocillin—active against some *Pseudomonas* strains and other Gram-negative bacilli (plus some anaerobes and streptococci)

Suitable combinations include an aminoglycoside plus an 'anti-pseudomonas' penicillin, or an aminoglycoside plus a cephalosporin. A cephalosporin which is resistant to most Gram-negative beta-lactamases, such as cefuroxime or cefoxitin, plus an anti-pseudomonas penicillin might also be suitable.

Most authorities prefer to use an aminoglycoside in the combination and this is usually gentamicin. The parenteral doses for an adult with normal renal function are as follows: a loading dose of 160–240 mg and then 120–160 mg 8-hourly maintenance doses during the first 36 hours. Doses should be adjusted as necessary according to the results of serum gentamicin assays. Peak serum gentamicin levels 0·5–1 hour after the dose should preferably exceed 8·0 mg/l, but the trough level 8 hours after the dose should preferably not exceed 2·0 mg/l. Repeated checks of gentamicin levels will be necessary. (*See* pp. 55, 91.)

Carbenicillin is probably still the most widely used antibiotic in blind combination with gentamicin. The usual dose is 5 g, intravenously and 6-hourly. If *Pseudomonas aeruginosa* strains resistant to carbenicillin but sensitive to one of the other penicillins, such as ticarcillin, mezlocillin or azlocillin, are a frequent cause of infection in a hospital, a change to one of these other penicillins could be considered instead of carbenicillin. Tobramycin may also be preferred to gentamicin in such a hospital as it may have slightly higher activity against *Pseudomonas* than gentamicin; a combination of tobramycin plus azlocillin could be considered.

Gentamicin, or another aminoglycoside, plus a cephalosporin is often clinically effective, but carries a risk of synergic nephrotoxicity; daily checks on renal function as well as aminoglycoside assays are necessary. The more recent cephalosporins, such as cefuroxime, are probably less nephrotoxic than the early cephalosporins, such as cephalothin. If the patient develops impaired renal function, the doses should be reduced accordingly and an alternative drug, such as mezlocillin, might be considered to replace the cephalosporin in the combination.

Amikacin should be reserved for blind treatment of possible infections by Gram-negative bacilli resistant to gentamicin or tobramycin, such as some gentamicin-resistant *Klebsiella* or *Serratia* strains and this might be applicable in some units that have had recent infections due to these organisms (provided of course sensitivity to amikacin had been demonstrated).

Subsequent Treatment and Management of 'Non-responders'

If the patient responds to initial therapy and culture results confirm that the infecting organisms are sensitive to the combination, the treatment should be continued for at least 4 or 5 days after the pyrexia has disappeared. The treatment may need to be changed according to culture and sensitivity results. The problem of a patient not responding to the antibiotic treatment has already been discussed. As mentioned, in a susceptible patient with possible lung infection the diagnosis of unusual opportunist organisms should be considered. Alternative explanations for an apparent non-response include the possibility of (1) a cryptic collection of 'pus' which might require drainage, (2) superinfection by antibiotic-resistant organisms, (3) administration of inadequate doses of drugs or (4) profound granulocytopenia.

Granulocyte transfusions have proved especially useful in some patients with acute myeloid leukaemia and persistent severe neutropenia (less than 500 granulocytes per mm^3) who developed Gram-negative septicaemia responding poorly to antibiotic therapy during cytotoxic drug treatment. Fresh granulocytes are available to treat a few patients only and should be considered in addition to antibiotics in carefully selected 'non-responding' patients who are likely to suffer persistent neutropenia, providing that the bone marrow can be expected to recover eventually.

Antituberculous drugs should be especially considered empirically in non-responding PUO cases who have been persistently immunosuppressed, including recipients of renal transplants, especially if fever presents longer than a week. If chest lesions are present in an acute non-responding immunosuppressed patient, then erythromycin should also be considered for treating possible Legionnaires' disease.

Anti-fungal Chemotherapy

Fungal infections of the lungs (mainly *Aspergillus* or *Cryptococcus*), central nervous system, heart or other sites most frequently have an insidious onset in patients with lymphomas or prolonged immunosuppression and treatment is often only considered when the disease is well advanced with fatal consequences. Early recognition of the possibility of fungal infection and 'blind' empirical anti-fungal treatment is usually necessary without confirming the diagnosis microbiologically.

The polyene anti-fungal drug amphotericin B is still the best agent to use for treating aspergillus, cryptococcal and candida systemic infections and is also given in 'blind' anti-fungal chemotherapy. An intravenous infusion in 5% dextrose is necessary, usually starting with a daily dose in an adult of 1·0 mg and increasing the dose progressively to 0·6 mg/kg/day during the next fortnight. Some authorities recommend simultaneous mannitol administration to reduce the chances of nephrotoxicity developing. Febrile and other unwanted effects are common, but usually it is necessary to continue the treatment unless serious toxic effects develop. Combined treatment with amphotericin B and 5-fluorocytosine has been recommended for treating some serious yeast infections, e.g. *Candida albicans* oesophageal and bronchial infections with candidaemia, in an immunosuppressed patient. Specialist advice from experts with extensive experience in treating serious fungal infections should be sought at an early stage.

Anti-viral Chemotherapy

Acute pneumonitis or disseminated lesions caused by varicella-zoster or herpes simplex viruses in immunosuppressed patients or patients with lymphoma are rapidly fatal and require urgent systemic anti-viral chemotherapy. Adenine arabinoside (Ara-A) has sometimes been effective but is likely to be superseded by acycloguanosine (('Acylovir') which has recently produced dramatic clinical improvement in some patients. Herpes simplex encephalitis is often difficult to treat effectively (*see* Chapter 10).

Cytomegalovirus is a frequent cause of infection in immunosuppressed patients, but is usually associated with infection of only mild to moderate severity. However, anti-viral treatment may be indicated for some patients who have suspected severe cytomegalovirus pneumonitis or disseminated disease as these conditions may be fatal. Adenine arabinoside has less effect against cytomegalovirus than against herpes simplex, but is occasionally effective in patients with cytomegalovirus infection.

Anti-pneumocystis Chemotherapy

Prompt 'blind' anti-pneumocystis chemotherapy is occasionally indicated when interstitial pneumonitis is clinically and radiologically suspected. This is most likely to arise in children with acute lymphoblastic leukaemia, lymphoma patients and recipients of transplants receiving prolonged immunosuppression. Pentamidine is often effective but is a toxic drug. Cotrimoxazole, given in high dosage, has now replaced pentamidine and is effective provided treatment is started in the early stages of the disease.

Anti-strongyloides Chemotherapy

Thiabendazole has been used successfully to treat pulmonary strongyloidiasis in immunosuppressed patients but may not be effective unless treatment is started early in the infection.

PREVENTION OF OPPORTUNISTIC INFECTIONS

Any impairment of general host defences by treatment is kept under regular review so that the lowest dosage of immunosuppressive drugs, such as steroids, are used for the shortest possible duration that is compatible with effective treatment of the non-infective condition. Measures to prevent hospital acquired infections are discussed in Chapter 24. The main preventive measures include:

1. High standards of asepsis and antisepsis

Special care is necessary to avoid infection when putting up intravenous infusions, inserting CVP lines, performing peritoneal dialysis or other forms of instrumentation.

2. Agreed antimicrobial drug policy

a. Systemic drugs

The use of systemic broad spectrum antibiotics in special units should be reduced to a minimum. 'Prophylaxis' with antibiotics, such as ampicillin plus cloxacillin, is not indicated and may lead to an increased incidence of *Klebsiella* and other Gram-negative infections. However, a few authorities have suggested the use of cotrimoxazole for the prophylaxis of bacterial infections in neutropenic leukaemic patients and this antibiotic has also been recommended for the prophylaxis of pneumocystis infections in a unit with an unusually high prevalence of such infections. Constant bacteriological monitoring of the pathogens isolated from clinical specimens from patients in special units is necessary with particular attention to the current antibiotic sensitivity patterns. It may be necessary to temporarily 'ban' the use of certain antibiotics in a special unit which are associated with a high incidence of antibiotic resistance in the unit.

b. Oral non-absorbable drugs

Administration of oral non-absorbable drugs may help to prevent septicaemia and anorectal abscesses in patients during the treatment of acute leukaemia while severe neutropenia is occurring. Various mixtures have been recommended including a combination of polymyxin, paromomycin, vancomycin and nystatin (used in the U.S.A. in 1968) and FRACON (a combination of framycetin, colistin and nystatin, used in Britain in 1977). These oral drugs (occasionally supplemented by sterile topical antiseptics, such as chlorhexidine, applied to the external surfaces including the perineum and lower genital tract in the female) are given to reduce the gut flora which is the usual source of 'self-infections' in patients with granulocyte counts less than 500 per mm^3. These non-absorbable drugs are probably of most use when the severe neutropenia is expected to be prolonged. Oral non-absorbable drugs have been successfully used for a similar purpose in certain transplant recipient patients who have been given severe immunosuppressive treatment.

c. Prophylactic anti-tuberculous or anti-helminth drugs

In persistently immunosuppressed patients who are known to have had TB in the past, or who have come from a strongyloides endemic geographical area, there is a reasonable indication for prophylaxis with anti-tuberculous drugs or thiabendazole, respectively.

3. Protective isolation

A single room is preferable for leukaemic or transplant patients expected to develop severe neutropenia during treatment and protective isolation procedures are desirable (as indicated in Appendix II, Chapter 24).

The hospital staff attending the compromised patient should not also nurse other patients with TB or varicella-zoster infections, unless they are definitely known to have immunity to these infections. These infected patients should be adequately separated from compromised patients. If an accidental contact occurs between the susceptible compromised patient and a person with measles or varicella-zoster infection, prophylaxis with the appropriate immunoglobulin should immediately be given.

Patients who have severe and persistent immunodeficiency states or who are being immunosuppressed, including irradiated and immunosuppressed recipients of bone marrow transplants, may require complete positive pressure 'Trexler Tent' isolation together with sterilized food, pharmaceuticals and other items (*see* Selwyn, 1980). Patients with malignant disease who are having anticancer chemotherapy should not be given salads or uncooked vegetables which may be a source of Gram-negative bacilli that may colonize the gut.

4. Active immunization

Vaccines against *Pseudomonas aeruginosa* have shown encouraging results in trials with burns patients. It is possible that active immunization with Gram-negative polysaccharide or lipid antigens may be of value for certain patients before they are given immunosuppressive treatment. Such immunization may protect them subsequently from developing serious Gram-negative infections, but this is only a speculative possibility at present.

Further Reading

Bennet J. V. and Brachman P. S., ed. (1979) *Hospital Infections*. New York, Little Brown.
Editorial (1978) Infection prevention in acute leukaemia. *Lancet* **2**, 769.
Editorial (1980) Granulocytopenia and septicaemia. *Br. Med. J.* **281**, 1091.
Editorial (1980) Pneumonia during the treatment of acute leukaemia. *Br. Med. J.* **281**, 1235.
Houang E. T., Lovett I. S., Thompson F. D. et al. (1980) *Nocardia asteroides* infection—a transmissible disease. *J. Hosp. Infection* **1**, 31–40.
Jameson B. (1980) *Pneumocystis carinii* pneumonitis. *J. Hosp. Infection* **1**, 103–105.
Rogers T. (1980) Problems with cytomegalovirus in hospital practice. *J. Hosp. Infection* **1**, 281.
Selwyn S. (1980) Protective isolation: what are our priorities? *J. Hosp. Infection* **1**, 5–9.
Wardale E. N. (1980) Granulocytopenia and infections. *Br. Med. J.* **281**, 1567.
Weller I. V. D., Copland P. and Gabriel R. (1981) *Strongyloides stercoralis* infection in renal transplant recipients. *Br. Med. J.* **282**, 524.

Chapter 7

Obstetric, perinatal and neonatal infections

INFECTIONS IN PREGNANCY

Infections in pregnancy may cause spontaneous abortion, premature labour, still birth, perinatal or congenital infection. The risks to the foetus or newborn infant from infection are far greater than the risks to the mother since the incidence of serious puerperal sepsis and other maternal infections, such as pyelonephritis, has greatly declined during the last 35 years. Much larger numbers of low birth weight infants are born each year compared with even 20 years ago. These now survive with the help of special care baby units. However, they are highly susceptible to serious infection because of their immature phagocytic, humoral and cellular immune defence mechanisms. The IgM immunoglobulin starts to be produced from about 20 weeks of foetal life but IgG immunoglobulin is entirely derived from the mother by the transplacental route.

Infections in Early Pregnancy

Spontaneous abortion can result following maternal infection due to many viruses including rubella, influenza, mumps, measles and Coxsackie A16 viruses. Bacterial infections are rarely implicated although *Listeria monocytogenes* can cause abortion (or the delivery of a still-born infant). Protozoal infections, such as toxoplasmosis, only rarely cause abortion in Britain.

Up to the early 1960s in Britain, septic abortions occurred mainly as a result of the work of criminal back-street abortionists. These have fortunately become rare since the introduction of the reformed law on abortion. The causative organisms include *Clostridium welchii*, and other anaerobes (*see* Chapter 9). The aerobic organisms also causing septic abortion are the same as those causing puerperal sepsis (*see below*).

Asymptomatic bacteriuria of pregnancy occurs in about 5% of pregnant women attending the antenatal clinic where the urine should be routinely screened in early pregnancy. These infections can develop into severe pyelitis of pregnancy in up to about one-third of the cases unless promptly treated (*see* Chapter 19).

Intra-uterine infections due to the 'TORCH' group of organisms (*Toxoplasma gondii*, rubella virus, cytomegalovirus and herpes simplex virus) can result in congenital malformations especially when infections occur in early pregnancy. Organogenesis is completed mainly during the first trimester and maximum embryological development occurs in the first 6 weeks of pregnancy. The earlier that infection occurs, the more likely it is that multiple serious congenital malformations will result. Rubella virus can also cause selective congenital defects in later pregnancy, between the 4th and 6th months, such as 8th cranial nerve damage leading to deafness. These intra-uterine infections, and also congenital syphilis, are described in a section on congenital infections below.

Infections in Late Pregnancy

Mothers with heart disease may occasionally develop infective endocarditis before, during or shortly after labour. Streptococci are the main causative organisms, including viridans streptococci and enterococci (endocarditis is discussed in Chapter 18).

The foetus or neonate is at risk when intra-uterine infections are acquired in late pregnancy either by the transplacental route or by ascending infection from the maternal genital tract. Intra-uterine infections that may be acquired by the transplacental route include varicella-zoster, hepatitis B, Coxsackie B and vaccinial infections. The latter infection should never occur since not only is smallpox vaccination particularly contraindicated in a pregnant woman, but there is no point in giving it since smallpox has been eradicated.

Intra-uterine infections acquired by the ascending route include those due to bacteria colonizing the vagina or perineum, such as Lancefield group B haemolytic streptococci, *E.coli*, *Klebsiella*, *Proteus*, *Bacteroides* and staphylococci. Other infections acquired by this route include those due to *Listeria monocytogenes*, herpes simplex virus and *Mycoplasma hominis*. Chorioamnionitis due to these organisms may cause a maternal pyrexial illness possibly associated with positive blood or high vaginal cultures, and the pregnancy then often ends prematurely with the delivery of either a stillbirth or a sick neonate who may have acute respiratory distress. The risks of chorioamnionitis developing are greatly increased when the membranes have been ruptured for more than 24–48 hours. The range of organisms that may cause infections in association with prolonged ruptured membranes is so vast that rational guidance for effective antibiotic prophylaxis in this situation is difficult.

PERINATAL INFECTIONS

The effects on the foetus of perinatal infection are likely to be greatest when the pregnancy has not reached full term, especially between the 26th and the 36th week. Perinatal infection can result from an infection acquired in late pregnancy or during labour and delivery. The consequences of perinatal infection for the infant are likely to be more serious when the birth weight of the infant is less than 1000–1500 g. The organisms that can infect the infant during birth from the genital tract or perineum are similar to those already mentioned for later intra-uterine infection via the ascending route. In addition, there are some sexually transmissible organisms that may cause infection including *Neisseria gonorrhoeae*, *Chlamydia trachomatis* (TRIC) agent and herpes simplex type II (*see Table 7.1* and *see also* Ophthalmia neonatorum, in Chapter 11).

The most common serious causes of perinatal infection in low birth weight infants are Lancefield group B haemolytic streptococci and Gram-negative bacilli, especially *E. coli*. Other Gram-negative bacilli which may cause perinatal

Main organisms	Neonatal infection			Routes of infection include			
				Pregnancy		Labour and delivery: From genital tract/perineum	Post-natal: From other neonates, hospital staff and environment
	'Early onset'	'Late onset'	Main sites infected include	Trans-placental	Ascending		
E. coli, *Klebsiella* and other Gram-negative bacilli	+		Blood, lungs umbilical stump		+	+	
		+	Blood, meninges, umbilical stump, urinary tract			+	+
Enteropathogenic strains of *E. coli*: *Salmonella*, *Campylobacter*, *Shigella*		+	Gastro-intestinal tract and blood			+	+
Lancefield group B streptococci	+		Blood, lungs, umbilical stump		+	+	
		+	Meninges, blood			+	+
Staph. aureus		+	Skin, umbilical cord, eye, blood, bone and joints, lungs				+
Neisseria gonorrhoeae	+		Eye			+	
Treponema pallidum	+	+	Multi-system (*see* Congenital syphilis)	+			
Listeria monocytogenes	+		Blood, lungs, meninges		+	+	

'Early onset' during first 4 or 5 days of life.
'Late onset' after 4 or 5 days.

infections include *Klebsiella aerogenes* and *Pseudomonas aeruginosa* which are more likely to be associated with the giving of broad spectrum antibiotics, such as ampicillin, to the mother.

The Lancefield group B haemolytic streptococcus (also known as *Strep. agalactiae*) has increasingly been found to cause perinatal infections during the last 15 years when larger numbers of low birth weight infants have been delivered. Lancefield group B streptococci and *E. coli* together cause more sepsis and deaths in infants during the first week of life than any other organisms. The highest perinatal mortality rate, about 43%, is associated with serious sepsis due to Lancefield group B streptococci. Early onset infections due to Lancefield group B streptococci and Gram-negative bacilli are characterized by septicaemia and typically the infective process involves many parts of the body including the lungs and umbilical cord stump. The neonate shows signs of being unwell, even during the first 24 hours of life. Early onset Lancefield group B streptococcal infection may sometimes present as acute respiratory distress syndrome.

NEONATAL AND CONGENITAL INFECTIONS

Neonatal Infections due to Lancefield Group B Haemolytic Streptococci and Gram-negative Bacilli

Early onset infections due to Lancefield group B streptococci and Gram-negative bacilli have been described above in perinatal infections. After the fourth day of life, 'late onset' neonatal infections due to these organisms may appear. The source of the organisms in late onset infections need not necessarily be the maternal perineal or genital tract flora. The source may be the already infected neonates in a baby unit or the hands of hospital staff which transmit these infections from one neonate to the next. Occasionally moist contaminated equipment, such as baby incubators which are humidified or baby resuscitation equipment, is the source of infection in a common source outbreak due to *Pseudomonas aeruginosa* or other Gram-negative bacilli. Late onset serious Lancefield group B streptococcal or Gram-negative infection is often characterized by the development of meningitis (*see* Neonatal meningitis, in Chapter 10).

Neonatal Staphylococcal Infections

Staphylococcus aureus is a frequent cause of minor neonatal sepsis and occasionally is associated with more serious infections. During the 1950s and early 1960s, this organism was much more often the cause of moderately severe sepsis and occasionally caused fatal staphylococcal pneumonia or septicaemia. Outbreaks of neonatal sepsis were common in nurseries due to phage group I *Staph. aureus* strains, such as the '80/81' phage type strain, which were characteristically penicillin resistant. These outbreaks have become much less evident during the past 15 years. When they occur phage typing of the epidemic strains, which are usually resistant to penicillin only, shows phage types other than the 80/81 type. It seems probable that there has been a decline in the virulence of *Staph. aureus* strains, but other factors to control and treat staphylococcal sepsis in nurseries have also contributed to the reduced incidence of staphylococcal infections.

More than 30% neonates become colonized normally by *Staph. aureus* during the first week of life. The first sites to become colonized include the umbilicus, groin, nose, axillae and wrists. One advantage of encouraging close contact between the mother and infant during the first 24–48 hours after birth is that the infant may become colonized with a staphylococcus that the mother might be carrying rather than a hospital nursery staphylococcus. Handling of the neonate by the hospital staff should be reduced to a minimum.

Clinical features of neonatal *Staph. aureus* infections include multiple skin pustules appearing after the third day of life, 'sticky' eye, and less often an infected umbilical stump or breast abscess. More serious staphylococcal infections are uncommon and include pneumonia, osteomyelitis, septic arthritis, and septicaemia. Other serious staphylococcal neonatal problems include pemphigus neonatorum and the scalded skin syndrome, but these are fortunately rare. The latter syndrome, also known as Ritter's disease, is produced by a toxin that is secreted by certain phage group II strains of *Staph. aureus*, such as some type 71 strains, and the toxin splits the epidermis causing 'toxic epidermal necrolysis'. Outbreaks of Ritter's disease in nurseries can be associated with a high neonatal mortality rate. A frequent maternal complication of neonatal colonization of the nose by a hospital nursery strain of *Staph. aureus* is breast abscess. The organism may enter a traumatized nipple during breast feeding and the mother may not present with the breast abscess until many days or weeks after the birth of the infant.

Treatment of minor pustules with systemic antibiotics is not indicated but topical application of anti-staphylococcal substances such as 'triple dye' or hexachlorophane may be useful. When more marked sepsis occurs, such as sticky eye or umbilical sepsis, swabs should be collected. For more serious illness, blood cultures are necessary before the start of prompt 'blind' treatment with systemic cloxacillin or flucloxacillin. Virtually all the staphylococcal strains are resistant to penicillin but sensitive to cloxacillin. If an outbreak is suspected the strains of *Staph. aureus* isolated may be sent to a reference laboratory by the microbiologist for phage typing. Isolation of infected infants is important and in the event of an outbreak the unit may have to be temporarily closed.

Prevention of neonatal staphylococcal infections is more likely to be achieved in nurseries that are not overcrowded and where the hospital staff use good hand washing and aseptic techniques. Further useful protection for normal birth weight infants is possible by applying hexachlorophane powder routinely to the umbilicus, groins and axillae daily from birth (*see* Chapter 25). Some hospital nurseries also include a routine topical application of chlorhexidine cream to the nose of each neonate but usually this is not carried out unless an outbreak has recently occurred.

Other Neonatal Infections

These include urinary tract infections, gastro-enteritis and meningitis (*see* Chapters 10, 14 and 19). *E. coli* is the most common causative organism.

Neonatal gastro-enteritis

Gastro-enteritis is an important infection in both the neonatal period and throughout infancy since serious water and electrolyte depletion may result with possibly fatal consequences; the problem is particularly great in the underdeveloped world today. The causative organisms in neonates include enteropathogenic strains of *E. coli* or toxigenic strains of *E. coli, Salmonella* and *Campylobacter*. In contrast, rotaviruses do not usually appear to cause clinically significant gastro-enteritis episodes in neonates although they are important in later infancy. Dangerous outbreaks of gastro-enteritis may occasionally occur in maternity units and nurseries due to epidemic strains of the above bacteria. Salmonella outbreaks have sometimes started after a mother has been admitted with asymptomatic convalescent carriage of a food-poisoning strain of *Salmonella*, such as *Salmonella enteritidis*. Her infant may develop salmonella gastro-enteritis soon after birth and the infection may be transmitted by the hands of staff to other neonates in the unit. It is not practical to screen all pregnant mothers for salmonella carriage when they are admitted to a maternity unit.

Breast feeding

As with other infections the effects of gastro-enteritis are particularly serious in low birth weight neonates and some protection against infection should be given through the administration of fresh human breast milk. Breast feeding rather than the feeding of artificial milk in a bottle should be routinely encouraged to give the neonate some protection against infections, particularly gastro-enteritis. Human breast milk contains immunoglobulins, especially IgA, which in conjunction with the other constituents of complement, transferrin, and lysozyme, are active against Gram-negative bacilli. The high lactose content of human milk also encourages the growth of lactobacilli which results in acid faeces and an intestinal environment which discourages the multiplication of any strains of pathogenic *E. coli* which may be introduced. In some centres, pooled expressed breast milk is administered to low birth weight infants only after it has been gently pasteurized to remove any contaminating potential pathogens, such as *Klebsiella*, without destroying the antibacterial constituents; other centres have claimed that the maximum benefit from fresh human breast milk can only be obtained with unheated milk (*see also* p. 280 in Chapter 14).

Microbiological Investigations

Many infected neonates develop only non-specific clinical features possibly suggestive of infection, such as lethargy, poor feeding, irritability, vomiting, jaundice or episodes of apnoea. In infants with these features, prompt bacteriological investigations before the start of an immediate blind antibiotic treatment are essential. Investigations should include the taking of blood cultures, swabs of umbilicus, skin, eye or any septic site, faeces for culture, and the microscopy and culture of urine and cerebrospinal fluid. When pus is present, a Gram-strain of this can frequently give a rapid indication of the likely causative group of organisms; predominant numerous Gram-positive cocci could suggest the possibility of a Lancefield group B haemolytic streptococcus or *Staphylococcus aureus* infection. However, the results of microscopy and culture of skin sites are often difficult to interpret in practice since colonization of the neonatal skin by streptococci, staphylococci and Gram-negative bacilli is also common and difficult to distinguish in the laboratory from infection due to these same organisms.

Antibiotic Treatment of Serious Neonatal Infections

Blind antibiotic treatment for neonates with suspected serious 'early onset' infections with Lancefield group B streptococci or Gram-negative bacilli should be urgently started as soon as the cultures have been collected, a combination of benzylpenicillin and gentamicin being suitable in most units.

Special baby care units which accommodate low birth weight infants often have cross-infection problems causing 'late onset' infections with multiple antibiotic-resistant strains of *E. coli, Klebsiella aerogenes, Pseudomonas* or other Gram-negative bacilli. However, gentamicin would usually also be suitable for treating these infections although penicillin should be added in case of late onset Lancefield group B streptococcal infections. The antibiotic sensitivity patterns of bacterial strains encountered in each hospital unit must be taken into account when determining a blind antibiotic treatment policy. Gentamicin-resistant strains of Gram-negative bacilli are now becoming more common in a few hospitals and, in this situation, the use of one of the more recent cephalosporins such as cefuroxime may be indicated. In one well-known maternity hospital, mecillinam has proved useful in recent years for treating neonates who are not thought to have early onset Lancefield group B streptococcal infections and where only less severe infections are suspected; typically Gram-negative infections are the most common type of late onset infections that require blind treatment. However, *Pseudomonas aeruginosa*, which is always resistant to mecillinam but usually sensitive to gentamicin, is very rarely a cause of infection in that hospital. *Pseudomonas aeruginosa* infections are infrequent in most hospital neonatal units, but, when they occur, they are often associated with a high mortality rate unless effectively treated in the early stages. Cloxacillin is only necessary for blind therapy if *Staph. aureus* infection is suspected on clinical or epidemiological grounds.

If meningitis is suspected from abnormal CSF microscopic findings in a sick neonate, blind treatment with chloramphenicol is usually indicated although high dosage benzylpenicillin should also be started if Gram-positive cocci (possibly Lancefield group B streptococci) were seen in the Gram-stained CSF deposit. The dosage of chloramphenicol can be adjusted so that 'the grey baby syndrome' does not occur while giving effective levels of drug against the infecting organism. Assays of chloramphenicol in CSF and serum are helpful (*see* Chapter 10).

Rational specific antibiotic treatment only becomes possible once a microbiological diagnosis has been made and the antibiotic sensitivity test results on the infecting pathogen(s) are known. When gentamicin or other aminoglycoside drugs are used, serum assays of the antibiotic are desirable to check that effective levels are achieved and to adjust the dosage according to the results of assay.

Necrotizing enterocolitis

This condition is rare and occurs mainly in low birth weight neonates following intensive care management in special care baby units. The infant with necrotizing enterocolitis (typically a pre-term baby in its second or third week of life) presents with vomiting, abdominal distension and blood in the faeces. A straight X-ray of the abdomen shows signs of gas in the wall of the bowel (pneumatosis intestinalis) or within the portal venous system. In severe cases, the child is shocked with septicaemia and peritonitis. Findings at operation or post-mortem are ischaemic necrosis and ulceration of the bowel wall particularly in the ileo-caecal region.

The cause is not known although it seems likely that a microbial agent is one of the aetiological factors. Various anaerobes may play a role, particularly *Clostridium* species, but this is uncertain. Epidemics have sometimes occurred suggestive of a microbial cause.

Treatment is empirical and includes intravenous fluids, gastric suction and a combination of penicillin, metronidazole and gentamicin. Surgery on the bowel is also sometimes necessary. The condition is frequently fatal.

Prevention of Neonatal Infections

General measures to reduce cross infection in neonatal units have already been mentioned briefly, the main measure being frequent hand washing by staff and the use of good aseptic techniques. For high risk areas, such as special care baby units, an antiseptic preparation for the hands of staff, such as an alcoholic chlorhexidine solution or chlorhexidine detergent, is recommended. The usefulness of human breast milk has been discussed above.

Specific preventative measures for infections that have not been so far discussed include precautions against hepatitis B, gonococcal ophthalmia neonatorum, herpes simplex infection and varicella-zoster.

Anti-hepatitis B immunoglobulin may be necessary for neonates born to mothers who have had hepatitis B around the time of delivery and some mothers who are HBsAg positive. This immunoglobulin needs to be given to the infant during the 48 hours after delivery to be effective in the prevention of liver disease (*see* Chapter 15).

Gonococcal ophthalmia was prevented by the instillation of silver nitrate eye drops soon after birth but this measure is not worth while today as the condition is relatively rare. However, when a mother is known to have had recent gonorrhoea, this measure could be considered in addition to antibiotic treatment of the maternal infection. Possibly this measure may become more important in the future if ophthalmia neonatorum is more often caused by penicillinase-producing strains of gonococci.

Herpes simplex type II is an increasingly common cause of infection and ulceration of the female genital tract but is only rarely associated with serious disseminated disease, encephalitis or hepatitis in infants in Britain. Serious neonatal herpetic disease has been mainly reported from the U.S.A. However, when genital herpes simplex infection is apparent, especially primary infection, near the time of delivery the protection of the neonate against herpetic infection should be considered by performing a Caesarean section. This method of delivery of the infant reduces the chance of infection but does not eliminate this possibility altogether.

Varicella-zoster infection in pregnancy may cause disastrous congenital infection and if a susceptible mother has contact with a case of chickenpox or shingles she should be given hyperimmune anti-varicella-zoster immunoglobulin as soon as possible after the contact (*see* Chapter 20).

Congenital Infections

Foetal infection due to *Treponema pallidum*, rubella virus, cytomegalovirus or *Toxoplasma gondii* may follow intra-uterine infection. Transplacental spread of the organisms to affect the foetus may occur when there has been maternal bloodstream infection (as described in Infections in pregnancy *above*). Once foetal infection occurs due to these organisms, there are possible consequences of an abortion, stillbirth or congenital infection. These and other congenital infections are included in *Table 7.2*.

Table 7.2. Congenital infections

		Routes of infection include	
Main causative organisms include	*Associated infection*	*Intra-uterine infection via transplacental route?*	*Organisms from mother shortly before* or during delivery?*
Treponema pallidum	Congenital syphilis	Yes	
Rubella virus	Congenital rubella	Yes	
Cytomegalovirus	Congenital cytomegalovirus disease	Yes	
Toxoplasma gondii	Congenital toxoplasmosis	Yes	
Hepatitis B	Congenital hepatitis B infection	Yes (possible)	Yes (usually)
Herpes simplex (type II usually)	Neonatal herpes simplex infection		Yes
Varicella-zoster virus	Congenital varicella infection	Yes	Yes
Listeria monocytogenes	Listeriosis		Yes
Neisseria gonorrhoeae	Ophthalmia neonatorum		Yes
Chlamydia trachomatis (TRIC agent)	Ophthalmia neonatorum and neonatal pneumonia		Yes
Candida albicans	Neonatal oral thrush		Yes

* Viruses, such as varicella-zoster, may also infect foetus at this time via transplacental route.

Congenital syphilis

Treponema pallidum can affect many different sites of the body. The clinical features may appear early in neonatal life or later, often between the ages of 5 and 15 years. With the advent of routine antenatal serological screening for syphilis and treatment with penicillin this condition has become very rare in Britain today.

Clinical features in the neonate may include skin lesions such as a generalized maculo-papular rash, raised moist muco-cutaneous lesions, 'snuffles', hepato-splenomegaly, lymphadenopathy, periostitis, osteochondritis and failure to thrive.

Later presentations of congenital syphilis may include interstitial keratitis, sequelae of central nervous system infection, such as mental deficiency and 8th nerve deafness, anterior tibial periostitis, gummata in skin and mucous membranes, and Hutchinson's teeth (peg-shaped upper permanent incisors), bone and cartilage destruction, leading for example to a saddle-shaped nose.

Congenital rubella

Rubella occurring during the 1st month of pregnancy causes foetal damage in 60–80% of cases, while in the 3rd month this risk falls to 10–20%, and in the 4th month to less than 10%. Multiple congenital defects usually result from rubella infection occurring during the first 10 weeks of pregnancy. An isolated congenital 8th cranial nerve lesion is a complication of rubella infection occurring at about the 16th week of pregnancy.

Characteristic clinical features of congenital rubella include cataracts and other ocular defects, 8th cranial nerve deafness, congenital heart lesions, such as patent ductus arteriosus and ventricular septal defect, low birth weight, failure to thrive, hepatosplenomegaly, thrombocytopenic purpura, microcephaly and mental retardation. Unfortunately, there is a continuing incidence of congenital rubella in Britain today; there are many susceptible women who should be offered rubella immunization (*see Fig. 7.1, Fig. 7.2* and Rubella, in Chapter 8).

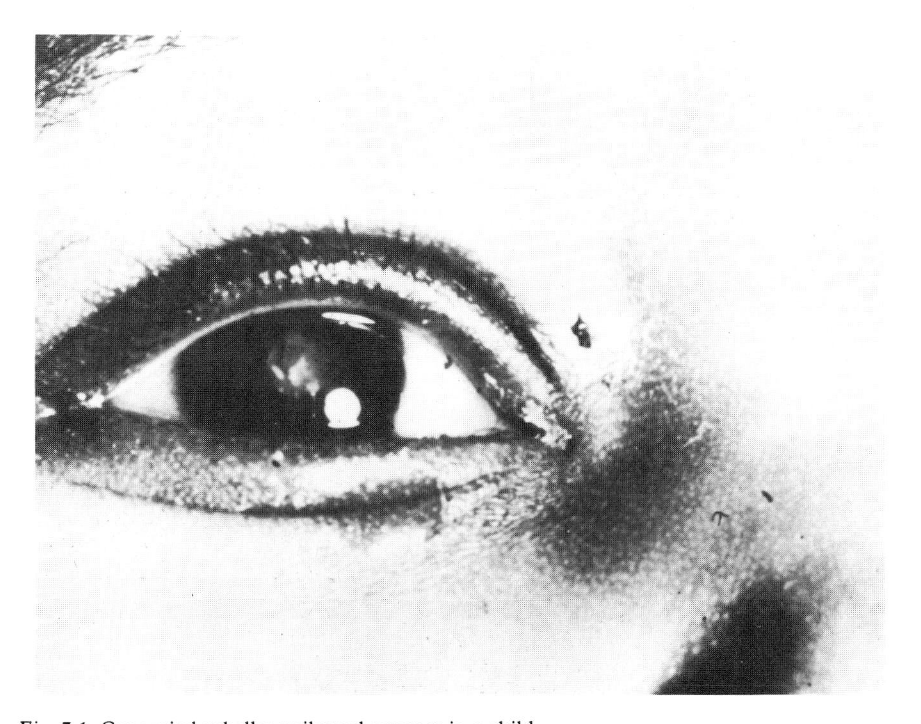

Fig. 7.1. Congenital rubella: unilateral cataract in a child.

Congenital cytomegalovirus disease

Cytomegalovirus is excreted in the urine by about 3% of apparently healthy pregnant women and by about 1% of newborn infants. Most babies with congenital infection show no harmful effects but serious disease may result in a minority of cases, especially of the central nervous system. Stern showed that cytomegalovirus was a much more frequent cause of severe mental retardation than rubella or toxoplasmosis.

Clinical features of congenital cytomegalovirus infection may include jaundice, hepatosplenomegaly, thrombocytopenic purpura, anaemia, spasticity, microcephaly, ophthalmic defects and mental retardation.

Congenital toxoplasmosis

Clinical features of congenital toxoplasmosis characteristically include choroidoretinitis and encephalitis.

There is a 10% mortality rate approximately, but survivors often show serious sequelae which may include hydrocephalus, intra-cranial calcification, mental retardation and impaired vision.

Microbiological investigations

In practice, serological investigations are usually of greater value than attempts at isolation of the organism causing congenital infection although both methods may be attempted in individual patients. Three general principles apply to serological diagnosis of congenital infections:

1. Maternal and infant serum samples should be tested simultaneously as soon as possible after birth and the antibody investigations should be repeated at appropriate intervals. When there is no active congenital infection, the infant's antibody titres progressively fall during the first few months of life,

Table 7.3. Microbiological investigations for the diagnosis of congenital syphilis, rubella, cytomegalovirus and toxoplasmosis

Congenital infection	*Screening tests on mother's and infant's sera*	*Further specific investigations when screening tests are positive*
Syphilis	VDRL and TPHA	FTA including IgM-specific FTA test on infant's serum
Rubella	Rubella HAI	IgM-specific rubella HAI test or IgM-specific rubella fluorescent antibody test on infant's serum
Cytomegalovirus (CMV)	CMV CFT	IgM-specific CMV fluorescent antibody test on infant's serum
Toxoplasma	Toxoplasma dye test	IgM-specific Toxoplasma fluorescent antibody test on infant's serum

VDRL	VD Reference Laboratory antibody test.
TPHA	*Treponema pallidum* haemagglutination antibody test.
Rubella HAI	Rubella haemagglutination antibody inhibition test.
FTA	Fluorescent treponemal antibody
CFT	Complement fixation antibody test.

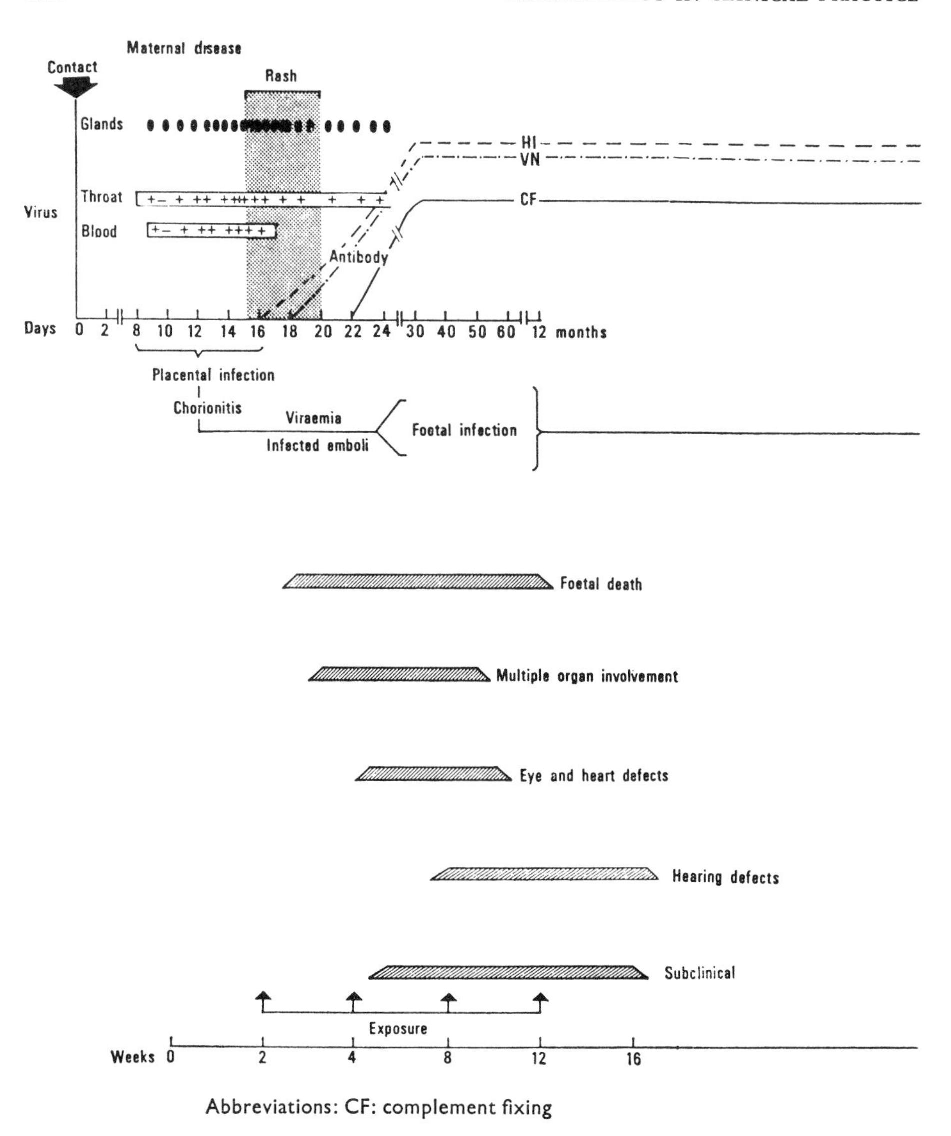

Abbreviations: CF: complement fixing

compared with the mother's antibody titres, due to the gradual disappearance of maternal antibody from the infant's serum. However, if there is active congenital infection the antibody titres of the infant may not fall during the first month of life and instead rising titres may be demonstrated.

2. IgM immunoglobulin determinations performed on the neonate's serum may give valuable evidence of congenital infection. The total IgM fraction may be raised >18 mg %, but of greater diagnostic importance is the frequent finding of raised specific IgM antibodies against rubella, *Treponema pallidum*, cytomegalovirus or *Toxoplasma*.

Examples of these tests are included in *Table 7.3*.

Fig. 7.2. Various stages in the pathogenesis of rubella infection in the mother and foetus, and also the clinical and immunological response of the foetus in relation to gestational age.

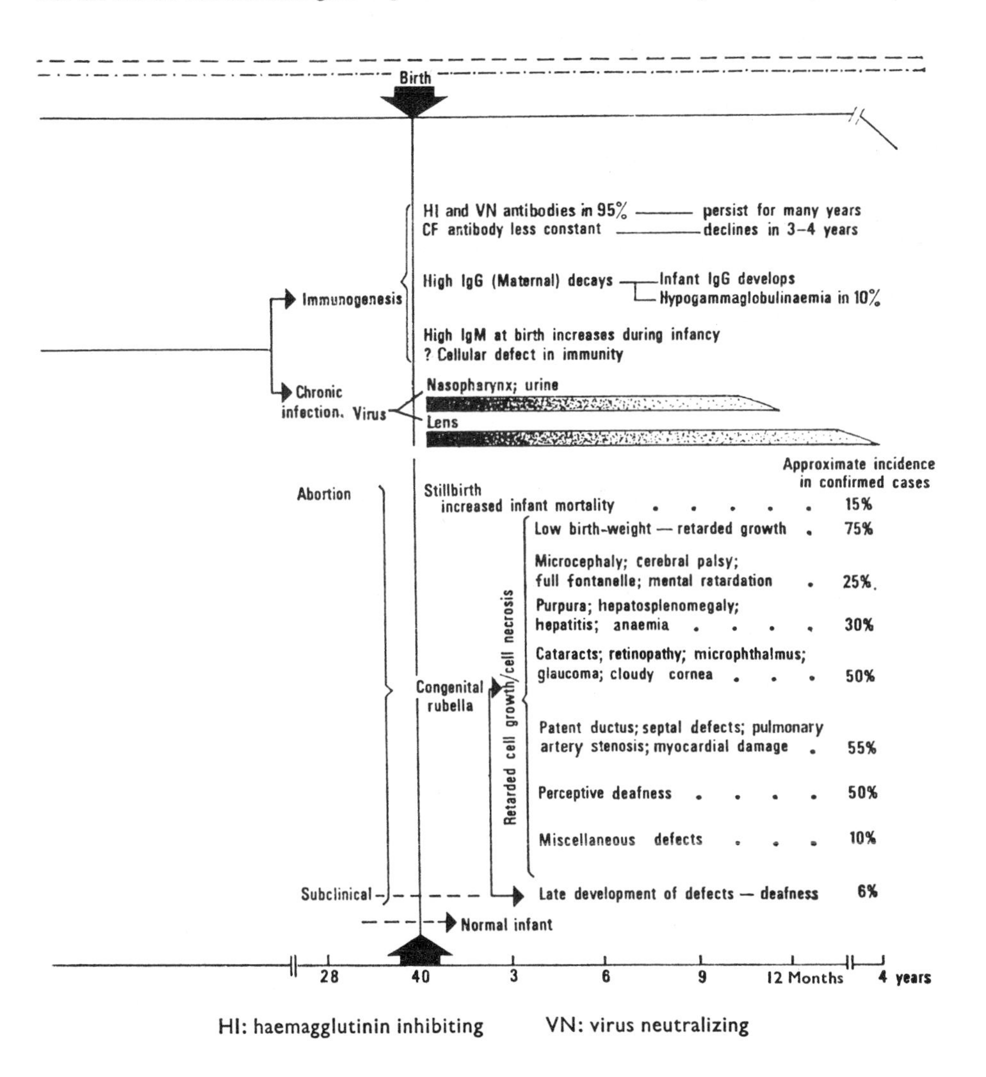

HI: haemagglutinin inhibiting VN: virus neutralizing

3. Routine screening tests for the detection of the appropriate antibody should be performed in the first instance on the mother's and infant's sera. If these tests are negative there is little point in proceeding with further serological investigations against these organisms.

   Detailed examples of the appropriate investigations are included in *Table 7.3*.

Treatment and prevention of congenital infections

Congenital syphilis can be treated effectively by a course of parenteral penicillin. Unfortunately the other congenital infections mentioned above cannot be treated effectively at present. Termination of the pregnancy must be considered when rubella is acquired during the first trimester.

Routine antenatal serological screening for syphilis is essential so that syphilis in pregnancy can be detected at an early stage. When syphilis is discovered adequate penicillin treatment is given to prevent congenital infection.

Rubella immunization should be given to all schoolgirls between the ages of 11 and 13 years and to non-pregnant sero-negative fertile females who must avoid pregnancy for at least 3 months following immunization. If this practice were more widely performed than at present, it is likely that the incidence of congenital rubella would become greatly reduced.

Congenital toxoplasmosis cannot be prevented at present. A suggestion that pregnant women should avoid cats is unlikely to be helpful.

Work is in progress to develop a vaccine against cytomegalovirus.

PUERPERAL SEPSIS AND POST-PARTUM PYREXIA

Puerperal sepsis, caused mainly by *Streptococcus pyogenes*, was a major cause of maternal deaths in the nineteenth and early twentieth centuries. About 100 years ago, Semmelweis showed how hospital attendants could spread the infection by their hands, and his observations helped to lay the foundations of good aseptic and antiseptic techniques in obstetrics.

After the introduction of sulphonamides in the 1930s and penicillin in the 1940s the disease has fortunately become rare although a few avoidable deaths in young mothers due to streptococcal puerperal sepsis have occurred in Britain during the last 20 years. *Strep. pyogenes* (Lancefield group A haemolytic streptococcus) has the ability to spread rapidly in the soft tissues of the genital tract and can cause a fatal septicaemia within 24–48 hours of the start of the illness.

Other organisms that may cause puerperal sepsis include anaerobes, such as *Clostridium welchii*, *Bacteroides* species and anaerobic cocci, and occasionally in mixed aerobic and anaerobic infections, Gram-negative aerobic bacilli such as *E. coli*. *Staph. aureus* can cause infection also but this is unusual.

Puerperal pyrexia and constitutional upset together with possibly offensive lochia are clinical features suggestive of puerperal sepsis. In practice, puerperal pyrexia should always be investigated by collecting high vaginal swabs and, in ill patients, blood cultures are also necessary. As soon as the cultures have been collected, blind antibiotic treatment with benzylpenicillin combined with metronidazole will usually be effective against the streptococcal and anaerobic causes of puerperal sepsis. However, penicillinase-producing strains of Gram-negative bacilli, such as ampicillin-resistant strains of *E. coli*, may be present and reduce the effectiveness of penicillin against streptococci. In ill patients, gentamicin could be added to the penicillin plus metronidazole blind initial therapy. A suitable alternative blind combination would be a cephalosporin plus metronidazole. Rational specific therapy can be given when the results of cultures and antibiotic sensitivities become available.

The source of the *Streptococcus pyogenes* infection could be from the nose, throat or skin of an attendant of the mother during labour, especially if the attendant has had a recent or current streptococcal infection. Hospital staff working in maternity units who develop a sore throat should not continue work until swabs of the throat and nose are negative for streptococci. The patient's own faecal flora is the usual source for the other main microbial causes of puerperal sepsis.

Post-partum pyrexia may be caused by puerperal sepsis due to the above bacteria but, during the last few years, *Mycoplasma hominis* has increasingly been demonstrated as a frequent cause. The mycoplasma organism can often be isolated from blood cultures providing that the subculture plates are incubated under moist conditions for at least 3 or 4 days. They are resistant to penicillins, cephalosporins and metronidazole, but are sensitive to tetracyclines. Tetracycline is usually clinically effective for post-partum pyrexia due to *Mycoplasma* but in the breast-feeding mother the length of the course must be kept to the minimum.

GYNAECOLOGICAL INFECTIONS

Microbial causes of vaginal discharge and pelvic inflammatory disease are described in Chapter 20. In recent years, 'new' infective gynaecological problems have become recognized including those associated with intra-uterine contraceptive devices, vaginal tampons and gynaecological surgery.

Infections Associated with Intra-uterine Devices

Plastic shield-type contraceptive devices that are inserted into the cervix have occasionally introduced the complication of chronic cervical and pelvic infection. Anaerobic organisms such as *Bacteroides* and anaerobic cocci are often prominent in the associated infection. Actinomycosis of the pelvic tissues has been found in a number of patients with these devices, whereas this infection is less likely when a copper contraceptive coil is used instead of the plastic device. Removal of the infected device, culture of the device and microbiological investigation of high vaginal and cervical swabs are indicated. Metronidazole is used to treat bacteroides infection and benzylpenicillin to treat actinomycosis, but surgery is also necessary when there is a large collection of pus or infected necrotic tissue in the pelvis. Copper devices, as well as plastic devices, can be secondarily infected by mixed vaginal flora, including anaerobes and, if gonococci are present, an attack of pelvic inflammatory disease may follow gonococcal infection.

Toxic Shock and Vaginal Tampons

In 1980 there were several published reports of shock associated with a febrile reaction and a rash developing in women who had used a vaginal tampon. Subsequently, it became apparent that in these women the vagina and tampon had become colonized by certain strains of *Staph. aureus* which produced a toxin that was responsible for the clinical syndrome. In most cases, there was spontaneous cure after removal of the tampon.

Gynaecological Surgery

Surgery on the female genital tract may become complicated by wound infection, due to non-sporing anaerobes as well as aerobic organisms (*see* Chapter 9), and also by the development of a hospital-acquired urinary tract infection, especially when an indwelling catheter has been inserted (*see also* Chapter 24).

Further Reading

Davies P. A. (1978) Use of antibiotics—treatment of neonatal bacterial infection. *Br. Med. J.* **2**, 676–679.

Drug and Therapeutics Bulletin (1980) Antibacterial chemotherapy in the newborn. Vol. 19, pp. 13–16.

Griffiths, P. (1981) Congenital cytomegalovirus infection. *Hospital Update*, Jan. 1981, pp. 35–42.

Hanshaw J. B. and Dudgeon J. A. (1978) *Viral Diseases of the Foetus and Newborn.* London, Saunders.

Hurley R., de Louvois J. and Drasar F. (ed.) (1979) Perinatal and neonatal infections. Proceedings of a Symposium held at Queen Charlotte's Hospital for Women, 9 June 1978. *J. Antimicrob. Chemother.*, Suppl. A, vol. 5.

Leading Article (1978) Preventing group B infections in babies. *Lancet* **2**, 1240.

Leading Article (1979) Premature rupture of the membranes. *Br. Med. J.* **1**, 1165–1166.

Platt R., Warren J. W., Edelin K. C. et al. (1980) Infection with *Mycoplasma hominis* in post-partum fever. *Lancet* **2**, 1217.

Siegel J. D. and McCracken G. H. (1981) Sepsis neonatorum. *N. Engl. J. Med.* **304**, 642.

Stern H. (1979) Intrauterine and perinatal cytomegalovirus infections. *J. Antimicrob. Chemother.*, Suppl. A, Vol. 5, 81–85.

Valman H. B. (1980) Bacterial infection in the newborn. *Br. Med. J.* **1**, 772–775.

Waterson A. P. (1979) Virus infections (other than rubella) during pregnancy. *Br. Med. J.* **2**, 564–566.

Chapter 8

Infections in children

Infections are very common in children and are responsible for a high proportion of the consultations in general practice. About 80% of illness in infants and children under 5 years old is due to infection. Of these infections approximately half are respiratory tract infections, about one-fifth are specific childhood fevers and about one-tenth infective diarrhoeas.

RESPIRATORY TRACT INFECTIONS

Numerous, recurrent 'colds' are very common in infants and children and these do not normally require antibiotic treatment. However, antibiotics are nearly always indicated for the management of the other common conditions of sore throat, otitis media and sinusitis, even though these are often viral in origin, since the distinction from bacterial causes cannot be easily made in general practice (*see* Chapter 11).

Acute Laryngitis, Acute Epiglottitis and 'Croup'

An infant with croup (inspiratory stridor) may have either acute laryngitis or acute epiglottitis; in both cases the condition of the infant can rapidly deteriorate. 'Croup' may lead to airways obstruction, with hypoxia, and is a potentially fatal complication of laryngitis or epiglottitis. In children with acute epiglottitis the collection of a swab and examination of the throat and larynx is extremely hazardous and is only indicated if preparations are made to intubate or perform a tracheostomy if necessary; otherwise blood cultures only should be collected and then treatment started immediately with intravenous antibiotics and steroid therapy to reduce the swelling associated with the inflammation.

Haemophilus influenzae, capsulated Pittman type b strain, is the main bacterial cause of acute epiglottitis and croup, although diphtheria was also an important cause of croup in the past. Viruses cause most cases of acute laryngitis and croup, including respiratory syncytial virus and para-influenza viruses.

The choice of 'blind' antibiotic in this situation is straightforward—chloramphenicol. Ampicillin should not be given as many strains of Pittman type b *Haemophilus influenzae* are beta-lactamase producers and are, therefore, resistant to ampicillin. Subsequent treatment can be modified according to the results of the antibiotic sensitivity tests on any *Haemophilus* strain which is isolated from the blood cultures.

Acute Bronchiolitis

Sporadic cases and outbreaks of acute bronchiolitis occur in infants under 1 year old, mainly in the winter. Infants with this condition may develop cough, rapid respiratory rate and cyanosis. Intermittent positive pressure ventilation may be necessary for those infants who develop worsening respiratory distress.

Respiratory syncytial virus is the cause of acute bronchiolitis in about 70% of cases. Para-influenza viruses and adenoviruses are occasional causes. Severely ill infants may also have an associated bacterial infection and treatment with antibiotics, such as erythromycin or ampicillin plus cloxacillin, may be necessary.

Rapid diagnosis of a viral cause is possible using direct immunofluorescent techniques on naso-pharyngeal secretions and respiratory syncytial virus (RSV) can often be demonstrated within a few hours of admission. Cross infection can be prevented in the paediatric ward by isolation of the infant. Culture of RSV or para-influenza viruses is best performed by rapid inoculation of respiratory secretions of infants into tissue culture, ideally at the cot side.

Pneumonia

Viruses are important causes of pneumonia in children but, clinically, it is difficult to distinguish between a viral and bacterial cause of pneumonia in an infant (*see* Chapter 12). Frequent bacterial causes include *Strep. pneumoniae, Staph. aureus* and *Haemophilus influenzae*, Pittman capsulated type b. Antibiotics are always necessary for the treatment of pneumonia in case there is a bacterial aetiology. In older children, *Mycoplasma pneumoniae* is also a frequent cause of pneumonia. Recently, a few infants have been diagnosed as having a rare type of pneumonia due to the Gram-negative bacillus, *Legionella pneumophila* (Legionnaires' disease).

Infants with pneumonia normally require emergency admission into hospital. Blood cultures, a throat swab and preferably viral investigations of naso-pharyngeal secretions should be arranged just before the immediate administration of 'blind' antibiotic therapy. Ampicillin and cloxacillin are usually a satisfactory combination although a few cases of pneumonia due to penicillinase-producing strains of *Haemophilus influenzae* may not respond to this therapy. If there is a lack of response to this combination, mycoplasma infection or Legionnaires' disease is an important possibility and erythromycin should be started. When the cultures show infection by a penicillinase-producing *Haemophilus influenzae* strain, the treatment can be modified according to the antibiotic sensitivities of the isolate; cotrimoxazole or chloramphenicol may be indicated in this situation. When a chest radiograph suggests a staphylococcal cause, fusidic acid may be given together with the initial ampicillin and cloxacillin therapy. For severely ill infants, Gram-negative bacilli as well as Gram-positive cocci should be 'covered' from the outset and a combination of ampicillin plus cloxacillin plus gentamicin or erythromycin combined with gentamicin is suitable pending the results of microbiological investigations.

Cystic fibrosis

Pulmonary infection is a major and recurrent problem in children with cystic fibrosis. Many of these children die as a result of chronic lung infections. Regular postural drainage and physiotherapy are necessary to assist the drainage of bronchial secretions. *Staph. aureus* is the main organism that infects the lower respiratory tract and causes lung damage. Prevention of *Staph. aureus* infections during the first 1–2 years of life is especially important using anti-staphylococcal antibiotic prophylaxis. If the chest radiograph is normal, the child is well and there is no positive bacteriology, this prophylaxis may be discontinued after 1 year of age. In early childhood *Staph. aureus* infections are predominant but with repeated courses of antibiotic therapy, subsequent infections with multiple antibiotic-resistant organisms also develop. These latter organisms include *Pseudomonas aeruginosa*, often 'mucoid' strains. Occasionally *Haemophilus influenzae* and *Strep. pneumoniae* may also cause lung infection in these children.

The management of cystic fibrotic children with established chronic lower respiratory tract infections is a difficult problem and some general principles should be considered:

a. In many early cases, it is best to withhold antibiotic therapy till the major pathogens and antibiotic sensitivities are identified repeatedly in fresh sputum specimens.

b. Keep the children out of hospital as much as possible and reduce the risks of colonization by 'hospital' antibiotic-resistant Gram-negative bacilli, including *Pseudomonas*.

c. Avoid superinfection with antibiotic-resistant organisms for as long as possible by (i) not giving long term antibiotic prophylaxis whenever possible, except in infants under 2 years of age when continuous prophylaxis with flucloxacillin may be indicated (*see above*); (ii) not giving broad spectrum antibiotics such as ampicillin for the treatment except when absolutely necessary. Some centres in Scotland which have claimed to follow these two principles have a much lower percentage of their patients with cystic fibrosis colonized or infected by *Pseudomonas aeruginosa* than other centres.

d. Differentiate mucoid from non-mucoid strains of *Pseudomonas aeruginosa* isolated from the sputum; there is a suggestion that non-mucoid strains are less often associated with clinically significant infection than mucoid strains.

e. Avoid virus infections which may lead to secondary bacterial infection whenever possible; for example, check that the child has been immunized against measles. Annual immunization against influenza might also be justified.

f. Do not give antibiotic therapy until criteria are decided in advance for indicating clinical improvement otherwise the duration of treatment may be too long and superinfection leading to further lung damage may result. The criteria might include diminution in symptoms or signs, a fall in the pyrexia, radiological improvement, and a decrease in the purulence of the sputum. Eradication of the pathogen from the sputum is often not a realistic criterion.

The choice of antibiotics used depends on the results of microbiological investigations, which may include blood cultures in severe cases, and the above considerations. Cloxacillin, alone, or with fusidic acid, is often valuable for treating *Staph. aureus* infections. Tobramycin, often considered with carbenicillin, is useful for treating many infections due to *Pseudomonas aeruginosa*. Recently there have been newer drugs to consider instead of carbenicillin, such as ticarcillin, mezlocillin or azlocillin. It is too early to state whether these newer drugs are clinically more effective than carbenicillin for treating pseudomonas infection in cystic fibrotic children (*see also* Cystic fibrosis, in Chapter 12).

Tuberculosis

In recent years, tuberculosis has mainly affected infants in immigrant families and it is important to arrange for BCG to be administered at an earlier age than is normally recommended in many instances (*see* Chapter 13).

SPECIFIC CHILDHOOD FEVERS

A. Exanthemata

Acute infectious exanthemata are common in childhood and include measles, rubella and chickenpox. Scarlet fever is rare today. Following the incubation period, there is usually a prodromal period with fever and then the characteristic exantham (rash) appears.

Measles

The measles virus mainly infects mucous membranes of the respiratory tract and the skin. The disease is common to both pre-school and young schoolchildren.

Incubation period: usually 9–11 days.

Prodromal period: 4–5 days before the onset of the rash the child has fever and malaise and may develop a sore throat and cough. Characteristically 'Koplik's spots' may appear on the buccal mucosa between the first and third day of the prodromal period.

Rash: The rash usually starts about the fourth day of the illness behind the ears, on the forehead and around the mouth. The skin lesions are dusky red in colour and the florid maculo-papular rash rapidly spreads over the trunk and limbs. The duration of the rash is about 5 days.

Period of infectivity: Throughout the prodromal period and for up to 4 days after the first appearance of the rash.

Mode of transmission: Respiratory droplets or direct contact—measles is highly contagious.

Complications: *a. Acute local complications* include:

i. infection of the ears and secondary bacterial otitis media
ii. infection of the lungs—pneumonia due to the virus itself, or to secondary bacterial infection with staphylococci, *Strep. pyogenes* or pneumococci
iii. conjunctivitis

Haemorrhagic skin lesions, viraemia and severe respiratory tract infection are particularly likely in malnourished infants and, in Africa today, measles is still frequently a life-threatening infection.

b. CNS complications include:

i. post-measles encephalitis occurring about 10 days after the illness with a significant mortality rate

ii. sub-acute sclerosing panencephalitis (SSPE), a rare fatal complication presenting several years after the original measles infection

Microbiological diagnosis: Investigations not indicated normally. However, if an acute CNS complication is suspected paired sera should be sent for complement fixing antibodies to measles to be estimated. If SSPE is suspected, the measles antibody titres in the CSF are estimated also.

Treatment: Antibiotics are indicated when secondary complications, such as otitis media or pneumonia, occur.

Prophylaxis: Active immunization with a live attenuated vaccine is routinely recommended for infants aged 15 months (*see below*).

Passive immunization with pooled immunoglobulin may sometimes be indicated in susceptible contacts on a hospital ward where a case of measles has appeared.

Immunity: Following an attack of measles there is life-long immunity to the disease.

Rubella ('German measles')

The rubella virus causes a mild febrile illness with a faint rash which is only of importance because of the damage it may cause to the foetus when a mother contracts the infection during pregnancy. Children and adults of any age may become infected but rubella is most common in primary school children.

Incubation period: 10–21 days—usually about 18 days.

Prodromal period: There may be no prodromal period apparent or only a mild pyrexia during the 24 hours before the rash appears.

Rash: A pink macular rash on the face and trunk appears in a child who is generally well—the rash may only last for a day or possibly up to 3 days. In some cases, the rash is so mild that a 'subclinical' attack of rubella occurs.

Other features: At the same time as the rash, there may also be characteristically sub-occipital lymphadenopathy. In older children or adults, an arthralgia or polyarthritis affecting the hands or feet may appear. Rarely there is thrombocytopenia.

Period of infectivity: From a week before the rash to 5 days after the appearance of the rash. The disease is highly contagious.

Mode of transmission: Respiratory droplets or contact.

Microbiological diagnosis: Not normally necessary unless there is a possibility of contact with a pregnant woman, or as a pre-immunization check on immunity (*see below*). The main reason for performing rubella serology is in a pregnant mother who has had contact with a suspected case or has an illness compatible with rubella. Serum is required urgently from the mother for rubella haemagglutination inhibition test (rubella HAI). If the date of contact is clearly ascertained and the mother has significant rubella HAI titres present within a week of the contact, it is likely that she is already immune at the time of contact. However, if no significant antibody titre can be demonstrated within a week of contact, she is at risk of developing rubella and a follow-up is then necessary about 4 weeks later to see if a rising titre can be demonstrated. When more than a week has passed since the contact, it may be necessary to perform a rubella-specific IgM test in patients in whom rubella antibodies are present—a positive rubella-specific IgM result suggests recent rubella.

Complications:

a. Congenital rubella syndrome may complicate rubella acquired during the first 4 months of pregnancy in about a quarter of infants. If rubella is acquired during the first month of pregnancy, the risk of foetal malformation is between 60 and 80%. Termination of the pregnancy must be considered when rubella occurs during the 1st trimester (*see* Chapter 7).

b. Post-rubella encephalitis. A rare complication occurring about 10 days after the rash.

Treatment: None.

Prophylaxis in Britain: Active immunization of schoolgirls and non-pregnant, fertile females with a live attenuated rubella virus providing pregnancy is avoided for at least 3 months after the immunization (*see below*).

Chickenpox

Varicella-zoster virus causes chickenpox which is usually a mild disease in children; in adults the disease may be more severe. Infants with immunodeficiency syndrome may develop serious life-threatening complications (*see below*).

Incubation period: 12–21 days—usually about 14 days.

Prodromal period: The child may have malaise or low grade fever for a day before the rash appears.

Rash: Characteristically 'crops' of skin lesions first appear centrally on the trunk and face. Subsequently the proximal areas of the limbs may become affected. Each lesion is oval and starts as a macule which progresses to papules to vesicles. The vesicles develop into pustules which heal and crusts result. Successive crops of skin lesions may appear at different stages in various parts of the body over a period of about a week.

Other features: Fever may become marked during the first 2 or 3 days of the rash, but after this the temperature is usually normal and the child feels reasonably well.

Period of infectivity: From about 5 days before the rash to 6 days after the final stages of the rash. The disease is highly contagious during the first week after the onset of the rash.

Mode of transmission: Respiratory droplets, and direct contact. Air, clothing and other items contaminated with discharge from skin lesions of the patient may also be a source of infection to contacts. Infection may be contracted following contact with a case of 'shingles'.

Complications: In otherwise healthy children, complications are rare.

a. Post-varicella encephalitis, about 10 days after the rash.
b. Varicella pneumonia—more likely in adults and immunodeficient or immunosuppressed patients.
c. Secondary bacterial infection of skin lesions—especially if scratching of the lesions has occurred.
d. Disseminated varicella-zoster lesions, usually fatal, in a patient with leukaemia or immunosuppressed cases.

Shingles ('zoster')—in later adult life the varicella-zoster virus may become reactivated at its site in a dorsal root ganglion or cranial nerve and cause 'shingles' in a dermatome supplied by the nerve. Ophthalmic zoster can cause serious eye lesions as a complication.

Microbiological diagnosis: In a straightforward case of chickenpox in a child, the diagnosis is obvious on clinical grounds. In atypical cases, electron microscopy of fluid from the vesicle will show typical herpes viral particles. Serology is also possible using a varicella-zoster CFT.

Treatment: Anti-viral treatment is not indicated except when rare complications occur, such as varicella-zoster pneumonia in the immunosuppressed—systemic adenosine arabinoside or acycloguanosine ('Acyclovir') has been useful for treating these complications.

The main measure usually required is to keep the skin lesions clean, possibly using chlorhexidine solutions topically. If secondary bacterial infection with *Staph. aureus* or *Strep. pyogenes* occurs treatment with penicillin plus cloxacillin or erythromycin may be indicated.

Prophylaxis: Hyperimmune immunoglobulin against varicella-zoster should be given to susceptible contacts who are pregnant, immunodeficient or immunosuppressed.

Scarlet fever

Scarlet fever is rare, probably mainly due to the great decline in virulent strains of *Strep. pyogenes*, the causative organism, which produce the erythrogenic toxin. The toxin is responsible for the exantham. Sporadic cases and outbreaks of scarlet fever may occur amongst children.

Pharyngeal infection due to *Strep. pyogenes* in scarlet fever can be complicated by both direct and indirect complications (*see* Sore throat, in Chapter 11).

Incubation period: Usually 2–4 days.

Prodromal period: In severe cases, there may be an initial period of 1–2 days with sore throat, headache, marked fever, flushed cheeks and serious constitutional upset.

Rash: Within 1–2 days of the onset of the illness, a punctate erythematous rash appears characteristically on the trunk, proximal chest and on the neck where it joins the flush of the cheeks. The rash typically blanches. The face around the mouth remains pale—circumoral pallor. After about a week, the skin begins to desquamate.

Other features: A ‘strawberry’ tongue may be apparent during the first couple of days of the illness when prominent red papillae show through a white ‘fur’ on the tongue. Cervical lymphadenopathy may also become noticeable.

Period of infectivity: For up to 21 days after the onset of the illness, reduced to about 1 day after the start of penicillin therapy.

Mode of transmission: Respiratory droplets.

Complications: Septicaemia and myocarditis were acute life-threatening complications in the past. Otitis media, quinsy, rheumatic fever and acute nephritis are other possible complications (*see* Streptococcal sore throat, in Chapter 11).

Diagnosis: A throat swab yields *Strep. pyogenes* but the diagnosis is on clinical grounds.

Treatment: Benzylpenicillin injections for the first 48 hours followed by penicillin V orally for 10 days. Erythromycin is recommended for any penicillin-allergic patients.

B. Other Childhood Fevers

Other childhood infectious diseases include mumps and whooping cough. Diphtheria is fortunately very rare in developed countries.

Mumps

The mumps virus causes infection most often between the ages of 4 and 14 years.

Incubation period: 12–28 days—usually about 18 days.

Main clinical features: Pain and swelling in the region of one parotid gland, accompanied by some fever, is the characteristic initial presenting feature. About 5 days later, the other parotid gland may become affected while the swelling in the first gland has mainly subsided. In most children, the infection is mild and the swellings in the salivary glands have disappeared within a fortnight. Occasionally, there is no obvious swelling of the parotid glands during an infection.

Period of infectivity: From 1–3 days before the parotid swelling to about 7 days after all swelling has disappeared.

Mode of transmission: Respiratory droplets.

Complications:
a. CNS complications—aseptic meningitis or encephalitis is an uncommon complication. The prognosis is usually excellent.
b. Orchitis—a complication in about 20% post-pubertal males, may rarely result in sterility.
c. Pancreatitis—a very rare complication.

Diagnosis: *Culture of virus*
The mumps virus can sometimes be isolated from a swab taken from the buccal outlet of the parotid gland duct. The swab is broken off into viral transport medium. However, this is rarely necessary in a straightforward case of mumps parotitis. The virus can occasionally be isolated from the CSF of patients with mumps meningitis.
Serological investigations
These may be useful in aseptic meningitis or encephalitis; mumps S and V CFT antibodies become positive and at least a four-fold rising titre can generally be demonstrated using paired sera (*see* Chapter 10).

Prevention: In the U.S.A., a live attenuated mumps vaccine is sometimes given often alone or together with measles and/or rubella vaccine. In Britain, there are considerable doubts about the wisdom of introducing a 'new' immunization against an essentially mild disease.

Whooping Cough (Pertussis)

Whooping cough is a common and potentially serious infectious disease affecting infants and young children. The causative organisms are *Bordetella pertussis* (>90% of cases) and *Bordetella parapertussis*. Certain viruses, such as respiratory syncytial virus, para-influenza viruses and adenoviruses, and *Mycoplasma pneumoniae* may occasionally cause respiratory conditions that may initially be confused with whooping cough. There is infection of the ciliated respiratory epithelium of the tracheo-bronchial tract. Inflammation is associated with the endotoxin of the bordetella organisms.

Incubation period: 5–14 days—usually about 8 days.

Main clinical features: Characteristically there are three main stages in the disease, each stage lasting from about 1–3 weeks. The catarrhal stage is usually shorter than the spasmodic stage.

1. *Catarrhal stage*

Fever and dry cough becoming worse at night. Infants often have a running nose and a lot of sneezing. The child is particularly infectious during the catarrhal stage.

2. *Spasmodic (or paroxysmal) stage*

Clinically it is difficult to diagnose pertussis until the spasmodic stage has started. There are paroxysms of coughing—each paroxysm consists of a series of coughs followed by a whoop as air is inhaled through the narrowed glottis. Vomiting often accompanies a paroxysm and the child may show exhaustion when there have been many paroxysms.

3. *Recovery stage*

The paroxysms become less frequent, the child sleeps better and there is less vomiting. At the end of the recovery stage, the cough has disappeared.

Period of infectivity: For up to 3 weeks after the onset of symptoms, probably shortened if erythromycin is given in the early stages.

Mode of transmission: Respiratory droplets.

Complications: The disease is most severe in infants less than 1 year old, especially if less than 6 months old and the mortality rate is highest in these young infants. The serious complications which may lead to death include:

a. Bronchopneumonia, partly due to secondary infection—pneumococci and *Haemophilus* are amongst the bacteria implicated. The pneumonia is sometimes severe and difficult to treat effectively with antibiotics.

b. Atelectasis—occasionally leading to bronchiectasis.

c. Cerebral—convulsions may occur at the end of a paroxysm of coughing. Serious brain damage resulting in hemiplegia may occur rarely.

Other complications include pressure effects of paroxysms leading to haemorrhage such as conjunctival haemorrhage or epistaxis. A small frenal ulcer may appear on the tongue in the earlier stages of the disease as a pressure effect from coughing.

Diagnosis: An attempt to obtain a microbiological diagnosis should be made whenever whooping cough is suspected clinically—the diagnosis may not always be clear on clinical grounds. From the epidemiological point of view it is important to make the correct diagnosis.

Culture

There are many potential microbiological difficulties in confirming the diagnosis. The first problem is the collection of good specimens as early on in the disease as possible—soon after the start of the classic paroxysmal stage all the cultures for *Bordetella* may become negative. The bordetella organism is a fragile short Gram-negative bacillus which needs to be cultured on special media where toxic substances are effectively neutralized. Effective media incorporate potato extracts or charcoal to help neutralize these substances. Either Bordet–Gengou or Lacey's medium is used to isolate *Bordetella pertussis*. These media also contain various growth factors and antibiotics are also added, such as penicillin, to suppress the normal mouth flora. Freshly prepared media are necessary for good results.

The special media should be inoculated directly with the swabs collected from the patient. Per-nasal swabs yield more positive results than post-nasal swabs but the highest yield of positive results is obtained by culturing both per-nasal and post-nasal swabs.

If direct inoculation of the pertussis media is not possible, a suitable transport medium is essential. The best transport medium is probably Lacey's pertussis transport medium. Positive results are occasionally possible using Stuart's transport medium containing charcoal.

The plates are heavily streaked with the swabs and are incubated in a moist aerobic atmosphere with carbon dioxide for 24–72 hours.

Characteristic 'pearly' colonies are looked for and agglutination tests are carried out on suspicious colonies. With good techniques, the *Bordetella* organisms can be isolated from 30–50% of cases of suspected pertussis.

Blood tests

Lymphocytosis is usually a prominent feature of pertussis. A complement fixation test may show rising titres in the third week of the disease but is only available at specialized centres.

Treatment: There is still no clear evidence that an antibiotic is clinically effective against *Bordetella pertussis* infection although antibiotics, such as chloramphenicol, may cause some clinical improvement in cases complicated by severe broncho-pneumonia. Erythromycin possibly attenuates the disease if started early enough and may shorten the period of infectivity.

Prevention: Immunization of infants from an early age is recommended routinely (*see* Immunization *below*). There is a suggestion that chemoprophylaxis with erythromycin is effective for child contacts in a family where another sibling has developed pertussis. However, recent trials of this type of chemoprophylaxis have produced disappointing results.

Epidemiology: Whooping cough is endemic in Britain, sporadic cases occurring every year. Outbreaks are common, usually during the winter. The outbreaks used to be at 2-year intervals but recently have been at 3–4-year intervals. A great decline in the incidence of pertussis was seen in the decade 1950–1960, probably associated with widespread immunization against the disease. In the late 1970s, there was a great increase in the incidence of the disease; in 1977 and 1978 large epidemics occurred. This increase was almost certainly related to the decreasing administration of pertussis vaccine (*see* Immunization *below*).

Close contacts in the home are especially liable to be infected. Long-term carriage of the organism does not often occur. Isolation of cases in residential nurseries may help to limit spread.

Diphtheria

Diphtheria is a serious infectious disease, mainly affecting infants over 1 year old, children and young adults. Due mainly to widespread immunization, the disease is rare in Britain today but it is more common in some parts of the world, e.g. Iran and Brazil. In the tropics, cutaneous diphtheria may occur. The causative organism is *Corynebacterium diphtheriae*, of which there are three main types, *mitis*, *intermedius* and *gravis*. The really important feature of an isolate of *C. diphtheriae* is whether it is able to produce toxin rather than what type it is. There are many harmless non-toxigenic strains of *C. diphtheriae* which are not infrequently carried in the throat.

Sites of infection

The pharynx, larynx and nose are the main sites of infection, but occasionally the skin, genital tract and other sites may become infected. The mucous membrane of the pharynx is the most frequent site of infection and a severe sore throat results. Necrotic changes occur so that a 'false' membrane is formed consisting of diphtheria bacilli, fibrin, leucocytes, red cells and epithelial cells. The membrane is most commonly found in the tonsillar region but may extend across the nasopharynx to involve the uvula and also down to the larynx. The membrane affecting the larynx may lead to the direct complication of croup and respiratory obstruction which may be life-threatening.

Diphtheria exotoxin

The potentially fatal indirect complications of diphtheria are entirely due to the release of diphtheria exotoxin into the blood and lymphatics by the organism. Toxin production by the *Corynebacterium diphtheriae* organism occurs when the organism is lysogenized by an appropriate β-phage and the toxin production is optimal when there is an optimal concentration of iron present at the site of infection. The exotoxin is a low molecular weight protein which is heat labile and highly active. Lethal effects may be produced by microgram amounts of the toxin. Unlike tetanus toxin, the diphtheria toxin is antigenic and there is usually some immunity after an attack of diphtheria. Formalin treatment of the toxin converts it into the highly antigenic, but non-toxic, toxoid which is used for active immunization. The diphtheria toxin is partially neutralized by anti-toxin and passive immunization is the mainstay of treatment of the disease. Schick testing was used in the past to determine whether an individual was susceptible or immune to diphtheria. Toxin was injected intracutaneously into one arm while a heat-treated toxin control was injected into the other arm. A positive result appeared as a reaction around the test toxin injection and showed that the individual was susceptible to infection and needed active immunization.

Incubation period: Usually 2–5 days, but 1–7 days possible.

Main clinical features: Faucial diphtheria may have an insidious onset or else a severe sore throat accompanied by serious constitutional upset may occur. The membrane is characteristically firmly adherent and bleeding occurs when there is an attempt to remove it. Oedema of the neck tissues and cervical lymphadenopathy may occur, causing a 'bull neck' appearance. The pulse rate is often rapid.

Period of infectivity: Up to 2–3 weeks after the onset of the disease—shorter if antibiotics are given.

Mode of transmission: Respiratory droplets and direct contact.

Complications: Direct: laryngeal croup (*above*).

Indirect:

a. Neurological—polyneuritis affecting the cranial or peripheral nerves. Cranial nerve lesions can cause paralysis of the soft palate and regurgitation of fluids. Diaphragmatic and limb paralysis could also occur.

b. Cardiovascular—shock may result from the toxaemia, myocarditis, bundle branch block or other effects of disturbances to the conducting fibres of the heart.

c. Renal—toxic changes are frequently manifest by albuminuria.

Other complications include broncho-pneumonia and otitis media.

Diagnosis: Clinical diagnosis is urgently necessary and treatment is based entirely on this rather than on time-consuming laboratory investigations. Laboratory diagnosis is particularly useful epidemiologically and a throat swab is cultured on blood agar, selective tellurite media and enriched Loeffler's medium. (After incubation, an Albert's stain can be performed on the culture from the Loeffler's slope to look for metachromatic granules in diphtheria bacilli, but this procedure is of limited value as the granules do not necessarily correlate with toxin production.) Suspicious grey-black colonies on tellurite media are investigated by Gram-stain, His's sugar fermentation tests and the ability to split urea. When these tests indicate the likely presence of *Corynebacterium diphtheriae* organisms, urgent tests for toxin production are set up.

a. The Elek plate test: Precipitin lines form in an agar plate between antitoxin, which diffuses from a filter paper strip soaked in diphtheria antitoxin, and toxin produced by streaks of growth of any toxigenic strains of *C. diphtheriae* which are placed at right angles to the antitoxin strip. This test needs careful controls and some experience to work optimally (*see Fig. 8.1*).

b. Guinea-pig inoculation tests: These are often more reliable than the Elek plate test and are always advisable when the Elek plate is apparently negative. Two animals are injected intraperitoneally with the test organism and one is protected with antitoxin beforehand. If the unprotected guinea-pig dies this indicates toxin production.

Prevention: Routine immunization with diphtheria toxoid is very effective at preventing the disease (*see* Immunization *below*).

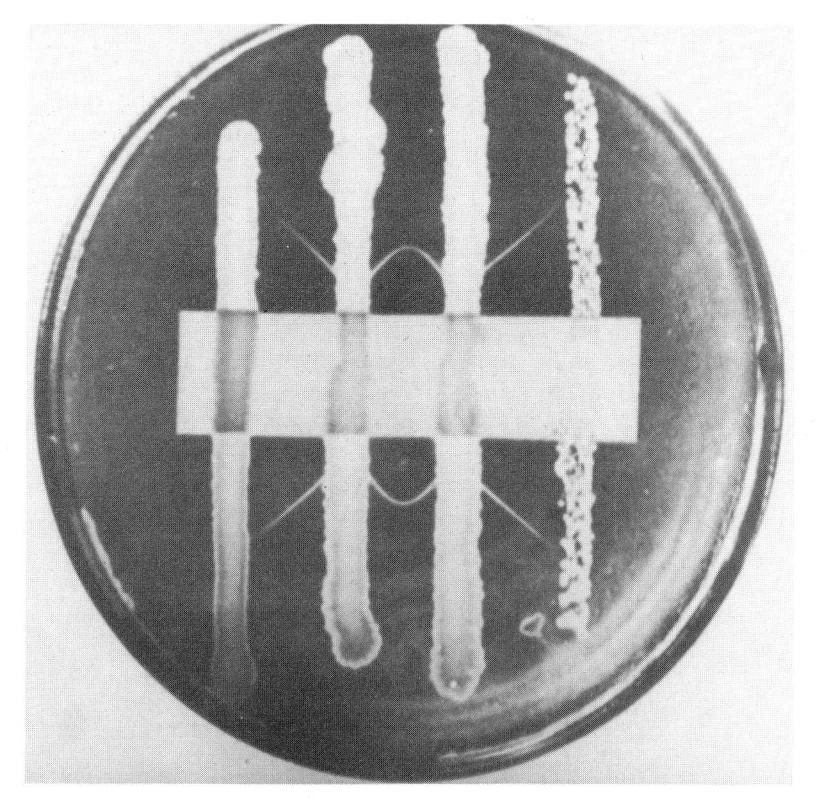

Fig. 8.1. Elek plate test for toxigenic *C. diphtheriae.*

Management of suspected case and contacts

Antitoxin treatment should be started as soon as the diagnosis is suspected clinically and the patient is strictly isolated. In Britain, the Medical Officer for Environmental Health should be notified immediately. A throat and nose swab are collected from the patient so that the laboratory may confirm the diagnosis and the patient is then started on penicillin, or if allergic to penicillin, erythromycin treatment. The antibiotics are only an ancillary aspect of treatment, but are especially useful in reducing the period of infectivity of the disease. Contacts are investigated for signs of the disease and for carriage of the organism and chemoprophylaxis can be considered for close susceptible contacts by administration of oral erythromycin. Immunization of susceptible contacts is also carried out. Asymptomatic carriers of toxigenic strains of *C. diphtheriae* must be looked for during outbreaks of the disease as these carriers may help to spread the organism. They must be isolated and treated.

SOME OTHER INFECTIONS IN CHILDHOOD

Gastro-intestinal Tract Infections

Gastro-enteritis in children in Britain is often associated with rotavirus, campylobacter or salmonella infection but enteropathogenic strains of *E. coli* may also be the causative organisms in infants under 3 years old. Sonnei dysentery is most frequent amongst infants of pre-school age (gastro-enteritis, dysentery and other causes of diarrhoea are discussed further in Chapter 14). Worm infestations are relatively common in children in most countries and, in Britain, threadworms are especially common in young children (*see* Chapter 23).

Urinary Tract Infections

Urinary tract infection occurs in 0·1–5·0% of children and the incidence increases with age. It mainly affects females and the majority of cases are asymptomatic, although some infants have febrile illnesses. However, the symptoms are often non-specific and the diagnosis of urinary tract infection may be missed unless urine cultures are carried out. The recognition of urinary tract infections in children is important since recurrent infections may occur, and result in decreased renal growth and impaired renal function (*see* Chapter 19).

Infections of the Central Nervous System

Bacterial meningitis is uncommon, but is much more frequent in infants and children under 5 years old than in adults. More than two-thirds of the cases are caused by the three primary pathogens, *Neisseria meningitidis, Haemophilus influenzae* and *Strep. pneumoniae*. *Haemophilus influenzae* (capsulated type b strains) causes meningitis almost entirely in infants and children. Viral meningitis, which is far more common than bacterial meningitis, also occurs more frequently in children than adults (*see* Chapter 10). Febrile convulsions is also a problem encountered in infants but, in most instances, there is no clear microbiological explanation for this clinical condition which may be associated with a wide range of febrile illnesses. In occasional cases there is underlying disease of the central nervous system.

Skin, Bone and Joint Infections

Skin, bone and joint infections are more frequent in children than adults and are most frequently associated with *Staph. aureus* or *Strep. pyogenes* infections (*see* Chapters 16 and 17). A few children suffer from recurrent or persistent skin infections, because they have a congenital or acquired immunodeficiency syndrome or defect of their white blood cells.

CONGENITAL IMMUNODEFICIENCY AND IMPAIRED RESISTANCE TO INFECTION

'Physiological' immune deficiency of an extreme kind is an increasingly important problem due to the increased numbers of births of live premature low birth weight infants (*see* Perinatal and neonatal infection, in Chapter 7). The full-term normal-birth-weight infant also has greatly limited production of immunoglobulins, such as IgG, for a period of up to 3–6 months and maternal antibodies help to protect the infant for this period. For a few organisms, such as measles virus, maternal antibodies might still be effective in the infant up to about 1 year.

Recurrent, severe or persistent infection or 'opportunistic infection' in an infant may rarely be due to a congenital ('primary') immunodeficiency syndrome or a congenital defect of polymorphs or macrophages. However, such infections are more often due to acquired or secondary immunodeficiencies. Such secondary immunodeficiencies may result from severe malnutrition, malabsorption, or nephrotic syndrome (these are associated with IgG immunoglobulin deficiency), or with malignant disease or its immunosuppressive treatment. Lymphomas and leukaemia together with their treatment are often associated with impaired 'cellular immunity' or severe neutropenia. Virus infections such as measles may cause transient impaired cellular immunity. The type of infection problem encountered depends on the particular defect present in the host's defences (*Table 8.1*), the age of the child and the epidemiological circumstances. Opportunistic infections are further discussed in Chapter 6.

Congenital Immunodeficiency Diseases

The immunodeficiency diseases may involve the humoral antibody response or the cellular immune response alone or a combination of both; in some congenital diseases the details of the types of immunodeficiency present are unknown. When the immunological stem cells are affected combined deficiency results, when the B-lymphocyte cell function is affected there is a defect in humoral antibody response and when the T-lymphocyte cell function is mainly affected there is an impaired cellular immune response (*Table 8.1*). The skin and mucous membranes of the respiratory or intestinal tracts are the main sites of recurrent infections in immunodeficient children. Failure to thrive and diarrhoea are occasionally presenting features in infants.

Bruton-type hypogammaglobulinaemia

B-lymphocyte production is defective in boys with this condition which is inherited as an X-linked recessive disease. There is a decreased number of plasma cells and poor development of the lymphoid follicles in lymph nodes and in other collections of lymphoid tissue, such as in the alimentary tract. Persistently low levels of serum immunoglobulins (IgG, IgM, IgA or combinations of these) are characteristic and there is a poor antibody response to infecting bacteria. Arthritis may occur in some children possibly as a complication of intestinal infection.

Hypogammaglobulinaemia with B-lymphocytes

Recurrent bacterial infections associated with hypogammaglobulinaemia in children of either sex may be due to this condition. The plasma cells are less obviously deficient than in Bruton-type hypogammaglobulinaemia and although B-lymphocytes are present they do not proliferate properly in response to bacterial antigenic stimulation. Treatment with repeated administration of immunoglobulins can be attempted for both this condition and Bruton-type hypogammaglobulinaemia.

Di George syndrome

This syndrome arises from a fault in the embryological development of the third and fourth branchial pouches so that there is poor or absent development of the

Table 8.1. Congenital immunodeficiency diseases

Disease	Type of impaired immune response			Examples of associated infections				
						Viral infections		
	'Delayed hyper-sensitivity' greatly impaired?*	*Humoral antibody response greatly impaired?*	*Main abnormal cell line*	*Recurrent bacterial infections*	*Infections due to 'intracellular' bacteria*	(i) *Prolonged viraemia*	(ii) *Persistent intracellular virus multiplication*	*Fungal/protozoal infections*
Bruton-type hypogamma-globulinaemia	—	Yes	B-lymphocyte	Staphylococcal Streptococcal *Salmonella* and other Gram-negative infections	—	E.g. polio vaccinia	—	—
Hypogamma-globulinaemia with B-lymphocytes	—	Yes	B-lymphocyte	Similar to Bruton-type deficiency	—	Similar to Bruton-type deficiency	—	—
Di George syndrome	Yes	—	T-lymphocyte	—	*M. tuberculosis* *Listeria* *S. typhi* Excessive or disseminated BCG infection	—	Measles, vari-cella-zoster, herpes simplex, vaccinial complications	Systemic fungal infections, e.g. *Candida* Protozoal infections, e.g. *Pneumo-cystis*
Swiss-type hypogamma-globulinaemia	Yes	Yes	B- and T-lympho-cyte, and stem cell	Combination of patterns of infection seen with both Bruton-type and Di George immuno-deficiency diseases				

* Cellular immune response

thymus and para-thyroid glands. There is apparently normal lymphoid tissue and the serum immunoglobulins are normal but the T-lymphocytes are deficient due to thymic agenesis. Treatment can be attempted with a thymic transplant.

Swiss-type hypogammaglobulinaemia

Extreme combined types of immunodeficiency occur in infants with this rare syndrome which is probably due to stem cell deficiency. Serum immunoglobulins are absent and the cellular immunity response is very poor. Infections of all types are serious in these children and death usually occurs before the age of 20 years. The thymic tissue is deficient and Hassall's corpuscles are absent. A few infants may be saved by treatment with a bone marrow transplant. There are small lymph nodes which lack follicles, lymphocytes and plasma cells.

Nezelof syndrome

This is similar to combined immunodeficiency of the Swiss type except that normal levels of one or more serum immunoglobulins are present especially IgM. The disease is more gradually fatal than with the Swiss-type immunodeficiency.

Wiskott-Aldrich syndrome

The thymus is small and deficient in Hassall's corpuscles in this sex-linked recessive condition of infants. The T-lymphocytes are mainly affected; the thymus dependent para-cortical areas of the lymph nodes are deficient in small lymphocytes and the cellular immune response is greatly impaired. The serum level of IgG immunoglobulin is normal but the IgM level is low. IgA levels are raised. Characteristically these infants have eczema, thrombocytopenia and recurrent pyogenic infections of the skin and upper respiratory tract.

Ataxia-telangiectasia

Infants with this rare congenital condition have defective T-cell function and impaired cellular immune response. Sometimes IgA deficiency is also present and occasionally other immunoglobulin levels are reduced. Repeated upper or lower respiratory tract infections are frequent and eventually infection by antibiotic-resistant strains of bacteria may occur.

Chronic mucocutaneous candidiasis

Chronic, extensive and repeated *Candida albicans* infection of the skin and mucous membranes might be associated with a specific type of defect of cellular immune response to *Candida* species. Possibly ancillary factors associated with proper functioning of the T-cells (such as macrophage inhibition factors and ferrous iron) are lacking in children with this condition. Extensive skin granulomas due to candida infection have occasionally been treated effectively by the administration of lymphocyte 'transfer factor'.

Congenital Defects Associated with Decreased Intracellular Killing or Phagocytosis of Organisms

Chronic granulomatous disease

This disease of infants is typically inherited as an X-linked recessive defect and is characterized clinically by recurrent attacks of suppurative lymphadenitis, skin sepsis, osteomyelitis or abscesses in the respiratory tract, liver or spleen. Death usually occurs in childhood. The neutrophils and macrophages in this condition phagocytose bacteria but have impaired killing mechanisms for certain types of bacteria once these are inside the white cells. Catalase-positive bacteria, such as *Staph. aureus* or *Staph epidermidis*, are especially able to resist the lysosome-killing mechanisms of neutrophils in these patients. Other bacteria that may cause infection include *Serratia marcescens* and *Nocardia asteroides*.

Normal neutrophils characteristically show a 'respiratory burst' of activity during the phagocytosis and killing of many bacteria. This killing of bacteria, which is less efficient under anaerobic conditions, is dependent on an oxidase system that involves a complex electron transport chain, the coenzyme NAD and the production of 'superoxide'. In chronic granulomatous disease, there is no apparent activity of this oxidase system. The lack of activity may be associated with different enzyme deficiencies (e.g. glutathione peroxidase deficiency).

Abnormal neutrophil function in this disease is apparent when the nitroblue tetrazolium dye test (NBT) is carried out on the blood of these patients. The dye is normally reduced by enzyme mechanisms—during the production of 'superoxide' in the vacuoles of the neutrophils—to black formazan. In chronic granulomatous disease there is markedly decreased reduction of nitroblue tetrazolium dye during phagocytosis. The NBT test is thus characteristically negative in this disease while phagocytosis itself is apparently normal.

Chediak-Higashi syndrome

In this syndrome there is characteristically neutropenia, normal phagocytosis but decreased killing of intracellular bacteria. An intrinsic neutrophil chemotactic defect is also apparent.

Defective phagocytosis and chemotaxis

Opsonins are of vital importance for promoting the phagocytosis of organisms and these are often lacking in the immunoglobulin deficiencies mentioned above.

Chemotaxis of neutrophils to sites of infection is dependent on complement activation as well as antigen–antibody interactions. Rare cases of a demonstrable deficiency of complement factors C_3 or C_5 have been described where chemotaxis was greatly impaired and resistance to infection was reduced.

IMMUNIZATION

Immunization procedures have greatly contributed to the decline in incidence of many serious infectious diseases in developed countries. Smallpox is the first disease to become extinct as a result of the W.H.O. campaign using smallpox vaccine.

General Principles

There are many factors that affect the value of particular immunization procedures and these include:

1. Seriousness of the disease

The disease should be potentially serious enough to warrant the development of a vaccine.

2. Safety of the vaccine

The vaccine itself should not cause serious unwanted effects; certainly the risks associated with the immunization must be much less than the risks associated with acquiring the disease.

3. Routine or selective immunization?

Ideally the immunization should benefit both the community and the individual; in most situations where 'routine' immunizations are recommended this is the case. However, rubella immunization is an example of a possible exception: rubella is a mild disease to the individual child or adult and the sole reason for recommending its use in fertile females is to protect as yet unborn children from developing congenital malformations. This is one reason why rubella immunization is not recommended in boys in Britain, although this is carried out in the U.S.A. In order to effectively protect the community against the spread of a potentially serious disease, such as poliomyelitis, it is important that there is an adequate uptake of the routinely recommended polio immunization and that the great majority of the population should have been actively immunized against the disease.

Some immunizations are justifiably recommended for selective use only to benefit particular individuals. Yellow fever immunization need only be considered to protect a traveller from Britain who is visiting an endemic region in Africa or South America; only the individual benefits here. If the individual travels from Africa to India, it is also in the interests of the community in India that he is immunized against yellow fever since there is a theoretical possibility that mosquitoes in India could spread the disease to the community there. Rabies and anthrax vaccinations are good examples of selectively recommended immunizations to individuals in certain high risk situations where the individual, rather than the community, benefits from the immunization.

Since smallpox has been eradicated, there is no justification for vaccination with vaccinial virus and only harm to the individual and his/her contacts, who may develop vaccinial lesions, may result.

4. Effectiveness of the vaccine

The immunization procedure should give effective protection against the disease. The effectiveness of a vaccine depends on several main factors including the following:

a. Suitable protective antigens

The vaccine should include suitable 'protective antigens' that stimulate an immune response which prevents disease occurring. Diphtheria and tetanus immunizations use toxoids which are prepared from modified exotoxins; these protective antigens included in the toxoids stimulate the production of relevant antitoxin antibodies which are effective in preventing disease without necessarily preventing infection by *C. diphtheriae* or *Cl. tetani* organisms. Many viral vaccines stimulate the production of serum-neutralizing antibodies which limit or prevent viraemia so that invasive complications of viral infection are prevented, such as with rubella or poliomyelitis vaccines. In recent years, purified influenza vaccines have been manufactured which consist of pure haemagglutinin and neuraminidase influenza 'protective' antigens. BCG vaccine produces suitable protective antigens during multiplication in vivo which stimulate a 'delayed hypersensitivity' cellular immune response. This response is useful in preventing or attenuating subsequent infection due to *Mycobacterium tuberculosis.*

The vaccines have to be kept under constant review since there may be a need to change the antigens when the antigenic constituents of the 'wild' strains of organisms change; this is especially the case with whooping cough and influenza vaccines.

b. Adequate potency and stability

The dose of protective antigen must be adequate and the vaccine should be stable on storage. The success of the campaign to eradicate smallpox depended on the development of a freeze-dried smallpox vaccine which could be stored and reconstituted for use in potent form in the tropics.

c. Adjuvants

An increase in the immune response can sometimes be achieved by giving a substance unrelated to the vaccine at the same time—such as aluminium salts with tetanus toxoid. Pertussis vaccine itself acts as an adjuvant to tetanus and diphtheria toxoids in 'triple antigen'.

d. Repetition of the doses and 'dead' or 'live' vaccines

Ideally only one dose of a vaccine would be necessary—but effective immunity can only be obtained after one dose with some 'live' vaccines. Multiplication of the organism results in a prolonged antigenic stimulus (and also the possible formation of new 'protective' antigens in vivo). A single dose of attenuated 17 D yellow fever virus vaccine gives solid immunity for over 10 years. Dead vaccines or toxoids need to be given at spaced intervals repeatedly to generate good secondary immune responses which result in effective immunity.

Potential disadvantages of live compared to dead vaccines include the risk that batches of live vaccine may cause some harmful effects associated with infection due to the live vaccine itself. Polio live vaccines rarely can cause a poliomyelitis-like illness in non-immunized contacts of the patient who is immunized. Current live rubella vaccines may possibly harm the foetus and are to be avoided in pregnancy. Similarly smallpox vaccination, measles and yellow fever virus vaccinations during pregnancy could harm the foetus. In patients with impaired immunity, live vaccines can cause serious infective complications and even death, as with BCG or smallpox vaccinations in immunosuppressed patients or patients with lymphomas.

e. Age of the patient
To confer maximum useful immunity each vaccine needs to be given at an age when protection is most necessary while still being effective. Pertussis immunization needs to be given as early as possible since the mortality of pertussis is greatest in infants less than 6 months old, but the immunoglobulin production of infants is not fully developed until 3–6 months old. Maternal antibody is present for between 3 months and 1 year; measles vaccination given before 1 year may not be effective since interference from maternal antibody might result.

Harmful effects of vaccines may also be more likely at certain ages; diphtheria immunization is best carried out in infancy when it is a relatively safe procedure and the protective effect of the vaccine is most desirable. If primary immunization is necessary after 10 years of age, CNS complications become more likely.

f. Duration of immunity
Booster doses may be advisable after a primary course of immunizations for effective long-term prevention of some diseases such as tetanus and poliomyelitis.

g. Interference
Some live viral vaccines may interfere with each other, or they may be less effective when given while the patient has a viral infection, particularly because of the production of interferon. Live polio vaccines type 1, 2 and 3 may interfere with the multiplication of each other when they are administered simultaneously, which is why three repeated doses are necessary. The giving of vaccines should usually be avoided when the patient has an intercurrent infection.

5. Cost

In addition to being effective and safe the immunizations should preferably be cheap and this is especially important for underdeveloped countries.

Routine Immunization Schedule for Infants and Children

First year of life—'triple antigen' and polio immunization

Triple antigen consists of diphtheria and tetanus toxoids and the killed organisms of *Bordetella pertussis*. It is given by injection.

Polio vaccine consists of attenuated live polio virus types 1, 2 and 3. The dose of this Sabin polio vaccine is three drops orally. The administration of this live polio vaccine results in good local production of IgA protective antibody in the intestinal tract as well as effective circulating neutralizing antibodies in the serum. 'Herd' immunity as well as individual immunity may occur following administration of the live polio vaccine.

Timing of the doses of 'triple antigen' and polio vaccine

The first doses of triple antigen and polio vaccine are recommended at 3–6 months. The second doses of these immunizations are given at 6–8 weeks following the first doses. The third doses of triple antigen and polio vaccine are given at 4–6 months, following the second doses.

Recent problems with pertussis immunization

During 1976 and 1977, there was much publicity about possible neurological complications of pertussis vaccine, particularly encephalitis leading to permanent brain damage. The risks of these complications were often exaggerated in the media and a great fall in the 'uptake' of the vaccine and of routine immunizations generally resulted.

In 1978 large epidemics of pertussis occurred in Britain and this was almost certainly due to the decreased immunity in the infants associated with the abandonment of the pertussis vaccine.

The effectiveness of pertussis vaccines was demonstrated by the Medical Research Council trials in 1959; there was protection afforded against severe disease and the spread of *Bordetella pertussis* organisms to home contacts also became limited by immunization. However, *Bordetella pertussis* has the ability to vary ('modulate') its antigenic characters and the earlier strains which predominantly had 1,2 agglutinogens were replaced by strains with 1,3 agglutinogens in the late 1960s. Since the earlier vaccines lacked the 3 agglutinogen antigen, they became less effective. Modern vaccines include this antigen and provide a reasonable degree of protection against serious disease due to current strains of *Bordetella pertussis* while also helping to reduce the spread of the disease.

The risk of neurological complications with current pertussis vaccines is extremely small although the risk probably varies slightly with different commercial vaccines and different batches. The numbers of reactions to pertussis vaccine are reduced when the known contraindications are observed. Contraindications include evidence of a previous convulsion or of brain damage in a baby, a history of epilepsy or a neurological disorder in a parent or sibling, or the presence of a febrile illness at the time the baby is brought for immunization. Also, if there is a history of a previous reaction to triple antigen, the pertussis component should not be given again while further doses of diphtheria and tetanus toxoids may be given.

Adverse recent publicity about vaccines was also possibly indirectly responsible for the occurrence of several cases of polio in the late 1970s in Britain. Cases of diphtheria and tetanus still occur each year in Britain although these are fortunately rare. The importance of continuing with these routine immunizations in the first year of life needs to be constantly emphasized to the public.

Second year of life—measles vaccination

Measles vaccination is recommended at 12–15 months old. In early infancy, the child is usually protected by maternal antibodies. Measles vaccination with an attenuated live strain of the virus should be encouraged in order to reduce the incidence of the complications of measles which include otitis media, pneumonia and neurological complications (*see* Measles).

Since measles immunization was introduced in Britain, the incidence of measles generally has become much reduced. The vaccine itself is effective and safe, although the contraindications to immunization with live virus should be observed. These contraindications include leukaemia, steroid therapy and active tuberculosis.

School entry—booster doses of toxoids and polio vaccine

At about 4–5 years old, booster doses of diphtheria and tetanus toxoids and of polio vaccine are recommended.

At 11–13 years old—BCG immunization

Children should be Mantoux or Heaf skin tested at 11–13 years old and those with negative reactions should be offered BCG immunization to protect them against tuberculosis. BCG is the Bacille-Calmette-Guérin live attenuated strain of *Mycobacterium* which was originally derived from a bovine source.

In areas with a high relative incidence of tuberculosis, such as those with many immigrants from Asia, BCG can be given at 5 years instead of 13 years. In families at risk it may be advisable to give BCG immunization to newborn infants during the first week of life.

Medical Research Council trials have shown that, in Britain, the BCG immunization was effective in giving a high degree of long-lasting protection against invasive complications of tuberculosis, such as tuberculous meningitis, as well as moderately good protection against pulmonary tuberculosis.

BCG should not be given to patients with impaired cellular immunity such as immunosuppressed patients as disseminated potentially fatal infection due to the BCG organism may occur.

Rubella immunization

Girls of 11–13 years of age should be routinely given the live attenuated rubella virus vaccine without taking into account any possible past history of rubella. Screening the blood for antibodies is not indicated at this age. The purpose of immunization is to reduce the number of future cases of congenital rubella. The vaccine cannot be expected to stop the spread of rubella infection as the wild rubella virus may still spread among boys and from boys to mothers who have not had the vaccine or the disease previously.

In later life, females of child-bearing age are encouraged to have blood collected for rubella antibody screening. Sero-negative females should be given the rubella vaccine if they are not pregnant and take precautions to avoid pregnancy for 3 months after the rubella immunization. This type of procedure is easily carried out among young women attending family planning clinics or their general practitioners. Women attending ante-natal clinics are also screened for rubella antibodies and sero-negative women should be offered rubella vaccine immediately after the birth of the baby.

School-leaving age

A booster dose of tetanus toxoid and polio vaccine is recommended.

Smallpox vaccination contraindicated

As mentioned previously, smallpox vaccination with the live vaccinia virus is no longer indicated and there are serious risks associated with primary vaccinations including ectopic vaccinial lesions, disseminated vaccinia, vaccinia eczematum, vaccinia gangrenosum and vaccinial encephalitis. These complications are much more likely in immunodeficient or immunosuppressed patients, but occasionally can occur in apparently healthy individuals. No deaths or disease now occur in the world due to smallpox, since the disease was eradicated during the late 1970s. However, the 'message' about smallpox vaccination has not been appreciated widely enough in practice and even in 1980 there were serious vaccinial complications reported in patients in Britain who had received unnecessary smallpox vaccinations.

Influenza vaccines

Selectively recommended only for certain groups of individuals—including some elderly patients and those with known chronic lung or heart disease (*see* Chapter 12).

Immunization and Preventive Measures for Travellers

The recommendations for prevention of communicable diseases, including malaria in particular, vary each year (*see* Chapter 22). However, the following should be considered for travellers to the Middle East, Asia, Africa or South America.

1. *Typhoid immunization*—a course of two injections given 1 month apart with killed *Sal. typhi* organisms.
2. *Cholera immunization*—given at the same time as typhoid immunization, with killed *V. cholerae* organisms to give some protection for up to 4 months against both El Tor and classic cholera. This is important for the Middle East, Asia and Africa.

   Typhoid and cholera vaccines can be given intradermally and are probably associated with fewer side effects when given by this route than by the deep subcutaneous route.
3. *Polio vaccine booster dose.*
4. *Hepatitis A protection*—an injection of pooled immunoglobulin given during the week before departure will give some good protection against developing a serious attack of hepatitis A for a period of 3–6 months or longer and is strongly recommended.
5. *Malaria prophylaxis*—essential for many parts of Asia, Africa and Latin America (*see* Chapter 22).
6. *Yellow fever virus vaccine*—one dose injected only for visiting the highly endemic regions of Africa or Latin America.

Further Reading

Christie A. B. (1980) *Infectious Diseases: Epidemiology and Clinical Practice*, 3rd ed. Edinburgh, Churchill Livingstone.

D.H.S.S. (1977) *Immunisation against Communicable Diseases*, Letter CMD (77) 7 and Appendix.

*Dick G. (1978) *Immunisation*. London, Update Books.
Mandell G. L., Gordon Douglas R. and Bennett J. E. (ed.) (1979) *Principles and Practice of Infectious Disease (Secion B. 'Host Defense Mechanisms')*. New York, John Wiley.
Mearns M. (1980) Cystic fibrosis. *Prescribers Journal* **20**, 45.
Noah N. D. (1980) Vaccination today. *Br. J. Hosp. Med.* Dec. 1980, p. 533.
Shanson D. C., Rees T. and Sinclair L. (1979) Ear infection due to penicillin-resistant pneumococcus in an immunodeficient child. *Lancet* **2**, 956.
Soothill J., Hobbs J. R., Hitzig W. H. et al. (1968) Immunological deficiency syndromes. *Proc. Roy. Soc. Med.* **61**, 881.
Valman H. B. (1980) The first year of life, contraindications to immunisation. *Br. Med. J.* **1**, 1138–1139.

* Particularly recommended for further study by undergraduates.

Appendix to Chapter 8

List of infectious diseases notifiable in Britain

There is a statutory duty on the part of the clinician to notify the following infectious diseases to the 'proper officer'. In Britain this is the local Medical Officer for Environmental Health:

Acute encephalitis
Acute meningitis
Acute poliomyelitis
Anthrax
Cholera
Diphtheria
Dysentery
Food poisoning
Infective jaundice
Lassa fever
Leprosy
Leptospirosis
Malaria
Marburg disease
Measles
Ophthalmia neonatorum
Paratyphoid fever
Plague
Rabies
Relapsing fever
Salmonella gastro-enteritis (*see* Food poisoning)
Scarlet fever
Smallpox
Tetanus
Tuberculosis
Typhoid fever
Typhus
Viral haemorrhagic diseases
Whooping cough
Yellow fever

Chapter 9

Anaerobic infections

DEFINITION OF AN ANAEROBE

An anaerobe is a microbe that can only grow under anaerobic conditions. In the laboratory, an organism of which the identity is in doubt may be subcultured both anaerobically with added carbon dioxide and aerobically with added carbon dioxide, and the plates incubated for at least 5 days. A micro-aerophilic, carbon dioxide-dependent coccus may, for example, appear on the aerobic plate on the fifth day even though it was apparent on the anaerobic plate on the second day. A strict anaerobe will only grow on the anaerobic plate.

In practice, any bacterial isolate, which is sensitive to metronidazole on routine disc testing anaerobically, will also prove to be an anaerobe.

CLASSIFICATION OF ANAEROBES

A simple classification which has clinical relevance is to divide anaerobes into two groups: the non-sporing anaerobes and the spore-forming anaerobes. As infections due to non-sporing anaerobes are far more common today than infections due to the spore-forming organisms these are mentioned first.

1. Non-sporing Anaerobes

These organisms die quickly in an aerobic environment, as they do not form spores, and are also relatively easily killed by heat and chemical disinfectants.

a. Gram-negative non-sporing anaerobes include:

Bacteroides fragilis *Bacteroides melaninogenicus* Fusiform species	strictly anaerobic Gram-negative bacilli
Veillonella species	anaerobic Gram-negative cocci

b. Gram-positive non-sporing anaerobes include:

Anaerobic cocci	'peptococci' and 'peptostreptococci'
Propionibacteria	anaerobic diphtheroids—common skin contaminants (a rare cause of infection after neurosurgery or heart valve operations)
Actinomycetes israelii	anaerobic Gram-positive branching bacillus, the cause of actinomycosis (*see* Chapter 13)

Non-sporing anaerobes form an important part of the normal flora of man, especially in the mouth, large intestine, lower genital tract and skin (*Fig. 9.1*). *See also* Normal flora of intestine, in Chapter 14.

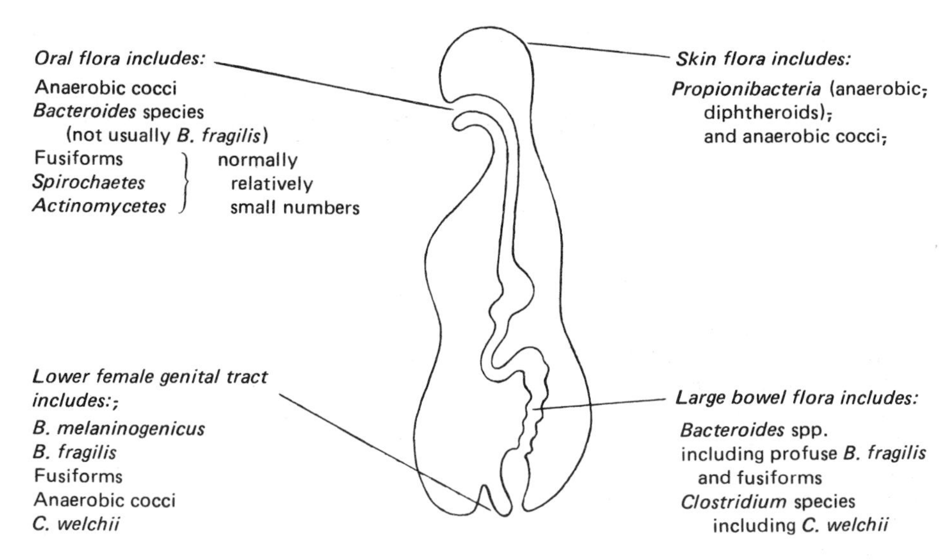

Fig 9.1. Anaerobes in the normal flora of man.

2. *Spore-forming Anaerobes*

Spore-forming anaerobes frequently form spores in 'hostile' environments and these spores may survive for many years. The spores resist drying, many chemical disinfectants and are not always killed by boiling water at 100 °C (*see* Chapter 25).

The spore-forming anaerobes consist of many species of clostridia, which are anaerobic Gram-positive bacilli. These include those which have saccharolytic biochemical characteristics, such as *Clostridium welchii* (*perfringens*) and those with proteolytic characteristics (such as the non-pathogenic *Clostridium sporogenes*). The ability to spread over the surface of a blood agar plate is characteristic of a large number of clostridial species including *Clostridium tetani* and *Clostridium oedematiens. Clostridium welchii*, however, is a non-spreading organism.

Clostridial species are commonly found in the environment in soil, dust, etc., as well as in the faecal flora of animals and man. Almost every person has *Clostridium welchii* in the faeces and some people also carry *Clostridium tetani* in the faeces. Spores of *Clostridium welchii* are often demonstrable on the normal skin between the waist and knees.

PREDISPOSING FACTORS FOR ANAEROBIC INFECTIONS

Anaerobic bacteria will not multiply in vivo to cause infection unless factors are present which lower the oxygen tension or which are associated with a lowering of the Eh (oxidation-reduction potential) through the production of reducing substances. These predisposing factors include:

1. *Trauma*—dead tissue, particulary in deep or extensive wounds.

2. *Foreign bodies*—e.g. clothing or soil inserted into a wound following an accident or war injury. (Modern surgery may involve insertion of a foreign body prosthesis, a prosthetic heart valve or knee joint for example, and these predispose to infections including anaerobic infection).
3. *Impaired blood supply*—e.g. ischaemic arterial disease affecting the foot or leg of a diabetic.
4. *Other organisms also present*—infection or colonization with other organisms is associated with lowering of the Eh, e.g. *E. coli* in an abdominal wound may encourage the growth of *Bacteroides fragilis*. Synergistic infection due to different organisms can also rarely cause extensive gangrene or ulceration although each organism alone cannot cause such necrotizing infection; Meleney's synergistic gangrene is an example, due to infection by a combination of *Staph. aureus* and micro-aerophilic or anaerobic streptococci.

NON-SPORING ANAEROBIC INFECTIONS

In addition to one or more of the above general factors which predispose to anaerobic infection, there is often some breach in the skin or mucosal surface. The causative organisms usually come from the normal flora colonizing these surfaces. Further possible predisposing factors for non-sporing anaerobic (NSA) infections are included in *Table 9.1*. Examples of autogenous NSA infections at different sites are included in *Table 9.2*. Sometimes more than one anaerobic species is implicated as a cause of infection at a particular site and aerobic organisms also often contribute to the severity of the infection.

Bacteroides infections are common following surgery on the colon, or perforation of an inflamed appendix. *Bacteroides fragilis* is usually co-existent with other bowel organisms in peritonitis or wound infections and is particularly important in causing collections of pus in the abdomen (subphrenic, pelvic, liver abscesses, etc.). Occasionally bacteroides bacteraemia may occur resulting in further complications (*Table 9.3*).

Table 9.1. Additional predisposing factors for non-sporing anaerobe infections

1. Surgery, or manipulations, trauma or disease at a site where non-sporing anaerobes are found in the normal flora
2. Debilitating conditions present
   e.g. malignancy
   diabetes mellitus
   alcoholism
   drug addiction
3. Decreased immunity
   e.g. steroid therapy
   cytotoxic drugs
   radiotherapy
4. Broad spectrum antibiotic therapy with ampicillin and aminoglycosides combinations may predispose to *Bacteroides fragilis* bacteraemia
5. Damaged tissues or the presence of a prosthesis at a site normally sterile may provide a suitable nidus for a metastatic infection to develop, e.g. bacteroides pyoarthrosis in a joint affected by rheumatoid arthritis, or bacteroides endocarditis affecting a prosthetic heart valve

These and other important NSA infections have also been referred to in other chapters where appropriate (e.g. Surgical sepsis, in Chapter 24; Brain abscess, in Chapter 10).

Investigations for the Diagnosis of Non-sporing Anaerobic Infections

Clinical suspicion of the presence of NSA infections and attempts to prevent them have become greatly increased during the last few years in Britain, the U.S.A. and other developed countries. This has resulted in microbiological diagnostic problems since drugs, such as metronidazole, are often used before specimens are collected; the anaerobes are then difficult to isolate from blood

Table 9.2. Autogenous infections associated with non-sporing anaerobes

Site	*Infections*	*Anaerobes*
Mouth	Vincent's infection; gingivitis	Fusiforms and spirochaetes
	Actinomycosis	*Actinomycetes israelii*
	Dental sepsis → anaerobic endocarditis as a rare complication	Anaerobic cocci and anaerobic Gram-negative bacilli
Ear and sinus	Chronic suppurative otitis media Sinusitis	*Bacteroides* species in a minority of cases (aerobes more frequent)
Lower respiratory tract	Aspiration pneumonia Bronchiectasis Lung abscess Empyema	Anaerobes from the mouth including fusiforms and anaerobic cocci; occasionally *Bacteroides fragilis*
Abdomen	Wound infection Abscesses or peritonitis associated with large bowel cancer, appendicitis, diverticulitis, and bowel surgery → bacteraemia complication	Faecal anaerobic bacteria—mainly *Bacteroides fragilis*
Skin, soft tissues	Infected diabetic ulcers, deep pressure sores; axillary abscesses; infected sebaceous cyst; Meleney's synergistic gangrene	Anaerobic cocci and various anaerobic Gram-negative bacilli
Female genital tract	Post-hysterectomy, and occasionally post-Caesarean section wound infections	Fusiforms, *Bacteroides melaninogenicus* *Bacteroides fragilis* Anaerobic cocci
	Pelvic actinomycosis in association with intra-uterine coil contraceptive device	*Actinomycetes israelii*
	Pyosalpinx Septic abortion* Bartholin's abscess	Fusiforms, *Bacteroides melaninogenicus* *Bacteroides fragilis* Anaerobic cocci

* *See also Clostridium welchii* gas gangrene.

Table 9.3. Complications of *Bacteroides fragilis* bacteraemia

Complication	*Incidence*	*Mortality rate*
1. Endotoxic shock	Common*	High
2. Renal failure	Common*	High
3. Endocarditis	Rare	High
4. Jaundice	Frequent	Low
5. Suppurative thrombophlebitis and embolism	Frequent	Moderate
6. Metastatic abscesses, e.g. in liver, lung, joints and bone, breast	Common	Varies with site

* Some authorities claim *E. coli* is much more often associated with Gram-negative shock and renal failure than *Bacteroides fragilis*.

cultures, pus, etc. Gas–liquid chromatography (GLC) is especially useful for the rapid diagnosis of anaerobic infection when pus or blood culture specimens are examined and, occasionally, this may give positive results even when metronidazole or other antibiotics have already been started (*see Fig. 9.2*). Multiple volatile fatty acids, such as butyric acid, isobutyric acid, valeric acid, isovaleric acid, succinic acid, propionic acid, etc., are often apparent in the GLC tracing and are diagnostic of an anaerobic infection.

Traditional laboratory methods for the diagnosis of anaerobic infections are still very important and, once a clinically relevant anaerobe has been isolated, the antibiotic sensitivity tests may help to modify the treatment. A simple summary of these basic laboratory methods is given in *Table 9.4*. One of the main problems is to distinguish colonization from infection. Points that have to be considered include the clinical condition of the patient, the nature of the wound or other site of isolation of the organism, the number of organisms isolated and the presence of pus. (*See also* Stokes and Ridgway, 1980.)

Treatment

Treatment is usually surgical drainage of the pus together with antibiotics active against anaerobes such as metronidazole or clindamycin. Clindamycin has become less popular in recent years as it has been closely associated with the serious complication of pseudo-membranous colitis. Penicillin drugs are active against the majority of anaerobes that cause infection above the diaphragm, such as fusiforms, anaerobic cocci and *Actinomycetes*, but are not active against the majority of anaerobes associated with infection below the diaphragm, especially *Bacteroides fragilis*. The latter organism is characteristically resistant to ampicillin, most cephalosporins and gentamicin, but usually sensitive to metronidazole, clindamycin and chloramphenicol. The last drug is especially useful for helping to treat anaerobic brain abscesses although metronidazole is now also very valuable for this purpose. Treatment of the aerobic organisms accompanying anaerobes in a mixed infection is also often necessary. Further details of treatment and prophylaxis are included in the relevant sections of other chapters.

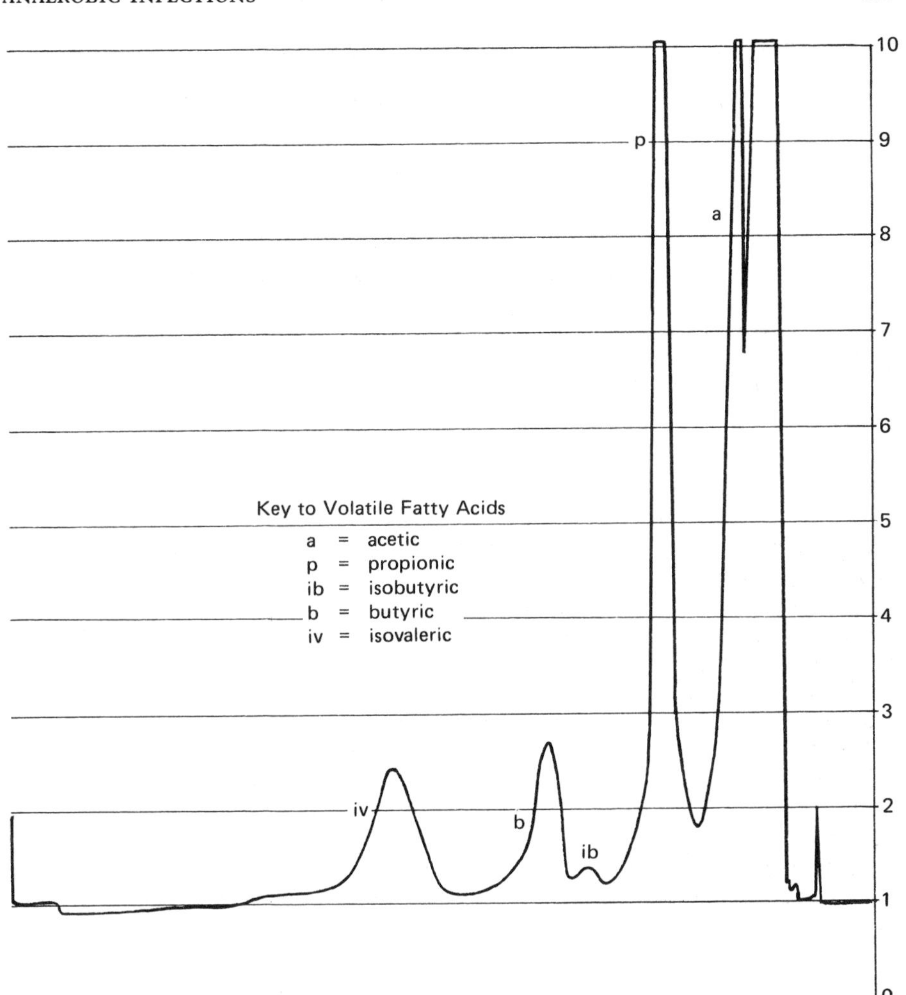

Fig. 9.2. Gas–liquid chromatography tracing indicating the presence of anaerobes in pus.

CLOSTRIDIAL INFECTIONS

Gas gangrene, clostridial septic abortion, clostridial food poisoning, clostridial necrotizing jejunitis, tetanus and pseudo-membranous colitis associated with *Clostridium difficile* infection are the main clostridial infections affecting man.

Gas Gangrene

Wounds associated with war injuries or accidental civilian trauma may become infected with clostridial spores which are widely distributed in the soil and environment. Spores of *Clostridium welchii* may often enter wounds from the patient's own faecal flora. Surgical wounds, especially after major or orthopaedic

Table 9.4. Summary of basic bacteriological methods for diagnosis of anaerobic infections

1. Specimen of pus rather than swab whenever possible and include anaerobic blood cultures, preferably before antibiotic therapy
2. Prompt transport to laboratory essential and transport media for swabs (e.g. Stuart's transport medium) are essential
3. *Macroscopic examination*:
   foul smelling pus characteristic
   ultraviolet light may show brick-red fluorescence suggesting *Bacteroides melaninogenicus* infection
4. *Microscopic examination*:
   Gram-stain especially helpful for clostridial infections and anaerobic coccal infections
   N.B. negative results possible even when profuse *Bacteroides fragilis* later isolated
5. *Gas–liquid chromatography*:
   increasingly helpful for rapid diagnosis of anaerobes in pus and blood cultures
6. *Direct culture*:
   only likely to succeed if prompt transport of good specimens to laboratory and if selective media used as well as blood agar for specimens of pus or wound swabs
   direct culture on fresh blood agar and kanamycin blood agar (preferably with added methadione and lysed blood)
   incubation in anaerobic jar (McIntosh and Fildes or GasPak jar) which includes adequate anaerobic controls (e.g. a non-toxigenic *Clostridium tetani* variant)
   all anaerobic cultures incubated for at least 2 days at 35–37 °C and preferably for up to 5 days with added 10% carbon dioxide
7. *Direct sensitivity test*:
   metronidazole disc on kanamycin blood agar often helpful
8. *Enrichment culture*:
   Robertson's cooked meat broth; thioglycollate media including Brewer's medium; iron nail, not yet rusted, in broth
   these liquid methods are sometimes difficult to interpret when positive; they are generally less significant than direct culture obtained on blood agar
   variations of these liquid media may be suitable for anaerobic blood culture

surgery around the hip joint or after leg amputations, may become complicated by post-operative gas gangrene. Rarely, a closed fracture may become infected following haematogenous spread of *Clostridium welchii* from the bowel.

Causative organisms

Three clostridial species are most often responsible for gas gangrene: *Clostridium welchii (perfringens)*—usual cause; *Clostridium oedematiens*, and *Clostridium septicum*; infrequently a fourth species, *Clostridium histolyticum*, is implicated.

Clinical features

Local signs suggestive of gas gangrene include myositis (brick-red discoloration of muscle), myonecrosis, oedema, gas formation (detected by palpable crepitus or on radiographs), and discoloration of the overlying skin which often presents with a mottled appearance.

In a classic case of gas gangrene, the patient is very unwell as a result of the severe toxaemia caused by the toxins secreted by the clostridia. This occurs with or without septicaemia and ensuing complications include shock, jaundice, severe haemolysis and acute renal failure. There is a high mortality rate.

Microbiological diagnosis

Pus, wound swabs and blood cultures are collected. A Gram-stain of the pus characteristically shows numerous Gram-positive bacilli which are thick, with a rectangular shape and without spores. *Clostridium welchii* is capsulated and occasionally capsules may be evident.

Cultures are set up but it is important not to wait for the results before starting treatment. When *Clostridium welchii* is the causative organism, anaerobic culture on blood agar yields characteristic haemolytic colonies after overnight incubation. The other clostridia, such as *Clostridium oedematiens*, require very strict anaerobic techniques for successful isolation.

Anaerobic sugar fermentation tests on the clostridial species help to identify the organism. Characteristically a 'stormy' clot reaction occurs in litmus milk with *Clostridium welchii*, although this is not a specific test. *Clostridium welchii* also typically shows a positive Nagler reaction.

Nagler Reaction

This reaction is demonstrated by a bacteriological plate containing lecithin (provided by egg yolk or serum) showing a zone of opacity around each *Clostridium welchii* colony, due to the release of triglyceride through the lecithinase activity of the alpha-toxin of the organism. If one side of the plate has specfic antitoxin applied to it before inoculation, no opacity is seen.

Treatment

Hyperbaric oxygen is useful for improving the general condition of the patient as this appears to neutralize some of the effects of the clostridial toxins. Surgery is then essential to remove infected and dead tissue together with general débridement. Penicillin is given to treat the clostridial infection together with other antibiotics, such as gentamicin, to treat accompanying Gram-negative infection or cloxacillin if *Staph. aureus* infection is present.

Prompt administration of antitoxin in high dosage against the appropriate clostridial species is also recommended by some authorities.

Prevention

Benzylpenicillin injections are essential to cover below knee or other leg amputations, especially in diabetics with ischaemic arterial disease. Iodine or iodophor compresses are also recommended as pre-op. skin disinfection for these operations. Adrenaline and other vasoconstrictive drugs should be avoided in the buttock.

Septic Abortion

Causative organisms: *Clostridium welchii* is very important; non-sporing anaerobes; coliforms, streptococci and rarely *Staph. aureus*. Mixtures of organisms are common.

In the past, severe toxaemia associated with *Clostridium welchii* uterine myonecrosis often gave a clinical picture similar to gas gangrene with a fatal outcome. Clostridial septic abortion used to occur associated with 'criminal' back-street abortions in Britain before the abortion law was reformed. This type of septic abortion is fortunately rare in Britain today. The microbiological diagnosis and management is similar to that outlined for gas gangrene.

Clostridial Food Poisoning and Jejunitis

See Chapter 14.

Tetanus ('Lockjaw')

This disease is now rare in Britain but is more common in developing countries. The main emphasis of the medical approach to tetanus is preventive; if all children were routinely immunized and booster doses of tetanus toxoid were given during later life, the disease could not occur at all.

Causative organism: *Clostridium tetani*
Incubation period: 3–21 days usually but can be up to several years after the original injury.

Main clinical features

Lockjaw due to trismus is a characteristic early feature of the disease. Muscular spasms may also characteristically cause dysphagia, 'risus sardonicus' of the face and opisthotonos. The spasms increase in frequency and duration often causing multiple injuries, and death results from exhaustion and respiratory failure.

The diagnosis is clinical but supporting microbiological evidence is occasionally possible.

Microbiology

When there is a wound present, a swab might reveal the classical drumstick bacilli on Gram and spore stains. However, the presence of *Clostridium tetani* in a wound could simply mean colonization of the wound by the organism and the diagnosis is mainly clinical.

Characteristics of the Clostridium tetani organism include:

a. 'Drumstick' bacillus, with terminal spore.
b. Spores very resistant. Autoclaving is essential to destroy spores in dressings, suture material, etc.

c. Spores ubiquitous in the soil and environment. The organism is usually present in the faeces of horses and many other mammals occasionally including man.
d. On strict anaerobic culture on blood agar the flagellated organism spreads in a thin film with a characteristic 'feathery' edge.
e. The powerful exotoxin released by the organism is entirely responsible for the clinical manifestations of the disease.
f. Mice injected with a cooked meat culture of the organism show tetanic spasms which can be prevented by tetanus antitoxin.
g. The exotoxin is not antigenic and, even if the patient recovers, a further attack of tetanus is possible in the future unless the patient is immunized with tetanus toxoid.
h. The organism is biochemically relatively inactive. Gelatin liquefaction in vitro is one of its few positive characteristics.
i. There is no local inflammation associated with the multiplication of *Clostridium tetani* in tissues.

Epidemiology

There are usually less than 100 new cases of tetanus each year reported in Britain. Most patients have a history of a previous wound, often trivial, which may have become contaminated by soil. Footballers, farm workers, gardeners, jockeys and children playing bare foot are amongst those in Britain especially at risk. Injuries associated with farm or traffic accidents in rural areas may become complicated by tetanus. In India and other countries, where cow dung may be placed on the umbilicus of a newborn baby, tetanus neonatorum is common. Sometimes, a chronically infected ear is the site of original infection—otogenic tetanus. Often no history of a previous wound is available—idiopathic tetanus.

Deep or penetrating lesions and wounds in avascular sites such as the sole of the foot are more likely to become complicated by tetanus than other injuries. Foreign bodies such as dirt, gravel or, particularly, a nail in the sole of the foot increase the chances of germination of the spores and active infection occurring.

Pathogenesis

After germination of the spores of *Clostridium tetani*, the vegetative organisms secrete the potent tetanus neurotoxin into the tissues. The toxin probably reaches the central nervous system in man by ascending the peripheral nerves to the spinal cord and medulla. The tetanus toxin is a protein with a great affinity for the presynaptic terminals of inhibitory spinal neurones in the anterior horns of the spinal cord. At these terminals the release of inhibitory neurotransmitter substances, such as glycine, is inhibited by the tetanus toxin and this leads to excessive activity of the alpha-motoneurones. This excessive activity results in the muscular spasms typical of tetanus.

Treatment of tetanus

As soon as tetanus is suspected clinically, specific treatment with human antitetanus immunoglobulin is started, the wound excised, and benzlpenicillin is also given. Other antibiotics may be advisable also to treat infection due to other organisms mixed in with the *Clostridium tetani*. Skilled intensive care unit management, preferably in a centre experienced in treating tetanus cases, is the main hope for the patient together with suitable administration of the tetanus antitoxin. The reported mortality rate varies between 0 and 60%; higher mortality rates tend to occur in centres with only a limited experience of treating the disease. For excellent recent reviews of this subject, *see* Edmondson (1980) and Warrell (1981).

Prevention of tetanus

Routine active immunization in infancy with a course of tetanus toxoid, usually as part of 'triple antigen', is the most essential general preventive step which needs to be taken. This should be followed by booster doses of tetanus toxoid every 5–10 years thereafter (*see* Immunization, in Chapter 8). Any person not actively immunized against tetanus should be encouraged to complete a course of toxoid injections.

Another general measure which is relevant to hospitals is adequate sterilization of dressings, suture materials, etc., to destroy any *Clostridium tetani* spores that might contaminate these items from the environment. In practice, this is done adequately and post-operative tetanus virtually never occurs in Britain today.

The main problem encountered in practice is the appropriate management of accidental wounds and the following measures may be necessary:

1. *Surgical toilet and débridement*
   This applies to all wounds. For minor abrasions or wounds on the hands, immediate hand washing may suffice. For major wounds, deep or penetrating puncture wounds, remove all dead tissue and any foreign bodies.
2. *Passive immunity*
   Immediate passive immunization with human hyperimmune tetanus immunoglobulin is a valuable prophylactic measure in patients with selected wounds who are considered non-immune to tetanus. Wounds which are selected include dirty or penetrating wounds or those which present to a medical attendant 6 hours after the injury.

   A non-immune person is defined as someone who either (*a*) has not had a complete course of tetanus toxoid immunizations in the past, (*b*) the immune status is unknown, or (*c*) the last dose of tetanus toxoid was more than 10 years previously.
3. *Antibiotics*
   Some patients have been given antibiotics prophylactically in the past without sufficient attention being paid to the immunological and surgical precautions necessary and subsequently these patients have died of tetanus. Antibiotics are useful but as an ancillary measure only in selected wounds (*see* Passive immunity *above*). Penicillin or ampicillin alone may not be suitable in some instances due to the accompanying presence of penicillinase-producing organisms in the wound. Cloxacillin and other antibiotics should be considered for other infecting organisms in the wound.

4. *Active immunity*
   a. All patients who present with a wound should be given a dose of tetanus toxoid unless there is definite evidence that a complete course of toxoid or a booster dose has been given during the previous year.
   b. Patients who are non-immune should be given the adsorbed tetanus toxoid into one arm at the same time as the human tetanus immunoglobulin is administered into the other arm. After the first dose of toxoid, subsequent repeat doses of toxoid are arranged to complete the course of active immunizations.
   c. Patients who have received tetanus toxoid between 5 and 10 years previously require one immediate booster dose of tetanus toxoid.

Pseudo-membranous Colitis

Pseudo-membranous colitis usually presents with acute profuse diarrhoea or collapse during or soon after a course of antibiotic therapy. There are characteristic mucosal changes apparent during sigmoidoscopic examination of the patient and the diagnosis can be confirmed by histological examination of a colonic mucosal biopsy specimen. In severe cases, there may be acute sloughing of the entire colon with a possible fatal outcome.

The antibiotics most often associated with this relatively rare but important condition include clindamycin, lincomycin, tetracyclines and ampicillin, but many other antibiotics have also been implicated at different times. Patients with previous bowel disease or those over the age of 60 years are predisposed to this condition and should not be given clindamycin or lincomycin, unless there is an exceptional indication for these drugs. If a patient develops diarrhoea due to an antibiotic the antibiotic should normally be stopped.

Faeces of patients with this condition characteristically contain a toxin which causes tissue culture changes that are neutralized by *Clostridium sordelli* antitoxin. In the last few years, it has become clear that the toxin associated with the pathogenesis of the disease is produced by *Clostridium difficile*; cross-antigenicity occurs with the toxin produced by *Clostridium sordelli*. The *Clostridium difficile* organisms can occasionally be isolated from the faeces of normal patients using selective media, but it is nearly always present in increased numbers in the faeces, together with its toxin, in patients suffering from pseudo-membranous colitis. This disease appears to be associated with a superinfection by *Clostridium difficile* strains which are toxigenic and resistant to the antibiotics that have been administered to the patient.

Treatment of the *Clostridium difficile* superinfection with oral vancomycin is usually effective (*see also* Chapter 14).

Further Reading

Edmondson R. J. (1980) Tetanus. *Br. J. Hosp. Med.* **23**, 596–602.
Ellis C. J. (1980) How should we use metronidazole? *J. Antimicrob. Chemother.* **6**, 305–307.
Leading Article (1980) Gas chromatographic diagnosis of infection. *Lancet* **2**, 513.

Phillips I. and Sussman M. (ed.) (1974) *Infection with Non-sporing Anaerobic Bacteria.* A Symposium of the British Society for Antimicrobial Chemotherapy. Edinburgh, Churchill Livingstone.

Stokes E. J. and Ridgway G. L. (1980) *Clinical Bacteriology*, 5th ed. London, Edward Arnold, pp. 60, 351.

*Warrell D. A. (1981) Tetanus. *Medicine International* **1**, 118–122.

Willis A. T. (1977) *Anaerobic Bacteriology: Clinical and Laboratory Practice*, 3rd ed. London, Butterworth.

* Particularly recommended for further study by undergraduates.

Chapter 10

Infections of the central nervous system

In Britain, viral meningitis is by far the commonest infection of the central nervous system. Bacterial meningitis is the next most frequent condition. Cerebral abscesses and viral encephalitis are rare.

MENINGITIS

Main Clinical Features and CSF Findings

The characteristic clinical features of acute meningitis include headache, irritability, fever and neck stiffness. Kernig's sign is often positive. Nausea, vomiting and the subsequent development of coma are also frequently seen. These features are typical in most adults. However, neonates, some children, the elderly and the immunosuppressed patients may develop meningitis without specific features suggesting central nervous system (CNS) infection.

Acute bacterial meningitis is a life-threatening infection which needs urgent specific treatment whereas viral meningitis is a less serious disease where spontaneous recovery generally occurs. Bacterial meningitis is generally associated with a purulent CSF whereas viruses are associated with 'aseptic meningitis' CSF findings (*Table 10.1*).

Causative Organisms

Viruses, bacteria, fungi and protozoa are the main groups of organisms that may cause meningitis (*Table 10.2*). Certain causative organisms, such as *Mycobacterium tuberculosis* or *Cryptococcus neoformans*, are associated with a more 'chronic' meningitis (*Table 10.1* and *see below*). Acute bacterial meningitis needs to be managed as a medical emergency and is considered first.

Bacterial Meningitis

In Britain, where meningitis is a notifiable disease, there are approximately 2000 cases of bacterial meningitis reported each year.

Primary bacterial meningitis most often arises through the spread of bacteria from the bloodstream to the meninges and at the time of meningitis, bacteraemia is still usually present.

Secondary bacterial meningitis is much less common than primary meningitis and results from the direct spread of infection from infected ears, sinuses, congenital defects such as spina bifida, trauma or surgery.

Bacterial causes of meningitis are included in *Table 10.2*. Three bacterial species cause more than 75% of all cases of bacterial meningitis and are known as the three 'primary pathogens':

Table 10.1. Characteristic CSF changes in meningitis and the differential diagnosis

Condition	*Appearance*	*Cells, $\times 10^6/l$ (per mm^3)*	*Gram-stain or immunoelectrophoresis or culture for pyogenic bacteria*	*Protein, g/l*	*Glucose, mmol/l*	*Main differential diagnosis*
Normal	Clear	0–5 lymphocytes*	Negative results	0·15–0·4‡	2·2–3·3§	—
'Purulent' meningitis	Turbid	100–2000 polymorphs†	Positive results	0·5–3·0	0–2·2	1. *Bacterial meningitis* 2. Amoebic meningitis 3. Cerebral abscess
'Aseptic' meningitis	Clear or slightly turbid	15–500 lymphocytes (polymorphs may predominate in the acute stage)	Negative results	0·5–1·0	Normal	1. *Viral meningitis* 2. Partially antibiotic‖ treated bacterial meningitis‖ 3. Leptospiral meningitis 4. Encephalitis 5. Brain abscess 6. TB/fungal meningitis
Tuberculous meningitis	Clear or slightly turbid; fibrin web may develop	30–500 lymphocytes plus polymorphs	Negative results (scanty acid-fast bacilli may be seen in a Ziehl-Neelsen stained smear)	1·0–6·0	0–2·2	1. *TB meningitis* 2. Brain abscess 3. Cryptococcal meningitis

* In a neonate, up to 30×10^6 cells/litre, mainly polymorphs.
† A few cases of pyogenic meningitis may have $5–100 \times 10^6$/l polymorphs.
‡ In a neonate, protein concentration up to 1·5 g/l.
§ Approximately 60% of blood glucose level.
‖ Glucose level could be reduced.

Table 10.2. Some causative organisms of meningitis

Bacteria		*Viruses*	*Fungi*	*Protozoa*
1. *Gram-stainable*: *Neisseria meningitidis* *Haemophilus influenzae* *Streptococcus pneumoniae*	three 'primary pathogens'	*a. Enteroviruses* Echo Coxsackie, A and B Polio	*a. Yeasts*: *Cryptococcus neoformans* *Candida* species	*Amoebae*: *Naegleria* *Hartmanella*
E. coli, other coliforms Group B haemolytic streptococcus *Staphylocossus epidermidis* *Listeria monocytogenes* *Salmonella* species *Pseudomonas* species 'Low-grade pathogens', such as flavobacteria and *B. cereus*	causes affecting mainly neonates	*b. Paramyxovirus*: Mumps *c. Herpesviruses*: Herpes simplex Varicella-zoster *d. Adenoviruses* *e. Arboviruses*: Louping-ill	*b. Filamentous* *Aspergillus* species Mucor	
Staphylococci and streptococci *Streptococcus pneumoniae* Coliforms *Pseudomonas aeruginosa* Anaerobes	causes following trauma or surgery			
2. *Acid fast*: *Mycobacterium tuberculosis*				
3. *Spirochaetes*: *Leptospira interrogans var. canicola* *Leptospira icterohaemorrhagiae* *Treponema pallidum*				

1. *Neisseria meningitidis*
2. *Haemophilus influenzae* (capsulated, Pittman type b)
3. *Streptococcus pneumoniae*

The meningococcus is the most common of the three primary pathogens in Britain and *Haemophilus* is the second most common. In the U.S.A., *Haemophilus* is the most common cause of meningitis in infants.

Bacterial causative organisms and the relationship with age

Children develop meningitis and die of the disease much more often than adults. Over two-thirds of all cases of bacterial meningitis are children less than 5 years old. The main associations between some important bacterial causes of meningitis and the ages of affected patients are summarized below:

Meningococcus	all ages, most cases seen in children and adolescents
Haemophilus	more than 80% cases less than 5 years old, rarely seen before 3 months or after 12 years old
Pneumococcus	all ages, most common at extremes of life—in infants less than 2 years old and in the elderly
Escherichia coli	commonest cause of meningitis in neonates, rarely a cause after infancy
Group B haemolytic streptococcus	a frequent cause of meningitis in neonates only
Listeria monocytogenes	an uncommon cause of meningitis in neonates, although a patient at any age may become infected when an immunodeficient condition is present

Meningococcal meningitis

Causative organism

Neisseria meningitidis, a Gram-negative intracellular diplococcus. There are three main serological types—A, B and C.

Epidemiology

The meningococcus is carried asymptomatically in the nasopharynx of 2–25% people and is spread from person to person by respiratory droplets. The carriage rates are highest in children, and in circumstances of overcrowding. High carriage rates are often found amongst the inmates of institutions, such as military barracks or boarding schools.

Meningitis occurs after the organism invades the bloodstream from the nasopharynx, to reach the meninges. Meningitis is a rare event compared with the incidence of meningococcal carriage in the community.

In Britain, meningococcal meningitis is most common in the first quarter of each year. Most of the cases are sporadic, with only the close family contacts, especially children, at risk of acquiring the disease in the home. Epidemics are uncommon and occur mainly in residential schools. The majority of meningococcal infections in Britain are due to the group B serotype. Widespread epidemics repeatedly occur in Africa and Brazil, due to meningococci of serogroup A or C, and cause many deaths.

Incubation period

The usual incubation period is from 1 to 3 days.

Clinical features

Characteristically there is a sudden onset of the disease, starting with a sore throat or headache and rapidly progressing within several hours to drowsiness and signs of meningitis (*see* p. 167).

A haemorrhagic skin rash is often present, associated with an accompanying septicaemia, during the first 18 hours of the illness (*see Fig. 10.1*). Many patients have widespread petechiae. About 30% of patients may present with a fulminating meningococcal septicaemia and these patients frequently develop numerous large ecchymoses and gangrenous skin lesions. The fulminating cases often develop complications associated with disseminated intravascular coagulation, Gram-negative shock and acute renal failure. There may be bleeding into many

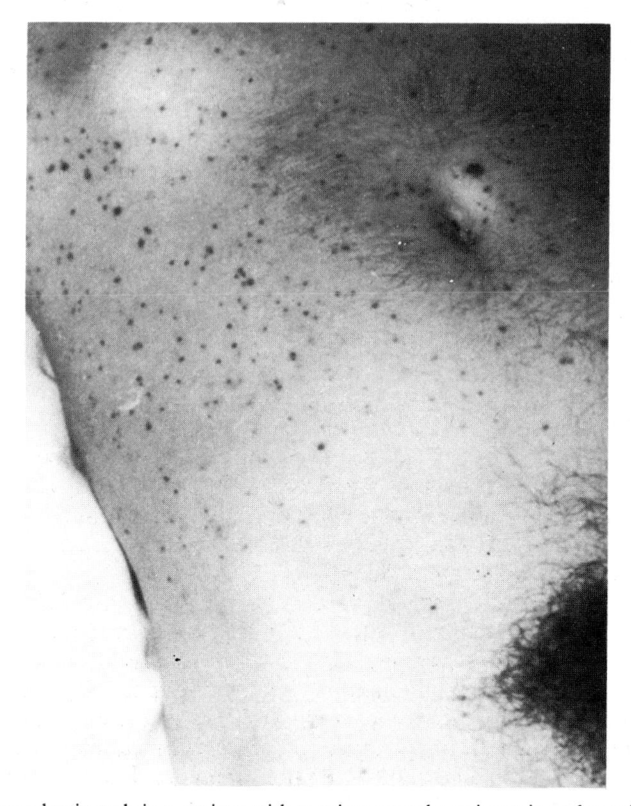

Fig. 10.1. Haemorrhagic rash in a patient with meningococcal septicaemia and meningitis.

different organs including the brain and adrenal glands. When the latter occurs, usually as a terminal event, an acute Addisonian crisis may develop as part of the Waterhouse-Friderichsen syndrome. Fulminating septicaemia cases often die within 24–36 hours of being apparently well and may never reach hospital alive.

The majority of meningococcal infections are associated with features of both meningitis and septicaemia but cases with apparent meningitis only or septicaemia only also occur. The overall mortality of all cases of acute meningococcal infection is about 10%.

A small number of patients may develop subacute or chronic allergic complications including arthritis, cutaneous vasculitis, episcleritis or pericarditis, probably due to immune complex disease.

Microbiological investigations

CSF and blood cultures should both be collected, where possible, before antibiotics are given. The organism is sometimes isolated from the blood cultures when the CSF culture is negative.

The meningococcus is extremely fragile and it is often not possible to isolate the organism from the CSF. For the best results of cultures, it is important that the warm CSF is transported immediately to the laboratory for culture. The CSF *deposit* is promptly cultured on chocolate and blood agar in moist conditions with added carbon dioxide. Culture of the CSF is essential even when the CSF is clear and colourless.

The CSF is usually purulent, frankly turbid with over 100 polymorph white cells per mm^3 (*Table 10.1*), but very occasionally is only slightly turbid or clear.

An urgent Gram-stain on the CSF deposit characteristically shows Gram-negative diplococci, some intracellular and some in an extracellular location. The numbers of cocci seen varies a lot; frequently large numbers of pus cells are apparent with only a few cocci and, rarely, a few white cells are seen with numerous cocci present.

Immunoelectrophoresis for the detection of meningococcal polysaccharide antigen in the CSF has been more useful for the rapid microbial diagnosis of meningitis due to meningococcal serotype A or C than the B serotype which is endemic in Britain. However, improved antisera against group B meningococci have recently become available which should improve the usefulness of this test.

Immediate antibiotic sensitivity tests are included to penicillin and chloramphenicol, using the CSF deposit, and to sulphonamides where special antibiotic sensitivity media must be employed.

Antimicrobial treatment

Approximately 10% of meningococcal strains in Britain are resistant to sulphonamides, but all meningococcal strains throughout the world continue to be fully sensitive to benzylpenicillin.

It is vital that therapy should not be delayed in suspected cases of meningococcal meningitis either because of delay in transport of the patient to hospital or while awaiting the results of investigations carried out in hospital. Urgent penicillin treatment is necessary to reduce the risk of death and is often best started in the patient's home as soon as the diagnosis is clinically suspected.

In hospital, intravenous benzylpenicillin should be given as soon as the cultures have been collected, giving 30 mg/kg body weight 4-hourly, for 10 days.

Individuals who are hypersensitive to penicillin can be successfully treated with chloramphenicol, 15 mg/kg body weight 6-hourly, while awaiting the results of sensitivity tests. Sulphonamides alone may be used subsequently instead of chloramphenicol if the tests show that the strain is sensitive to sulphonamides.

Once a good clinical response starts, it usually proceeds rapidly during treatment to a complete recovery without any sequelae.

Prophylaxis

Close contacts, especially children in the family, room-mates and pre-school children in day nurseries, should be given immediate chemoprophylaxis to protect them against meningococcal infection. Swabs of contacts are not necessary and prophylaxis should not be delayed for the results of antibiotic sensitivity tests. Rifampicin is usually the most appropriate drug which is given by mouth for 2 days; the dosage suggested is 5 mg/kg, b.d., for infants aged 3 months to 1 year, 10 mg/kg b.d. for children aged 1–12 years and 600 mg, b.d., for children older than 12 years and for adults. Medical and nursing staff attending the patient do not usually require prophylaxis (exceptions include intimate contact with pharyngeal secretions which may occur, for example, during mouth-to-mouth resuscitation or the insertion of an endotracheal tube).

There are only a few drugs which can eliminate nasopharyngeal carriage of meningococci and these include sulphadiazine, rifampicin and minocycline, but do not include penicillins. Sulphadiazine used to be the drug of choice, but as 10–25% of meningococci are resistant to sulphonamides in many countries, including Britain, this drug is usually no longer appropriate. However, when an epidemic meningococcal strain is known to be sensitive to sulphonamides, the best prophylactic drug is sulphadiazine. (Minocycline frequently causes side effects, including vertigo.)

A group A meningococcal vaccine is under investigation in Brazil and the results so far suggest that the vaccine doses have a worthwhile effect against Group A meningococcal infection.

Haemophilus meningitis

Causative organism

Haemophilus influenzae, capsulated Pittman type b. This is a pleomorphic Gram-negative cocco-bacillus which requires both X and V factors for successful culture in the laboratory as demonstrated by 'satellitism' tests.

Epidemiology

Haemophilus influenzae, capsulated type b, commonly colonizes the respiratory tract of infants and frequently causes respiratory tract infections in young children. Occasionally, the organism may invade the bloodstream and cause infection at other sites including the meninges. Only sporadic cases of the disease are seen.

During the first few months of life, maternal antibody in the infant's blood provides some protection against the development of haemophilus bacteraemia and meningitis. Cases of haemophilus meningitis mainly occur in children from 3 months old to 5 years old, with a peak incidence at about 2 years. This age relationship is probably explained by the increasing prevalence of significant antibody titres against the haemophilus capsular antigen after 2 years of age; by 12 years of age nearly all children have specific antibodies present in the serum which protects them against infection.

Clinical presentation

The incubation period is long, about 5 days, and the onset of meningitis is usually much more insidious compared with meningitis due to the meningococcus or pneumococcus.

Predominant early clinical features include nausea, vomiting and a febrile illness with possible respiratory symptoms. Subsequently headache, irritability and the other features of meningitis gradually become evident. There is no skin rash.

Complications are more likely to develop if antibiotic therapy is delayed or is not appropriate. These include subdural effusions, cerebral and cranial nerve palsies (including the eighth nerve leading to deafness). Death is less frequent than with the meningococcus or pneumococcus and the overall mortality rate is now about 5%.

Microbiological investigations

Both CSF and blood cultures should be collected before the start of antibiotic therapy. Blood cultures are occasionally positive when the CSF culture is negative.

The CSF is characteristically purulent with a high polymorph count (*see Table 10.1*) and pleomorphic Gram-negative cocco-bacilli are usually seen in the Gram-stain of the centrifuged deposit.

Culture of the CSF deposit on chocolate agar in a CO_2 atmosphere typically yields growth of the capsulated Pittman type b *Haemophilus influenzae*.

Immunoelectrophoresis methods may be useful for detecting the capsular b type antigen of the organism in the CSF or serum of a patient who has already been given antibiotics and also to give rapid confirmatory identification of a short Gram-negative bacillus seen in a Gram-stain of the CSF.

Antibiotic sensitivity tests to ampicillin, sulphonamides, trimethoprim and chloramphenicol are included. (A chromogenic test for detecting β-lactamase production is useful for the investigation of strains showing a reduced inhibition zone with a 2-µg ampicillin disc. Cefuroxime and cefotaxime may also be tested when ampicillin-resistant strains are suspected.)

Antimicrobial treatment

Chloramphenicol is still the drug of choice for the treatment of *Haemophilus influenzae* meningitis given as 50–100 mg/kg/day for 10 days to children. This drug is generally bacteriostatic but, in the CSF, is bactericidal to *Haemophilus*. It is highly effective in the treatment of haemophilus meningitis and is associated with a very low relapse rate. Nearly all *Haemophilus* strains are sensitive to chloramphenicol in Britain.

Ampicillin-resistant strains of Pittman type b *Haemophilus influenzae*, due to plasmid-mediated β-lactamase production, have become increasingly recognized in recent years and between 7 and 12% of strains in Britain, depending on the area, are ampicillin resistant. When ampicillin is used to treat infections due to sensitive strains, high intravenous doses are necessary, at least 150 mg/kg/day given in divided 4-hourly doses for 10 days. The relapse rate is higher following ampicillin than with chloramphenicol treatment of haemophilus meningitis.

Pneumococcal meningitis

Causative organism

Streptococcus pneumoniae, a capsulated Gram-positive diplococcus. The capsule is closely associated with the virulence of the organism and there are numerous different antigenic capsular types. The pneumococcus is a common cause of respiratory tract infections both in children and adults.

Epidemiology and pathogenesis

Certain capsular serotypes of the pneumococcus, such as type III, are particularly associated with invasion of the bloodstream and meningitis complicating a pneumococcal pneumonia or other respiratory tract infection. Bacteraemia and meningitis are most likely to occur in infants less than 3 years old, adults over 60 years old, and those with debilitation, malnutrition or alcoholism. Antibodies to the capsular antigens act as opsonins which facilitate the phagocytosis of pneumococci. The majority of young and middle-aged adults have serum antibodies against a wide range of different pneumococcal serotypes.

Direct spread of pneumococcal infection may occur from an infected middle ear or sinus to involve the meninges, particularly in young infants.

Rarely recurrent pneumococcal meningitis is seen in a patient and there is nearly always an anatomical predisposing factor present such as a hairline fracture through the base of the skull or the temporal bone, or a congenital abnormality. This predisposing factor is responsible for a communication between the nasal passages or ear and the meninges. Occasionally, there is an obvious CSF leak through the nose (rhinorrhoea) or ear.

Clinical features

Characteristically the features of meningitis are of acute onset and drowsiness appears rapidly. Within several hours, many patients become comatose. There is no skin rash.

The pneumococcus should be immediately suspected in the elderly as this is the most common cause of meningitis in this age group. It can also be strongly suspected clinically when meningitis of sudden onset supervenes in an infant with otitis media.

Complications with cranial nerve damage, intra-ventricular adhesions and intra-cranial loculations of pus may occur. Death is common, particularly when antibiotic treatment is started only after coma has occurred. The mortality rate of pneumococcal meningitis is about 30%—much higher than for meningococcal meningitis.

Microbiological investigations

Both CSF and blood cultures should be collected, as for the other major bacterial causes of meningitis. The CSF is purulent (*Table 10.1*) and an urgent Gram-stain of the CSF deposit usually shows large numbers of typical Gram-positive diplococci. Culture of the CSF on blood agar shows next day the typical alpha-haemolytic *Strep. pneumoniae* (draughtsman colonies, sensitive to optochin). Antibiotic sensitivity tests to penicillin, sulphonamides, trimethoprim and chloramphenicol are included.

Immunoelectrophoresis of the CSF and serum is usually positive for pneumococcal antigen and this test may give useful rapid results, particularly when previous antibiotics have been given.

Antimicrobial treatment

In Britain, nearly all strains of *Strep. pneumoniae* are fully sensitive to penicillin. Massive frequent intravenous doses of benzylpenicillin should be given as early on in the disease as possible. In an adult, 1·2 g (2 MU) every 2 hours is initially recommended. In children 60 mg/kg body weight, 4-hourly, intravenously is recommended. Treatment may need to be continued for more than 10 days in some patients.

Chloramphenicol, 1 g 4-hourly, can be given to an adult who is allergic to penicillin. In children the total daily dose is 50–100 mg/kg.

Prophylaxis

Known predisposing factors, such as a structural defect in the ear, may be corrected surgically. Prompt treatment of otitis media, pneumonia and other respiratory infections may greatly help to reduce the incidence of pneumococcal meningitis, especially in infants.

A polyvalent pneumococcal polysaccharide vaccine has recently been introduced which stimulates antibody production against the main capsular serotypes of pneumococci likely to be encountered in North America or Britain. Its role in the prophylaxis of pneumococcal meningitis is uncertain at present.

Blind Management of a Child (not a Neonate) or Adult with Suspected Acute Bacterial Meningitis

When a general practitioner suspects acute bacterial meningitis clinically in the patient's home and a delay of more than 1 hour is anticipated before the patient can be admitted to hospital, an injection of benzylpenicillin should be given immediately. The benefit of earlier treatment of possible meningococcal or pneumococcal meningitis outweighs the disadvantage of causing negative cultures during subsequent investigations.

As soon as the immediate lumbar puncture and blood cultures have been performed on a patient admitted to hospital with suspected acute bacterial meningitis, a 2-MU dose of benzylpenicillin should be given intravenously without waiting for the results of the investigations. However, if turbid CSF is seen at lumbar puncture, intrathecal penicillin should *not* be given; there are no clear advantages in giving intrathecal penicillin, but there are dangers of causing paraplegia or death when an overdose of intrathecal penicillin is accidentally administered.

If urgent CSF investigations fail to reveal the cause of the meningitis in a child, 'blind' therapy should be continued with a combination of benzylpenicillin to treat meningococcal and pneumococcal meningitis, and chloramphenicol to treat haemophilus meningitis.

In an adult, haemophilus meningitis is rare, and blind treatment with benzylpenicillin alone, 2 MU intravenously every 2 hours, should be given.

If the patient is allergic to penicillin, chloramphenicol may be given.

Neonatal Meningitis

A neonate is more likely to develop meningitis during the first week of life than after this time, although there are a significant number of 'late onset' meningitis cases due to group B streptococci.

Neonatal meningitis carries a very high morbidity and mortality rate. The reasons why at least one-third of cases of neonatal meningitis die are well described by Davies (1977) and include:

1. The host defence mechanisms against infection are relatively poorly developed, particularly in low birth weight pre-term infants. There are low levels of circulating immunoglobulins and of complement.
2. It is difficult to diagnose meningitis clinically in the early stages in a neonate; only minor behavioural changes may indicate meningitis.
3. Infection may have started shortly before the birth of the neonate in some cases, especially with early onset group B streptococcal septicaemia and meningitis, and treatment started after birth may be too late to control a rapidly progressive infection in these cases.
4. Since the possible range of causative organisms is wide (*Table 10.2*) and it is difficult to predict the antibiotic sensitivity patterns of Gram-negative bacilli, there is a greater problem in suggesting effective blind therapeutic regimens than with older children.
5. Aminoglycosides, such as gentamicin, may need to be given for treating some cases of meningitis due to Gram-negative bacilli and these drugs, unlike chloramphenicol, do not penetrate the CSF well even when the meninges are inflamed. When given intrathecally by the lumbar route, aminoglycosides may not reach the affected areas.
6. Congenital abnormalities, such as myelomeningocoele or a dermal sinus when infected, provide a continuing potent source of central nervous system infection which cannot become eradicated by antimicrobial therapy alone.

Pathogenesis

E. coli, group B streptococci and other causative organisms may enter the bloodstream to subsequently infect the meninges from the colonized or localized infections of the umbilical stump, the respiratory tract, the urinary tract, the ear or other sites.

Direct infections of the central nervous system may result from an infected dermal sinus or myelomeningocoele.

Clinical features

Any neonate that is moderately unwell, particularly if febrile or feeding poorly, should have immediate investigations performed to exclude the possibility of meningitis or septicaemia. Other presenting features may include vomiting, lethargy, respiratory distress, jaundice or diarrhoea. The 'classic' signs of bulging fontanelle, altered consciousness and neck stiffness are late signs only and may not be present at all.

Bacteraemia is usually present at the same time as the meningitis.

A history of predisposing factors is often present including late complications in pregnancy such as premature rupture of membranes, a complicated forceps delivery or asphyxia at birth, a maternal genito-urinary tract infection and a pre-term delivery.

Infants, less than 1000-g weight, born after only 28–34 weeks of pregnancy, are much more likely to develop fatal group B streptococcal septicaemia and meningitis than full-term infants of normal birth weight. Death occurs in between 40 and 75% of cases.

Complications are common in spite of treatment amongst the survivors:

1. Handicap is usual. This may take the form of cerebral or cranial nerve palsies, epilepsy or mental deficiency.
2. Hydrocephalus often develops, due to obstruction of the foramina or aqueduct by purulent exudate, and needs to be recognized early and treated promptly by shunts.
3. Relapse of meningitis sometimes occurs due to persisting ventriculitis. This is particularly liable to occur if treatment is not given early and also treatment should be continued for a sufficient duration.
4. Reinfection is liable to occur when there is a congenital defect such as myelomeningocoele.

Causative organisms

Hundreds of different bacterial species have been reported at one time or another to cause neonatal meningitis. Some of the more important examples are included in *Table 10.2*. The three primary bacterial pathogens, which are important causes of meningitis later on in infancy and childhood, rarely cause neonatal meningitis.

A single bacterial species causes meningitis in the majority of cases, but occasionally simultaneous infection due to two or more different bacterial species occurs, particularly when there is a congenital defect.

Coliform organisms most frequently cause neonatal meningitis in Britain, followed by group B haemolytic streptococci. In some other countries, such as the U.S.A., the group B streptococcus has now displaced *E. coli* as the leading cause of neonatal meningitis.

E. coli and other Gram-negative bacilli

E. coli and other coliforms colonize the neonatal alimentary tract to form the normal faecal flora. When ampicillin or other antibiotics have been given to the mother for any reason shortly before the birth of the infant, it is possible for the neonate to become colonized with antibiotic-resistant strains of Gram-negative bacilli, such as *Klebsiella* species, from the mother's perineal flora. These coliforms may also colonize external surfaces of the neonate during or after bith, especially the umbilical stump, and sometimes cause frank sepsis at this site. Invasion of the bloodstream may occur from an infected umbilical stump, urinary or respiratory tract or from colonized sites in the nose or alimentary tract. Once the bloodstream has been invaded meningitis may develop.

Factors that increase the likelihood of Gram-negative bacteraemia and meningitis developing in a neonate include instrumentation, such as nasogastric intubation or umbilical vessel catheterization, and the presence of a condition which is associated with impaired host defences, such as low birth weight. A further factor is dependent on the type of *E. coli* strain which is present in the infant; over 75% of *E. coli* strains causing meningitis possess the K_1 capsular antigen which is associated with invasiveness of the organism.

Breast feeding of the neonate probably protects against the early *E. coli* colonization of the alimentary tract and against bloodstream invasion of the organism from the gut and other sites.

Careful attention to keep the umbilical site clean and dry using aseptic techniques may help to reduce umbilical sepsis rates and the incidence of Gram-negative meningitis.

Group B haemolytic streptococcus

The incidence of meningitis due to group B haemolytic streptococci is continuing to increase. This may be related in part to the increasing numbers of low birth weight infants being delivered and kept alive.

Up to about 25% of mothers asymptomatically carry the group B streptococcus in the lower genital tract or rectum and the great majority of infants born to these mothers develop no infective complications. The risk of serious infection developing is much higher in a pre-term low birth weight infant, although infection can occasionally occur in full-term infants of normal birth weight.

In the more common early onset group of infections type I, II and III group B streptococci can all cause rapidly progressive bacteraemia and meningitis which usually results in death within the first few days of life.

The less common late onset variety of meningitis with group B streptococcal meningitis usually develops between the second and fourth weeks of life, and has a more insidious onset. (These infections are usually due to a type III group B streptococcus.)

Other organisms

Organisms other than Gram-negative bacilli from the faecal flora or the group B streptococcus are relatively uncommon causes of neonatal meningitis and include:

a. Staphylococcus epidermidis
This coagulase-negative staphylococcus is associated with infections of the Spitz-Holter valve in infants with hydrocephalus. Infections of these shunts are not usually cured by antibiotics alone and the infected shunts need to be surgically removed.
b. Salmonella species
Food-poisoning *Salmonella* species, such as *Salmonella virchow*, are occasionally carried asymptomatically in the faeces of the mother at the time of the delivery of the neonate. If the neonate becomes colonized by *Salmonella*, invasive infection may follow and salmonella meningitis can develop which carries a high mortality rate. Outbreaks of salmonella infection can occur in a maternity unit and a number of babies may become infected (*see* Salmonella infections, in Chapter 14).
c. Listeria monocytogenes
This organism may occasionally colonize the maternal genital tract and subsequently cause a rare listeria neonatal bacteraemia and meningitis. Infection due to *Listeria* can also occur in older infants or adults, particularly if there is a predisposing host factor present such as a lymphoma or immunosuppression. The Gram-positive bacillus must not be mistaken for a 'diphtheroid' contaminant of a blood culture or CSF sample.

Cross-infection in baby units

Cross-infection with Gram-negative bacilli, staphylococci and group B streptococci may occur between neonates, particularly in a special care baby unit which accommodates 'high risk' infants. The cross-infection is often transmitted by the hands of staff and every effort is necessary to prevent this with good hand-washing techniques and other hygienic methods.

Microbiological investigations

CSF

A CSF sample should be collected from a neonate in whom meningitis is suspected at an early stage in the illness wherever possible.

Microscopy of the CSF for white cells is of less value than in older infants, since there is a wide overlap between the cell counts of low birth weight or high-risk infants without a central nervous system infection and those with meningitis.

The most useful investigations are the urgent Gram-stain of the CSF deposit and the culture of the CSF which need to be performed even when the CSF is clear and no white cells are seen.

When early CSF samples are culture negative, further CSF samples may need to be collected for culture depending on the clinical situation.

Antibiotic sensitivity tests are of course urgently carried out on any isolates.

Blood cultures

These should always be collected at a similar time to the CSF cultures and are usually positive in meningitis cases.

They should be taken from a peripheral vein rather than an umbilical catheter, since the umbilical region is often colonized by bacteria which may contaminate the blood cultures and cause 'false positives'.

Investigation of other sites

Swabs of the throat and nose, ear, umbilicus, and the collection of gastric aspirate, if available for culture during the first few days of life, might be helpful in low birth weight babies or those with respiratory distress to help predict which organisms may become responsible for subsequent bacteraemia and meningitis.

Antimicrobial treatment

Immediate 'blind' antibiotic treatment is necessary when neonatal meningitis is suspected and should be started as soon as the cultures have been collected.

A suitable 'blind' antibiotic combination is chloramphenicol plus benzylpenicillin. The chloramphenicol will treat nearly all strains of *E. coli* or other coliform species. The benzylpenicillin will be active against group B streptococci. *Pseudomonas aeruginosa* is resistant to this antibiotic combination, but meningitis due to this organism is fortunately rare. If *Pseudomonas* or chloramphenicol-resistant Gram-negative bacilli are known to be present in a baby unit or have been isolated from previous cultures of the neonate, gentamicin or tobramycin should also be given.

An urgent Gram-stain of the CSF may influence the choice and dosage of the subsequent doses of antibiotics. If Gram-positive cocci are seen in the CSF of a neonate, very high doses of benzylpenicillin should be given to treat assumed group B streptococcal infection. The chloramphenicol should be continued as well since this penetrates the CSF well and also has useful activity against the streptococci.

If Gram-negative bacilli are seen on the CSF Gram-stain, the penicillin can be stopped and treatment continued with chloramphenicol.

When the CSF and blood culture and sensitivity results are available the treatment may be changed accordingly if necessary:

1. *E. coli or other Gram-negative bacilli isolated*

When a coliform is isolated which is sensitive to chloramphenicol, the chloramphenicol is continued. The dosage of chloramphenicol should not be excessive to neonates so that the development of the grey syndrome, a possible complication of chloramphenicol therapy, is less likely. Assays of chloramphenicol in the CSF are desirable to ensure that adequate levels are achieved. Assays in blood should also be carried out to avoid overdosage, especially in premature babies. Ampicillin in high dosage may be given with the chloramphenicol for ampicillin-sensitive strains.

If the Gram-negative bacilli isolated are resistant to chloramphenicol, other antibiotics to which the organism is sensitive need to be given, preferably those which are likely to penetrate the CSF, such as sulphonamides and trimethoprim (*see Table 10.3*). The dose of cotrimoxazole needs to be reduced suitably so that there is less risk of blood dyscrasia developing (*see* Davies, 1977).

Table 10.3. Penetration of antimicrobial drugs into the CSF

Drug	Penetration into the CSF	
	1. When normal meninges	*2. When inflamed meninges*
Benzylpenicillin	Poor	Good
Ampicillin	Poor	Good
Chloramphenicol	Good	Good
Sulphonamides	Good	Good
Trimethoprim	Good	Good
Gentamicin	Poor	Poor
Streptomycin	Poor	Poor
Isoniazid	Good	Good
Rifampicin	Moderate	Good
Pyrazinamide	?	Good

Aminoglycosides, such as gentamicin or tobramycin, are necessary for treating infections due to multiple antibiotic-resistant strains of coliforms and *Pseudomonas aeruginosa*. These should be given systematically to treat septicaemia and intrathecally to treat meningitis. The levels of gentamicin in the CSF are greater after intra-ventricular than after spinal administration of intrathecal doses of the drug. However, there is a risk of haemorrhage or spread of infection arising from the intra-ventricular administration of gentamicin. Repeated intrathecal doses are necessary and frequent assays of gentamicin in the blood and CSF are desirable to check that adequate concentrations are being reached.

2. *Group B streptococci isolated*

High dose intravenous benzylpenicillin therapy, combined with chloramphenicol therapy, is suggested for treating group B streptococcal infections where the strain is sensitive to penicillin and chloramphenicol. Some authorities recommend treatment with benzylpenicillin alone provided that doses greater than 250 000 units/kg/day are given.

3. *Staph. epidermidis isolated*

The antibiotic sensitivity pattern of different strains of *Staph. epidermidis* varies considerably and many strains are resistant to penicillin and methicillin. A combination of cloxacillin and gentamicin, or cloxacillin and chloramphenicol, may be indicated depending on the results of sensitivity tests. Infected shunts will not usually be cured by antibiotics alone and need to be removed.

4. *Salmonellae isolated*

Chloramphenicol and ampicillin are generally the two most suitable drugs for treating salmonella meningitis, for strains sensitive to these antibiotics. Treatment may need to be prolonged.

5. *Listeria monocytogenes isolated*

Ampicillin, given in high dosage has cured cases of listeria meningitis. Occasionally it has been given together with either chloramphenicol or gentamicin, depending on the results of antibiotic sensitivity tests.

Duration of treatment

At least 2-week, and often much longer, courses of antibiotics are necessary to treat neonatal meningitis. When the duration of treatment is too short, relapses are more likely to occur.

Monitoring of treatment

The best indication of adequate chemotherapy is a good clinical response.

Repeated CSF cultures are necessary and it is desirable that at least three or four negative CSF cultures will be obtained.

Antibiotic assays in the CSF, including those where the inhibitory or killing power of the CSF is assayed against the patient's own isolate, are desirable to ensure that effective doses are being given.

Prevention

Factors that may help reduce the incidence of neonatal meningitis include:

a. The delivery of full-term normal birth weight infants where possible.

b. Good hygienic measures to prevent cross-infection in the neonatal unit.

c. Prompt recognition and treatment of maternal infections of the genito-urinary tract during the last stages of pregnancy and avoidance of prolonged ruptured membranes.

The administration of benzylpenicillin to the mother at the start of labour and to the infant at birth might help to prevent group B strepto-coccal infection when the delivery of a pre-term infant is expected, but this is controversial at present.

d. The urgent surgical correction of some congenital defects may help to prevent CNS infections.

Tuberculous Meningitis

Tuberculous meningitis is rare in Britain today affecting mainly young or middle-aged Asian immigrants.

Clinical features and complications

The early clinical features include general malaise, low grade fever, intermittent headaches and anorexia. A few weeks later confusion, oculomotor palsies, persistent headaches and neck stiffness may also appear. During the final phase of the disease increasing drowsiness, multiple cranial nerve palsies, hemiplegia and decerebral rigidity can develop, leading within a few more weeks to death.

Complications can persist amongst survivors, particularly if antituberculous chemotherapy is delayed because of the failure to diagnose the infection in the early stages. These complications include hydrocephalus, spinal block, epilepsy, deafness and vestibular dysfunction, and mental deficiency.

Acute miliary tuberculosis may be associated with the tuberculous meningitis in over half the cases. There may be signs of miliary TB on the chest radiograph and the retina should be examined for the presence of choroid tubercles. Most patients have a positive Mantoux skin test and a raised ESR but often these non-specific tests are unhelpful.

Causative organism

Mycobacterium tuberculosis (usually human type).

Microbiological investigations

CSF

As much CSF as can safely be collected is necessary for microscopy and culture for acid-fast bacilli. A prolonged search for tubercle bacilli is necessary in the CSF deposit. Often only scanty acid-fast bacilli are present.

Other changes in the CSF (*Table 10.1*) which are characteristic of the meningitis include:

i. Moderately high white cell count—up to 600/mm^3, predominantly lymphocytes but including some polymorphs.
ii. Raised protein, usually 80–500 mg %.
iii. Low glucose level in CSF—often zero—but in any case much lower than simultaneous blood glucose concentration.

Occasionally the CSF may initially appear normal, and then repeat CSF samples should be examined. The CSF is cultured on Lowenstein-Jensen media.

Antimicrobial treatment

Antituberculous drugs which penetrate the CSF are selected whenever possible (*Table 10.3*).

Isoniazid, pyrazinamide and rifampicin penetrate the CSF well and should be used together throughout the initial stages of treatment. Streptomycin may also be given initially in combination with the above three drugs, but then intrathecal administration is necessary to achieve therapeutic levels in the CSF. This use of intrathecal streptomycin is controversial.

Repeat CSF collections are necessary during treatment for examination for the white cell count, protein, glucose and acid-fast bacilli.

Over 75% of cases survive when effective antituberculous treatment is given but some survivors may be handicapped by complications (*see above*).

Leptospiral Meningitis

Clinical features of leptospirosis include fever, conjunctivitis, jaundice and meningitis. Nephritis is a common feature. (*See* Leptospirosis in Chapter 21.)

Causative organisms

i. *Leptospira interrogans* var. *canicola* infects puppies. Urine from the dog may infect children.
ii. *Leptospira icterohaemorrhagiae* may be contracted by sewer workers and others from infected rat urine.

Microbiological investigations

CSF

The CSF findings may suggest the presence of aseptic meningitis with a clear or mildly turbid CSF, 20–300 white cells per mm^3, mainly lymphocytes, and a normal glucose concentration.

Occasionally, motile *Leptospira* can be seen under dark-ground illumination of a fresh CSF sample. Culture of the CSF for *Leptospira* by inoculation of Korthoff's medium and intraperitoneal inoculations of mice may be carried out.

Blood and urine

Culture of blood and (alkalinized) urine for *Leptrospira* using Korthoff's medium can be attempted.

Serum

Paired sera should be collected to show a rising antibody titre against *Leptospira* species using a leptospiral complement fixation test.

Antimicrobial treatment

Benzylpenicillin may help to relieve symptoms but only when given early on in the illness. Most cases of leptospiral meningitis recover spontaneously.

Viral Meningitis

Young adults and children are most often affected.

Clinical features and pathogenesis

The clinical features of viral meningitis are similar to those of bacterial meningitis in the early stages. Later on, patients with viral meningitis are generally much less ill than those with bacterial meningitis and nearly all the patients recover spontaneously.

When the meningitis is due to an enterovirus there is frequently a bi-phasic illness. In the first phase there may be a mild headache, sore throat or 'flu'-like illness which accompanies a viraemia from the respiratory tract or intestine. About 1–2 weeks later the patient may present with the second phase of the illness when sufficient virus multiplication in the central nervous system causes the symptoms of meningitis or encephalitis. Between the two phases of illness, the patient may feel temporarily better. A few patients may develop the complications of lower motor neurone flaccid paralysis due to virus damage of anterior horn cells in the spinal cord. This complication occurs in a minority of cases infected with polioviruses or certain echo- or Coxsackie viruses.

Skin rashes may occasionally occur with echoviruses and sometimes vesicles appear with Coxsackie A infections.

Mumps, the other common virus infection associated with meningitis, may be suggested by the development of unilateral or bilateral parotitis in about 50% of cases.

Causative organisms

Important viral causes of meningitis are included in *Table 10.2*.

1. Enteroviruses

These picornaviruses are spread mainly by the faecal–oral route although respiratory spread is also possible.

a. Echo viruses

Echo (Enteric, Cytopathic, Human, Orphan) viruses are the most frequent causes of viral meningitis, particularly in spring and summer. There are over 30 different types.

b. Coxsackie viruses

Coxsackie A viruses (24 types) are frequent causes of meningitis. Coxsackie B viruses (6 types) may also cause meningitis.

c. Polioviruses

Polioviruses, types I, II or III, are important but rare causes of meningitis in Britain. Type I virus was associated with the most virulent form of the disease and paralysis in the past. Unfortunately, there has been a recent increase in the number of patients developing poliomyelitis in Britain due to decreasing numbers of children being immunized against the disease.

2. Mumps

Mumps virus, a paramyo (RNA) virus is the next most common cause of viral meningitis after enteroviruses. It is only rarely associated with any serious sequelae (*see* Encephalitis).

The virus is spread by respiratory droplets and the infection is most common in winter and spring.

3. Herpesviruses (DNA viruses)

a. Herpes simplex

Herpesvirus hominis is an uncommon cause of viral meningitis. In recent years, a few patients with severe genital herpes have developed aseptic meningitis as a complication.

b. Varicella-zoster

Shingles results from reactivation of the varicella-zoster virus in the dorsal root ganglia to cause skin lesions in one or more dermatomes and is not usually associated with meningitis. However, a few patients with severe infection may also develop aseptic meningitis.

4. Adenoviruses (DNA viruses)

Adenoviruses are infrequent causes of aseptic meningitis.

5. Arboviruses

Numerous different arboviruses (togaviruses) can cause meningitis or encephalitis.

The only arbovirus endemic in Britain is louping-ill, a tick-borne virus, which is a very rare cause of meningitis or encephalitis.

Microbiological investigations

Acute specimens collected as early on in the illness as possible need to be collected for virus isolation investigations.

CSF

The CSF shows characteristically a typical aseptic meningitis picture (*Table 10.1*). This includes a clear and colourless CSF, or any slightly opalescent CSF, with usually 50–200 white cells per mm^3, predominantly lymphocytes. In the first 24 hours of the meningitis there may occasionally be a predominance of polymorphs. The protein is 50–100 mg per 100 ml and the glucose is usually normal.

The CSF should be kept at −70 °C at night so that next day an attempt at virus isolation can be made. Echo, herpes simplex and other viruses are sometimes isolated from the CSF but the yield is relatively low.

Throat swabs

A throat swab broken off into viral transport medium should be collected for the attempted isolation of enteroviruses and mumps virus.

Faeces

A faeces sample is collected for virus isolation investigations, especially for enteroviruses.

Paired sera

An acute and convalescent serum should be collected so that neutralization antibody tests against any enterovirus isolated can be performed. A rising titre would help to confirm that the illness was due to the enterovirus isolated.

Mumps S and V antibodies can also be tested for in the sera. S antibody is detected soon after the start of infection and disappears quickly while V antibody persists after the infection. The demonstration of a high titre of S antibody indicates recent infection.

Prevention

The routine immunization schedule includes a course of immunizations using Sabin's live oral attenuated polioviruses I, II and III, and paralytic poliomyelitis can be almost totally prevented by the widespread administration of this vaccine. Contraindications to the giving of the vaccine are few and include pregnancy, steroid or immunosuppressive therapy and diseases such as lymphoma where the patient's immunity is impaired.

Fungal Meningitis

Cryptococcus neoformans meningitis is a rare type of opportunistic infection affecting mainly patients with sarcoidosis, lymphomas or those receiving immunosuppressive therapy. The patient may complain of recurrent worsening headaches. In a few cases there are also features of pulmonary cryptococcal infection.

Examination of the CSF may show no obvious abnormality, but usually a slight or moderate increase in the white cell count, mainly lymphocytes, is apparent. Negative staining of the CSF deposit, using indian ink or nigrosin, may reveal the typical capsulated yeasts which otherwise may become confused under the microscope with white or red cells. Culture of the CSF on blood agar for at least 5 days is necessary and, when the diagnosis is suspected clinically, the CSF should be cultured on Sabouraud's agar which gives more rapid results than blood agar.

A rapid immunological test to detect cryptococcal antigen in the CSF, using latex particles, is useful when the CSF microscopy is inconclusive.

Treatment with amphotericin B or in combination with 5-fluorocytosine is occasionally successful, but the disease carries a high mortality rate.

Protozoal Meningitis

Free-living amoebae, *Naegleria* or *Hartmanella* species, may multiply in stagnant warm fresh water in Australia, and other warm countries including Britain during a hot summer. Children or young adults who have been swimming or diving in contaminated water may develop amoebic meningitis or encephalitis. The organisms probably reach the meninges through the cribriform plate.

Clinically, the patient may present with acute or subacute meningitis and the CSF usually appears purulent and bloodstained. A wet preparation of the CSF should be examined on a warm stage (heated penny on a slide) and slowly motile trophozoites, about 10 μm diam., looked at for over a period of a few minutes. If the CSF is very thick it can be diluted first with sterile warm saline. (The amoeba can also be cultured using a medium containing *E. coli*.)

There is a high mortality rate but treatment should be attempted by giving amphotericin B.

ENCEPHALITIS

Encephalitis, inflammation of the brain, may occur at any age but most often affects children or young adults. Viruses cause the great majority of cases of encephalitis.

Clinical Features

Most patients have no symptoms or only mild illnesses, as with many viral infections. A minority of patients develop classic clinical features of encephalitis which include drowsiness, coma with more severe illness, confusion, personality changes, headache, fits and localized neurological signs such as hemiparesis, cranial nerve palsies, dysphasia and nystagmus.

The differential diagnosis often includes cerebral abscess, severe meningitis and intra-cranial haemorrhage.

Complications and death occur in many cases especially when the causative agent is herpes simplex, varicella-zoster or measles viruses. Complications in survivors include a permanent severe loss of memory, emotional disturbances, impairment of motor functions or loss of intellectual ability. Serious complications and death are less common with mumps encephalitis.

A history of a recent immunization or of a febrile illness during the preceding few weeks may be obtained in some cases of post-infectious encephalomyelitis.

Investigations which may help include an EEG which often shows diffuse slow activity, an isotopic brain scan and possibly carotid angiography. The use of computerized axial tomographic scans (CAT scans) may particularly help differentiate encephalitis from brain abscess, cerebral tumour, subarachnoid haemorrhage and cerebro-vascular disease. However, the most important investigations once the diagnosis is seriously suspected are those on the CSF and brain biopsy (*see* Microbiological investigations).

Causative Organisms

1. Viruses

Many viruses may cause an acute meningo-encephalitis (*see Table 10.4*). In Britain, herpes simplex is the most important cause of sporadic cases of encephalitis and other causes include mumps, enteroviruses, varicella-zoster and Epstein-Barr virus. Louping-ill virus, which is tick borne, may rarely cause encephalitis in Britain.

In North America, Africa, the Soviet Union, the Indian subcontinent, the Far East and Australia, scores of different anthropod-borne viruses may cause endemic or epidemic encephalitis. A few examples of toga viruses are included in *Table 10.4*.

Epidemics of encephalitis due to enteroviruses, particularly echoviruses, have rarely been reported in Britain, affecting mainly infants.

During an influenza epidemic a few cases are sometimes seen of encephalitis due to the influenza A virus.

Post-infectious encephalomyelitis is a rare complication of certain virus infections, such as measles or rubella, and may rarely follow immunization against a virus (or bacterial) disease (*see Table 10.4*). The disease probably results from an immunological reaction against nerve tissue as well as against microbiological antigens.

Herpes simplex

Herpes simplex, the most frequent cause of severe sporadic encephalitis, may cause encephalitis in previously apparently healthy individuals as well as in patients who have impaired host defences due to conditions, such as Hodgkin's disease. The poor prognosis of the disease is even worse in the patients with impaired immunity.

Patients with herpes encephalitis only occasionally show clinical evidence of herpes infection involving the skin, mouth or genitalia. In neonates, there may be evidence of more widespread viral infection.

Table 10.4. Some microbial causes of encephalitis, post-infectious encephalomyelitis and degenerative central nervous system diseases

Acute encephalitis		*Post-infectious encephalomyelitis*	*Degenerative diseases*
1. *Sporadic*	2. *Epidemic*		
Herpes simplex	*Toga (arbo-) viruses*: Eastern Equine (mosquito-borne)	Measles Rubella	Measles—Subacute Sclerosing Panencephalitis (SSPE)
Mumps	Western Equine (mosquito-borne)		
Varicella-zoster	Louping-ill (tick-borne)		
Epstein-Barr (glandular fever) Rabies	Japanese B (mosquito-borne) St Louis (mosquito-borne) Murray Valley (mosquito-borne)	Vaccinations against smallpox, measles, pertussis, and other microbial diseases	'Slow virus' of Kuru 'Slow virus' of Jacob-Creutzfeldt disease
	Enteroviruses: Coxsackie A and B Echo Polio (Influenza viruses)		JC virus—progressive multifocal leucoencephalopathy

The herpes simplex virus is particularly associated with a severe haemorrhagic necrotizing encephalitis affecting the temporal lobe. This may cause the patient to present clinically with the features of a space occupying lesion in the temporal lobe with many focal neurological signs and epilepsy is a common feature. The mortality rate is about 70% and may be reduced if the diagnosis is made early and prompt anti-viral therapy is given.

2. Non-viral causative organisms

Some bacterial species which may cause infection primarily at other sites, such as *Legionella pneumophila*, or cause meningitis, such as the meningococcus, may also occasionally cause an encephalitis (*Table 10.5*). A 'cerebritis' may precede the development of a pyogenic brain abscess.

Encephalitis is a rare complication of Q fever and *Mycoplasma pneumoniae* infections. It is also a complication of rickettsial diseases.

Toxoplasmosis is common throughout the world but infrequently involves encephalitis which runs a chronic course that is only rarely fatal. *Plasmodium falciparum*, the causative organism of malignant tertian malaria, may cause cerebral malaria which is frequently fatal. Trypanosomes may invade the central nervous system in Africa and cause sleeping sickness.

Cryptococcus neoformans and other fungi can cause meningo-encephalitis in immunocompromised patients with, for example, sarcoidosis or Hodgkin's disease or during steroid therapy (*Table 10.5*).

Helminths may rarely cause encephalopathies (*Table 10.5*).

Microbiological Investigations

CSF

Characteristically, the CSF shows a moderate lymphocytosis and rise in protein concentration but initially the CSF may appear normal.

In herpes simplex encephalitis, red cells are often found together with the lymphocytes.

The CSF may be examined microscopically for evidence of cryptococci or protozoa (*see* Fungal and protozoal meningitis) as well as bacterial infections. It should be cultured for both bacteria and viruses.

Brain biopsy

The urgent virological diagnosis of herpes simplex encephalitis is usually only possible by performing a brain biopsy. The biopsy material is examined by immunofluorescent staining techniques using antibody to herpes simplex and by electron microscopy. These microscopic methods enable the diagnosis to be made within a few hours. The inoculation of tissue cultures and sometimes animals may subsequently confirm the daignosis by yielding growth of the causative viruses.

Serology

A high antibody titre to herpes simplex virus in a single serum sample may suggest the presence of the infection, but only a rising titre demonstrated by

Table 10.5. Some non-viral microbial causes of encephalitis or encephalopathy

Bacteria	*Coxiella Rickettsiae Mycoplasma*	*Protozoa*	*Fungi*	*Helminths*
1. *Bacteria causing 'cerebritis' prior to the formation of a brain abscess*				
Streptococci	*Coxiella burnetii*	*Toxoplasma*	*Cryptococcus*	*T. solium*
Pneumococci	*Rickettsiae*	Plasmodia	*Aspergillus*	*Echinococcus*
Staphylococci	*Mycoplasma pneumoniae*	Trypanosomes	*Histoplasma*	*Trichinella*
Anaerobes		Amoebae		*Schistosoma*
Gram-negative bacilli				
2. *Encephalitis complicating Legionnaires' disease*				
Legionella pneumophila				
3. *Meningo-encephalitis due to*				
Meningococcus and other bacterial causes of meningitis				
Spirochaetes—*Treponema pallidum*				
Leptospira				

comparison with the titre in a later sample can provide more convincing evidence of active herpes infection. Serology is of retrospective value only for herpes infection and cannot influence the urgent management of the patient.

High antibody titres in an early serum to Q fever, rickettsiae, *Mycoplasma pneumoniae*, mumps, *Toxoplasma* or *Legionella pneumophila* may quickly help to point to the likely diagnosis. A serum sample collected 10–14 days later will be necessary to show a rising titre to antibody.

Other specimens

Isolations of the causative organism can be attempted from a throat swab in viral transport medium (enteroviruses, mumps), faeces (enteroviruses and parasites) and blood (arboviruses using animal inoculations).

Blood films and cultures may also be collected for investigation of protozoal and bacterial causes of encephalitis/cerebritis.

Antimicrobial Therapy

Anti-viral drugs given parenterally in the early stages of herpes simplex encephalitis may improve the chances of recovery from the disease. Idoxuridine proved to be disappointing and cytosine arabinoside was only slightly better than idoxuridine. Adenine arabinoside has occasionally been effective but is likely that the best results will be achieved using the new drug acycloguanosine (acyclovir).

Varicella-zoster encephalitis, which rarely complicates ophthalmic zoster, may be treated in a similar way to herpes simplex encephalitis. In addition, hyper-immune zoster immunoglobulin should be given urgently.

Q fever or *Mycoplasma* encephalitis should be treated by parental tetracycline therapy. Rickettsial encephalitis may be effectively treated by chloramphenicol.

Toxoplasma encephalitis should be treated as early as possible by a combination of pyrimethamine and sulphadimidine. An alternative combination is spiramycin and sulphadimidine.

Prevention

Post-infectious encephalomyelitis complicating smallpox vaccination is totally avoidable now by never giving the vaccine as smallpox has been eradicated. Contraindications to pertussis immunization should be observed (*see* Immunization, in Chapter 8, p. 150).

An immunodeficient patient who has had contact with chickenpox or zoster should be given immediate prophylaxis with hyperimmune zoster immunoglobulin.

Rabies*—see* Chapter 21

Subacute Sclerosing Panencephalitis (SSPE)

This rare complication of persistent measles infection, which is rapidly fatal once diagnosed, generally presents in a child or adolescent. Characteristically there is intellectual impairment and the development of progressive jerking movements. Very high titres of measles antibody are typically found in the CSF and serum.

'Slow Virus' Infections of the Central Nervous System

'Slow viruses' are difficult to isolate, have long incubation periods and are associated with long, chronic, progressive degenerative diseases of the central nervous system which are severe and usually fatal.

In man, slow virus diseases are Kuru, affecting cannabilistic tribes in New Guinea, and Jacob–Creutzfeldt disease which very rarely occurs in Britain. In animals, slow virus diseases include the Aleutian disease of mink and scrapie in sheep.

Cerebellar symptoms as well as symptoms arising from the degeneration of the spinal cord are prominent features of the slow virus diseases.

The causative agents of Kuru and Jacob–Creutzfeldt diseases have been demonstrated by transmission experiments using chimpanzees.

CEREBRAL ABSCESSES

There has been a sharp decline in the incidence of brain abscesses over the last 35 years due to the antibiotic treatment of many of the acute infections, which previously became chronic and were sometimes complicated by the development of brain abscesses. Unfortunately, as the disease is rare and clinically often difficult to diagnose, many patients are diagnosed only in the late stages and develop permanent complications or die of the disease. The overall mortality rate of brain abscesses today varies between 15 and 40%.

Pathogenesis

An abscess may develop in the extra-dural, sub-dural or intracerebral sites (often near the junction of the cortex and subcortex). It may arise as the result of direct spread of infection from the ear or sinuses or from an external source following accidental trauma or surgery. Alternatively, the abscess may result from the haematogenous spread from a distant site of infection such as the lungs (bronchiectasis/emphysema), bones (osteomyelitis) or heart (endocarditis).

Chronic infections of the ear, sinuses, lungs and other sites are much more likely to become complicated by brain abscess formation than by acute infections.

Clinical Features

The main early clinical features are those of the general signs of systemic infection including pyrexia, and minor neurological symptoms or signs. Only minor neck stiffness or a vague personality change may be apparent. More severe features may develop including hemiparesis, cerebellar syndrome, visual field defects and papilloedema. Other features which may be present also during the later stages are fits and coma.

Some patients have no pyrexia and only neurological features are apparent. Occasionally a cerebral abscess may masquerade as a worsening 'cerebrovascular accident'.

A patient diagnosed as a case of meningitis may occasionally have a cerebral abscess present also. The latter may be suggested clinically by the presence of a focal neurological sign or raised intra-cranial pressure.

A history of known predisposing factors of brain abscess should be particularly noted, as with known chronic middle ear infection or sinusitis, chronic bronchiectasis, or congenital heart disease associated with right to left shunt.

General investigations for brain abscesses include an EEG, and an urgent CAT scan. The patient should be immediately transferred to a nerosurgical centre once the diagnosis is suspected clinically.

Causative Organisms

The pattern of bacterial species which cause brain abscesses varies with the site of the original source of infection (*see* de Louvois et al., 1977).

1. Otogenic source

In about 50% of patients the chronically infected middle ear is the source of infection and especially for temporal lobe or cerebellar abscesses. Non-sporing anaerobes, particularly *Bacteroides fragilis*, predominate in intra-cranial pus and are usually mixed with aerobic Gram-negative bacilli such as *E. coli*, *Proteus*, or *Klebsiella* species.

Streptococci or staphylococci are isolated sometimes.

2. Sinus source

Sinusitis is often associated with frontal lobe abscesses. The pus usually yields pure growth of streptococcal species, particularly *Strep. milleri*, or pneumococci.

3. Accidental or surgical trauma

Gram-positive organisms predominate in the intra-cranial pus in this situation, mainly *Staph. aureus*. Occasionally coagulase-negative staphylococci or propionibacteria may be implicated.

4. Chest sources of infection

Streptococci, including *Strep. milleri*, pneumococci and staphylococci may invade the blood from a respiratory or cardiac source of infection and cause a metastatic brain abscess.

Microbiological Investigations

Pus

A sample of pus aspirated from the brain for bacteriology before the start of antibiotic therapy is the most vital investigation.

The pus should be transported in a plain sterile container and a further sample should be put into thioglycollate broth in the operating theatre; both samples should be transported to the laboratory as quickly as possible. A Gram-stain of the pus will often give an immediate clue as to the likely infecting organisms. In the laboratory, the pus should be cultured within 1 hour of collection on to a wide range of aerobic and anaerobic blood agar media, with and without antibiotic selective agents such as neomycin or nalidixic acid, in 10% CO_2 aerobically and anaerobically (*see* de Louvois et al., 1977; and Ingram et al., 1977). Prolonged cultures may be necessary. Antibiotic sensitivity tests on the isolates will help the rational subsequent therapy.

CSF

When there is a strong clinical suspicion of brain abscess, a lumbar puncture may be contraindicated as the patient's condition may worsen if the intra-cranial pressure is greatly raised due to the space occupying lesion.

If the diagnosis is more doubtful and it is clinically considered safe to perform a lumbar puncture, the examination of a small quantity of CSF may show:

i. No abnormality—especially for the more deeply situated abscesses
   or
ii. clear or opalescent CSF with a moderate number of white cells consisting of both lymphocytes and polymorphs
   or
iii. frankly turbid CSF with a high polymorph count.

A Gram-stain of the CSF should be performed as well as aerobic and anaerobic cultures. The CSF deposit should also be inoculated into thioglycollate broth. *Bacteroides fragilis* isolated from CSF is more likely to be associated with brain abscess than meningitis.

Blood cultures

Blood cultures may be positive in cases of systemic or respiratory infection due to *Staph. aureus* or pneumococci and help to point to the likely causative organism of a metastatic brain abscess.

Anaerobes or streptococci may also occasionally be isolated from the blood of patients with advanced brain abscess lesions arising from ear or sinus infections.

Other specimens for culture

Swabs of pus from a discharging ear and sputum from a patient with bronchiectasis may give indirect clues as to the likely causative organisms present in a brain abscess.

Antimicrobial Therapy

Urgent drainage of the pus and repeated aspirations of the pus are of major importance in the treatment of the patient and, initially, systemic antimicrobial therapy is of secondary importance. Local instillation of chloramphenicol is advisable.

In order to obtain rapid resolution of the remaining infection after drainage and to avoid relapse, effective chemotherapy is necessary. The choice of drugs depends partly on the source of infection.

a. Otogenic source

i. Metronidazole, 400–600 mg 8-hourly, orally or intravenously will effectively treat the bacteroides infections that are usually present. This drug penetrates the intra-cranial pus well.

ii. Chloramphenicol should initially be used in high dosage, such as 1 g 6-hourly in an adult, to obtain adequate concentrations of drug at the site of infection, and this will be active against many aerobic organisms which are mixed in with *Bacteroides*. There is also some activity against *Bacteroides*.

iii. Benzylpenicillin may be added to the above, particularly when there is evidence of streptococcal infection.

b. Sinuses

Benzylpenicillin, 16–24 MU per day intravenously, is the usual mainstay of diagnosis here since streptococci are the predominant pathogens.

c. Trauma or surgery

Fusidic acid penetrates the intra-cranial pus well and should be used in this situation where staphylococci often cause brain abscess. The drug should be considered with another antistaphylococcal drug given in high dosage, such as cloxacillin, for treating infections due to penicillinase-producing *Staph. aureus*. If the *Staph. aureus* is resistant to penicillin and fusidic acid, but sensitive to lincomycin or chloramphenicol, these drugs may be used. When the *Staph. aureus* is sensitive to both penicillin and fusidic acid a combination of these two drugs should be given.

d. Unknown source

A combination of penicillin, chloramphenicol and metronidazole should be used to treat a brain abscess where the source of infection is unknown, while waiting for the results of bacteriological investigations on the intra-cranial pus.

In all cases, the treatment is appropriately modified once the antibiotic sensitivities of isolates from the pus are known.

EXTRA-DURAL SPINAL ABSCESS

An extra-dural spinal abscess can cause acute paraplegia unless promptly treated in the early stages with appropriate antibiotics. The causative organism is usually *Staph. aureus*. The staphylococcus may have reached the spinal site by metastatic spread from a focus of infection elsewhere such as in the lungs, skin or bones. There may be acute spinal tenderness, fever and a raised white blood count. Blood cultures should be collected and 'blind' treatment then started immediately with a combination of benzylpenicillin, cloxacillin and fusidic acid.

Urgent surgical drainage of the abscess may be necessary in advanced cases or in those who do not quickly respond to antibiotic therapy.

GUILLAIN-BARRÉ SYNDROME

This syndrome, also known as infectious polyneuritis, is characterized by CSF findings of a high protein concentration, up to 1200 mg per 100 ml, and a clear CSF with a normal white cell count.

Typical clinical features include paraesthesiae and weakness in the limbs of acute onset which sometimes progress to paraplegia. These features may follow various infections including glandular fever and *Mycoplasma pneumoniae* respiratory tract infection.

Investigations for the causes of aseptic meningitis, including polio, are indicated (*see* previous section). Other tests that may help diagnose the cause include a Paul-Bunnell and *Mycoplasma pneumoniae* complement fixation tests on paired sera.

There is usually no specific therapy unless mycoplasma infection is diagnosed when tetracycline may be given. Most cases gradually resolve spontaneously.

CONGENITAL CENTRAL NERVOUS SYSTEM INFECTIONS

Congenital neonatal infections result from intra-uterine infection or from infections acquired from the maternal genito-urinary tract during birth. The central nervous system is usually only one of a number of sites affected (*see* Chapter 7).

Causative Organisms

Viruses	**Comments**
1. Cytomegalovirus	the most frequent infective cause of congenital mental deficiency
2. Rubella	eighth cranial nerve damage, cerebral palsy, etc.
3. Herpes simplex	neonatal herpes encephalitis (*see* previous section)

Bacteria	
1. *Treponema pallidum*	congenital syphilis—central nervous system infection may not be clinically evident until much later
2. Group B haemolytic streptococcus	*See above* Neonatal bacterial meningitis
3. *Listeria monocytogenes*	

Protozoal	
Toxoplasma gondii	intracerebral calcification, ventriculitis, microcephaly or hydrocephaly, and mental deficiency

(Congenital infections are discussed in Chapter 7, p. 119.)

Further Reading

Begent R. (1977) Opportunistic infections of the CNS. *Br. J. Hosp. Med.* **18**, 402–411.
Davies Pamela A. (1977) Neonatal bacterial meningitis. *Br. J. Hosp. Med.* **18**, 425–434.
de Louvois J., Gortvai P. and Hurley R. (1977) Antibiotic treatment of abscesses of the central nervous system. *Br. Med. J.* **2**, 985.
Hambleton G. and Davies P. A. (1975) Bacterial meningitis: some aspects of diagnosis and treatment. *Arch. Dis. Child.* **50**, 674–683.
Ingham H. R., Selkon J. B. and Roxby C. M. (1977) Bacteriological study of otogenic cerebral abscesses: chemotherapeutic role of metronidazole. *Br. Med. J.* **2**, 991.
Legg N. J. (1979) Intracerebral abscess. *Br. J. Hosp. Med.* **22**, 608–614.
McCracken G. H. and Mize S. G. (1980) Intraventricular gentamicin in meningitis. *Lancet* **2**, 252–253.
Warren R. E. and Roberton N. R. C. (1980) Intraventricular gentamicin in meningitis. *Lancet* **2**, 252.

Chapter 11

'ENT' and eye infections

EAR, NOSE AND THROAT INFECTIONS

Normal Flora of the Upper Respiratory Tract

Many different bacterial species normally colonize the mouth and main examples are included in *Table 11.1,1*. Host defence mechanisms, including those associated with the ciliated epithelium in the nose and sinuses, lysozyme in saliva and IgA and other immunoglobulins in mucous secretions or serum, may help to reduce the incidence of infections due to respiratory pathogens (*see also* p. 142, Section on Immune deficiency, in Chapter 8). The normal mouth flora probably contributes to the prevention of attachment of exogenous pathogens to the mucosa. Nevertheless, certain 'respiratory pathogens' are sometimes carried asymptomatically in the mouth or nose of healthy individuals (*see Table 11.1,2*). The administration of broad spectrum antibiotics may greatly disturb the normal flora and predispose to colonization by organisms which are not normally evident in the mouth (*Table 11.1,3*); ultimately this might result in superinfections, such as thrush (*see* p. 206).

Table 11.1. Normal flora of upper respiratory tract (throat or nose)

1. *Bacteria carried in the majority of people*	
Streptococcus viridans	
Neisseria spp.	
Diphtheroids	
Anaerobic cocci, fusiforms and *Bacteroides*	
2. *'Respiratory bacterial pathogens' that may be carried asymptomatically*	
Streptococcus pyogenes	(2–5% carriage rate)
Streptococcus pneumoniae	
Haemophilus influenzae	
Corynebacterium diphtheriae	(less than 0·1% carriage rate)
3. *Organisms sometimes associated with transient colonization secondary to antibiotic therapy*	
Coliforms—Klebsiella spp., *E. coli*, etc.	
Pseudomonas spp.	
Candida albicans	

Frequency of Upper Respiratory Tract Infections in Relationship to Age

Upper respiratory tract infections are extremely common in infants and young school children. An average pre-school child is said to have about six upper respiratory tract infections a year. Most of the infections are of viral aetiology and occur in winter. Bacterial infections are also very common in young children. The relationship between age and infections due to viruses, *Streptococcus pneumoniae, Haemophilus influenzae*, capsulated Pittman type b strains, *Bordetella pertussis* and other organisms affecting the upper respiratory tract are mainly discussed in Chapters 8 and 10. The Eustachian tubes in infants are relatively wider and more horizontal than in adults; this might partly explain the greater incidence of acute otitis media in infants since the causative organisms may spread directly from the throat to the middle ear via the Eustachian tube. Older children and adults usually have good immunity to a wide range of respiratory pathogens but the 'common cold' continues to be prevalent in these age groups. Sinusitis frequently occurs in adults and children.

The 'Common Cold' (Coryza)

Clinical features

The incubation period is usually between 2 and 4 days and the main clinical features include nasal discharge, sneezing and sore throat. Some patients are febrile and also complain of headache. The peak incidence of this most common of all infectious diseases is in children aged 2–7 years, but colds are common at most ages. The symptoms have usually disappeared within a week.

Causative organisms

Rhinoviruses (over 100 serotypes) are by far the most common cause.

Other viruses also often cause colds including:

Coronaviruses
Respiratory syncytial virus
Para-influenza viruses (four types)
Coxsackieviruses A_{21} and B_3
Echoviruses types 11, 20
Adenoviruses

Bacteria may cause mild secondary bacterial infection in the later stages of a cold.

Investigation and treatment

Microbiological investigations and chemotherapy are not indicated. Antibiotic treatment may occasionally become advisable in certain patients with chronic bronchitis who develop a cold (*see* Chapter 12).

Sore Throat and Tonsillitis

Clinical features

Sore throat and tonsillitis are most common in young children. The main presenting features of tonsillitis in children under 3 years old include fever and a refusal to eat. Common presenting features of pharyngitis and tonsillitis in older children or young adults include sore throat, dysphagia and sometimes a painful cervical lymphadenopathy. On examination of the throat a purulent follicular tonsillitis may be seen. Frequently only a mild pharyngitis is observed without any pharyngeal exudate.

It is not possible clinically to distinguish between the common viral and bacterial causes of sore throat, even when purulent follicular tonsillitis is present, which is why bacteriology investigations should be carried out whenever possible.

Diphtheria should be suspected clinically when there is a membranous exudate present in the throat or when there is serious constitutional upset—urgent expert advice is then necessary. (Some laboratories still look routinely for *Corynebacterium diphtheriae* as well as *Streptococcus pyogenes* when culturing throat swabs from all patients with acute sore throat. However, the bacteriological investigations are of secondary importance to prompt clinical diagnosis and the administration of diphtheria antitoxin.) *See* Diphtheria, in Chapter 8.

Sore throat may be severe in glandular fever (infectious mononucleosis) and sometimes a thick white shaggy exudate is present on the tonsils. There may be marked constitutional upset followed by prolonged malaise.

Causative organisms

1. Viruses

These are the most frequent causative organisms of sore throat and include:

Adenoviruses (33 types causing pharyngitis and conjunctivitis)
Epstein-Barr virus—cause of glandular fever
Enteroviruses
Other viruses that cause the 'common cold' (mentioned above)
} common causes

Viruses causing childhood infectious diseases such as measles (prodromal stages)

Cytomegalovirus	may occasionally cause a Paul-Bunnell negative glandular fever type illness
Herpes simplex	may cause severe primary stomatitis in children. Recurrent secondary lesions may occur afterwards at the muco-cutaneous junctions (herpes labialis)

2. Bacteria

Streptococcus pyogenes (Lancefield group A beta-haemolytic streptococcus)—isolated from about 30% of patients with acute sore throat and is *the only common bacterial cause*

Beta-haemolytic streptococci belonging to Lancefield groups C or G—occasional causes

Corynebacterium diphtheriae
Corynebacterium ulcerans
} rare causes

Vincent's organisms	*Borrelia vincenti* (spirochaetes) and anaerobic Gram-negative fusiform bacilli, together may cause painful ulcers in the throat or an ulcerative gingivitis
Treponema pallidum	primary chancres may occur inside the mouth but sore throat is more frequently associated with secondary rather than primary syphilitic lesions

Neisseria gonorrhoeae	gonococcal pharyngitis should be considered in patients with possible sexually transmitted disease who have a history of recent oral intercourse

Bacteriological investigations

1. Throat swab

A Gram-stain of a throat swab may reveal numerous Vincent's organisms when Vincent's infection is clinically suspected. Microscopy is not carried out for the investigation of other bacterial infections.

The throat swab should be collected for the culture of streptococci before the start of antibiotic therapy. Care should be taken to sample the inflamed site and not to contaminate the swab by touching the other parts of the mouth. The swab should be put into Stuart's or other suitable transport medium if a delay of more than 1 hour is expected before the swab can be plated out on blood agar. If no beta-haemolytic streptococci are isolated after overnight incubation of the culture plate, viruses are the probable cause of the sore throat. However, if a bacitracin-sensitive beta-haemolytic streptococcus is isolated, it is likely that the sore throat is due to *Strep. pyogenes* (but *see* p. 518). Cultures for *C. diphtheriae* are essential when diphtheria is clinically suspected (*see* p. 140).

2. Nose swab

A nose swab should be collected in addition to a throat swab for culture for streptococci to see if there is nasal carriage of *Strep. pyogenes* as well as throat infection due to this organism. This is particularly necessary during a suspected outbreak and may be of epidemiological importance as *Strep. pyogenes* is more likely to spread when there is nasal carriage.

Virus isolation investigations

Virus isolation attempts are not indicated routinely. Exceptionally in an unusually severe case or during an unexplained outbreak of acute sore throats, virus isolation can be attempted by taking a throat swab from the inflamed lesions in the first couple of days of the infection. The swab should be put immediately into viral transport medium and sent at once to the laboratory.

Blood and serological tests

When glandular fever is suspected clinically a blood count in the acute stage will help to show whether there is a lymphocytosis and atypical lymphocytes present which are characteristic of this condition. Heterophile antibodies can also be looked for in the Paul-Bunnell test. This serological test may need to be repeated since it can take up to 3 months to become positive. When the patient has a glandular-fever-like illness and the Paul-Bunnell test is negative, other serological tests may be indicated to diagnose possible infection with cytomegalovirus (CMV complement fixation test) or *Toxoplasma* (Toxoplasma Dye Test) using paired sera.

Anti-streptolysin O (ASO) or anti-streptococcal DNAase B antibody titres should be estimated in the serum where evidence of recent streptococcal infection is sought and the throat swab culture result is negative. A rise in anti-streptococcal antibodies can be demonstrated using these tests in between 80 and 100% patients within 2–4 weeks of a previous *Strep. pyogenes* pharyngeal infection. These serological tests may be particularly indicated when possible indirect complications of *Strep. pyogenes* infection are suspected (*see below*).

Antibiotic treatment of sore throat and tonsillitis

If *Strep. pyogenes* is isolated from the patient penicillin should be given if the patient is not allergic to it. All strains of this organism are sensitive to penicillin. Treatment should be started with one or two intra-muscular doses of a mixture of benzylpenicillin and procaine penicillin followed by oral penicillin V for 10 days (*see also* Duration of therapy p. 49, in Chapter 3). Erythromycin is an alternative antibiotic especially suitable when the patient is allergic to penicillin.

In general practice, the results of bacteriological investigation are often not available and 'blind' antibiotic treatment of acute sore throat should be with penicillin or erythromycin (as for *Strep. pyogenes* above) on the assumption that there is a streptococcal cause present. Ampicillin or amoxycillin should not be given as these drugs are particularly likely to cause a rash when the patient's sore throat is due to glandular fever which may not be distinguished from streptococcal infection (as discussed above).

If there is clinical or bacteriological evidence for Vincent's infection, effective treatment with either metronidazole or penicillin can be given.

Complications of Strep. pyogenes Throat Infections

Strep. pyogenes can cause both direct and indirect complications.

1. Direct complications

a. *Peri-tonsillar abscess ('quinsy')*

Untreated streptococcal tonsillitis may become complicated by the development of a peri-tonsillar abscess but this is much less common than in the past. The abscess may require surgical drainage under penicillin cover.

b. *Otitis media*

This is discussed below.

c. *Scarlet fever*

Certain strains of *Strep. pyogenes* produce an erythrogenic toxin as a result of the presence of a particular lysogenic phage (*see* Scarlet fever, p. 134, in Chapter 8).

2. Indirect complications

a. *Rheumatic fever*

Rheumatic fever most often occurs in children aged 6–15 years, with a peak incidence at about 7 years old, but the disease is rarely seen in Britain today.

The decline in the incidence of the disease in developed countries is probably mainly due to an improvement in general living conditions.

Pathogenesis

The exact pathogenesis of rheumatic fever is unknown but there is no doubt that it is related to a previous *Strep. pyogenes* throat infection which occurs usually 2–4 weeks before the clinical onset of the disease. Antibodies develop to cell wall antigens of the streptococcus which cross react with the sarcolemma of human heart and other tissues. Characteristic rheumatic granulomata develop in connective tissue in many different sites in the body and, in the heart, these are known as Aschoff nodules. Rheumatic heart valvular disease can ultimately occur especially if there are repeated attacks of rheumatic fever. Certain children appear to have a genetic predisposition to developing rheumatic fever following *Strep. pyogenes* infection. They may develop repeat attacks of rheumatic fever following infection due to a wide range of M types of *Strep. pyogenes.*

Diagnosis

Major clinical features of rheumatic fever may include fleeting polyarthritis, evidence of myocarditis or pericarditis, chorea, subcutaneous nodules and erythema marginatum. Supporting laboratory evidence of a recent streptococcal infection is usually provided by demonstrating a rising serum ASO titre, or a raised ASO titre greater than 200 Todd units per ml. The diagnosis of rheumatic fever is unlikely if the ASO and anti-streptococcal (DNAase B) titres are not raised. Occasionally, *Strep. pyogenes* is also isolated from a throat swab but this is of little diagnostic value since this merely indicates streptococcal carriage.

Prophylaxis

Following the first attack of rheumatic fever, prophylaxis to prevent repeated episodes of rheumatic fever developing is effectively carried out by giving either monthly injections of benzathine penicillin or twice daily oral penicillin V. Penicillin prophylaxis against throat infections is necessary throughout childhood and the early teenage years.

b. Acute glomerulonephritis

Post-streptococcal acute glomerulonephritis characteristically affects children or young adults and usually occurs about 10 days after *Strep. pyogenes* infection.

Pathogenesis

This complication only follows infection due to a small number of 'nephritogenic' types of *Strep. pyogenes*, including M types 12, 1, 3, 4 and 25 when the site of infection is the throat. (Different M types, including M types 49 and 52, are implicated when nephritis follows streptococcal pyoderma; *see* Chapter 16, p. 308. The pathogenesis of the disease involves the deposition of circulating immune complexes in the glomerulus and there have been recent reports of streptococcal plasma membrane having been identified in affected glomeruli. Characteristically the serum complement components are reduced during the active stage of the disease, especially C_3. Activation of the complement and coagulation systems at the sites of deposition of the immune complexes in the glomeruli results in local tissue inflammation and histology of the lesions shows typical proliferative changes.

Diagnosis, prognosis and use of penicillin
Clinical features include haematuria and signs of acute nephritic syndrome. The prognosis is good in children—they usually recover completely. Subsequent serious complications, such as renal failure, may rarely occur and this is possibly more likely in adults. The serum ASO titre is usually elevated and a rising titre may be demonstrated after streptococcal throat infection (in contrast anti-DNAase B antibodies only are elevated after previous streptococcal skin infection). Penicillin may be given to treat any residual. *Strep. pyogenes* infection. Subsequent prophylaxis with penicillin is not indicated as it is unlikely that a repeat infection due to a nephritogenic type of *Strep. pyogenes* would occur.

c. *Streptococcal skin rashes*

Erythema nodosum, Henoch-Schönlein purpura and guttate psoriasis may result from the immune sequelae of previous streptococcal infection although there may also be other causes for these conditions. Erythema marginatum may occur as part of the rheumatic fever syndrome (*see above*).

Oral candidiasis ('Thrush')

Candida albicans is the main *Candida* species that causes an acute infection in neonates (*see* p. 119 in Chapter 7) and the elderly, with typical white plaques which are only loosely adherent, covering the tongue and other mouth surfaces.

The candida organisms may also behave as 'opportunists' in patients who have impaired immunity or severe debilitation due to malignancy or other causes especially when there has been recent antibiotic therapy. White plaques or erythematous lesions may form in the throat of these patients due to candida infection and occasionally these lesions may extend into the oesophagus in severe cases of infection.

Diagnosis of 'thrush' can usually be quickly confirmed by a Gram-stain of a throat swab of the lesion which shows typical budding Gram-positive yeast-like organisms. Culture of the swab on blood agar or Sabouraud's medium will yield growth of the causative *Candida* species after 24–48 hours, incubation at 35 °C.

Treatment with topical nystatin or amphotericin B lozenges is usually effective. Severe lesions in immunosuppressed patients may need treatment with a systemic anti-fungal drug, such as 5-fluorocytosine, miconazole or ketoconazole.

Acute Otitis Media

Acute otitis media is most common in infants and young children (*see* Age and upper repiratory infections *above*). The most frequent symptom is pain in the ear but the condition should be considered in any child with unexplained fever, diarrhoea or vomiting. The ear drum characteristically shows dilated vessels and in the later stages bulging of the drum and disappearance of the 'light reflex'. If the condition is not recognized and treated early, the drum may perforate. Rupture of the drum is followed by relief from the pain.

Causative organisms

Viruses cause acute otitis media in up to about 50% of cases, but it is not usually possible to distinguish clinically between a viral and bacterial cause; management of acute otitis media should be on the assumption that a bacterial cause is present.

Bacterial causes include:

Strep. pneumoniae
Haemophilus influenzae } the main causative bacteria
Strep. pyogenes
Staph. aureus

Mycoplasma pneumoniae may rarely cause acute bullous myringitis

Microbiological investigation

Gram-stain microscopy and culture of pus from the middle ear of a patient are feasible when a myringotomy is performed to drain pus but this is an infrequent situation.

Treatment

Amoxycillin is probably the best antibiotic at present for treating acute otitis media although large doses of penicillin V may also give satisfactory results. If the patient is allergic to penicillin, cotrimoxazole or erythromycin can be given. Cephalexin has failed to cure some patients with haemophilus otitis media (it is possible that cefaclor might produce better results as it is more active than cephalexin against *Haemophilus*). Beta-lactamase-producing strains of *H. influenzae*, which are resistant to amoxycillin (or ampicillin), cause otitis in a few patients. If there is no improvement in the ear drum after 2–3 days' treatment with amoxycillin, a change to cotrimoxazole should be considered. Antibiotic treatment should be continued for at least 10 days. Repeat examination of the drums is necessary before treatment is stopped. A few months later, there should preferably be further examination of the ears to detect possible complications.

Complications of acute otitis media

a. Chronic suppurative otitis media (CSOM)

This condition is more likely to occur when there has been no adequate treatment of attacks of acute otitis media. The patient has chronic discharge of pus through a perforation in the ear drum, and there is often some obvious loss of hearing present. The causative bacteria include those mentioned above for acute otitis media, especially *Staph. aureus* and *Strep. pneumoniae*, but Gram-negative bacilli are also important, such as *Proteus* spp., *Pseudomonas aeruginosa* and *Bacteroides* spp.

b. Other suppurative complications

These include mastoiditis, detected by tenderness or swelling behind the pinna, meningitis and otogenic brain abscess.

c. *Secretory otitis media ('glue ear')*

This condition may follow a previous attack of acute otitis media but sometimes the aetiology is uncertain. Characteristically, there is an effusion present in the middle ear, which is serous or mucinous, and there is fluctuating hearing loss. A persistent effusion may require drainage by performing a myringotomy and the insertion of a grommet may be indicated. Recurrent attacks of 'glue ear' may occur.

Otitis Externa

Clinical features include irritation in the outer ear and a scanty discharge. Infective causes include:

Staph. aureus	Bacterial
Proteus spp.	Bacterial
Pseudomonas aeruginosa	Bacterial
Aspergillus niger	Fungal
Candida albicans	Fungal

Recurrent superficial infections are common. Rarely, a 'malignant otitis externa' may occur in elderly diabetic patients associated with a deep infection of the cartilage and bone of the outer ear due to *Pseudomonas aeruginosa.*

Culture of an ear swab for bacterial and fungal organisms is desirable. Topical treatment with ear drops containing polymyxin or other antibiotics can be given according to the results of culture and antibiotic sensitivities. However, repeated topical application of antibiotics can result in the selection of antibiotic-resistant strains and agents such as neomycin are contraindicated if a perforated ear drum is present.

Acute Sinusitis

Clinical features include periodic facial pain and localized tenderness over the affected sinus. If the maxillary antrum is affected, a failure to trans-illuminate clearly may be demonstrated.

Causative organisms

These include the same three main bacteria that cause acute otitis media, but *Haemophilus influenzae* and *Strep. pneumoniae* appear to be much more frequent causes than *Strep. pyogenes.* Also many other organisms may cause sinusitis including anaerobes, viridans streptococci, *Staph. aureus* and viruses.

Microbiological investigation

Gram-stain microscopy and culture of pus aspirated from the affected sinus often reveals the causative bacteria and antibiotic sensitivities may help guide subsequent treatment.

Antibiotic treatment

Initial treatment with parenteral ampicillin followed by large doses of oral amoxycillin is recommended as 'blind' treatment for severe cases. Alternative drugs that may be effective include erythromycin or cotrimoxazole. If an anaerobe is isolated from the sinus fluid, metronidazole may be indicated.

Complications

Chronic sinusitis is the most frequent complication. Complications of osteomyelitis, meningitis or cerebral abscess may rarely develop especially in patients with frontal sinusitis.

Other Upper Respiratory Tract Infections

Acute epiglottitis and some other respiratory tract infections that mainly affect children are included in Chapter 8.

EYE INFECTIONS

Normal Flora

The conjunctiva is often lightly colonized with *Staph. epidermidis* and diphtheroids. Lysozyme and IgA present in lacrimal secretions help to protect the eye against infections.

Causative Organisms

1. Conjunctivitis, keratitis and cataract

a. Bacteria

Neisseria gonorrhoeae. Severe purulent conjunctivitis due to a gonococcus from the mother's genital tract classically occurs on the first or second day of life—ophthalmia neonatorum. Unless this is promptly treated, corneal damage may occur resulting in blindness in later life. Prophylaxis with silver nitrate eye drops is not indicated today.

Staphylococcus aureus. 'Sticky eye' in neonates due to *Staph. aureus* conjunctivitis usually occurs 5–10 days after birth. Sometimes this is associated with an outbreak of staphylococcal sepsis in a maternity unit. In later life autogenous infection can develop, the staphylococcus having been introduced into the eye from the patient's nose or skin by his/her fingers.

Haemophilus influenzae. Conjunctival infection due to *Haemophilus* can develop at any age, sporadically or as part of an outbreak.

Neisseria meningitidis
Streptococcus pneumoniae } rare causes of severe purulent conjunctivitis

Pseudomonas aeruginosa is an opportunist cause of serious eye infection following trauma to the eye, the presence of a foreign body or operations on the eye. It may also occur when there is a defective immune response in a patient. This organism rarely causes harm to the healthy conjunctivae. Invasion of the eye and blindness can result as complications of the infection. Sources of *Pseudomonas* include contaminated multi-dose containers of eye drops, wet nail brushes and soap dishes. Prevention of infection involves use of single dose containers of sterile solutions and the elimination of other potential sources in the wards, theatre and eye out-patient department.

Treponema pallidum. Interstitial keratitis may develop as part of the congenital syphilis syndrome leading to blindness.

Leptospira. Conjunctivitis can occur as part of Weil's disease (*see* p. 406).

b. *Chlamydia*

'*Chlamydia trachomatis*'. Can cause trachoma inclusion conjunctivitis (TRIC) as a congenital infection in developed countries or trachoma in certain underdeveloped countries.

Congenital trachoma inclusion conjunctivitis is characterized by a follicular kerato-conjunctivitis developing 4–7 days after birth.

Chlamydia is an intracellular organism that requires at least a couple of cycles of reproduction, each lasting about 48 hours for a sufficient number of epithelial cells to be damaged to cause a clinically evident lesion. TRIC can also occur in later life, sometimes contracted in swimming pools. Often the infection is mild but severe kerato-conjunctivitis occasionally occurs and may result in corneal damage.

Trachoma is endemic in several African countries and the Middle East. The chlamydia organisms are spread from eye to eye by hands and a chronic follicular kerato-conjunctivitis occurs particularly involving the upper tarsal conjunctivae. In the later stages, a cicatricial entropion develops with inturned eye lashes which abrade the cornea. Secondary bacterial infection is common amongst these overcrowded and unhygienic conditions and this also contributes to the corneal scarring and development of blindness. More cases of blindness are due to *Chlamydia trachomatis* than to any other cause.

c. *Viruses*

Rubella. The virus is contracted during intra-uterine life and may cause congenital eye lesions, including cataracts (*see* p. 120).

Adenoviruses. Sporadic cases or outbreaks of non-purulent conjunctivitis may be caused by various adenoviruses often in association with pharyngitis. Occasionally the cornea is also infected.

Epidemic kerato-conjunctivitis, due to adenovirus type 8, is particularly associated with factories ('Shipyards eye') or hospitals where dust particles or manipulations on the eye (especially with a tonometer) can cause sufficient trauma to predispose to this viral infection.

Herpes simplex. An initially superficial corneal 'dendritic' ulcer may result from herpes simplex keratitis. This is more likely to occur in debilitated or immunosuppressed patients and the ulcer may extend and cause serious corneal damage, particularly when steroids are administered.

Varicella-zoster. The ophthalmic division of the trigeminal nerve is frequently involved with varicella-zoster and conjunctivitis is sometimes a presenting feature.

Vaccinia. Smallpox vaccination is only rarely necessary nowadays, so accidental inoculation of the eye with the vaccine is less likely to occur than in the past. Emergency prophylaxis involving treatment with methisazone and immunoglobin may be advised by a clinical virologist whose advice should be sought immediately.

d. Fungi

Fusarium, Candida and *Aspergillus* species may very rarely cause corneal ulcers with serious consequences. These infections may occur in some immunosuppressed patients or may follow operations on the cornea in immunologically normal patients.

e. Worms

In parts of Africa near freshwater rivers, *Onchocerca volvulus*, a filarial worm spread by a simulian fly, may be endemic and affected patients can develop a keratitis and other eye lesions which may cause 'river blindness' in later life (*see* p. 456).

Loa loa, another filarial helminth found in Africa, can involve the eye and cause serious eye lesions. Often no eye damage occurs but the worm crosses the eye deep to the conjunctiva (*see* p. 456).

2. Eyelid infections

Staphylococcus aureus is the main cause of eyelid infections: blepharitis, 'styes', are infections of the eyelash follicles.

3. Orbital and inner eye infections

A cellulitis of the skin around the eye or a spreading infection from adjacent sinuses can cause orbital cellulitis with possible further dangerous complications of inner eye infection or cavernous sinus thrombosis. A mixed infection is often present.

Bacterial causes include:

- *Staphylococcus aureus*
- *Streptococcus pyogenes*
- *Streptococcus pneumoniae*
- Diphtheroids
- *Streptococcus viridans*
- Coliforms and *Pseudomonas*
- *Haemophilus influenzae*
- Anaerobic cocci and *Bacteroides*

Endophthalmitis or panophthalmitis can result from spreading orbital cellulitis, progressive ulcerative kerato-conjunctivitis or direct penetrating injuries to the eye complicated by infection, particularly when a foreign body is present. Any of the above bacteria can be involved and pseudomonas infections are particularly difficult to treat effectively.

4. Choroido-retinitis

Viral:	Cytomegalovirus—congenital and acquired (immunosuppressed patients) Rubella—congenital
Protozoa:	*Toxoplasma gondii*
Helminths:	*Toxocara canis* and *catis* A granuloma due to *Toxocara* can be associated with a peripheral eosinophilia. This condition should not be mistaken for malignant retinoblastoma, which may give a similar ophthalmoscopic appearance, otherwise an eye may be unnecessarily enucleated (*see* p. 453).

Microbiology Investigations

1. Conjunctivitis, keratitis and cataract

a. Direct smears and inoculation of plates

Many eye pathogens such as the gonococcus or *Haemophilus* are delicate and special care is necessary to obtain satisfactory specimens for microbiology. Ideally a sterile platinum loop should be used to collect infected material from the conjunctival fornix and then this is immediately streaked onto warm chocolate agar and blood agar plates. This is the best method of culture. Smears for Gram-stain are collected at the same time. The plates are transferred to a moist carbon dioxide incubator and results are often available the following day.

A small serum-coated cotton-wool swab can be used instead of a loop to make direct smears and immediate inoculation of culture plates. Great care is necessary to avoid contamination of the swab with the skin flora of the eyelids during collection of the specimen.

b. Swab in Stuart's transport medium for bacterial cultures

If direct inoculation of the plates is impractical then the swab must be placed in appropriate transport medium. Dry swabs are of limited value for culture but may be useful for a Gram-stain. Both swabs should be sent promptly to the laboratory.

c. Conjunctival scrapings and cultures for Chlamydia

Superficial pus should be removed with a swab moistened in sterile saline and scrapings collected for Giemsa, iodine or fluorescent antibody stains to look for the characteristic chlamydial inclusion bodies in the epithelial cells.

Culture for *Chlamydia* is possible in some centres and the swab should first be placed in chlamydia transport medium. Treatment of clinically suspected chlamydial lesions should be started after collection of the swab without waiting for the results of culture.

d. Swab for virus isolation

When viral conjunctivitis is suspected clinically, particularly in outbreaks of infection, it may be advisable to do some virology investigations. These investigations are also indicated when a serious viral keratitis lesion is suspected.

i. A swab of the eye lesion is put into viral transport medium.
ii. A throat swab should also be collected and placed in viral transport medium, particularly when pharyngitis is also present and adenovirus infection is suspected.

e. *Mycological investigations*

Suitable scrapings should be collected by an ophthalmologist for microscopy and culture on Sabouraud's medium.

f. *Serology and blood films*

Syphilis and rubella serological tests are indicated when congenital lesions of the cornea or lens are suspected. Serology for filarial diseases may be rarely indicated in patients with suspected loiasis or onchocerciasis. Blood films to demonstrate the microfiliariae in these patients and skin snips may be helpful (*see* p. 323, Chapter 16 and p. 457, Chapter 23).

2. Eyelid infections

Swabs of eyelid lesions are not routinely indicated.

When recurrent 'styes' are causing a problem a nose swab as well as a swab of the lesion should be taken. If carriage of the same strain of *Staph. aureus* is demonstrated then it is possible that autogenous infection is occurring and a course of chlorhexidine nasal cream may be of value.

3. Orbital and inner eye infections

a. Blood cultures
b. Pus or swabs of discharging lesions of the eye for microscopy and culture

4. Choroido-retinitis

Serology for:

a. Rubella HAI antibodies—if IgM is positive this indicates congenital infection
b. CMV IgM fluorescent antibody tests are also necessary if the CFT is positive
c. Toxoplasma Dye Test
d. Toxocara fluorescent antibody test

Antimicrobial Treatment

1. Conjunctivitis and keratitis

The choice of initial therapy after the collection of specimens depends on the clinical clues as to the likely infecting organisms. In serious cases, the result of an urgent Gram-stain may be of help. Subsequent treatment depends on the results of culture and sensitivities. Chloramphenicol ointment should not be used in infection with *Chlamydia* or gonococci is suspected. Gonococcal conjunctivitis should be promptly treated locally and systemically with benzylpenicillin. Cefuroxime may be indicated when penicillinase-producing gonococcal strains are isolated.

Chlamydial conjunctivitis responds to tetracycline ointment and, in severe cases, systemic erythromycin is also indicated.

When herpes simplex keratitis is suspected local idoxuridine ointment is usually indicated. If there is an insufficient response, other agents such as acycloguanosine may be tried depending on the advice of the microbiologist and ophthalmologist.

Vaccinial lesions should be treated with topical idoxuridine and systemic antivaccinal immunoglobulin (oral methisazone may also be necessary).

2. Eyelid infections

Eyelid staphylococcal infections sometimes require surgical drainage and local neomycin ointment.

Systemic antibiotics like flucloxacillin should only be given in addition if the lesion is severe or associated with spread of infection constituting a risk of cavernous sinus thrombosis.

3. Orbital and inner eye infections

After the collection of specimens, 'blind' systemic treatment with benzylpenicillin, cloxacillin and gentamicin may be indicated. If there is doubtful allergy to penicillin, a cephalosporin may be used instead of penicillin plus cloxacillin. Erythromycin plus gentamicin may be given to a patient with a definite history of penicillin allergy.

Surgical intervention and local antibiotic therapy, depending on the results of culture and sensitivity, are also often necessary.

4. Choroido-retinitis

Unfortunately toxoplasma eye lesions often do not respond well to pyrimethamine and sulphonamide which might be tried in some cases.

Toxocariasis can be treated by diethylcarbamazine, but the eye lesions may not be affected.

Further Reading

Editorial (1978) Glue ear and grommets. *Br. Med. J.* **2**, 1247.

Editorial (1981) Secretory otitis media and grommets. *Br. Med. J.* **282**, 501.

Garrod L. P., Lambert H. P. and O'Grady F. (1981) Infections of the eye. In: *Antibiotic and Chemotherapy*, 5th ed. Edinburgh, Churchill Livingstone.

Ludman H. (1980) ABC of E.N.T.—pain in the ear. *Br. Med. J.* **281**, 1538.

Ludman H. (1981) ABC of E.N.T.—throat infections. *Br. Med. J.* **282**, 628.

Chapter 12

Infections of the lower respiratory tract

NORMAL FLORA OF THE LOWER RESPIRATORY TRACT

Host defence mechanisms normally remove any microbes which transiently invade the bronchial tract or lung alveoli in healthy people. These mechanisms, which normally keep the lower respiratory tract sterile, include mechanical clearance of microbes by the upward movement of mucus produced by the ciliated epithelium of the tracheo-bronchial tract, phagocytosis by polymorphs and macrophages, and the local production of lysozyme, interferon and secretory IgA.

The bronchial tract may become persistently colonized by organisms, including *Haemophilus influenzae* and *Strep. pneumoniae*, when the host defence mechanisms are defective because of damage to the bronchial tract or lungs, due, for example, to advanced chronic bronchitis. The patient is then predisposed to developing recurrent or severe lower respiratory tract infections.

ACUTE TRACHEO-BRONCHITIS

Viruses, such as rhinoviruses, influenza or para-influenza viruses, cause most acute infections of the trachea or bronchi. Secondary bacterial infection may occasionally follow, especially by *Strep. pneumoniae* or *Haemophilus influenzae*. *Staph. aureus* is a possible but infrequent secondary infecting organism. Microbiological investigations are not usually indicated.

Antibiotic treatment of secondary bacterial infection with either ampicillin (or amoxycillin), cotrimoxazole or erythromycin is usually satisfactory. When there has been a recent influenza epidemic ampicillin (or amoxycillin) might not be suitable if there is secondary infection by penicillinase-producing strains of *Staph, aureus*.

INFECTIVE EXACERBATIONS OF CHRONIC BRONCHITIS

Microbial Causes

Viruses often cause acute infective exacerbations of chronic bronchitis, particularly rhino- and para-influenza viruses, in chronic bronchitic patients who have young children living in their homes. Occasionally, the viral infection becomes complicated by secondary bacterial infection.

Bacterial causes of infective exacerbations are relevant when chronic bronchitic patients produce muco-purulent sputum (yellow or green sputum) instead of the usual mucoid sputum. *Haemophilus influenzae* is probably the most important bacterial cause (*Table 12.1*). This organism may sometimes be isolated in small numbers from an early morning mucoid sputum sample and in these

Table 12.1. Microbial cause of infective exacerbations of chronic bronchitis

	Chronic bronchitis cases	
Organism	*Early disease*	*Advanced disease*
Haemophilus influenzae	+ + + +	+ + + +
Strep. pneumoniae	+ + +	+ + +
Viruses	+ +	+ +
Mycoplasma pneumoniae	+	+
Staph. aureus		+
Coliforms (some resistant to ampicillin and other antibiotics)		+
Pseudomonas		+
Non-sporing anaerobes		+

+ + + + Very common cause.
+ + + Common cause.
+ + Frequent cause.
+ Occasional cause.

circumstances may only indicate colonization. The indirect evidence that *Haemophilus influenzae* is also a major cause of infective exacerbations includes the following:

i. The purulence of sputum is strongly associated with large numbers of *H. influenzae* in sputum.
ii. The purulence decreases with antibiotic treatment appropriate for *H. influenzae*.
iii. Clinical improvement usually coincides with the eradication of *H. influenzae*.
iv. Serum precipitins to *H. influenzae* (H_1 and H_2, after absorption) are present in high titre in 70% patients with muco-purulent chronic bronchitis compared with 8% controls.

Strep. pneumoniae and other bacteria may also cause infective exacerbations (*Table 12.1*). Patients with advanced disease have often had repeated courses of antibiotics and may therefore become infected by antibiotic-resistant strains of bacteria, such as *Haemophilus* strains resistant to ampicillin or cotrimoxazole, *Klebsiella* (resistant to ampicillin) and *Pseudomonas* (resistant to several antibiotics).

Microbiological Investigations

Most patients with infective exacerbations of chronic bronchitis do not need any microbiological investigations since the two main bacterial pathogens are *Haemophilus influenzae* and *Strep. pneumoniae* and their antibiotic susceptibility patterns are reasonably predictable. Also, it is usually impractical for suitable sputum specimens to be sent to the laboratory promptly from patients seen in general practice.

Investigations may be worthwhile in a few patients with advanced disease who develop severe infective exacerbations. These patients may be at risk of developing serious pneumonia due to one of the less frequent and also antibiotic-resistant pathogens. They are often admitted to hospital and then the collection of sputum, preferably before the start of antibiotics, is easily arranged (*see also* Sputum microbiology, in Pneumonia *below*).

Treatment

Patients with chronic bronchitis are best given some antibiotics to keep at home and instructed to start a course as soon as the sputum becomes purulent. For most patients, one of the following courses would be expected to be effective for treating infective exacerbations due to *H. influenzae* or *Strep. pneumoniae*:

i. Ampicillin (before meals), 500 mg, 6-hourly, orally for 5–7 days, OR
   Amoxycillin, 250–500 mg, 8-hourly, orally for 5–7 days
ii. Cotrimoxazole (before meals), 2 tablets, b.d., for 5–7 days
iii. Oxytetracycline (before meals, not with milk which reduces its absorption), 250 mg, 6-hourly, orally for 5–7 days, OR
   Doxycycline, orally, 100 mg, once daily

When there is a history of possible penicillin allergy, tetracycline or cotrimoxazole can be given. Oral cephalosporins such as cephalexin or cephradine are not very active against many *H. influenzae* strains although cefaclor is reasonably active. Erythromycin is only moderately active against *H. influenzae*, and its place in the treatment of infective exacerbations is uncertain; it may have a special use for treating 'persisters' after ampicillin is given.

Patients with advanced disease who have a severe infective exacerbation should have sputum microbiology performed before prompt 'blind' antibiotics are started. In this situation, parenteral ampicillin, 1 g, 6-hourly, intramuscularly (or intravenous cotrimoxazole) may be indicated. A few patients may not respond to the initial chemotherapy because of antibiotic resistance to the drug selected. Cefuroxime is another alternative which, unlike ampicillin, would also be active against penicillinase-producing *Staph. aureus* strains. Cefuroxime and cefamandole are recently developed parenteral cephalosporins which are highly active against *H. influenzae* strains including the few ampicillin-resistant strains. The dosage usually recommended for cefuroxime is 750 mg, 8-hourly, intra-muscularly or intravenously.

Prevention

Patients are generally advised not to smoke, to avoid going out in cold or foggy weather and to have influenza immunizations.

Those patients who develop frequent infective exacerbations each winter may be given continuous chemoprophylaxis in the winter months, especially if they have advanced chest disease. Ampicillin is not usually recommended for this purpose because of the possible development of gastro-intestinal or other side effects. Oxytetracycline, 250 mg, 6-hourly, or 500 mg, b.d., orally may reduce the number of infective exacerbations when given continuously during the winter months. However, in areas where there is a high incidence of tetracycline resistance in *Strep. pneumoniae* or *H. influenzae* strains this drug should not be given. Cotrimoxazole, 2 tablets, b.d., may also be useful as continuous prophylaxis for up to 3 months, but a few patients may develop skin rashes or rarely haematological complications.

The best course of action for most patients with severe chronic bronchitis is to start a suitable 5-day course of antibiotic (*see* Treatment *above*) within 24 hours of developing purulent sputum. Continuous prophylaxis should probably only be considered for a small minority of patients where the latter approach has proved unsuccessful.

INFLUENZA

Causative Organisms

Myxoviruses—Influenza A, B and C (*see Fig. 12.1*).

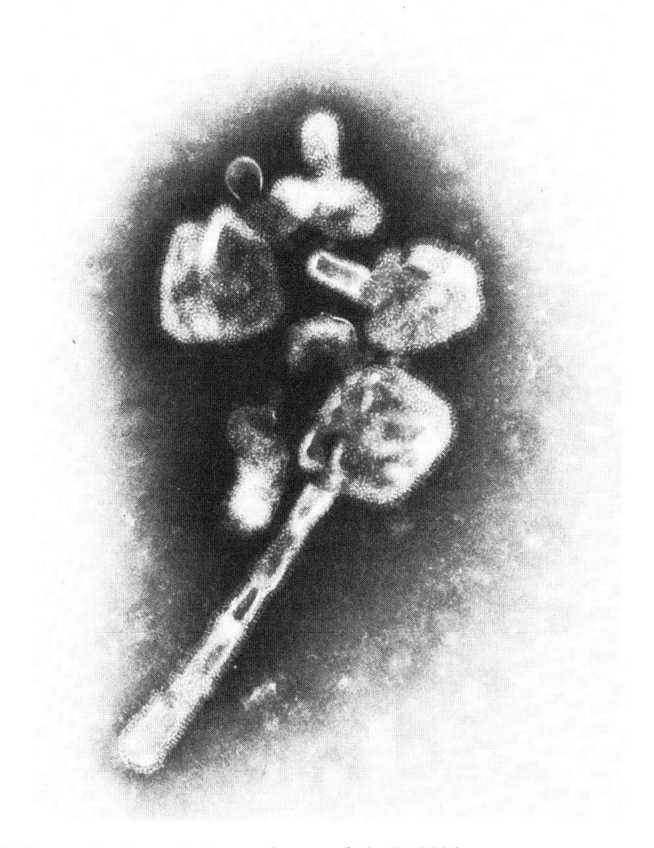

Fig. 12.1. Influenza A virus, electron micrograph.(× 86 000.)

Epidemiology

Influenza remains an unconquered infectious disease and its epidemiological characteristics are difficult to predict accurately.

Influenza A

Pandemics due to 'new' influenza A virus strains that show major antigenic change (antigenic 'shift') in the haemagglutinin (H) and neuraminidase (N) surface antigens occur approximately every 10 years. The major antigenic 'shifts' in influenza A viruses have been:

1945–1957 H_1N_1 influenza A viruses
1957–1968 H_2N_2 influenza A viruses (Asian influenza/57)
1968–1980s H_3N_2 influenza A viruses (Hong Kong/68)

Influenza A viruses mainly affect man but may also cause infection in a wide range of mammals and birds; new strains might emerge during passage between mammals, birds and dense human populations in China or Asia. When antigenic shift occurs, the pandemic lasts from about 1 month to 4 months and, thereafter, a smaller number of cases occur during the subsequent years. Minor changes in the surface antigens, known as antigenic 'drift', occur every year and vary slightly in different parts of the world. Examples of current H_3N_2 influenza A viruses that may cause infection in Britain include A/Texas/1/77 and A/Bangkok/1/79.

H_1N_1 influenza A viruses unexpectedly caused a fresh outbreak of infection around the world in 1977–1979 after an absence of about 20 years. Patients affected were mainly young people under the age of 26 years who had no immunity to the H_1N_1 type. This re-emergence of H_1N_1 viruses first occurred in 1977 in China and then affected Russia and Europe from 1978 to 1979 ('Russian' influenza). During 1980–1981 some patients were still having influenza due to the H_1N_1 strain such as the A/U.S.S.R./90/77 strain or the A/Brazil/11/78 variant. Small influenza A epidemics usually occur each year or every other year mainly during the winter months.

Influenza B

Influenza B viruses cause small epidemics, usually of mild influenza, every 2–3 years in institutions, affecting mainly children and young people. Minor 'drift', and rarely 'shift', occurs amongst the surface antigens of influenza B viruses. Current influenza B virus strains in Britain include the B/Singapore/222/79 variant and the antigenically slightly different previous B/Hong Kong virus strains of 1972.

Influenza C

Influenza C viruses cause mild sporadic infection only.

Mode of Transmission

All the influenza viruses are transmitted by respiratory droplets during sneezing or coughing and during close contact. Like other respiratory viruses, they can probably be spread by the hands or by fomites contaminated by respiratory secretions from a patient. Spread may be rapid amongst susceptible individuals.

Incubation Period and Pathogenesis

The incubation period is 1–3 days. The virus multiplies in the epithelium of the upper and lower respiratory tract damaging the ciliated mucosa of the trachea and bronchi. The multiplication stimulates the production of interferon, local IgA and systemic serum antibodies which are active against the haemagglutinin and other surface antigens of influenza virus. These latter defence mechanisms gradually help the patient to overcome the infection. In a few patients, the virus may directly infect the alveoli and cause an intense rapidly fatal alveolitis.

Clinical Features

Classically 'flu' has an abrupt onset with fever, headache, malaise and cough. The cough is usually non-productive and associated with acute tracheitis or bronchitis. There may also be muscle aches, loss of appetite and a sore throat. Symptoms usually subside within 4 days but there may be tiredness and some depression for a few days afterwards. A great majority of influenza illnesses are due to influenza A viruses.

Complications

Secondary bacterial infection frequently complicates influenza in the elderly or those with previous chest disease, including patients with chronic bronchitis although it may also occur in previously healthy young people. The main bacterial pathogens are *Staph. aureus*, *Strep. pneumoniae, Strep. pyogenes* and *Haemophilus influenzae*. Pneumonia due to *Staph. aureus*, or less frequently *Strep. pyogenes*, may be rapidly progressive and can kill a patient within a few days in spite of antibiotic treatment.

Primary influenza virus pneumonia is a less frequent complication than secondary bacterial infection but is even more lethal. The patient's condition can suddenly worsen and typically this is followed by severe respiratory distress and cyanosis. Death may occur within a few hours or within a day of the onset of this complication. The lungs are characteristically congested and oedematous, the tracheo-bronchial ciliated epithelium is desquamated and the mucosa is hyperaemic. Pneumonitis is usually viral without significant bacterial infection.

Other uncommon complications include: myocarditis, pericarditis, encephalitis and polyneuropathy.

Microbiological Diagnosis

Patients with severe influenzal illnesses requiring hospital admission or patients involved in an institutional outbreak of influenza should have specimens collected for virological and bacteriological investigations. A Gram-stain of sputum may give a rapid indication of secondary infection, for example with *Staph. aureus*.

Virological investigations include:

1. Virus isolation and rapid diagnosis

A throat swab, or naso-pharyngeal washing, is collected and transported in viral transport medium and inoculated into monkey kidney tissue. After incubation, the multiplication of a myxovirus in the tissue culture may be indicated by haemabsorption of human group O red cells. An alternative but less frequently used method is inoculation into a chick embryo amniotic cavity. Once a presumptive influenza virus has been isolated, it can be typed using known haemagglutin inhibition antisera.

Rapid virological diagnosis is also possible using direct immunofluorescent techniques on respiratory secretions (or post-mortem material) from the patient.

2. Serology

An acute serum and a convalescent serum collected 10–14 days later are simultaneously tested by an influenza A complement fixation test to detect a greater than four-fold rise in antibody titre. An influenza B complement fixation test is usually carried out at the same time.

An influenza haemagglutination inhibition test may be performed instead of the complement fixation test but this test is strain specific whereas the complement fixation test is group specific (either group A or B influenza). This test is therefore only really applicable during an epidemic due to one known strain of influenza.

Treatment

General measures such as bedrest and aspirin are usually sufficient.

If bacterial complications arise in general practice, prompt treatment with an antibiotic, such as cotrimoxazole, that is active against *Staph. aureus*, *Strep. pneumoniae* and *Haemophilus influenzae* should be given. Patients with severe bacterial complications usually require urgent hospital admission, sputum and blood cultures, and prompt parenteral antibiotics—intravenous high dose cloxacillin and ampicillin—may be necessary.

When a patient is admitted with suspected influenza, isolation of the patient is indicated to prevent spread of infection to others.

Prevention

Immunization against influenza is mainly recommended in patients with known chest or heart disease and in elderly patients. The influenza virus strains included in the killed vaccine should include currently prevalent strains. In 1980–1981, these included strains of influenza A(H_3N_2, H_1N_1) and influenza B. The vaccine is given by subcutaneous or intra-muscular injection, preferably in September to give protection during the winter months. Ideally, a second dose should be given 4–6 weeks after the first dose, especially in younger people with chest disease. This may give up to about 60% protection against influenza. When a new influenza A strain is detected by the World Health Organization (W.H.O.), there may be time to produce a modified recombinant vaccine containing the appropriate protective haemagglutinin antigens before the new strain reaches Europe. Rarely, serious complications of influenza vaccine may occur such as the Guillain-Barré syndrome which followed the use of the 'swine influenza vaccine' in the U.S.A. during the late 1970s.

Adamantadine is an expensive anti-viral drug with activity against influenza A viruses. If given to contacts of a patient with influenza A_2 successful prophylaxis against infection may be achieved.

PARA-INFLUENZA

Para-influenza viruses I–IV usually cause upper respiratory tract infections or tracheitis in adults, of less severity than influenza viruses. These viruses may cause serious lower respiratory tract infections in infants and infections by para-influenza virus type III are specially likely to result in croup in small infants (*see* Chapter 8). The investigation of para-influenza is similar to influenza; serological tests are also available using complement fixation antigens of para-influenza types I and III.

PNEUMONIA

Clinical Features

The characteristic symptoms of pneumonia include cough, pleuritic chest pain and fever. The cough is often non-productive in the early stages of bacterial pneumonia but, subsequently, there is characteristic production of muco-purulent yellow or green sputum. Patients with atypical pneumonia characteristically have a dry cough. Physical signs of pneumonia include diminished movement on the infected side and crepitations. Sometimes an associated pleural effusion is present. The chest radiograph usually shows signs of consolidation but abnormal physical signs and radiological changes may be absent or minimal in the early stages.

Pneumonias due to bacteria are more acute and of greater severity than atypical pneumonias due to *Mycoplasma* or other organisms, but sometimes these causes are indistinguishable clinically. Pulmonary tuberculosis may also occasionally present clinically as an acute pneumonia.

Clinical Clues to the Causative Organisms

The following factors need to be considered:

a. General practice or hospital patient?

Streptococcus pneumoniae is by far the most frequent cause of pneumonia in both general practice and hospital patients (*Table 12.2*). There are approximately 80 pneumococcal serotypes related to the capsular polysaccharide antigens. *Strep. pneumoniae* type III is an especially virulent organism and is frequently associated with severe pneumonia and bacteraemia. In general practice, pneumococci are the probable cause in at least one-third of patients presenting with pneumonia. Pneumococcal pneumonia is most often seen in association with 'secondary causes' where there is a factor present predisposing to pneumonia, such as old age, impaired respiratory defences against infection because of previous chest disease, influenza, aspiration of vomit or alcoholism, and chronic hepatic or renal disease. However, pneumococci may also cause 'primary' pneumonias in previously healthy people. In the past, classical pneumococcal

Table 12.2. Causes of pneumonia acquired outside or inside hospital

Types of pneumonia	*General practice patient*		*Hospital patient (nearly all 'secondary')*
	'Primary'★	*'Secondary'*†	
1. *Bacterial pneumonias*, e.g.			
Strep. pneumoniae	Common	Common	Common
Staph. aureus	Rare	Occasional	Occasional (o)
Haemophilus influenzae	Rare	Occasional	Occasional (o)
Coliforms, e.g. *Klebsiella*	Rare	Rare	Occasional (o)
Pseudomonas aeruginosa	—	Rare	Occasional (o)
Anaerobes, e.g. *Bacteroides*	—	Rare	Occasional (o)
2. *Legionnaires' disease*			
Legionella pneumophila	Rare	Occasional	Rare (o)
3. *Tuberculosis*			
Mycobacterium tuberculosis	Rare	Occasional	Rare (o)
4. *Primary atypical pneumonia*			
Mycoplasma pneumoniae	Common	Occasional	Rare
Chlamydia B (psittacosis)	Occasional	Rare	Rare
Coxiella burnetti (Q fever)	Rare	Rare	Rare
5. *Viruses*			
Influenza A	Rare	—	—
Respiratory syncytial virus	Rare		
Para-influenza viruses	Rare		
Adenoviruses	Rare		
Measles	Rare	Rare (o)	Rare (o) (except outbreaks)
Varicella-zoster	Rare	Rare (o)	
6. *Other viruses, protozoa, fungi and worms*	—	Rare (o)	Rare (o)

(o) Includes 'opportunistic infections'.
★ Patients who are previously healthy.
† Patients who are debilitated, elderly or have some specific predisposing factor for pneumonia.

lobar pneumonia was common and this was followed by either 'crisis' or 'lysis'. Recovery after a pneumococcal lobar pneumonia was followed by immunity to the infecting capsular serotype, but a fatal pneumococcal pneumonia could subsequently occur due to a different serotype. This classical type of lobar pneumonia is very uncommon today compared with broncho-pneumonia which is also most often caused by the pneumococcus. Complications of pneumococcal pneumonia include empyema and meningitis. Death most often occurs in elderly and debilitated patients.

Staphylococcus aureus is more likely to cause pneumonia in hospital patients, except when there is an influenza epidemic in the general community. It is also an important secondary cause of pneumonia in heroin addicts and in infants with rare congenital disorders of the host defences, such as chronic granulomatous disease. Complications include multiple lung abscesses, empyema and septicaemia. Death may occur rapidly in patients who have had recent influenza.

Haemophilus influenzae (non-capsulated) strains, often mixed with *Strep. pneumoniae*, are occasional causes of secondary pneumonia in chronic bronchitic patients.

Coliforms or *Pseudomonas* are only rare causes of pneumonia in general practice patients, and are mainly seen in alcoholic patients who have aspirated vomit. In hospital patients they may occasionally be important causes (*see* Intensive care unit and other relevant sections, in Chapters 24 and 6). In the U.S.A., 'Friedländer's *Klebsiella* is an important primary cause of pneumonia in patients outside hospital but this is rare in Britain.

Anaerobes, usually mixed with other organisms either from the upper respiratory tract or from the intestine, may contribute in the cause of severe aspiration pneumonia and also of pneumonia in patients who have an obstructive cause such as an inhaled foreign body (e.g. a peanut).

Other important causes of pneumonia in general practice include the causes of primary atypical pneumonia, especially *Mycoplasma pneumoniae* and *Chlamydia psittaci* and also *Legionella pneumophila*, the cause of Legionnaires' disease. The characteristic clinical features of atypical pneumonia include unproductive cough and remittent fever, without marked physical signs in the chest. The blood count shows no leucocytosis whereas in many cases of bacterial pneumonia there is a leucocytosis present. The chest radiograph usually shows patchy consolidation.

Tuberculosis may rarely present as acute pneumonia and this is most frequent in immigrants or elderly men.

Viruses are rarely the primary cause of pneumonia and when they do cause pneumonia, it is mainly in infants or immunocompromised patients.

b. Age

Strep. pneumoniae is an important bacterial cause of pneumonia at all ages but is overwhelmingly the predominant causative organism in elderly patients. The mortality rate of pneumococcal pneumonia is greatest in patients over 70 years old. *Staph. aureus* is also an important but uncommon cause in infants.

Mycoplasma pneumoniae is a common cause of pneumonia in children and young people.

Legionella pneumophila is most often a cause of serious pneumonia in patients over 45 years old.

Haemophilus influenzae, Pittman capsular type b, is a rare cause of pneumonia and mainly occurs in infants.

Viruses such as respiratory syncytial virus, para-influenza viruses or adenoviruses are frequent causes of pneumonitis in infants. (*See also* Respiratory infections and Childhood fevers, in Chapter 8.)

Chlamydia trachomatis, which may be acquired by an infant from an infected mother during birth, has mainly been reported in the U.S.A. as causing pneumonia in the neonatal period.

c. Occupation and pets

Previous recent close contact with birds, such as turkeys, ducks, parrots and budgerigars, should raise the possibility of ornithosis or psittacosis. However, a history of recent contact with birds is only obtained in about one-third of affected patients.

Contact with cattle or sheep, or drinking unpasteurized milk, should raise the possibility of Q fever. If the patient's occupation involves handling a lot of raw meat or animal products, Q fever should be considered.

A microbiology worker who develops pneumonia may have acquired psittacosis or tuberculosis while handling sputum specimens.

If the patient works with air-conditioning apparatus, such as evaporative condensers or cooling towers, humidifier or shower apparatus, the possibility of Legionnaires' disease should be strongly considered.

d. The geography and season

Patients who have developed a 'flu'-like illness leading to pneumonia during or soon after a recent visit to a hotel in Benidorm, Spain, or other warm holiday resorts, may have Legionnaires' disease.

Legionnaires' disease is endemic in Britain, but appears to be most frequently acquired in the summer months whereas pneumococcal pneumonias most often occur in winter. Certain cities such as Nottingham and others in the North of England and Scotland appear to have a greater incidence of Legionnaires' disease than cities in South East England, such as London.

e. Unresolving pneumonia

Patients who have already been given some antibiotic therapy and who have an 'unresolving' pneumonia may not have received optimal antibiotic treatment. For example, tetracycline may have been given for pneumonia which was due to a tetracycline-resistant strain of pneumococcus, but there are other possible causes including:

i. *Primary atypical pneumonias*
These would not respond to penicillin, ampicillin or cephalosporins, for example. The causative organisms include *Mycoplasma pneumoniae,* psittacosis agent and *Coxiella burnetii.* These atypical pneumonias may respond to tetracyclines or possibly erythromycin.

ii. *Legionnaires' disease*
This may not respond to treatment with beta-lactam antibiotics or aminoglycosides but might respond to erythromycin or tetracycline.

iii. *Secondary infection associated with an obstructed respiratory tract*
Bacterial infection associated with a blocked bronchus due for example to an inhaled foreign body or a carcinoma of the bronchus.

iv. *Tuberculosis*
This is especially possible in immigrants, elderly males and immunocompromised patients.

f. Opportunistic conditions

Predisposing factors for opportunistic pneumonias include: severe previous lower respiratory tract disease, serious general debilitation, intensive care unit management, broad spectrum antibiotic therapy, steroids and cytotoxic drug treatments, instrumentation and immunodeficiency diseases.

Causative organisms include:

i. Gram-negative bacilli—*Klebsiella*, *Pseudomonas*, *Serratia*, other coliforms, and *Legionella*
ii. Tubercle bacilli
iii. Fungi—*Aspergillus*, *Cryptococcus*, mucor, *Histoplasma*
iv. Viruses—cytomegalovirus, varicella-zoster, herpes simplex, measles
v. Protozoa—*Pneumocystis carinii*
vi. Worms—*Strongyloides*

(*See* Chapters 24 and 6.)

Microbiological Investigations of Pneumonia

Investigations are indicated in all patients with severe pneumonia.

Collection and transport of specimens

a. Sputum for microscopy culture and antibiotic sensitivities

i. Salivary samples are unsuitable.
ii. Muco-purulent or purulent sputum should be collected before the start of antibiotics.
iii. A physiotherapist can help to collect a good specimen when the patient has difficulty in producing one.
iv. Sputum must reach the laboratory within 2 hours of collection otherwise overgrowth by Gram-negative bacilli may occur. Also, if transport is delayed, probable pathogens, such as *Haemophilus* and *Pneumococcus*, might die.
v. Trans-tracheal aspiration is particularly useful for a diagnosis of anaerobic or other unusual lung infections, as there is less contamination by oral flora. This is more frequently performed in the U.S.A. but not in Britain possibly because of rare complications associated with the procedure. It should probably be used more often for investigation of serious pneumonia.
vi. If bronchoscopy is performed any purulent secretions should be collected.
vii. More invasive techniques may be justified for the investigation of opportunistic lung infections (*see* Chapter 6).

b. Pleural fluid for microscopy culture and antibiotic sensitivities

Collect in a sterile bottle containing citrate for microscopy and in another sterile bottle for culture.

c. Sputum, blood and urine for pneumococcal antigen

These tests for pneumococcal antigen are carried out by immunoelectrophoresis and are especially useful when antibiotics have already been started.

d. Blood cultures

Collect one, or preferably two sets, from all patients with pneumonia before the start of antibiotics.

e. Paired sera

Acute serum should be collected when the patient has been admitted to hospital with pneumonia and convalescent serum 10 days later when primary atypical pneumonia or Legionnaires' disease is suspected. Also, these serological tests are useful when fungal, influenza or cytomegalovirus lung infections are considered. A third serum is collected for legionella fluorescent antibody tests a few weeks later, as occasionally specimens collected earlier in the disease do not show a raised titre.

f. Blood for white blood cell count

Total white blood count and differential film may be useful for distinguishing severe bacterial pneumonias from non-bacterial pneumonias and Legionnaires' disease; the former usually have raised total white count and neutrophilia often greater than 12 000 white cells per mm^3.

g. Cold agglutinins

These are useful when atypical mycoplasma pneumonia is suspected as approximately 50% of patients may give positive results.

Methods of sputum culture

Fresh sputum is cultured after initial homogenization to reduce the risk of sampling errors. A 'dilution' method of sputum culture is preferred to give a semi-quantitative idea of the numbers of organisms present and to dilute out small numbers of mouth commensals, present in a fresh sample. The diluted homogenized sputum specimen is routinely cultured on blood agar and chocolate agar for up to 48 hours in a moist aerobic atmosphere with 5–10% carbon dioxide added.

Interpretation of results

1. When no previous chemotherapy

a. Sputum microscopy and culture

i. *Gram-stain*	rapid results possible
Pneumococcal pneumonia	suggested by numerous Gram-positive diplococci + pus cells (*see Fig. 12.2*)
Staphylococcal pneumonia	suggested by numerous Gram-positive cocci in clusters + pus cells
Gram-negative pneumonia	suggested by numerous Gram-negative bacilli + pus cells in fresh sample

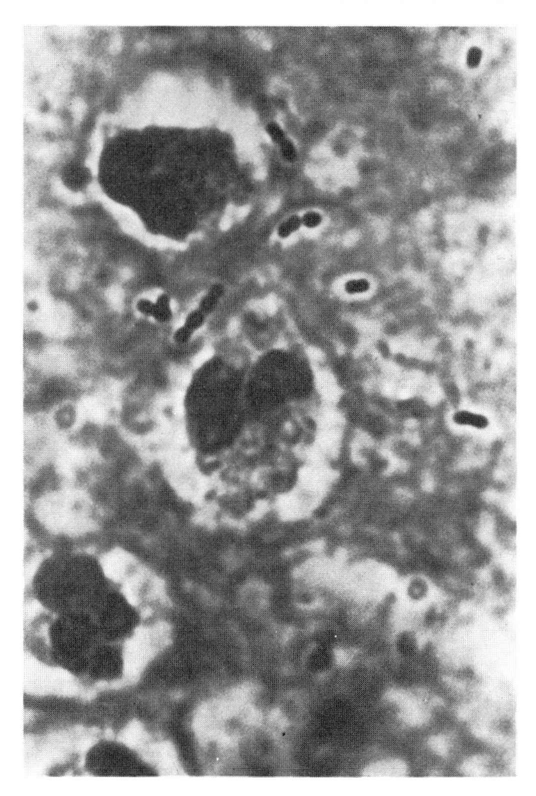

Fig. 12.2. Gram-stained smear of sputum from a patient with pneumococcal pneumonia.

In practice Gram-stain of sputum often only gives equivocal results.

ii. *Culture* — the result is available after 24–48 hours. A heavy predominant growth of pneumococci, staphylococci or *Haemophilus* is likely to be clinically significant

Gram-negative pneumonia: in hospital practice there are frequently delays in transport of sputum. The following points should be checked:

α. that the result is a heavy growth of coliforms, *Klebsiella* or *Pseudomonas* obtained from a fresh sputum specimen collected before antibiotic therapy.

β. that pus cells and many Gram-negative bacilli are apparent in the Gram-stain. However, pus cells may not be present in a trap specimen from some patients in intensive care unit or from specimens from severely neutropenic patients.

The limitations of sputum culture investigations can be summarized as problems due to sampling errors, contamination of sputum by oral flora, overgrowth of Gram-negative bacilli and yeasts especially when there has been previous antibiotics given, and poor survival of some respiratory pathogens in sputum.

b. Blood culture, pleural fluid

Blood cultures are sometimes more valuable than sputum culture. In pneumococcal pneumonia, about 30% of patients may have pneumococci isolated from the blood cultures. When there is staphylococcal, *Haemophilus* or Gram-negative pneumonia, blood cultures frequently yield growth of the causative organism. Pleural fluid is valuable: any organisms seen in the Gram-stain or isolated on culture are likely to be clinically significant.

An immunoelectrophoresis test for pneumococcal antigen can also be included when a pleural fluid specimen is available.

2. When chemotherapy has already been started

a. Sputum microscopy and culture

This is extremely limited in value and highly misleading results may be obtained:

i. Recognized respiratory pathogens may be damaged by the antibiotic increasing the likelihood of negative results for pneumococci, staphylococci or *Haemophilus*.

ii. Gram-negative bacilli—*Klebsiella, Pseudomonas,* coliforms—are common in the saliva of hospital patients and these are selected out by antibiotics to become predominant in the mouth flora that contaminates the sputum specimen.

iii. Candida overgrowth is also common in patients receiving antibiotics—this is nearly always not indicative of candida pneumonia which is exceedingly rare. It more likely reflects colonization or candida infection in the upper respiratory tract.

In rare instances, it is essential to culture sputum samples from patients already receiving antibiotics, especially in intensive care unit patients, but these investigations should only be performed where there is close collaboration between the clinician and microbiologist.

b. Blood culture

Blood cultures are almost always negative when collected from patients with pneumonia already receiving antibiotics.

c. Microbial antigen tests by counter-current immunoelectrophoresis on sputum, blood and urine

Pneumococcal antigen can often be detected when pneumococci are not found in sputum or blood and this suggests a pneumococcal cause for the pneumonia.

3. Specific serological tests

Rising titres of antibody, four-fold or greater, suggest active infection due to the respective organisms:

a. Complement fixation tests

These are carried out against antigens of *Mycoplasma pneumoniae*, psittacosis organism, *Coxiella burnettii,* influenza A and B.

b. Fluorescent antibody tests

This is carried out against *Legionella pneumophila,* the cause of Legionnaires' disease, using a specific legionella yolk sac antigen and titres greater than 1/128 suggest the diagnosis although preferably a rising antibody titre should also be demonstrated.

Treatment of Pneumonia

1. Blind treatment in general practice

Most adults will need an antibiotic active against pneumococci and if the patient has had chronic bronchitis the antibiotic should also be active against *Haemophilus*. In both situations oral amoxycillin or ampicillin would be suitable (*Table 12.3*). *Staph. aureus* need only usually be considered as a cause during an influenza epidemic and then a combination of amoxycillin and flucloxacillin would be preferable. In patients allergic to penicillin, erythromycin would be a suitable alternative to this combination.

If there is a possibility that the patient may have a mycoplasma pneumonia or a pneumococcal pneumonia, erythromycin is probably the best choice especially in a young person. The duration of treatment suggested is usually 7–10 days.

Patients with severe pneumonia or unresolving pneumonia should be urgently admitted to hospital for microbiological and radiological investigations and prompt parenteral antibiotic therapy.

2. Treatment of a patient who is admitted to hospital with pneumonia

Microbiological investigations can give rapid valuable assistance in the management of a patient with severe pneumonia. An urgent Gram-stain showing large numbers of characteristic Gram-positive diplococci indicates the need for immediate benzylpenicillin injections for pneumococcal infection. Numerous clusters of Gram-positive cocci indicate the need for high dose anti-staphylococcal treatment as well as anti-pneumococcal treatment (benzylpenicillin plus flucloxacillin plus fusidic acid.) Sometimes a positive pneumococcal antigen immunoelectrophoresis result can be obtained from sputum or serum or both within a few hours of admission and this would also indicate the need for benzylpenicillin treatment. However, in the majority of situations, clearcut useful bacteriological information is not available.

Blind treatment of 'primary' pneumonias

A young adult with a moderately severe primary pneumonia can usually be treated satisfactorily with erythromycin to treat possible pneumococcal, mycoplasma and legionella causes. However, it has been suggested that a combination of benzylpenicillin plus intravenous erythromycin should be considered in this situation (*see* Miller, 1981). An older patient with a primary pneumonia can usually be treated by benzylpenicillin alone (to cover pneumococcal infection) provided there has been no likelihood of *Legionella* or of recent influenza or staphylococcal infection. For treatment of pneumonia in children, *see* p. 128.

Blind treatment of 'secondary' pneumonias

An adult with possible secondary pneumonia, for example a chronic bronchitic patient who develops pneumonia after a possible viral infection needs ampicillin (or amoxycillin) plus flucloxacillin to cover pneumococcal, haemophilus and staphylococcal infection. An alternative would be injections of cefuroxime which would also treat these infections. Erythromycin might also be suitable but a few strains of *Haemophilus* might not be fully sensitive to it.

If a patient has aspirated material, then a combination of ampicillin (to treat pneumococcal and haemophilus infection), gentamicin (to treat Klebsiella and other coliform infection) and metronidazole (to treat anaerobic infection) would be advisable. Alternatively cefuroxime plus metronidazole would be suitable.

Blind treatment of pneumonias of 'unknown origin'

For patients admitted with a very severe pneumonia of uncertain cause, an initial combination of high dose intravenous erythromycin lactobionate together with benzylpenicillin plus gentamicin would be reasonable. This would cover infections due to pneumococci (erythromycin and benzylpenicillin), staphylococci (erythromycin plus gentamicin), anaerobic organisms (erythromycin plus penicillin), *Klebsiella* (gentamicin), *Legionella* (erythromycin) and *Mycoplasma* (erythromycin).

Subsequent treatment depends on clinical progress and the results of radiological and microbiological investigations including antibiotic sensitivity test results. If serological tests suggest psittacosis or Q fever as the cause of pneumonia, tetracyclines are usually indicated. Treatment is continued for at least 2–3 days after the patient has become afebrile and for a minimum period of 1 week.

3. Treatment of a patient who develops pneumonia in hospital or who acquires an opportunistic lung infection

Pneumonias that are acquired in hospital may be pneumococcal or staphylococcal, especially in an elderly patient who has recently had an operation. They may also be due to Gram-negative bacilli or a wide range of other organisms. This subject is fully discussed in Chapters 24 and 6.

Prevention of Pneumonia

Prevention of pneumonia in the general population depends on non-specific measures such as a high standard of living with good housing and nutrition, antipollution measures, avoidance of cigarette smoking and of excessive consumption of alcohol.

More specific measures include the immunization of children against pertussis and measles, and immunization of selected patients including those with chronic broncho-pulmonary disease against influenza. The prompt antibiotic treatment of an infective exacerbation of chronic bronchitis is important.

Recently a polyvalent pneumococcal vaccine has been introduced which may prove useful for preventing pneumococcal chest infections in patients with known predisposing factors. This vaccine is still under evaluation.

LEGIONNAIRES' DISEASE

Legionnaires' disease is a newly recognized type of pneumonia due to an unusual Gram-negative bacillus *Legionella pneumophila*. The disease became recognized

Table 12.3. Initial antibiotic therapy of pneumonia (*also see text*)

Likely causative organism	*Antibiotic*	*Dose (adult)*	*Comments*
Streptococcus pneumoniae	Benzylpenicillin	1–2 MU i.m. 6-hourly (first choice)	Almost all strains sensitive to penicillin
	Amoxycillin	500 mg–1 g 8-hourly (second choice)	
	Erythromycin	500 mg o./i.v. 600 mg 6-hourly	*Alternatives if allergy to penicillins present* and when parenteral treatment necessary
	or		
	Cotrimoxazole	2 tablets o. 12- or 8-hourly	
		or	
	or	10 ml infusion i.v. 12-hourly	
	Cefuroxime	750 mg i.m. 6-hourly	
	Tetracycline*	500 mg o. 6-hourly	Many pneumococcal strains resistant to tetracycline in some areas
Staphylococcus aureus	Flucloxacillin	1–2 g o./i.m./i.v. 6-hourly	Penicillinase destroys penicillin and ampicillin but not flucloxacillin—most strains are penicillinase producers
	plus		
	Fusidic acid	500 mg o./i.v. 8-hourly	Fusidic acid is a valuable agent—should not be used alone because resistance may then develop rapidly
	plus		
	Benzylpenicillin	1 MU i.v. 6-hourly	Benzylpenicillin is added in case pneumococcal infection is also present
	Erythromycin	1 g o./i.v. 6-hourly	*Alternatives if allergy to penicillins*
	plus		
	Fusidic acid	500 mg o./i.v. 8-hourly	
	Cefuroxime*	750 mg i.m. 6-hourly	
Haemophilus influenzae	Amoxycillin	500 mg o. 8-hourly (first choice)	*Haemophilus* strains resistant to ampicillin or amoxycillin are rare in adults
	or		
	Ampicillin	500 mg o./i.m./i.v. 6-hourly	
	Cotrimoxazole	2 tablets o. 12- or 8-hourly	*Alternatives if allergy to penicillins* Strains resistant to trimethoprim occasionally occur in bronchitic patients
	Cefuroxime*	750 mg i.m./i.v. 8-hourly	Cefuroxime also useful—when resistance to other agents suspected, especially β-lactamase-producing *H. influenzae* strains in infants

Table 12.3.

Likely causative organism	*Antibiotic*	*Dose (adult)*	*Comments*
Coliforms including *Klebsiella*	Gentamicin† or Cefuroxime	80–120 mg i.m./i.v. 8-hourly or 750 mg–1·5 g i.m./i.v. 8-hourly	Gentamicin assays necessary. Maintenance doses depend on state of renal function
Pseudomonas aeruginosa	Tobramycin plus Carbenicillin	120 mg i.m./i.v. 8-hourly 5 g i.v. infusion 6-hourly	Tobramycin assays necessary. Dose régime influenced by state of renal function
Anaerobic infection	Metronidazole	400 mg o. 8-hourly	
Legionnaires' disease	Erythromycin or Tetracycline	1·5–2·5 g i.v. 6-hourly (first choice) 500 mg o. 6-hourly (second choice)	
Primary atypical pneumonia—*Mycoplasma pneumoniae*	Tetracycline or Erythromycin	500 mg o. 6-hourly 500 mg o. 6-hourly	
Psittacosis agent, *Coxiella burnettii*	Tetracycline	500 mg o. 6-hourly	
Acute tuberculous pneumonia	Rifampicin plus Isoniazid plus Streptomycin	600 mg o. daily 100 mg o. 8-hourly 500 mg i.m. 12-hourly	Ethambutol is an alternative for streptomycin but streptomycin injections may be used initially for an acutely ill case

o., orally.
i.m., intra-muscular.
i.v., intravenous.

*Do not use cefuroxime if definite allergy to penicillin.
†An antibiotic active against pneumococci should also be added, such as erythromycin.

following a large explosive outbreak of febrile illness and pneumonia with many fatalities among war veterans (Legionnaires) who attended their convention in the Bellevue-Stratford Hotel, Philadelphia, U.S.A., during July 1976. The Communicable Disease Center (C.D.C.), Atlanta, isolated the causative Gram-negative bacillus from the lungs of fatal cases. One reason why the organism had not been previously recognized was that it did not appear clearly as a Gram-stainable bacillus in tissues and silver stains were required to see it. After the organism was isolated, using guinea-pigs and chick embryos, it ultimately grew on a special culture medium; Gram-stains of colonies then showed a Gram-negative bacillus.

Epidemiology

Epidemiologically the original Philadelphia outbreak was clearly associated with air-borne spread. The incubation period was about 5 days. There is no evidence of case-to-case spread. Pneumonitis follows the inhalation of air contaminated by water that contains legionella bacilli and people have become infected from contaminated air-conditioning systems and from shower mixers. There have been many outbreaks in the United States, mainly in the summer, and outbreaks have since been recognized in many other parts of the world. Retrospectively, it is clear that the disease has existed for a long time.

In the general population it is probable that *Legionella pneumophila* causes between 1 and 3% of microbiologically undiagnosed pneumonias. Previously fit and young people who have become infected may only suffer a mild disease. Patients who are over 45 years, who smoke many cigarettes, or who have previous chest disease are at most risk of developing severe Legionnaires' disease with a mortality rate of greater than 15%. Men appear to be twice as frequently affected as women and most of the cases are sporadic. Fatal outbreaks of Legionnaires' disease have been described in hotels in Benidorm, Spain, and in hospitals in the U.S.A. and Britain.

Clinical Features

Clinical features of severe Legionnaires' disease include an initial 'flu'-like illness, dry cough, and mental confusion, psychiatric or neurological features in about 50% of patients. By the time the patient is admitted to the hospital, chest radiograph evidence of consolidation is usually apparent (*see Fig. 12.3*). There may be non-distinctive changes only initially, such as bilateral patchy basal consolidation. Occasionally, radiograph changes of lobar pneumonia are seen. A characteristic of the disease radiologically is that the consolidation may affect new areas of lung and rapidly progress, sometimes with the original areas of consolidation disappearing. Frequently, patients have already received antibiotics before admission and, even when they have received high dose ampicillin plus cloxacillin for 48 hours in hospital, there is not any clinical improvement. The general condition may deteriorate rapidly and intensive care unit management becomes necessary, often because of respiratory failure. The patients' conscious state may also deteriorate. Laboratory features include a lymphocyte count of less than $1{\cdot}0 \times 10^9$ per litre, a serum sodium less than 130 mmol per litre, a serum albumin less than 20 g per litre and raised serum aminotransferases. Many organs are characteristically affected by severe Legionnaires' disease.

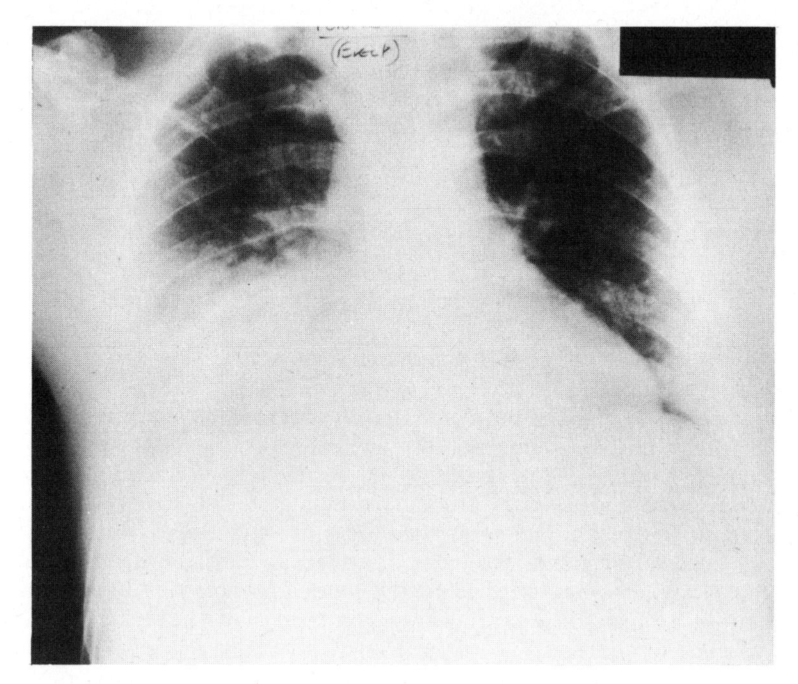

Fig. 12.3. Legionnaires' disease—chest radiograph.

Skeletal muscle is often affected and a raised serum creatine phosphokinase is characteristic. Renal failure and also liver involvement leading to hepatic failure, respiratory failure and cardiovascular collapse may occur.

Microbiological Diagnosis

Specific microbiological diagnosis is usually made by showing a four-fold rising titre of serum immunofluorescent antibody to *Legionella* in paired sera and a titre $\geqslant 1/128$ using specific legionella yolk sac antigen. There are six serotypes of *Legionella* and this yolk sac antigen usually uses serotype I, which is satisfactory for a majority of the cases. Improved culture media have also become available and it may become possible in the future to isolate the organism routinely from blood cultures, bronchial washings, pleural aspirate as well as sputum (when this is produced). However, at the present time, the mainstay of diagnosis is serological and the results are usually not available in time to influence the early management of the patient. In fatal cases, the organism is sometimes seen intracellularly in macrophages in the lungs using silver stains, immunofluorescence or electron microscopy.

Antibiotic Treatment

Erythromycin, tetracycline and rifampicin have greater activity against *Legionella* than many other antibiotics. However, the drug of choice is probably erythromycin and, when Legionnaires' disease is suspected, clinically high doses of erythromycin should be given intravenously, preferably at least 1·5 g 6-hourly in the initial stages. In patients who do not appear to respond to this treatment, the addition of rifampicin should be considered. Treatment should be continued for at least 3 weeks to avoid a relapse.

ASPERGILLUS BRONCHO-PULMONARY DISEASES

Spores of *Aspergillus fumigatus* and other *Aspergillus* species are about 3 μm in diameter and may be inhaled to reach most parts of the lower respiratory tract including the alveoli.

The four main types of aspergillus diseases include:

1. *Asthma*
   Some patients with eosinophils in the sputum have an allergy to *Aspergillus* which may be responsible for the asthma. These patients have a type I (reagin IgE antibody) hypersensitivity response to the *Aspergillus*.
2. *Allergic broncho-pulmonary aspergillosis*
   Spores of *Aspergillus clavatus*, *fumigatus* or other aspergilli reaching the lungs or lower bronchial tract may stimulate an extrinsic allergic bronchio-alveolitis which may be due to a type I and type III hypersensitivity reaction. This condition sometimes occurs in malt workers.
   Clinical features include asthma and chronic cough with sputum production. Recurrent illnesses with low-grade fever and eosinophilia may occur. Bronchi may become obstructed by mucus plugs containing aspergillus hyphae. Bronchiectasis may also occasionally complicate the disease.
3. *Aspergilloma*
   Aspergillus fumigatus, *Aspergillus flavus* or other aspergilli can cause a chronic infection in a damaged area of lung, usually a healed post-tuberculous cavity. The cavity characteristically becomes filled by a ball of fungus known as a mycetoma. On the chest radiograph, the aspergilloma may appear characteristically as a dense opacity with a translucent halo above it. Patients may develop cough and haemoptysis; in a few patients there may be massive bleeding. There is often a type III immune response to the *Aspergillus* with fever and constitutional upset. Occasionally, secondary bacterial infection of the aspergilloma occurs associated with the production of purulent sputum.
4. *Disseminated aspergillosis*
   Invasive lung infection by *Aspergillus* is discussed in Chapter 6.

Microbiological Investigations

Sputum microscopy and culture

Mucous plugs in the sputum stained by silver stains may show the aspergillus hyphae in patients with allergic broncho-pulmonary aspergillosis. Culture of sputum for *Aspergillus* is carried out on Sabouraud's medium, but aspergillus colonies may also sometimes be seen on blood agar cultures. Scanty colonies of aspergilli can occasionally be cultured from the sputum of patients with non-fungal diseases, due to 'contamination' or transient colonization of the upper respiratory tract by small numbers of aspergillus spores. However, *Aspergillus* may be repeatedly isolated from sputum specimens, often in only small amounts, from a patient with an aspergilloma.

Negative fungal cultures of sputum may be obtained in patients with all four types of aspergillus broncho-pulmonary disease.

Serological tests

Aspergillus agar gel precipitin tests are strongly positive in greater than 90% of patients with aspergilloma. There are frequently multiple precipitin lines present.

In allergic broncho-plumonary aspergillosis, positive precipitin lines are obtained in about 75% of patients.

Patients with asthma or disseminated aspergillosis usually have negative or only very weak aspergillus precipitins present.

Skin tests

Skin tests using aspergillus antigens are usually positive in patients with allergic asthma due to *Aspergillus* and in patients with allergic broncho-pulmonary aspergillosis. The skin tests are usually negative in patients with a simple aspergilloma.

Treatment

Treatment of the allergy without the use of anti-fungal drugs is sufficient in patients with asthma or allergic broncho-pulmonary aspergillosis. In the latter condition, long-term steroid treatment is often necessary.

Amphotericin B is not usually indicated in the treatment of aspergilloma unless there is evidence of co-existent dissemination of *Aspergillus*. When problems with massive recurrent haemoptysis arise, surgical resection of the mycetoma may be indicated.

Systemic amphotericin B is necessary for the treatment of disseminated aspergillosis.

FARMER'S LUNG

Clinical Features

This condition predominantly affects male farm workers who have worked with mouldy hay. The characteristic clinical features include episodic attacks of cough and breathlessness occurring several hours after exposure to the hay. Many patients also have wheezy symptoms and may expectorate sputum. Some patients have fevers and generalized aches.

The chest radiograph usually shows scattered nodular shadows and, in advanced cases, fibrosis of the upper lungs may be apparent. Characteristically, there is a reduced vital capacity and impaired gas transfer when respiratory function tests are performed.

Pathogenesis

The disease is caused by an extrinsic allergic alveolitis (type III hypersensitivity reaction) that follows the chronic inhalation of the dust of mouldy hay.

Thermophilic actinomyces, such as *Micropolyspora faeni* and *Thermoactinomyces vulgaris*, multiply in warm moist hay that becomes mouldy. Exposure to mouldy hay is more likely to occur during the winter months when stored hay is used most. Inhalation of the spores of the thermophilic actinomycetes in the dust may occur just on walking into a shed containing the mouldy hay and is then followed by an attack of acute respiratory symptoms.

Microbiological Diagnosis

Serum from about 80% of patients with farmer's lung contains precipitating antibodies to the thermophilic actinomycete antigens.

Treatment and Prevention

There is no specific antimicrobial treatment indicated, but steroids may be necessary in some patients with acute symptoms.

Prevention of further attacks may be possible by avoiding contact with dust from mouldy hay. If hay is kept as dry as possible there is less risk of it becoming mouldy and causing disease.

BRONCHIECTASIS

Bronchiectasis is defined as chronic dilatation of the bronchi. Collections of necrotic material and bronchial secretions in the dilated bronchi may result in inflammation, secondary bacterial infection and fibrosis of an associated area of lung. Recurrent or persistent lower respiratory tract infections are frequent.

Clinical features include cough, occasional haemoptysis and the production of profuse purulent sputum during acute episodes of respiratory infection. The chest radiograph may show cystic changes with fluid levels in patients with gross disease.

Possible causes of bronchiectasis include damaged bronchi from childhood infections such as pertussis, measles or tuberculosis, bronchial obstruction due to the inhalation of a foreign body (such as a peanut in a child), cystic fibrosis, recurrent pulmonary infections associated with hypogammaglobulinaemia, allergic broncho-pulmonary aspergillosis or a rare congenital cause, e.g. Kartagener's syndrome where dextrocardia and sinusitis may be associated with bronchiectasis.

Infections are the main complications of bronchiectasis: infective episodes of bronchitis, recurrent pneumonia, empyema, lung abscess and cerebral abscess. Other complications of severe chronic bronchiectasis include massive haemoptysis, respiratory failure and cor pulmonale, and amyloidosis

Microbiological Investigations

Sputum microscopy and culture during an acute respiratory infection are desirable with fresh sputum collected before antibiotics are started. If there is a severe infection, blood cultures should also be collected.

The sputum should be cultured both aerobically and anaerobically from these patients. The most frequent pathogens isolated include:

1. *Haemophilus influenzae*
2. *Streptococcus pneumoniae*
3. *Staph. aureus*
4. Anaerobes, including *Bacteroides* species and anaerobic cocci
5. 'Coliforms', such as *Klebsiella*, and *Pseudomonas aeruginosa*
6. *Aspergillus fumigatus*, in patients with allergic broncho-pulmonary aspergillosis

Often mixtures of pathogens are demonstrated, such as *Haemophilus* plus pneumococci or coliforms plus anaerobes. Anaerobes are particularly likely to be relevant in patients with gross bronchiectasis who produce putrid sputum.

Treatment

Postural drainage and appropriate physiotherapy is usually necessary to treat severe respiratory infections associated with bronchiectasis.

Rational antibiotic treatment must be based on the results of sputum microscopy, culture and antibiotic sensitivity test results.

Haemophilus influenzae infection usually responds to amoxycillin, 500 mg orally, 6-hourly, but if an ampicillin-resistant strain is isolated, other antibiotics such as tetracycline (or doxycycline), cotrimoxazole or possibly cefuroxime or cefaclor may be suitable instead. Some patients who have had many recurrent haemophilus respiratory infections treated by cotrimoxazole may become infected by cotrimoxazole-resistant strains of *Haemophilus*.

Infections with *Strep. pneumoniae* should be treated by benzylpenicillin (although amoxycillin would also be suitable). When *Staph. aureus* is isolated, flucloxacillin, 500 mg orally, 6-hourly, is appropriate.

Anaerobic infections usually respond to a course of metronidazole but another antibiotic would be necessary at the same time to treat any aerobic pathogens that are also isolated.

Occasionally patients with severe disease and confirmed *Pseudomonas aeruginosa* infections require intravenous tobramycin, plus carbenicillin or another anti-pseudomonas penicillin depending on the results of antibiotic sensitivity tests.

In most instances, a 10-day course of antibiotics is sufficient.

Prevention

Bronchiectasis has become less common since the incidence of childhood infections due to pertussis, and measles has declined in association with routine immunization policy. Effective antibiotic treatment of bacterial chest infections has also helped to prevent this disease.

CYSTIC FIBROSIS

Staph. aureus is the main cause of chest infections in children with cystic fibrosis (*see* Respiratory tract infections, in Chapter 8, p. 128).

Many children survive until adulthood and similar principles of management, as in childhood, continue to be necessary including postural drainage, physiotherapy and antibiotic treatment of each respiratory infection as soon as fresh sputum specimens for culture have been collected. Whenever possible, at least 3 sputum samples should be collected before treatment. In older patients *Pseudomonas aeruginosa* is usually isolated from the sputum as the respiratory tract is often persistently colonized by this organism. *Pseudomonas* may be clinically significant at the time of a worsening infection of the respiratory tract and may require treatment with an aminoglycoside combined with an anti-pseudomonas penicillin but occasionally, however, *Haemophilus* or *Staphylococcus* is mixed with *Pseudomonas* but may not be isolated from the sputum because of technical difficulties. Empirical treatment for staphylococcal or haemophilus infection with flucloxacillin or cotrimoxazole, respectively, may be justified.

Aerosols of antibiotics may have a therapeutic role in certain patients. This method of treatment is still under evaluation.

LUNG ABSCESS

Lung abscess may develop following a localized lung infection due especially to *Staph. aureus* or, rarely, *Klebsiella* species (especially the Friedländer's type of *Klebsiella*). Drug addicts and patients who develop influenza A infections are most often at risk of developing staphylococcal lung infection leading to multiple lung abscesses. Secondary bacterial infection of the lung behind a bronchial obstruction due to a foreign body or neoplasm may rapidly lead to a lung abscess where anaerobes, such as *Bacteroides necrophorus*, become important. *Entamoeba histolytica* is also a rare cause mainly affecting immigrants (amoebic lung abscess).

Clinically the patient may have a swinging pyrexia and respiratory symptoms, but the diagnosis is usually suggested by the typical chest radiograph appearance with cavitated lesions.

Microbiological Investigations

Sputum and blood cultures are collected. If an obstruction is suspected and bronchoscopy is performed, then direct culture of the bronchial secretions may be possible. Anaerobic and aerobic cultures of the specimens are necessary. A serum amoebic fluorescent antibody test can be carried out if amoebic lung abscess is suspected.

Treatment

Postural drainage and intensive antibiotic treatment is usually successful if there is not an obstruction present requiring surgical treatment. In a few patients not responding to antibiotic therapy open surgical drainage of an abscess may become necessary.

Whenever possible, the choice of antibiotic should be based on the results of culture and antibiotic sensitivities of pathogens isolated from the sputum or blood. High-dose flucloxacillin plus fusidic acid may be suitable for treating staphylococcal lung abscess, and cefuroxime or gentamicin for treating a klebsiella abscess. Metronidazole plus penicillin should be given to patients with suspected anaerobic lung abscess (e.g. in patients with a possible obstruction) and to others who are not responding to the initial treatment given, even when no anaerobes are isolated from clinical specimens.

Metronidazole is also appropriate for treating rare lung abscesses due to *E. histolytica*.

EMPYEMA

Empyema, or pus in the pleural cavity, may be a result of a previous episode of pneumonia. The organisms isolated from empyema pus may include *Strep. pneumoniae*, *Staph. aureus*, anaerobes, Gram-negative bacilli, *Strep. milleri* or mycobacteria. Microbiological diagnosis is usually easy since the pus is examined by Gram-stain, acid-fast stains for rapid presumptive diagnosis of tuberculous empyema, and cultured anaerobically and aerobically. Antibiotic treatment usually depends on the results of anti-microbial sensitivity tests but is secondary, of course, to drainage of the pus.

Further Reading

Ashford R. F., Edmonds M. E., Lant A. F. et al. (1978) Legionnaires' disease: first case in London. *J. R. Soc. Med.* **71**, 778–779.

Gardner P. S. (1971) Acute respiratory virus infections of childhood. In Banatvala J. E. (ed.) *Current Problems in Clinical Virology*. Edinburgh, Churchill Livingstone.

Hodson M. E. (1978) Today's treatment. Diseases of the respiratory system. Bronchiectasis and cystic fibrosis. *Br. Med. J.* **1**, 971–973.

Lambert H. P. and Stern H. (1972) Infective factors in exacerbations of bronchitis and asthma. *Br. Med. J.* **3**, 323–327.

Leading Article (1981) *Legionella* and amoebae. *Lancet* **1**, 703.

May J. R. (1975) Bronchitis. The Chemotherapy of Chronic Bronchitis. *Hospital Update,* March 1975, pp. 217–223.

Mearns M. (1980) Cystic fibrosis. *Prescriber's Journal* **20**, 45–51.

Miller A. C. (1981) Erythromycin in Legionnaires' disease: a re-appraisal. *J. Antimicrob. Chemother.* **7**, 217–212.

Spencer R. C. and Philp J. R. (1973) Effect of previous antimicrobial therapy on bacteriological findings in patients with primary pneumonia. *Lancet* **2**, 349.

Stuart-Harris C. H. and Schild G. C. (1976) *Influenza: The Virus and the Disease.* London, Arnold.

Chapter 13

Mycobacterial and actinomycete infections

MYCOBACTERIAL INFECTIONS

Mycobacteria are seen as 2–4-μm long, red, acid-alcohol-fast bacilli in a Ziehl–Neelsen stain. *Mycobacterium tuberculosis* strains have abundant 'Wax D' and lipids in the cell wall and multiply intracellularly, in macrophages, as well as extracellularly. Infection with mycobacteria leads to a 'delayed hypersensitivity' type of immune response.

Mycobacterium tuberculosis and *Mycobacterium bovis* cause, respectively, 'human type' and 'bovine type' tuberculosis in man. Opportunist mycobacteria may also cause mycobacterial disease in man.

TUBERCULOSIS

Incidence

Tuberculosis is still very common in underdeveloped countries throughout the world, especially in Asia and Africa. The incidence of tuberculosis in Western Europe and North America has declined greatly due to improvements in housing, nutrition and specific preventive measures (*see* p. 251). However, in Britain today about 10 000 new cases are diagnosed and between 1000 and 1500 deaths occur as a result of the disease each year. It is most commonly seen in elderly men and in young or middle-aged Asian immigrants.

Natural History

The natural history of the disease is closely related to age. Characteristically 'primary' tuberculosis occurs in childhood, consisting of a subpleural 'Ghon' focus of infection, with associated regional infected lymph nodes in the mediastinum. Primary infection is usually accompanied by mild or no symptoms and is followed by spontaneous resolution. Complications of primary infection include: (*a*) haematogenous spread leading to miliary tuberculosis which may involve the lungs and non-pulmonary sites, such as bones, joints, meninges and kidneys, or (*b*) direct spread causing tuberculous bronchopneumonia.

Primary infection usually occurs after inhalation of infected droplet nuclei but can also occur after ingestion of milk containing tubercle bacilli. In the latter instance the disease acquired is usually bovine tuberculosis and it is the intestine which is primarily affected. Following primary infection the individual develops cellular immunity to tubercle bacilli. Characteristically, there is a relatively insusceptible period to tuberculosis between the ages of five and fifteen years.

'Post-primary' tuberculosis characteristically occurs in late adolescence and in adults following reactivation of a previous primary focus of infection or possibly repeat exposure to exogenous tubercle bacilli. Tubercle bacilli may survive in a dormant state in macrophages for a long period, following primary infection, and, when an individual becomes 'stressed', for example, following a gastrectomy, the old tuberculous lesion can be reactivated causing a post-primary tuberculosis. The majority of serious tuberculosis lesions are associated with post-primary rather than primary tuberculosis.

Pulmonary Tuberculosis

About two-thirds of patients with clinical tuberculosis in Britain present with pulmonary tuberculosis. The most characteristic sites of infection in post-primary tuberculosis are in the apical regions of the lower lobes or in the upper lobes of the lungs. Cavitation is most characteristic in post-primary tuberculosis, but spread of infection to involve the pleura may also result in pleural effusion. Tuberculous pleural effusion can also occur in children in association with early primary infection.

When the cavitating lesions in the lungs communicate with the bronchial tree, tubercle bacilli are expectorated in the sputum and become contained in respiratory droplet nuclei which are expelled during coughing. The patient has then developed 'open' tuberculosis and contacts may be infected by inhaling the tubercle bacilli contained in the droplet nuclei.

Predisposing factors to the development of pulmonary tuberculosis include malnutrition, alcoholism, old age, immunodeficiency or immunosuppression, and exposure to dust and silica as occurs in miners. Clinical features include respiratory symptoms such as chronic cough or haemoptysis and general symptoms such as malaise, loss of weight, or pyrexia with occasional 'night sweats'. Chest radiograph changes are frequently suggestive of pulmonary tuberculosis but, in miliary tuberculosis involving the lungs, it is possible to have an apparently normal chest radiograph. Pulmonary TB should be especially considered in patients with the above known predisposing conditions and in all those patients who have an unresolving pneumonia.

Cavitating lesions in the lungs are due to human type tubercle bacilli in more than 98% of the cases. 'Opportunist' mycobacteria cause 1–2% of cases of clinical pulmonary tuberculosis and are important as they are usually resistant to some commonly used antituberculous drugs (*see below*).

Non-pulmonary Tuberculosis

This is at least ten times more common in immigrants than in non-immigrants in Britain today. One main site of infection is usually involved, but occasionally multiple non-pulmonary sites may be involved as part of miliary tuberculosis. Both *M. tuberculosis* and *M. bovis* may cause non-pulmonary tuberculosis. However, the great majority of these infections in Britain are 'human type' caused by *M. tuberculosis*. Non-pulmonary tuberculous conditions include:

1. Tuberculous lymph glands

Tuberculous lymph glands are the most common type of non-pulmonary tuberculosis. At least 25% of reported new cases of tuberculosis in Britain present with this condition. Cervical lymphadenitis due to tuberculosis infection characteristically presents, as firm, discrete, painless, enlarged neck lymph glands. Occasionally a diffuse swelling in the neck is apparent instead of discrete lymphadenopathy and this 'cold abscess' results from confluent caseation of the glands.

2. Genito-urinary tuberculosis

'Sterile pyuria', haematuria, malaise or pyrexia are some of the possible manifestations of tuberculous urinary tract infection. Female genital tract tuberculosis may present with infertility, pelvic pain and menorrhagia or amenorrhoea.

3. Tuberculosis of bone and joints

Tuberculosis of the spine or of the digits is still occasionally seen in Britain although tuberculosis of the hip joint is rare (*see* Chapter 17).

4. Tuberculous meningitis

Tuberculous infection of the central nervous system is rare. The disease carries a high morbidity and mortality rate in spite of antituberculous therapy. This is due in part to an insidious onset and failure of prompt diagnosis (*see* Chapter 10).

5. Other tuberculous infections

Tuberculosis can affect virtually any site in the body and uncommon presentations are particularly liable to occur in the immigrant population. Subcutaneous 'cold abscesses' may occur without obvious associated underlying tuberculous gland or bone and joint infections. (*See also* pp. 81, 305.)

Miliary Tuberculosis

In the past miliary tuberculosis was most often a complication of primary pulmonary TB in infants. This rare disseminated form of tuberculosis is most often diagnosed today in immunosuppressed patients, the elderly and immigrants.

Laboratory Diagnosis of Tuberculosis

Collection of specimens

The numbers of acid-fast bacilli in clinical specimens from TB patients are often low even when there are obvious clinical or pathological features of tuberculosis present. Many acid-fast bacilli need to be present in the specimen for a reasonable chance of successful culture. Therefore, a large specimen volume is preferable and multiple specimens rather than a single specimen are collected where possible, before the start of anti-tuberculous therapy. Early morning specimens of sputum or urine are likely to be more concentrated and therefore contain more acid-fast bacilli than specimens collected later in the day. Specimens required for investigation of suspected TB at different sites include:

1. *Pulmonary tuberculosis*
a. Sputum, early morning specimens, on three successive days.
b. Pleural biopsy and aspiration if a pleural effusion is present.
c. Laryngeal swabs × 3 and gastric washings, when the patient has not produced suitable sputum specimens. However, every effort should be made to collect good sputum specimens, possibly with the help of a physiotherapist.
d. Biopsy specimens of lung or bronchial mucosa collected while performing fibre-optic bronchoscopy.

2. *Non-pulmonary tuberculosis*
a. The whole of the early morning specimen of urine on three successive days when TB of the urinary tract or miliary TB is suspected.
b. Pus or tissue rather than a swab is always necessary when tuberculosis of soft or other tissues is suspected. Lymph node biopsy specimens may be sent initially, but when a node is surgically excised the whole of the node is preferable to a biopsy specimen. The specimens should be collected into a dry sterile container for microbiology. A separate portion of lymph node should also be sent in formol saline for histological examination.
c. Liver and bone marrow biopsy specimens are indicated when miliary TB is suspected especially in patients with chronic pyrexia of unknown origin (*see* Chapter 4).
d. Peritoneal biopsy specimens collected during laparotomy are necessary when TB peritonitis is suspected.
e. CSF—as large a volume as it is practical and safe to collect is necessary for investigation when TB meningitis is suspected. Repeat samples are usually desirable.

Safety aspects

To comply with the recommendations contained in the *Howie Code of Practice*, the specimens are handled only in an approved B1 safety cabinet which is placed in a suitable separate room. The manipulation of cultures of tubercle bacilli are particularly dangerous and these manipulations are reduced to a minimum. Most laboratories send the cultures to reference centres for sensitivity testing to antituberculous drugs. Only laboratory staff who are 'Mantoux' positive should handle the specimens.

Microbiological investigations of specimens

A negative microscopy or culture result does not exclude mycobacterial infection since there may only be a few acid-fast bacilli present in the lesion. Other evidence including negative histological evidence is often necessary for 'excluding' TB. False negative results are especially frequent in non-pulmonary TB, and in pulmonary TB where a lesion does not communicate freely with the bronchial passages. Non-pathogenic commensal or environmental acid-fast bacilli may be seen or cultured during investigation of gastric washings, urine, faeces and sputum. In a few instances, laboratory errors have occurred due to the presence of environmental acid-fast bacilli, such as *Mycobacterium kansasii* or *M. xenopei*, in specimen containers, taps, stains or slides. (However, these environmental bacteria may also cause infections—*see below.)* Cross-contamination of the laboratory slides and equipment with *M. tuberculosis* and other pathogenic mycobacteria, between specimens may also inadvertently occur unless strict precautions are taken.

Microscopy

Rapid laboratory diagnosis of a mycobacterial infection depends on finding acid-fast bacilli during the microscopy of sputum, pus, tissue or CSF. Microscopy for acid-fast bacilli is not usually indicated in urine, gastric washings or faeces since false positives associated with mycobacteria from the normal flora may occur, as mentioned above, which could cause confusion. Direct smears of sputum, pus and other specimens may be adequate for investigation for acid-fast bacilli but, when CSF, pleural or joint fluids are examined, concentration by centrifugation and placing the deposit on a small area of slide are necessary. The Ziehl–Neelsen stain is still widely used consisting of a heated strong carbol–fuchsin stain followed by decolourization with acid and alcohol and counterstaining with malachite green or methylene blue (*see* Chapter 2, p. 29). When Ziehl–Neelsen films are examined, a prolonged search for at least 10 minutes is usually necessary before a specimen is accepted as being negative on microscopy. However, for rapid scanning of smears for acid-fast bacilli the fluorescent auramine phenol acid-fast stain is recommended using a microscope with an ultraviolet light source and a low power objective lens.

'Screening' microscopy

One specimen of sputum that is sent for 'routine' microscopy and culture is also routinely examined for acid-fast bacilli (although this has not been requested), since a few cases of TB are diagnosed by the laboratory which otherwise would be 'missed' by the clinician. This screening procedure is particularly worthwhile in parts of Britain with a high incidence of TB.

Culture

The main steps necessary for the culture of specimens for mycobacteria include:

1. Collection of adequate quantities of relevant specimens.
2. Concentration of the specimens, e.g. culture of pooled centrifuged deposits from the whole of three early morning specimens of urine. Prior liquefaction of certain specimens, such as sputum, is necessary before centrifugation.
3. Decontamination of specimens which contain normal flora or other bacteria. Sputum, urine, gastric washings and other specimens often contain bacteria, such as streptococci and coliforms, which may contaminate the culture media. The degree of contamination will be less if fresh specimens

are transported quickly to the laboratory and refrigerated until culture for acid-fast bacilli can be carried out.

'Ordinary' culture will give an indication of the degree of contamination present. Specimens which are heavily contaminated may need a more vigorous decontamination process than specimens which only contain scanty contaminants. In the Petroff decontamination method, the specimen is treated with 4% sodium hydroxide, diluted, centrifuged and neutralized; the sodium hydroxide can kill the mycobacteria as well as the contaminants if the duration of treatment is too long. Neutralization of the specimen is often carried out today by culture on acid egg media (which are modifications of Lowenstein-Jensen media). Malachite green and antibacterial agents, such as nalidixic acid, are sometimes included in the media as selective agents since decontamination prior to culture is often not completely effective. Alternative decontamination methods to the Petroff method are available including a sodium triphosphate method.

4. Incubation of culture media at 32 °C and at 42 °C as well as at 35 °C is necessary (*see* Opportunist mycobacteria *below*). Culture for up to 12 weeks is preferable. Both *M. tuberculosis* and *M. bovis* characteristically grow on Lowenstein-Jensen media (LJ media) at 35–37 °C after about six weeks incubation. When there are many organisms present on the media the characteristic buff colonies can sometimes be seen after only two weeks incubation, but occasionally when very few organisms are present no colonies may be apparent until 8–12 weeks incubation. *M. tuberculosis* often grows best when LJ medium contains suitable concentrates of glycerol while the growth of *M. bovis* is stimulated by pyruvate in the medium.
5. Suspected mycobacterial colonies are examined by Ziehl-Neelsen stains to check that they are acid-fast bacilli. The cultural characteristics are then tested in the dark and also on exposure to light, as well as at different temperatures and on different media (*see below*). In TB reference laboratories, detailed biochemical identification tests are usually performed, such as the niacin test, and, at the same time, antituberculous drug sensitivity tests are carried out.

Antituberculous drug sensitivities

Drug sensitivity tests are of most value in patients who have had a relapse or a repeat infective episode, or who come from a developing country where there is a high incidence of drug resistance. Drug sensitivities are performed by incorporating a range of concentrations of different antituberculous drugs into Lowenstein-Jensen media and comparing the growth of each test strain with known drug-sensitive control strains. The results are usually expressed as drug resistance ratios; when the ratio is greater than 4:1 this indicates that the test strain requires more than four times the concentration of drug than the control strain to inhibit it and that the test strain is resistant to that drug.

Guinea-pig inoculation

Inoculation of guinea-pigs is not any more sensitive than modern culture methods and it is rarely necessary nowadays to use a guinea-pig for mycobacteria isolation. However, the use of guinea-pigs, in addition to egg media cultures, may be considered for the isolation of tubercle bacilli from important surgical specimens such as peritoneal biopsies and bone biopsies. Guinea-pigs are no longer necessary for the isolation of tubercle bacilli from uterine curettings.

Skin testing for tuberculin hypersensitivity

Skin tests are used to find evidence of a 'delayed hypersensitivity' type of reaction to mycobacteria. In the Mantoux test, 0·1 ml of a standardized concentration of either 'old tuberculin' or 'purified protein derivative' (PPD) is injected intradermally into the forearm using a 1·0-ml syringe and needle. The usual dilution of standardized antigen suspension used is 1/1000 equivalent to (10 Tuberculin Units), but when TB is strongly suspected, a start should be made with a 1/10 000 dilution (equivalent to 1 Tuberculin Unit). Patients who have tuberculosis may react strongly to the skin test and develop an inflamed indurated lesion which might ulcerate. When there is no reaction to the weaker dilutions, the 1/100 dilution (equivalent to 100 Tuberculin Units) may be used. This could be necessary when screening for immunity acquired by past contact with TB or previous BCG administration. Some reports suggest that old tuberculin may give more reliable results than PPD, but this would depend on the particular batches of antigens used. The Heaf test is more convenient to use than the Mantoux test when a large number of people need to be screened for evidence of tuberculin hypersensitivity. In the Heaf test a standardized suspension of PPD is applied undiluted over the skin surface and a metal Heaf gun is used to make multiple punctures at the skin site. (Attention must be paid to decontamination of the gun in between patients.) The results of both the Mantoux or Heaf test are best read at about three days (the Mantoux test may become positive and readable at two days). A positive Mantoux test is characterized by an area of induration greater than 5 mm diameter in a 72-hour period, and a positive Heaf test by the appearance at three days of at least four papules at the multiple puncture sites. The Mantoux or Heaf tests are more reliable than the Tine test which is similar to the Heaf test, but uses a disposable applicator instead of a metal gun.

Interpretation of skin tests

Interpretation of the results of tuberculin skin tests depends on the incidence of mycobacterial infections in the geographical area in which the patient is living, the age of the patient and general factors affecting the immunity of the patient. In Britain, the percentage of the population giving positive tuberculin skin tests has declined greatly during the last 30 years and this is associated with the decline in the incidence of tuberculosis. Thirty years ago, a positive tuberculin skin test was not usually helpful diagnostically as it often merely indicated past infection or contact with mycobacteria. Today a positive result in a young British person who has not had previous BCG immunization is often suggestive of tuberculous infection. A positive Mantoux test in a child aged 5 years or younger is particularly suspicious of active TB, even if this is the only positive specific finding in the child, and chemoprophylaxis with an antituberculous drug such as isoniazid is usually indicated. Some authorities would use two antituberculous drugs in combination in this situation. In an older person, conversion from a known previous negative to a positive result, without intervening immunization, is also strongly suggestive of tuberculous infection and antituberculous drug therapy is again indicated.

A negative reaction may occur if the disease has only been present for less than six weeks or the patient has overwhelming TB or tuberculous peritonitis. A transient 'false' negative result may occur when there has been a recent or current viral infection such as measles (measles 'anergy'). Conversion of a positive Mantoux to a persistently negative Mantoux test may also occur if the patient subsequently develops decreased cellular immunity in association with sarcoidosis, Hodgkin's disease or immunosuppressive therapy.

Trials of antituberculous therapy

Some patients with a chronic PUO, or other clinical features suggestive of TB, may have no positive microbiological or pathological evidence of TB and in these patients a trial of antituberculous drug therapy may be considered as a diagnostic measure. A response to treatment is not always forthcoming in 2 weeks and at least 3 weeks' drug therapy may be necessary (*see* Chapter 4). Para-aminosalicylic acid (PAS) acid and isoniazid are a good combination for the purpose of trial therapy since these drugs have no significant action against other organisms. PAS may produce unacceptable gastro-intestinal side effects and a suitable alternative combination is ethambutol plus isoniazid.

Treatment

The decision to start treatment is often made on the basis of clinical and radiological evidence of tuberculosis in a seriously ill patient who has negative microscopy results for acid-fast bacilli. In all patients, prolonged therapy under close supervision is necessary. A blind combination of drugs is selected at the start of treatment; very occasionally the drugs may need to be changed when the results of the sensitivity tests become known (*see* Drug sensitivities, in Investigation *above*).

First-line antituberculous drugs

These include rifampicin, isoniazid and ethambutol. *p*-Aminosalicylic acid and streptomycin are much less frequently used today. The chance of resistant mutants emerging to a drug are greatly reduced when a combination of at least two drugs to which the strain is sensitive are used. Initial blind 'triple therapy' is used on the basis that the organism is likely to be sensitive to at least two of the drugs used. Less than 4% of new isolates of *M. tuberculosis* are resistant to a first-line antituberculous drug in Britain and this most frequently occurs with isoniazid. Occasional strains of *M. tuberculosis* isolated from patients from the Middle East and Asian countries are resistant to two or more of the first line antituberculous drugs.

Second line antituberculous drugs

Second line antituberculous drugs are mainly considered when the organism cultured is resistant to one or more of the first line antituberculous drugs, since they are associated with a high incidence of side effects and toxicity. Examples include cycloserine and kanamycin. Pyrazinamide is a less toxic second line drug which has been used in combination to treat tuberculous meningitis and also in combined therapy during ultra-short courses of treatment of pulmonary tuberculosis.

Chemotherapy for Pulmonary Tuberculosis

Traditional standard triple therapy 20 years ago consisted of PAS plus isoniazid plus streptomycin, given for 3 months which was followed by 15 months' dual therapy with PAS plus isoniazid. PAS caused many gastro-intestinal side effects and often was not well tolerated by patients; this drug is only rarely used today in Britain.

Rifampicin helps greatly to shorten the length of treatment required due to its potent and rapid bactericidal action against tubercle bacilli. Today standard triple therapy for the treatment of pulmonary tuberculosis usually consists of 600 mg rifampicin, 300 mg isoniazid, and 25 mg/kg ethambutol daily* given orally for the first two months of treatment. Streptomycin injections are occasionally used instead of ethambutol, especially if there are visual field defects present before the start of the therapy. Continuation therapy with the two drugs, rifampicin and isoniazid, is usually given for a further seven months, so that a total of nine months antituberculous therapy is given. Shorter courses of drug combinations including pyrazinamide, which has great 'sterilizing' properties, are under evaluation.

Examination of the sputum for acid-fast bacilli in smears and cultures is indicated each month until the smears are negative, and then every few months. A great increase in the numbers of acid-fast bacilli seen in the sputum during treatment (apart from the first month) might indicate non-compliance of the patient or the development of drug resistance. Rarely there may be a different explanation such as inadequate absorption of the drug in association with a malabsorption disease of the intestine. Chest radiographs do not show obvious improvement often until a few months have passed and they are of limited value compared to sputum microbiology for monitoring progress.

Chemotherapy for non-pulmonary tuberculosis

Chemotherapy, similar to that described for pulmonary tuberculosis, is usually effective in patients with non-pulmonary tuberculosis. Antituberculous drugs are always indicated for the treatment of tuberculous lymph glands whether surgery is carried out or not. Genito-urinary and orthopaedic TB is also effectively treated by the standard 9-month course of antituberculous drugs. TB meningitis is more difficult to treat effectively than other types of non-pulmonary TB (*see* Chapter 10).

Unwanted effects of anti-TB drugs

Febrile drug reaction, rashes, eosinophilia, lymphadenopathy and liver damage may all occur with many anti-TB drugs including rifampicin. Rifampicin is

*Doses stated are for adults.

particularly associated with hepatotoxicity, but a transient elevation of aminotransferases is not sufficient reason for stopping the drug. Severe liver damage occurs rarely, however, and in a few patients the drug may have to be stopped. Isoniazid is occasionally associated with peripheral neuropathy, but simultaneous pyridoxine administration helps to prevent this. Rarely, isoniazid may also be associated with significant liver damage. Ethambutol is started only after a check is made that the visual fields are satisfactory, since retrobulbar neuritis has been reported. If the vision becomes affected during treatment the ethambutol must be stopped immediately. Streptomycin is much less often used than in the past and its main toxic effect is on the 8th cranial nerve; serum streptomycin assays are necessary especially when there is impaired renal function or if the patient is elderly. The serum streptomycin level should be less than 3 mg/l at 24 hours after a daily injection, to reduce the chances of ototoxicity occurring.

Prevention of TB

Measures for the prevention of TB include:

1. General measures to maintain high living standards—good housing, nutrition, efficient health services, etc.
2. Public health measures to control bovine TB include the tuberculin testing of herds, slaughter of infected animals and pasteurization of milk. Recently badgers have been shown to be a potential reservoir of *M. bovis* in England and in some areas infected badgers have been slaughtered.
3. Recognition of new cases of TB, using clinical methods and selective radiography, is probably the most important specific measure in Britain today. Selective radiography is considered in groups with a high incidence of TB, such as immigrants, the elderly, and people in lodging houses, prisons and mental hospitals. The isolation of patients with untreated open pulmonary TB is necessary until (*a*) at least 2 weeks of anti-TB therapy have been given, when the anti-TB therapy includes rifampicin in combination with other drugs, or (*b*) until the smears of sputum have become negative for acid-fast bacilli. When smears are still strongly positive after 2 weeks' therapy, longer isolation might be necessary after discussion with the consultant microbiologist. Close supervision of each patient is essential to ensure that effective treatment is given and to recognize a relapse if this should occur.
4. Follow up of the contacts of each new patient with open TB is necessary using tuberculin skin testing, radiography as well as repeat clinical examination.

   Chemoprophylaxis for tuberculin-positive contacts amongst children or previously tuberculin-negative persons who become tuberculin positive may also be required.
5. Immunization of children with BCG is routinely recommended between the ages of 11–13 years (*see* Chapter 8). Immunization outside these age groups is carried out in selected groups including tuberculin-negative immigrants, contacts of known TB cases and health service personnel, including technicians working in microbiology laboratories.

OPPORTUNIST MYCOBACTERIA

Many mycobacterial species survive for long periods in the soil, water or dust and these species are known as the 'opportunist' mycobacteria or 'environmental' mycobacteria. Other synonyms include 'atypical' or 'anonymous' mycobacteria. Some of the opportunist mycobacterial species, such as *Mycobacterium phlei* or *Mycobacterium smegmatis*, behave as saprophytic organisms only, while other opportunist mycobacteria, such as *Mycobacterium kansasii*, may occasionally cause disease in man. Occasionally these mycobacteria may occur in the normal flora of man in sites such as the intestines, perineal skin and skin of the genitalia. *Mycobacterium smegmatis* is an example of a saprophytic mycobacterium that may colonize the external genitalia and contaminate urine specimens. The isolation of an opportunist mycobacterial species from a patient does not necessarily indicate disease due to that organism whereas the isolation of *M. tuberculosis* or *M. bovis* from a clinical specimen virtually always indicates tuberculosis.

Classification and Clinical Significance of Opportunist Mycobacteria

The opportunist mycobacteria used to be classified according to the 'Runyon groups', but other systems are in use in Britain today which depend on microbiological characteristics, such as the production of pigment, growth at different temperatures, speed of growth, oxygen preference and Tween hydrolysis. Examples are included in *Table 13.1*.

Opportunist mycobacteria are responsible for about 1·5% of newly diagnosed pulmonary 'TB type' infections in Britain. (The clinical and radiological features are indistinguishable from those due to *M. tuberculosis*.) *M. kansasii* is the most frequently isolated opportunist mycobacterial species from these patients. However, *M. kansasii* may occasionally be found as a saprophyte in the environment in sites such as water taps and in the soil. This species especially causes pulmonary 'TB type' lesions in patients predisposed to opportunistic infections and is most commonly a cause of this disease in miners and other patients with previously damaged lungs who have been exposed to dust. *M. kansasii* is an example of a 'slow-growing' opportunist mycobacterial species. Certain other opportunist mycobacteria, such as *M. avium-intracellulare*, which are strongly associated with clinical infections are also slow growing on Lowenstein-Jensen medium. The growth of many clinically significant opportunist mycobacteria which are slow growers on Lowenstein-Jensen medium, is less luxurious when compared with the growth of *M. tuberculosis*. This is known as a 'dysgonic' growth as compared with 'eugonic' growth seen with *M. tuberculosis*. In contrast, the saprophytes *M. phleii* and *M. smegmatis* grow rapidly within one or two weeks on Lowenstein-Jensen medium and also grow on ordinary media such as nutrient agar.

A clinically important feature of opportunist mycobacteria is that the majority of strains are resistant to at least one first line antituberculous drug, usually isoniazid, and they are frequently also resistant to other drugs. Rational treatment greatly depends on the results of drug sensitivity tests. The source of infection with opportunist mycobacteria is from the environment only. This contrasts with *M. tuberculosis* where human case-to-case transmission occurs.

Table 13.1. Some opportunist mycobacteria compared with *M. tuberculosis* and *M. bovis*

Organism	Pigment	*Growth at* 32°C	37°C	42°C	*Associated diseases*
*M. tuberculosis**	Non-chromogen (buff)	−	+	−	Tuberculosis
M. bovis†‡	Non-chromogen (buff)	−	+	−	Tuberculosis
M. kansasii	Photochromogen (orange pigment in light)	+	+	−	Pulmonary 'TB'
M. marinum	Photochromogen (orange pigment in light)	+	±	−	Skin granulomas
M. avium-intracellulare (Battey bacillus)	Non-chromogen (buff)	−	+	+	i. Pulmonary 'TB' ii. 'TB' lymph-adenitis
M. scrofulaceum	Scotochromogen (yellow pigment in dark)	±	+	+	'TB' cervical lymphadenitis
M. ulcerans	Cream	+	−	−	Buruli ulcer (East Africa)

* Positive niacin test.
† Negative niacin test.
‡ *M. africanum* also isolated in recent years from some immigrants with TB in Britain—this species probably related to *M. bovis*.

Skin Disease due to Opportunist Mycobacteria

M. chelonei and *M. fortuitum* occasionally cause subcutaneous abscesses following skin trauma. *M. marinum* may cause skin granulomas in swimmers or in tropical fish tank enthusiasts. Buruli ulcer, due to *M. ulcerans*, mainly occurs in East Africa and affects exposed surfaces of the limbs. The *M. ulcerans* organism infects subcutaneous tissues to form a spreading granulomatous nodule which eventually causes ulceration. Excision of the nodule in an early stage and treatment with rifampicin may prevent an ulcer forming. Secondary infection of a Buruli ulcer may become complicated by fibrosis and limb deformities may result.

Interpretation of an Opportunist Mycobacterial Isolate from a Clinical Specimen

When an opportunist mycobacterial species is isolated from a clinical specimen the following criteria need to be considered before the organism is regarded as clinically significant:

1. Has the organism been isolated repeatedly from the patient? If this has been demonstrated on at least a few different occasions from the same type of specimen, the chances are greatly increased of a causal relationship with disease rather than transient contamination from the normal flora or the environment.

2. Has the organism been cultured from a site that is normally sterile? In such sites the isolation on only one occasion is probably significant.
3. Has the organism been previously known to be associated with the type of clinical lesion present? *M. chelonei* has, for example, been described in the patients who have subcutaneous abscesses associated with trauma or injections. When it is isolated from a patient in these circumstances it is likely to be of great significance.
4. Are many acid-fast bacilli demonstrable in microscopy of the specimen? If so, the large numbers may indicate greater clinical significance than when only scanty organisms are seen, although it would still be preferable if this could be demonstrated in more than one specimen (*see* (1) *above*).
5. Can cellular immunity to the mycobacterial species isolated be demonstrated by appropriate skin tests? Patients with disease due to opportunist mycobacteria may have a Mantoux test, with standard PPD, only weakly positive. When skin testing is performed using mycobacterial antigens related to the species that has been isolated, there is often a much stronger reaction to the PPD derived from the relevant species. An example of such a PPD that is available is the one derived from *M. avium-intracellulare.*

LEPROSY

Leprosy is caused by *Mycobacterium leprae* (Hansen's bacillus) which is the only known mycobacterial species that still has not been successfully cultured in vitro. The organism prefers to grow near the cooler body surfaces in man. It can also be experimentally cultured in vivo in the foot pads of immunosuppressed mice and in the nine-banded armadillo.

Epidemiology and Control

The disease is only weakly infectious. Prolonged close contact is usually required such as may occur when a contact habitually sleeps in the same room as a leper under overcrowded circumstances. Spread may occur by contact with respiratory droplets from the nasal discharge of a lepromatous leper. Immigrants have imported the disease into Britain during this century but no indigenous cases of leprosy have been reported during this time. There are about 12 million patients with leprosy in the world, and countries in S. America, Asia and Africa are mainly affected. The incidence of the disease may not decline in endemic areas until cases are more frequently recognized and treated effectively. There is no need to isolate leprosy patients. Antilepromatous drugs should be given as soon as possible to newly recognized cases of lepromatous leprosy and within weeks or months the bacilli in the nasal discharge become non-viable.

Immune Responses to M. leprae and Clinical Features

Cell-mediated immunity

The cell-mediated immune response is most important for the eventual possible elimination of *M. leprae* from lesions. Patients with good cell-mediated immune response to the organism suffer from lesions in skin, nerves or skeletal muscle characterized by numerous lymphocytes and relatively few organisms. This is seen in tuberculoid leprosy. In contrast, patients with little cell-mediated immune response to the organism have lesions which are invaded by numerous acid-fast bacilli (*Table 13.2*). This occurs in classical lepromatous leprosy which is the least common form of the disease. In between these two characteristic extremes of immune response, there is a whole spectrum of intermediate immune responses with the clinical manifestations of borderline leprosy in the centre of the spectrum.

Table 13.2. Skin lesions and immune responses resulting from *M. leprae* infection

Type of leprosy	*Skin lesion*	*Cell-mediated immune response and degree of lymphocytic infiltration of lesions*	*Humoral antibody response*	*Numbers of acid-fast bacilli present in lesion*
Tuberculoid (T)	Single or few macular or depigmented lesions with central anaesthetic area	+ + +*	− or ±	− or ±
Borderline (B)	Lesions with features intermediate between T and L types (some lesions anaesthetic, others not anaesthetic)	+ or + +	+ +	+
Lepromatous (L)	Many erythematous or granulomatous lesions	−	+ + +	+ + +

* Associated with a strongly positive lepromin skin test in tuberculoid leprosy only.

Humoral immune responses

Serum antibodies to mycobacterial antigens, and also auto-antibodies, are frequently demonstrable in patients with lepromatous leprosy and borderline leprosy (*Table 13.2*). Sometimes, circulating immune complexes result from the humoral antibody response to *M. leprae* infection and inflammatory reactions may occur affecting skin and nerve tissue. Erythema nodosum leprosum (ENL) may be one clinical manifestation of this immune complex process. A false positive WR may occur and is an example of a non-specific auto-antibody response to *M. leprae* infection.

Tuberculoid leprosy

Patients with tuberculoid leprosy characteristically have depigmented anaesthetic skin lesions (*Fig. 13.1*). These are associated with a good cellular immune response to *M. leprae* (*Table 13.2*). They are frequently seen on the arms as a small solitary lesion. Some muscle weakness, as well as loss of sensation, may be demonstrable in the area served by an affected peripheral nerve, which is sometimes thickened, but the nerve lesions in tuberculoid leprosy are not usually serious. The lepromin skin test is usually strongly positive (*Table 13.2*). (However, this test is of prognostic rather than of diagnostic value.)

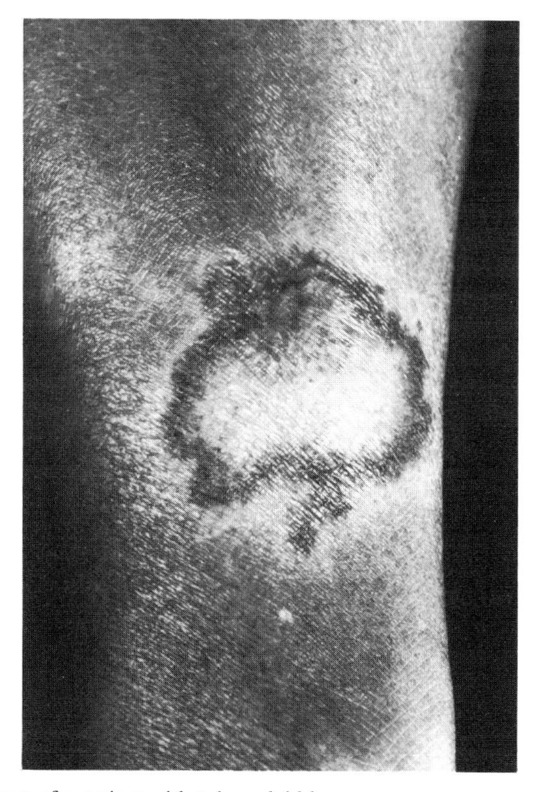

Fig. 13.1. Forearm of a patient with tuberculoid leprosy.

Borderline leprosy

Patients with borderline leprosy have both a cell-mediated and a humoral antibody response to *M. leprae* and marked inflammatory responses may be evident in the skin and nerve tissues. The lesions affecting the nerves are more severe in patients with borderline leprosy than with the other types of leprosy. In borderline leprosy, the loss of sensation and lower motor neurone palsies can result in injury, skin ulceration, secondary infection and auto-amputation of toes, fingers, and limb extremities.

Lepromatous leprosy

The nose may be congested and discharging in patients with lepromatous leprosy. The discharge contains many acid-fast bacilli. Secondary infection and ulceration of the nose and face may occur. As a result of these complications affecting the face, there may be a collapsed nasal septum and blindness from eye lesions. A few patients with advanced lepromatous leprosy may show a classical 'leontine' facies with a combination of thickened skin, granulomatous lesions and a collapsed nasal septum.

Diagnosis

The majority of patients present with skin lesions to a dermatologist and once the diagnosis is clinically suspected a split skin biopsy of the lesion should be carried out as described in the D.H.S.S. (1977) circular, *Memorandum on Leprosy*. A modified Ziehl-Neelsen acid-fast stain may only show scanty or no acid-fast bacilli in a skin biopsy from a patient with tuberculoid leprosy, but the histological features, which include a heavy lymphocytic skin infiltration, are characteristic. Lepromatous cases are only rarely seen in developed countries and in these cases numerous acid-fast bacilli are usually seen in skin biopsy specimens taken from a skin lesion, or the ear lobes, and also in the scrapings of the nasal septum. Some of the acid-fast bacilli may be inside mononuclear cells ('leprae cells').

The numbers of acid-fast bacilli apparent in a skin lesion from a lepromatous or borderline case can be counted in a standardized way during oil immersion microscopy to give a 'bacterial index'. The proportion of the bacilli which are evenly stained, or are of normal length, compared with abnormal bacilli is also noted. The long and evenly stained bacilli are likely to be viable and the 'morphological index' refers to the percentage of these viable bacilli present. When treatment of borderline or lepromatous leprosy is monitored by the laboratory, the morphological index gradually decreases even though the 'bacterial index' may stay roughly the same for many months.

The peripheral nerves in all types of leprosy are affected and the ulnar nerve behind the elbow is characteristically thickened. Occasionally biopsies of peripheral nerves or skeletal muscles are indicated and may reveal histological change and acid-fast bacilli characteristic of leprosy.

Notification

All new cases of leprosy are notifiable in Britain.

Treatment

Dapsone, a bacteriostatic drug, has been the traditional and relatively cheap treatment of leprosy for many years. Most leprosy bacilli probably become non-viable after about six months of dapsone treatment. However, dapsone resistance may emerge during treatment and occasionally this has been demonstrated by culture of the patient's strain of *M. leprae* in vivo. Rifampicin is a bactericidal drug which may cause many *M. leprae* bacilli to become non-viable within a few weeks of treatment, but if this drug is used alone resistance to it may also develop. A combination of dapsone with another active drug, such as rifampicin, is preferable during the first few months of treatment to decrease the chances of drug resistance developing and also to obtain a more rapid response. The main disadvantage of rifampicin is its high cost.

In developing countries it is particularly important that the lepromatous and borderline cases are treated; some mild tuberculoid leprosy cases may not require treatment.

Inflammatory reactions may occur during treatment, possibly in association with circulating immune complexes, and clofazimine is especially useful as an anti-inflammatory drug to reduce the incidence of these reactions.

ACTINOMYCETE INFECTIONS

Actinomycete organisms are Gram-positive branching bacilli. Aerobic actinomycetes include *Nocardia asteroides* and other *Nocardia* species. *Nocardia* are typically weakly acid-fast and have a Gram-positive beaded cocco-bacillary branching appearance on microscopy. Other actinomycetes are strictly anaerobic and include *Actinomyces israelii,* which is a Gram-positive branching bacillus without acid-fast staining characteristics.

Nocardia Infections

These are uncommon in Britain. Chronic nocardia lesions may occur in warmer climates and affect the subcutaneous tissues with sinus formation, an example being Madura foot (*see* Chapter 16). *Nocardia asteroides* is an organism which grows in a few days aerobically on blood agar. It is found in the environment and is occasionally inhaled or ingested by immunosuppressed or immunodeficient patients. It may then behave as an opportunist organism causing chest infection, brain abscess, renal infection or intestinal infection and can cause fatal disease (*see* Chapter 24). Cotrimoxazole and erythromycin have been used to treat some patients with nocardiasis.

Actinomycosis

Actinomycosis is caused by *Actinomyces israelii* although an ancillary bacillus may sometimes contribute to the pathogenesis *Actinobacillus actinomycetemcomitans.* Characteristically in actinomycosis infections, sulphur granules are apparent in the pus, sinus formation often occurs and the infections do not involve the lymphatics. The infection is probably endogenous in most patients and the causative organism may be found in small numbers in the normal mouth. Cervicofacial, pulmonary and abdominal are the three most common types of actinomycosis, in that order. The cervicofacial type mays start after an operation on the jaw or after trauma and is often first noted clinically as an indurated swelling or as a suppurative lesion with sinus formation in the neck. If neglected, the disease may spread extensively to involve the bones of the jaw or the face. Pulmonary actinomycosis may ultimately involve the chest wall with multiple discharging sinuses. Abdominal actinomycosis starts in the caecum or appendix and spreads to involve adjacent tissues in the abdomen; discharging sinuses through the abdominal wall may become apparent. Portal spread of infection to involve the liver may also occur.

Less commonly actinomycosis may involve other sites of the body including the lacrimal gland and the pelvic tissues in a woman (*see* Chapter 7).

Laboratory Diagnosis

Laboratory diagnosis depends on obtaining pus or infected tissue rather than culturing swabs from the affected sites. If a lot of pus is available, some can be washed in a Petri dish and yellow 'sulphur granules' may be seen. A granule, if seen, should be selected for Gram-stain and anaerobic culture. A Gram-stain of the pus may reveal a typical branching Gram-positive filamentous bacillus which appears as a pseudo-mycelium and Gram-negative 'clubs' might also be seen.

Prolonged anaerobic culture of an adequate specimen on blood agar for up to 10 days, with added CO_2, may result in a growth of the typical breadcrumb or 'molar tooth' colonies of *Actinomyces israelii*

Treatment

Penicillin is effective for the treatment of cervicofacial actinomycosis. Tetracyclines are sometimes recommended in patients who are penicillin allergic and this drug is also often active against the actinobacillus organism.

Actinomycosis may require penicillin treatment for 3–12 months as well as possible surgery. Another drug, such as streptomycin or cotrimoxazole, may be added initially if the actinobacillus is also demonstrated.

Further Reading

*Bryceson A. (1981) Leprosy. *International Medicine* **1**, 123–126.

D.H.S.S. (1977) *Memorandum on Leprosy*. London, H.M.S.O.

D.H.S.S. (1978) Health Services Management and Control of TB. NHS employees—Limitations of X-ray examinations. Circular HC(78/3) London, H.M.S.O.

Findlay J. M., Stevenson D. K., Addison N. V. et al. (1979) Tuberculosis of the gastrointestinal tract in Bradford, 1967–77. *J. R. Soc. Med.* **72**, 587.

Grange J. M. (1979) The changing tubercle. *Br. J. Hosp. Med.* **22**, 540–548.

Leading Article (1980) Isolation of patients with pulmonary tuberculosis. *Br. Med. J.* **281**, 962.

*Leading Article (1980) BCG in Britain. *Br. Med. J.* **281**, 825.

*McNicol M. W. (1979) Pulmonary tuberculosis. *Medicine,* 3rd series, 1194–1199.

Millar T. W. and Horner N. W. (1979) Tuberculosis in immunosuppressed patients. *Lancet* **1**, 1176.

Rook G. A. (1976) Immune responses to mycobacteria in mice and men. *Proc. R. Soc. Med.* **69**, 442.

Stokes E. J. and Ridgway G. (1980) *Clinical Bacteriology*. London, Arnold.

* Particularly recommended for further study by undergraduates.

Chapter 14

Infections of the gastro-intestinal tract

NORMAL FLORA OF THE GASTRO-INTESTINAL TRACT

Anaerobes are predominant in the normal flora of the mouth and in the intestines from the ileo-caecal valve to the rectum. The different species of anaerobe above the diaphragm, such as fusiforms, are more often penicillin sensitive than those found below the diaphragm, such as *Bacteroides fragilis*. In the colon, *Bacteroides fragilis* is about 100 times more numerous than *E. coli*, and present at 10^{10}–10^{11} organisms per gram faeces. Other organisms in the normal faecal flora may include various 'coliforms', such as *Klebsiella* and *Proteus* species, *Clostridium welchii* and *Strep. faecalis* (*see Fig. 9.1,* Chapter 9).

Organisms present in food and drink are often killed by the acid produced by the stomach. The dose of pathogens, such as *Salmonella*, required to initiate an infection is reduced when a person has hypo/achlorhydria.

WATER AS A VEHICLE OF INFECTION

Many infections of the gastro-intestinal tract are spread by faecally contaminated water which is used for drinking, washing or cleaning teeth, especially in underdeveloped countries (*Table 14.1*). Public health measures to introduce modern sewage disposal systems that are completely separate from water supplies have dramatically reduced the incidence of enteric fever and cholera in

Table 14.1. Some waterborne enteric pathogens

Organisms	*Disease*
1. *Bacteria*	
Salmonella typhi / *Salmonella paratyphi* A, B, C	Enteric fever
Vibrio cholerae—'Classical' and 'El Tor' biotypes	Cholera
Shigella species	Bacillary dysentery
2. *Viruses*	
Hepatitis A	Infectious hepatitis
3. *Protozoa*	
Giardia lamblia	Giardiasis
Entamoeba histolytica	Amoebic dysentery
4. *Worms*	
Schistosoma haematobium / *Schistosoma mansoni* / *Schistosoma japonicum*	Schistosomiasis

the developed world. However, even in developed countries, shellfish and oysters are sometimes contaminated by polluted tidal waters and cause enteric infections. Mussels and oysters may each filter several litres of polluted sea water each day and, therefore, greatly concentrate enteric pathogens, such as *Salmonella typhi* or hepatitis A virus. Shellfish are best cleansed before consumption by placing them in tanks to filter purified water.

ENTERIC FEVER

Enteric fever includes typhoid and paratyphoid fevers.

Typhoid Fever

The usual incubation period is 10–14 days.

Pathogenesis

The infective oral dose of *Salmonella typhi*, the causative organism, required to cause disease is between 10^5 and 10^8 organisms in human volunteers. Virulence surface antigen (Vi antigen) may inhibit killing of the organism by phagocytosis. Invasion of the small intestinal mucosa by *S. typhi* is followed by multiplication in the mesenteric lymph glands (*Fig. 14.1*). During the later stages of the incubation period, the organism localizes in the reticulo-endothelial system (RES) and gall bladder. Septicaemia later results from the release of organisms from the RES into the blood. The start of septicaemia coincides with the onset of fever.

Clinical features

Fever is the predominant clinical feature during the first 10 days of illness. When a person is febrile and has recently travelled abroad, typhoid (and malaria) must be suspected. Common symptoms during the first week of the fever include malaise, headache, non-productive cough, constipation, abdominal pain and mental confusion. Occasionally delerium, catatonia or other neuropsychiatric features may also occur.

By the second week, the causative organism, *Salmonella typhi,* has started to cause localized lesions in the Peyers patches (submucosal lymphoid tissue) of the small intestine and diarrhoea frequently commences. Physical signs of relative bradycardia, abdominal rose spots or splenomegaly occur in a minority of patients. Many patients show a leucopenia. The organism often persists intracellularly in macrophages and this may help to protect it from the humoral antibody defence mechanisms and, incidentally, also against some antibiotics.

Complications of typhoid may occur between 2 and 5 weeks after the onset of the illness, including intestinal perforation, intestinal haemorrhage, myocarditis, osteomyelitis and meningitis. Death occurs in about 10% of patients not receiving antibiotics.

Relapses of typhoid fever occur after an initial recovery in about 10% of patients. The severity of the illness is usually much less during the relapse than in the original illness.

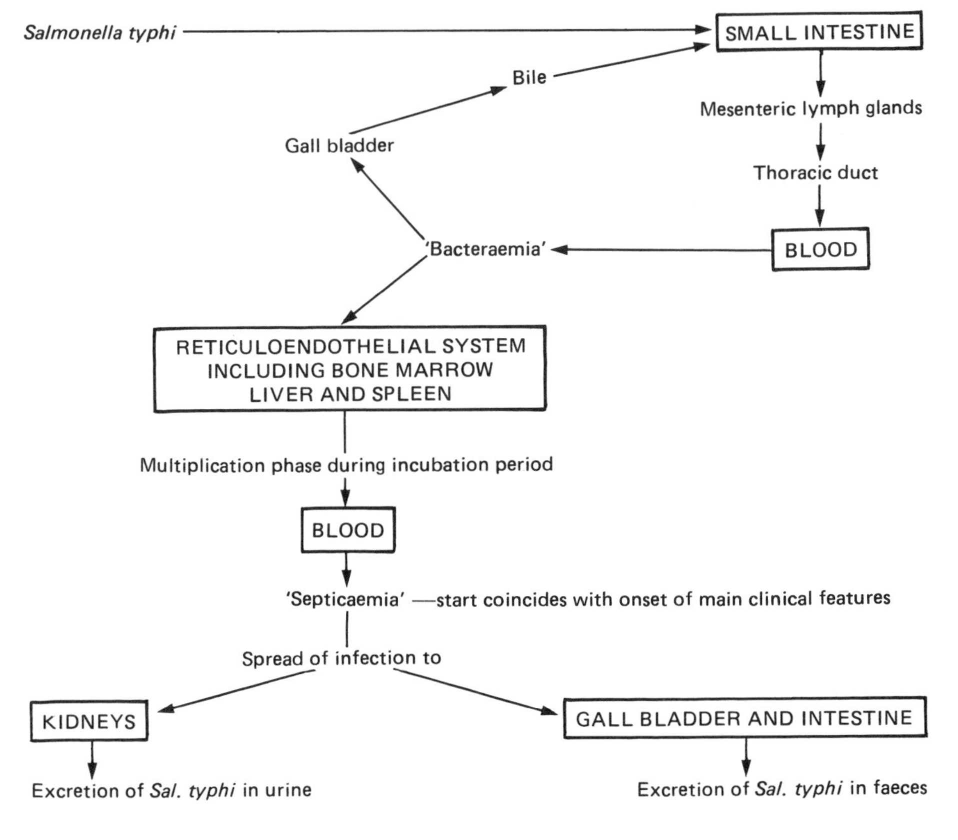

Fig. 14.1. Pathogenesis of typhoid fever.

Carriage state

Permanent faecal carriage, or, less often, urinary excretion of *Salmonella typhi* following the illness occurs in up to 5% of patients. Prolonged faecal carriage may be associated with persistence of infection in the biliary tract.

Microbiological investigations

Blood cultures and bone marrow culture

Salmonella typhi is isolated from the blood cultures of over 90% of patients with typhoid fever during the first week of the illness. Three sets of blood cultures should be collected and these are preferably taken just as the temperature starts to rise. Blood cultures are also frequently positive during the second to third week of the illness.

A blood clot culture may occasionally yield the causative organism when broth cultures are negative. Bone marrow culture is rarely worthwhile, but may be carried out if bone marrow biopsy is performed in a patient with PUO to investigate the possibility of other diagnoses such as leishmaniasis.

Culture of faeces and urine

The collection of faeces may not be possible during the early stages of the illness when the patient is often constipated and a rectal swab is then necessary. A specimen of faeces is always preferable to a rectal swab for culture and should be collected as soon as practicable. At least three faecal samples on different days should be cultured.

The chances of isolating *Salmonella typhi* from faeces and urine increases during the second and third weeks of the illness. One urine sample for salmonella culture is sent together with the other initial samples for culture and further urine samples are only collected when the early cultures are negative.

Widal test

In this test the serum agglutinin titres to the 'O' and 'H' antigens of *S. typhi*, *S. paratyphi* A and B are estimated. The Widal test is often unreliable, gives delayed results and is only of occasional use in patients with negative cultures. An 'acute' serum collected on the day of admission of the patient to hospital and a further serum sample collected 10–14 days later are necessary to demonstrate at least a four-fold rise in the agglutination antibody titres to the 'O' antigen of *Salmonella typhi* which would suggest typhoid fever. A single raised *S. typhi* 'O' agglutinin titre of 1/160 or greater during the first two or three weeks of illness may also be suggestive of typhoid fever. A four-fold rise in *S. typhi* 'O' antibodies can only be demonstrated in about 50% of untreated patients and about 25% of patients who are treated with antibiotics. The serum agglutinins to *S. typhi* 'H' antigens are generally of little use in diagnosis.

There are often great problems in interpreting the Widal test results in patients who have previously had TAB immunization and in those who live in endemic typhoid areas when raised antibody titres are commonly found which do not represent current enteric fever. Raised antibody titres can also occasionally result from antigenic cross-reactions during other infections and non-specifically in other illnesses, such as liver disease, when 'anamnestic reactions' may occur.

Investigations for typhoid carriers

In the past, the serum Vi-antibody test was used to screen waterboard employees for possible *Salmonella typhi* carriage but this practice has been abandoned. About 30% of typhoid carriers do not have Vi-antibody titres greater than 1 in 5. (Also most people with raised Vi-antibody titres are not *S. typhi* carriers—these antibodies are probably a result of cross-reactions with the capsular antigens of coliforms.)

There are two types of carriage, convalescent and permanent, which are detected by cultures.

a. Faeces culture

During convalescence, a patient recovering from typhoid may excrete *Salmonella typhi* for 1–3 months. Six consecutive negative stool cultures should normally be obtained before the patient's carriage state is declared ended. Ten consecutive negatives should be obtained before a food handler resumes work. About 3 months after the illness, less than 10% of patients are typhoid carriers. Chronic carriage for greater than 1 year after the acute illness is most likely in patients with biliary tract disease. Permanent carriage can develop in up to 5% patients, but may be difficult to detect since excretion of the organism in these asymptomatic carriers is often intermittent. Many repeat faeces samples for culture are necessary. The investigation and managements of these cases must follow discussions between the clinician, Medical Officer for Environmental Health (MOEH) and microbiologist.

b. Other cultures

Culture of urine and bile may occasionally reveal the typhoid carriage state when faeces cultures are negative. Bile may be collected by duodenal aspiration or during surgery.

Epidemiology of typhoid fever

a. Endemic areas

Typhoid is common in many parts of the Middle East, Africa, Asia and Latin America. The disease frequently occurs in several Mediterranean countries. Over three-quarters of typhoid patients seen in Britain contract their disease abroad, mainly from the Indian subcontinent and the Far East.

b. The 'host'

Man is the only known host for *Salmonella typhi*.

c. Spread of the disease

Human faeces or urine containing *Salmonella typhi* are the main sources of the disease. These sources may contaminate 'vehicles of infection' through poor sanitation or by the hands of infected persons. Water is the main vehicle of infection and this may contaminate food items such as fruit, vegetables, sea foods, such as oysters and mussels (*see* p. 260), and canned foods when water contaminates the can (as happened in South America when contaminated water entered corned beef cans that were cooled in water from a polluted river).

Contaminated hands or flies can cause a wide range of foods and milk to become vehicles of infection. The most infamous food handler who was a typhoid carrier was 'Typhoid Mary', a cook who worked in America and caused numerous cases of typhoid. The oral dose of organisms required to cause disease is much less with *Salmonella typhi* than with 'food-poisoning' *Salmonella* species. The infective dose may also be reduced in patients with previous gastro-intestinal disease.

d. Notification

The 'Proper Officer' (the M.O.E.H. in England and Wales) must be notified of any typhoid case. An investigation of possible contacts can then be started if necessary.

e. Isolation of patients

A patient with suspected typhoid must be barrier nursed, preferably in a single isolation room in hospital. Particular care is necessary for the safe disposal of excreta (*see* Stool/needle/urine isolation procedures, in Chapter 24).

f. Investigation of an outbreak

When two or more cases of typhoid appear to be connected epidemiologically, a search is immediately started by the 'Proper Officer' and microbiologist to identify the source and vehicles of infection. The source is always a typhoid case or carrier who has contaminated one or more vehicles of infection (in (*c*) *above*). The contacts of the patients are investigated and 'possible vehicles' cultured.

In developed countries where typhoid is infrequently contracted, the use of sewer swabs (Moore's swabs) may help to trace the person who is excreting *Salmonella typhi*.

Each isolate of *Salmonella typhi* is 'Vi' phage typed which is of help in confirming the connection of a source and vehicles of infection with the patients involved in the outbreak. Certain 'Vi' phage types of *S. typhi* are associated with endemic typhoid in a particular geographical area, e.g. phage type 28 is associated with the Indian subcontinent.

g. Prevention and immunization

Public health measures involving modern sewage disposal methods and separate chlorinated drinking water supplies, washing of hands after going to the toilet, and good hygienic practices involving the preparation and storage of food are all important in preventing the spread of the disease in the community.

Immunization with typhoid bacilli, killed by either acetone or heat and phenol, affords useful protection to an individual against the development of a serious illness but the protection is incomplete. The monovalent typhoid vaccine, BP is probably preferable to the 'TAB' vaccine since the presence of paratyphi A and B bacilli in the latter preparation increases the risk of side effects while conferring doubtful immunity against paratyphoid. Two injections of vaccine, given a month apart, give the best protection. The intradermal vaccine is associated with less side effects (slight constitutional upset and a localized arm reaction) than the subcutaneous vaccine.

Antibiotic treatment

a. Typhoid fever

When the patient presents in the early stages of the disease, it is usually safe to collect samples for culture over a few days before starting antibiotic treatment. For patients where the diagnosis is clinically strongly suspected, it is then often desirable to start treatment without waiting for a positive culture result. Where the diagnosis is in doubt, it is probably preferable to wait for the results of microbiology investigations and to have further discussions with the clinical microbiologist.

In all cases with positive cultures the antibiotic sensitivity results to chloramphenicol, ampicillin, trimethoprim, sulphonamides and mecillinam should be considered.

Effective antibiotic therapy can be expected to reduce the mortality rate to between 2 and 8%. However, the incidence of perforation and relapse is not affected by antibiotic therapy.

Chloramphenicol

Most physicians still consider chloramphenicol to be the drug of choice for treating typhoid. The usual initial adult dose is 500 mg 4-hourly orally. The temperature of the patient may not become normal until after a few days of treatment and an occasional positive blood culture can still occur without any 'sinister' consequences. When the temperature is normal the dose can be reduced to 500 mg 6-hourly and treatment continued for a total of two weeks.

If chloramphenicol needs to be given parenterally, much better blood levels of the drug occur after intravenous than intra-muscular administration.

The main disadvantage of chloramphenicol is, of course, a small risk of bone marrow aplasia, which is why the drug is reserved for systemic use for treating life-threatening infections only.

In Mexico and the Far East, the emergence of chloramphenicol-resistant strains of *Salmonella typhi* has limited its usefulness in the treatment of patients involved in recent outbreaks.

Cotrimoxazole

Good results of treatment of typhoid have been obtained using cotrimoxazole, but this drug should be given parenterally and in high doses at the beginning of treatment. The treatment is then continued orally with 4 tablets, later reducing to 2 tablets twice daily for a total of 2–3 weeks.

Some authorities feel that for fully antibiotic sensitive strains, this treatment may replace chloramphenicol in the future since it is associated with a lesser risk of fatal blood dyscrasia. Cotrimoxazole can also be given to patients allergic to penicillin drugs.

Ampicillin and amoxycillin

Ampicillin gives slightly less good results compared with chloramphenicol. Amoxycillin, 500 mg 6-hourly is effective for treating typhoid.

Mecillinam

Mecillinam, used alone, is less effective than chloramphenicol or cotrimoxazole. (Possibly when used in combination with amoxycillin a very good therapeutic effect could be obtained but this has yet to be demonstrated.)

b. Carriage

'Convalescent' carriers do not normally require any antibiotic treatment. Effective treatment of the chronic typhoid carriage state by antibiotics alone is difficult. Ampicillin is superior to chloramphenicol for treating *S. typhi* carriage. Amoxycillin, 1 g 6-hourly for 3 months is sometimes curative. Choleocystectomy is effective in eradicating the chronic carriage state in about three-quarters of cases. This operation is mainly considered when there are gallstones, and antibiotics have failed and the patient is considered to be a grave risk to the community, a situation which is fortunately rare in Britain.

Paratyphoid Fevers

Paratyphoid B due to *Salmonella paratyphi B* is still the main paratyphi *Salmonella* in Britain, although increasing numbers of patients have entered the country from abroad with enteric fever due to *Salmonella paratyphi A* in recent years. Only a few patients in Britain are seen with infections due to *Salmonella paratyphi C*.

The clinical features and complications are usually less serious in paratyphoid than typhoid, although some patients may develop severe enteric fever.

The investigation, epidemiology and treatment is similar to that described for typhoid.

There is no evidence that the *Salmonella paratyphi A* and *B* killed organisms in TAB vaccine afford any protection against paratyphoid.

GASTRO-ENTERITIS AND FOOD POISONING

Gastro-enteritis in older children and adults may occur sporadically or in epidemic form and is often assocated with food poisoning. Food-poisoning cases are reported more frequently in the summer, when raised ambient temperatures encourage the growth of pathogens in contaminated food, and at the festive periods such as Christmas when an increased consumption of turkey occurs.

Causative Organisms of Food Poisoning

Each causative organism of food poisoning is associated with a characteristic incubation period and typical clinical features (*Table 14.2*). In Britain, there has been an increasing reported incidence of food poisoning in recent years and the causative organisms have included, in order of frequency, *Salmonella typhimurium* and other *Salmonella* species, *Campylobacter jejuni, Clostridium perfringens (welchii), Staph. aureus, Bacillus cereus* and *Vibrio parahaemolyticus*. The great majority of cases of food poisoning have been caused by either *Salmonella* or *Campylobacter* species.

Salmonella Gastro-enteritis and Septicaemia

Salmonellae are the commonest known cause of gastro-enteritis. There were over 9000 reported cases of salmonella food poisoning in England and Wales during 1979. The 'enteric fever' salmonellae do not generally cause gastro-enteritis except for certain strains of *Salmonella paratyphi B*. There are over 700 'food-poisoning' *Salmonella* species that cause gastro-enteritis and common examples in Britain include *Salmonella typhimurium, Salmonella hadar, Salmonella enteritidis, Salmonella virchow* and *Salmonella agona*. *Salmonella typhimurium* is often found in the intestines of a wide range of mammals, reptiles and birds including poultry, cattle, pigs, tortoises and pigeons. Some other *Salmonella* species are more closely associated with a particular animal host, e.g. *Salmonella dublin* is associated with cattle. Poultry is the single most important source of infection for salmonella gastro-enteritis in man and all the food-poisoning salmonella examples mentioned, except *Salmonella dublin*, frequently contaminate chickens and turkeys.

Clinical manifestations

The clinical spectrum of illness due to 'food poisoning' *Salmonella* species is very wide, ranging from no symptoms to fatal Gram-negative shock. Most illnesses

Table 14.2. Bacterial causes, pathogenesis and characteristic clinical features of food poisoning*

Organism	*Pathogenesis*	*Incubation period, h*	Clinical features					
			Vomiting	*Diarrhoea*	*Abdominal pain*	*Prostration*	*Pyrexia*	*Other*
Salmonellae	Multiplication of orgs in small & large intestines causing epithelial cell damage	16–48	Slight	Moderate	Frequently present	Possibly in later stages	Often present	Bloodstained faeces in up to 25% cases
Staph. aureus	Heat stable enterotoxin in food	1–6	Profuse	Slight	Absent	Often severe	Absent	
Clostridium perfringens	Multiplication of orgs & release of enterotoxin in gut during sporulation	12–24	Absent	Moderate	Colicky pains commonly present	Slight	Absent	
Campylobacter jejuni	Multiplication of orgs & ? release of enterotoxin in gut	16–48	Slight	Often profuse	Often severe	Often severe	Often present	Bloodstained faeces often
Vibrio parahaemolyticus	Multiplication of orgs & release of cholera-like enterotoxin in gut?	6–36	Moderate	Moderate	Frequently present	Slight	Absent	
Bacillus cereus	Emetic enterotoxin in food	0·5–6	Profuse	Slight	Absent	Moderately severe	Absent	
Clostridium botulinum	Heat labile, potent neurotoxin in food	12–72	Slight	Absent	Absent	Severe	Absent	Nausea, vertigo, aphonia, respiratory paralysis and death can occur

* Food poisoning due to any of these causes is notifiable.
Main clinical feature/s are those that are in boxes.

consist of diarrhoea with slight constitutional upset, lasting for 1–3 days (*Table 14.2*). The diarrhoea may be severe, causing serious dehydration, in occasional patients, particularly the elderly. The differential diagnosis of patients with severe diarrhoea and blood in the faeces also includes acute dysentery or campylobacter enteritis. These patients often have colonic as well as small intestinal salmonella infection.

Abdominal pain is usually slight but can be severe and the patient may present as an 'acute abdomen' to surgeons, particularly when there is no obvious diarrhoea. Salmonella infections are frequently clinically confused with acute appendicitis.

Salmonella 'bacteraemia'

Bacteraemia sometimes accompanies salmonella gastro-intestinal infection and may be asymptomatic or clinically obvious (*see* Septicaemia *below*.) Infection at sites outside the gastro-intestinal tract may subsequently develop and, occasionally, patients present with these distant site infections without an obvious previous history of gastro-enteritis. Examples include salmonella bone and joint infections, especially in patients with sickle cell disease (*see* Chapter 17), meningitis, skin infection, splenic abscess, pyelonephritis and, very rarely, pneumonia and endocarditis. These invasive complications are more likely when there is a predisposing host factor present, such as a prosthesis in a joint or heart, impaired host immunity, and extremes of age.

Salmonella 'septicaemia'

Septicaemia frequently develops in patients with severe salmonella gastro-intestinal infection particularly in infants, elderly and debilitated patients. Clinically septicaemia should be suspected whenever there is severe constitutional upset or persistent fever accompanying the gastro-enteritis. Any 'food-poisoning' *Salmonella* species may cause septicaemia but several species are said to be more invasive than others including *Salmonella dublin* and *Salmonella choleraesuis* (the latter species, associated with hogs, has a particular predilection for bones and joints and is much more common in America than Britain). The mortality rate of salmonella septicaemia is highest in the elderly and debilitated. Metastatic infective complications may occur (*see* preceding paragraph).

Salmonella carriage

Asymptomatic faecal carriage of *Salmonella* usually follows an attack of gastro-enteritis and often lasts for up to six weeks (or longer).

Microbiological investigations

Three samples of faeces, any suspected food that may still be available, and blood cultures in infants and others with severe infections, are collected for salmonella investigation. Media used for isolating *Salmonella* from faeces include the selective media Desoxycholate Citrate Agar (DCA), Bismuth Sulphite Agar

(Wilson and Blair's medium), and the enrichment liquid medium Selenite F. Biochemical and serological tests on suspicious non-lactose fermenting colonies help to identify the particular *Salmonella* species implicated in an incident. Phage typing is a useful epidemiological tool for some of the more common *Salmonella* species, such as *Salmonella typhimurium*.

Epidemiology

Salmonella infections are notifiable (as food poisoning) in Britain. The peak incidence is in the summer. There are numerous Salmonella species (*see* p. 267).

Salmonella gastroenteritis is common throughout the world and, in recent years, has been increasing in incidence in many countries because of modern developments in animal husbandry and the food industry. Commonly involved foods include poultry (especially chickens and turkeys), meat, sausages and, in some countries, eggs. Salmonellae are frequently present in these raw foods, originating in the intestines of the animals. Inadequate cooking, cross contamination between raw food and cooked foods, and unsatisfactory storage of cooked foods can result in ingestion of an infective dose of the organisms.

The intensive 'battery' rearing of poultry and recycling of feeds facilitates the spread of salmonellae. A 'new' *Salmonella* species can be imported and emerge rapidly as a major cause of food poisoning. This happened recently when *Salmonella agona*—contaminated fishmeal was imported from Peru for feeding chickens in Britain; this previously unknown *Salmonella* species in Britain rapidly became a leading cause of salmonella gastro-enteritis in the United Kingdom. New methods of packaging and the distribution of deep frozen poultry, that requires adequate thawing before cooking, have contributed to the increase in salmonella infections.

There are four main patterns of food-poisoning salmonella incidents:

a. Sporadic cases or small family outbreaks
These incidents commonly involve a lack of adequate food hygiene in the kitchen arising from the handling of raw poultry, sausages, beef or pork, or inadequate cooking (*see* Food hygiene *below*). Occasionally the animal source is a pet, such as a dog, terrapin or tortoise, or pet food.

b. Contaminated food at a restaurant, hotel, reception or hospital
A brief explosive outbreak can follow the consumption of a poisoned meal such as a cold turkey contaminated with *Salmonella enteritidis*. Cross contamination between raw meat or poultry and the cooked turkey may have typically occurred and the cooked contaminated turkey may have been left out at room temperature for some time before consumption.

c. Single source widely distributed
Frequent sporadic cases in households and small outbreaks over a long period of time associated with a particular *Salmonella* species (e.g. *Salmonella virchow*) may result from the country-wide distribution of a contaminated single source; for example, a large contaminated batch of deep-frozen chickens from a particular supplier.

d. Institutional spread by direct contact
In hospitals, geriatric and children's homes and other institutions an explosive outbreak may originate from the kitchen (as in (*b*) *above*) but further cases of spread may occur by direct spread by hands.

Occasionally the salmonella outbreak originates from a patient who is a salmonella carrier. This is particularly the case in a maternity department when a mother is admitted who subsequently is shown to be the source of a salmonella outbreak amongst the neonates. Serious outbreaks in hospitals have required the closure of many wards, departments or whole hospitals until the outbreak has been brought under control.

In hospitals, all suspected cases of gastro-enteritis or diarrhoea of unexplained origin must be isolated, and also any mother with recent gastro-intestinal symptoms, until the faeces cultures results are negative.

Food hygiene

Since farm animals and poultry are the main sources of salmonellae, public health measures to reduce the spread of salmonellae are necessary on the farms, in abbattoirs, packing factories and in butchers. The pasteurization of milk and of pooled egg products also reduces the incidence of salmonellosis. In the kitchen, it is safest to assume that all raw poultry and meats are contaminated with salmonellae and to apply careful food hygiene. Essential measures include adequate thawing of deep frozen foods, storage of uncooked foods at 4 °C, adequate cooking of foods, storage of cooked foods separate from raw foods at 4 °C, and meticulous care to avoid contamination of cooked foods by contact with any surface, utensil or hand that is contaminated with raw food. Proper washing and drying of the hands after defaecation is of course necessary.

Food handlers who become carriers of food-poisoning salmonellae are usually victims rather than causes of salmonella outbreaks. The risk to the community is probably low provided the food handler follows meticulous hand washing and food hygiene techniques and does not have diarrhoea. Certainly the risk is much less than the risk with *Salmonella typhi* which is enormously more important. However, once carriage becomes known, the safest and recommended practice is to take the carrier off his/her food-handling duties until six consecutive negative faecal samples have been obtained.

Antibiotic treatment of 'food-poisoning' salmonella infections

Antibiotics are not indicated for the treatment of mild gastro-enteritis or asymptomatic carriage. The evidence available shows that antibiotics do not cause relief of the symptoms and in fact prolong the duration of carriage.

However, when there is severe constitutional upset, high fever or other evidence of severe illness or septicaemia, antibiotics are promptly required, particularly in infants, and geriatric, debilitated and immunosuppressed patients.

Choice of antibiotic

Chloramphenicol is recommended for the 'blind' treatment of seriously ill patients with suspected salmonella septicaemia in Britain. Antibiotic sensitivity test results in vitro are necessary to guide rational subsequent therapy. Unfortunately, many *Salmonella* strains in the world are multiple antibiotic resistant due to the possession of R factors (*see* Chapter 3 on Antibiotics). There is sometimes a poor correlation between sensitivity in vitro and effect in vivo for some antibiotics. For sensitive strains, ampicillin and chloramphenicol are most valuable. A combination of mecillinam and ampicillin has occasionally proved useful for treating severe salmonella infections. Cotrimoxazole has also occasionally been used successfully to treat salmonellosis.

Limitations of antibiotic therapy

When there is a salmonella abscess, or infection of a prosthesis, surgical drainage or removal of the infected prosthesis under appropriate antibiotic cover is usually essential.

Staph. aureus Gastro-enteritis

Symptoms of vomiting and prostration usually occur within a few hours of eating food containing staphylococcal toxin (*Table 14.2*).

Epidemiology

Staph. aureus can multiply at room temperature in contaminated foods which are rich in carbohydrates and also in salty foods, as the organism is relatively resistant to sodium chloride. The main foods incriminated are dairy foods, such as custards, cream cakes and trifles, cooked cold meat or poultry dishes and seafoods, such as prawns. Enterotoxin-producing phage types of strains of *Staph. aureus* from the food handler's nose, hands or septic skin lesions can contaminate these dishes, multiply when foods are not stored properly and can subsequently cause intoxication. The toxin is resistant to heat and may survive cooking.

Microbial investigations

In most patients the diagnosis is unconfirmed. Occasionally a typical phage group III *Staph. aureus* strain such as phage type 42 (that is shown by a reference laboratory to be producing enterotoxin A) can be isolated from vomit or faeces or suspected food using salt-containing media and MacConkey's agar.

Detection of the heat-stable enterotoxin in the clinical samples of food is sometimes possible using column chromatography and immunoprecipitation techniques in reference centres.

When there is an outbreak phage typing of *Staph. aureus* strains isolated from food handlers, food or patients may help to explain the epidemiology.

Prevention

Good hand washing, keeping the hands away from the nose, not handling food when there is skin sepsis and good food hygiene (*above*).

Clostridium welchii Gastro-enteritis

Clinical features and incubation period (*see Table 14.2*)

Outbreaks occur mainly in institutions where food is cooked in bulk.

Epidemiology and pathogenesis

Main foods incriminated include minced meat dishes, stews and cooked meats, such as sliced lamb, which are left to simmer or are re-heated. The disease is caused by ingestion of large numbers of *Clostridium welchii*. The organism releases enterotoxin in the bowel lumen during sporulation.

Microbial investigations

Anaerobic culture of faeces on neomycin blood agar shows numerous non-haemolytic *Clostridium welchii* colonies (normal faeces has only small number of *Clostridium welchii* in comparison). Further tests are necessary to show that the strain isolated is an enterotoxin-producing type A type. Some strains are associated with heat-resistant spores and can be isolated from inoculated cooked meat that has been heated to 100 °C for 30 minutes.

Treatment

No antibiotics indicated.

Prevention

Care not to keep cooked meat at 20–50 °C and avoidance of reheating meat and bulk cooking where possible (*see also* Food hygiene and salmonellae).

Campylobacter Gastro-enteritis

Adult patients and older children sometimes have an unpleasant protracted illness due to *Campylobacter jejuni*. A prodromal febrile phase lasting for 1–4 days, accompanied by headache and limb pains, precedes a diarrhoeal phase that often lasts for up to 1 or 2 weeks. Severe abdominal pains often accompany the diarrhoea which may be bloodstained (*see Table 14.2*). Septicaemia sometimes occurs and, rarely, death.

This condition became recognized as an important pathogen in Britain in 1977 and it has been claimed that it is a more frequent cause of acute diarrhoea than the other bacterial pathogens. In many young children there is mild diarrhoea only.

Epidemiology

Most cases are sporadic but food-poisoning outbreaks have occurred. The epidemiology appears to be similar to that for salmonellae with poultry foods as the main source of infection. Infection can also follow contact with animals including dogs. Infection may also be associated with the consumption of unpasteurized milk.

Microbiological investigation

The organism, a micro-aerophilic S-shaped vibrio (*see Fig. 14.2*) can be easily isolated from faeces using a selective medium containing vancomycin, polymyxin and trimethoprim which is incubated in a low oxygen concentration with 10% CO_2 at 40–43 °C. The plates must be incubated for at least 48 hours.

Blood cultures should also be collected from the more severely affected patients.

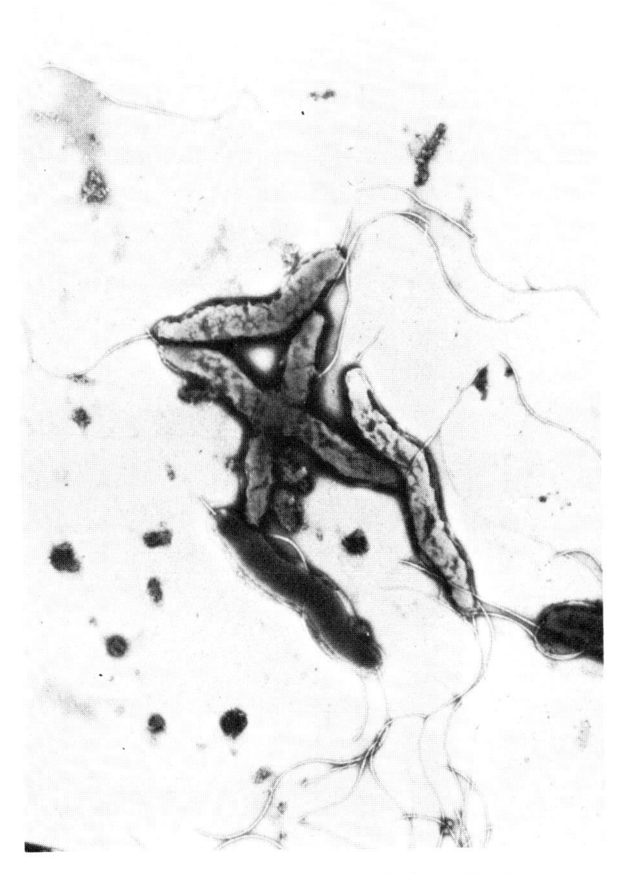

Fig. 14.2. Campylobacter jejuni—electron micrograph. (× 16 500.)

Antibiotic treatment

Nearly all strains of *Campylobacter*, on sensitivity testing, are sensitive to erythromycin.

Erythromycin stearate, 500 mg, 6-hourly, should be given for one week to patients with severe symptoms of diarrhoea and to those with constitutional upset. Occasionally a repeat course of treatment may be necessary in a few patients who suffer relapses.

Prevention

Similar to *Salmonella*.

Vibrio Parahaemolyticus

In addition to S.E. Asia, cases of *Vibrio parahaemolyticus* have been described off warm waters in America and South West England (*see Table 14.2* for incubation period and clinical features). Symptoms usually disappear after 1–2 days.

Epidemiology

Seafood harvested from warm waters may be contaminated by large numbers of vibrios, especially in S.E. Asia. Cross contamination between raw and cooked sea foods can occur. Main foods incriminated include raw and cooked sea foods (prawns, crab, shellfish and oysters). In 1979, there were only less than a dozen reported cases of food poisoning due to *Vibrio parahaemolyticus* in Britain.

Microbiology investigations

Faeces from symptomatic patients inoculated on to TCBS media show large numbers of the vibrio colonies.

Prevention

Care not to cross contaminate raw and cooked sea foods and to eat only cooked sea foods from endemic areas.

Bacillus cereus

Food poisoning incidents are sometimes traced to a Chinese restaurant (*see Table 14.2*). Aerobic spore-forming organisms are common in air and dust. Contamination of boiled rice and multiplication occurs when the rice is left out in warm conditions. There is usually a history of re-heating of the rice, especially by frying. Quick frying does not kill all the *B. cereus* organisms and enterotoxin in the fried rice subsequently causes intoxication. Two different toxins are produced by *B. cereus* but most of the food-poisoning incidents in Britain have been associated with the heat stable emetic toxin.

Microbiology investigations

Symptomatic patients often have large numbers of bacillus organisms in the faeces. The bacillus is isolated from faeces using blood agar and heated and unheated inoculated cooked meats.

Prevention

Boiled rice should be promptly refrigerated if not eaten or discarded.

Clostridium botulinum

Incubation period, pathogenesis and clinical features (*see Table 14.2*). The exotoxin acts by preventing the production or release of acetylcholine from nerve endings, so that neurotransmission at synapses is interfered with, resulting in flaccid paralysis.

Epidemiology

The most recent fatal British cases occurred from a contaminated tin of red salmon. Fortunately the disease is very rare. The main foods incriminated are home-preserved foods (other than fruit) and smoked foods, such as trout. Spores of *Cl. botulinum* from the environment may contaminate meat, fish or vegetable dishes and multiply under anaerobic conditions, such as may be found in a can. The organism is also sometimes found in freshwater fish caught in certain areas. Intoxication, due to powerful exotoxins from the organism, follows ingestion of the contaminated food. The Medical Officer for Environmental Health must be urgently notified. Anaerobic cultures of food and patient samples are carried out by public health laboratories with care as the toxin is very lethal! A search for the A–E botulinum toxins is carried out.

Infant botulism

On rare occasions infants have been described who have developed signs of botulism and in whose stools the toxin and, sometimes, the infecting organism have been identified. The original source of the infection has been obscure (honey has been implicated in some cases). Characteristically, the infants present as 'floppy babies' with muscle weakness, constipation and weakening sucking ability. A few cases of 'cot death' might be attributable to this condition.

Prevention

Only fruit should be preserved in the house—the pH is too acid for the ubiquitous spores to germinate.

Stringent public health regulations ensure that cans of food are heated sufficiently to destroy any spores that may be present. (Some *Cl. botulinum* spores are relatively heat resistant.)

Cooked foods that reach 80 °C for 40 minutes would be free of toxin since the toxin is heat labile.

Treatment

Antitoxin to A, B and E *Clostridium botulinum* toxin is given as early in the disease as possible and when the risk of exposure is known, the antitoxin can be given prophylactically.

Scrombrotoxin Poisoning

This is characterized clinically by the development of nausea, aches and a transient rash shortly after consuming foods such as smoked mackerel. Marine microbes multiply in the fish before it is prepared for freezing and break down tryptophan to release histamine; the symptoms arise in association with histamine intoxication.

Yersinia Gastro-enteritis and Mesenteric Adenitis

Yersinia enterocolitica causes gastro-enteritis much more frequently in Scandinavia and Continental Europe than in Britain, where it appears to be rare. The organism is widespread in wild and domestic animals especially on the Continent. The gastro-enteritis is acute but usually resolves without treatment. Occasionally septicaemia, erythema nodosum, arthritis (*see* Chapter 17), mesenteric adenitis and terminal ileitis may occur.

Yersinia pseudotuberculosis may cause abdominal pain and fever, but this is rare in Britain. Diarrhoea due to this organism is unusual. The organism is an important cause of mesenteric adenitis that clinically may be confused with acute appendicitis. It is often found in the intestines of animals in Britain and Europe.

Microbiological investigations for ‘Yersinia

Faeces

Desoxycholate-citrate agar (includes culture at room temperature), only rarely of value in Britain.

Blood culture

Incubation at 24 °C may help.

Lymph nodes

Removed at surgery, characteristic histological appearance and the organism can occasionally be seen by immunofluorescence and occasionally isolated on culture or animal inoculation methods.

Serology

This is the mainstay of diagnosis; paired sera are sent for yersinia agglutinins to a reference laboratory to look for high and preferably rising titres.

Treatment

These yersinia infections are usually self limiting but tetracycline may be helpful for treating a severe infection.

ACUTE DIARRHOEA IN CHILDHOOD

Acute diarrhoea in childhood, with or without vomiting, is usually caused by infections of the gastro-intestinal tract but infections elsewhere and also non-infective causes may sometimes be implicated:

Infections at non-enteric sites include:

- Otitis media, Respiratory tract infections, Urinary tract infections — especially in infants
- Septicaemia, Meningitis — especially in neonates

Non-infective causes include:

- Intestinal obstruction due to surgical causes such as intussusception or stenosis
- Intestinal allergy to milk or food
- Intra-cranial lesions
- Drugs

Infections of the gastro-intestinal tract include:

I. *Infantile gastro-enteritis—'Characteristic' causative organisms include*:

1. *Escherichia coli* — *a.* Enteropathogenic strains
   b. Enterotoxigenic strains
   c. Invasive strains
2. Viruses — Rotavirus—predominantly
   Astrovirus and other viruses

These two major groups of pathogens cause gastro-enteritis mainly in infants and only occasionally in adults, so it is reasonable to state that these groups of organisms are 'characteristic' pathogens of infantile gastro-enteritis. However, many other organisms may also cause gastro-enterities in infants.

II. *Gastro-enteritis in infants—other causative organisms*

1. *Salmonella* species — mainly 'food-poisoning' species which can be associated with septicaemia and spread by faecal–oral route and direct contact in nurseries (*see above*)
   Typhoid and paratyphoid may also present as a febrile gastro-enteritis in infants
2. *Campylobacter jejuni* — generally milder infections in infants than older children (*see above*)
3. Shigellae — causes of bacillary dysentery—occasional outbreaks amongst infants (*see below*)
4. *Giardia lamblia* — important protazoal cause of acute and chronic diarrhoea (*see below*)
5. *Yersinia* — *Yersinia enterocolitica*—rare—more common in Scandinavia and Belgium (*see above*)
6. *Clostridium welchii*
7. *Staph. aureus*
8. *Vibrio-parahaemolyticus*
9. *Bacillus cereus*

(6–9) } rarely cause 'food poisoning' in infants—more common in older children and adults (*see above*)

INFANTILE GASTRO-ENTERITIS

Gastro-enteritis in infants is common in all countries. In developed countries it is usually of mild to moderate severity and associated with a much lower mortality rate than in underdeveloped countries. The mortality associated with gastro-enteritis is highest in the first year of life. Even in developed countries, such as Britain, some infants develop severe diarrhoea with gross dehydration that results in death. The risk of severe dehydration is greatest in small infants, particularly neonates and infants less than 6 months old. Severe gastro-enteritis is less frequent in breast-fed than in bottle-fed babies.

Escherichia coli Gastro-enteritis

a. Enteropathogenic strains

About 20 serotypes of enteropathogenic *E. coli* have been associated with outbreaks of infantile gastro-enteritis. Only very occasionally are sporadic cases involved. Infants up to 3 years old may be affected but enteritis due to these strains is more likely to be important in infants less than 1 year old. In Britain, most of the severe outbreaks have occurred in maternity hospitals or neonatal units, and examples of serotypes that were implicated include 025, 055, 0111, 0126, 0128 and 0142. During the last 30 years, there have been several outbreaks associated with high mortality but, during the intervening years, the disease has been generally mild. Therefore the behaviour of these enteropathogenic *E. coli* serotypes is somewhat unpredictable.

The pathogenesis of diarrhoea due to the enteropathogenic *E. coli* is unknown in infants. By analogy with veterinary work, it is probable that the acquisition of plasmids is important for a strain to become virulent but there is no obvious evidence of enterotoxin production or of invasion of the intestinal epithelium by virulent human enteropathogenic *E. coli*. Characteristics that are plasmid mediated and which appear important for virulence include an adherence factor (analogous to K88 antigen in *E. coli* in animals) for attachment to the small intestine mucosa and a colonizing factor which facilitates the spread of *E. coli* from the large bowel to the small bowel to cause enteritis.

b. Enterotoxigenic strains

In recent years, two types of toxin have been demonstrated to be produced by a limited number of *E. coli* serotypes (not the 'Enteropathogenic' *E. coli* serotypes). The toxins may stimulate the smaller intestine mucosa to produce a flux of water and electrolytes which enters the lumen of the intestine.

i. *Heat-labile enterotoxin (LT)*
   High-molecular-weight enterotoxin similar to that of *V. cholerae* which stimulates adenylate cyclase. In some infants, these *E. coli* enterotoxigenic strains may produce a severe cholera-like enteritis.

ii. *Heat-stable enterotoxin (ST)*
   Low-molecular-weight enterotoxin—mechanism of action not known.

The ability of an *E. coli* strain to produce enterotoxin is probably plasmid mediated and does not by itself necessarily confer enteropathogenicity.

Only a small number of infants have so far been shown to be infected by these enterotoxin strains in Britain and it is possible that they are of greater importance in other countries such as the U.S.A. and some underdeveloped countries.

c. Invasive strains

There have been some *E. coli* strains described that have been the cause of gastro-enteritis in infants, but which are not of enteropathogenic serotypes and are not enterotoxin producers. These strains appear to be capable of invading the intestinal mucosal cells to cause disease similar to shigellae.

Microbiological investigations

In Britain, *E. coli* strains isolated from the faeces of infants less than 3 years old who have gastro-enteritis are routinely serotyped to identify the traditional enteropathogenic *E. coli* serotypes.

When an outbreak occurs which is not due to a known enteropathogenic serotype, advice from a reference laboratory is desirable and possible enterotoxin producing strains can be looked for.

Preventive measures including breast feeding

The most important preventive measure is breast feeding; severe *E. coli* gastro-enteritis is very infrequent in babies who are exclusively breast fed up to the age of 6 months. Breast milk contains non-specific and specific antibodies, especially IgA, and lactoferrin that greatly reduce the chances of *E. coli* infections in the small intestine. The faeces of breast-fed infants usually contain numerous lactobacilli and are acid which helps to inhibit the growth of *E. coli*. (*see* p. 116.)

Meticulous care in the preparation of milk feeds of bottle-fed babies is necessary. When an infant develops diarrhoea, or is known to be a symptomless carrier, the infant should be isolated and barrier nursed, and removed from a ward where there are infants less than 3 years old. Outbreaks can be started by such an infected infant and infection can also be spread by an asymptomatic mother or member of staff who is carrying the organism. Once an outbreak starts, it may be difficult to prevent further cases; it is desirable that staff who prepare milk feeds do not handle babies or their excreta. The organism may survive on dust and fomites and extensive cleaning and disinfection of the unit is required. Strict hand washing and hygiene is of paramount importance. Closure of the unit until the outbreak is over is necessary.

Antibiotic treatment

Urgent replacement of water and electrolytic losses is the main treatment necessary. The place of antibiotics is very limited even for sensitive strains and many *E. coli* strains are resistant to more than one antibiotic. Most authorities are agreed that antibiotic administration does not relieve the symptoms of *E. coli* gastro-enteritis.

When septicaemia is suspected in an infant with *E. coli* enteritis systemic antibiotics are indicated and the rational choice depends on the results of the sensitivity tests of the epidemic strain.

Complication—lactose intolerance

Following an attack of *E. coli* gastro-enteritis, some infants develop a disaccharidase deficiency and lactose intolerance develops which may become clinically manifest as chronic diarrhoea.

Viral Causes of Infantile Gastro-enteritis

Viruses are more frequent than bacterial pathogens as causes of infantile gastro-enteritis in temperate climates.

Rotaviruses

Rotaviruses cause between 30 and 60% of gastro-enteritis illnesses in infants between the ages of 6 months and 3 years. They are uncommon causes of gastro-enteritis after 7 years of age when high serum antibody titres are usually found. However, a few outbreaks also involving older children and adults have been described where some of the patients have developed moderately severe symptoms. Neonatal rotavirus infection is common in some hospital nurseries but is usually associated with mild or no symptoms.

Gastro-enteritis due to rotaviruses usually presents as an acute diarrhoea of mild to moderate severity, lasting for up to a few days, and vomiting may also occur.

The incubation period is between 2 and 4 days and the infection is most common in the winter months.

Microbiological investigations

1. *Electron microscopy of faeces*
   In the acute phase of the illness large numbers of rotaviruses are seen during electron microscopy of the faeces (*see Fig. 14.3*).
2. *Serological examination of faecal material*
   Rotavirus antigens can be detected in the faeces using 'ELISA' techniques and these tests may soon become routinely available.

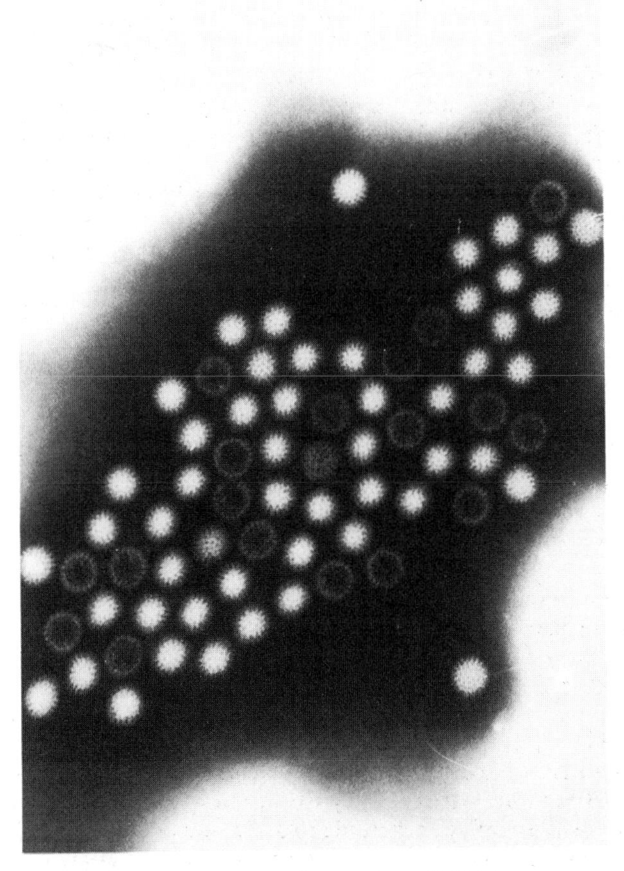

Fig. 14.3. Rotavirus in faeces—electron micrograph. (×85 000.)

Management

1. Replacement of fluid and electrolyte losses is necessary in infants with rotavirus gastro-enteritis until the enteritis resolves.
2. Strict isolation and barrier nursing of the affected infant is necessary in an attempt to prevent hospital outbreaks of rotavirus infection.

Prevention

Breast feeding probably protects against severe rotavirus enteritis.

Other viruses

Infantile gastro-enteritis due to astro-, calici-, adeno-, echo- and Norwalk agent viruses has occasionally been reported.

DYSENTERY

Dysentery is characterized by inflammation of the colon which clinically presents as diarrhoea with blood and mucus in the faeces. The differential diagnosis of acute dysentery type symptoms includes gastro-enteritis due to *Salmonella* or *Campylobacter* species. In Britain, the disease is generally much milder than in the tropics and clinically there is often diarrhoea without obvious blood or mucus in the faeces. There are two different aetiologies of dysentery—bacterial or amoebic.

Bacillary Dysentery

Shigella bacteria cause disease by invading the superficial colonic mucosa. They do not invade the blood or other organs except under rare circumstances (such as immunosuppression in a patient with Hodgkin's disease). Severe bacillary dysentery may be accompanied by constitutional upset manifest by malaise, fever and vomiting. Tenesmus is also occasionally present. Infants, who are frequently affected, may present clinically with convulsions or signs of meningeal irritation.

There are four important *Shigella* species:

1. *Shigella sonnei*
   This species causes over 90% of bacillary dysentery infections in Britain and is particularly associated with a mild type of dysentery which clinically is indistinguishable from gastro-enteritis.
   Strains of *Shigella sonnei* isolated from patients involved in an outbreak can be colicin typed to help in epidemiological studies.
2. *Shigella flexneri*
   In Britain, this species is the second most common cause of dysentery. Most cases of *Shigella flexneri* dysentery are of only mild to moderate severity, but in the tropics where *Shigella flexneri* is much more common, the dysentery is often more severe.
3. *Shigella boydii*
   Dysentery due to *Shigella boydii* is uncommon in Britain and most cases with this infection have recently travelled abroad.

4. *Shigella dysenteriae*
   The most severe forms of dysentery are associated with *Shigella dysenteriae* especially its subtype I, *Shigella shigae*, which also produces an enterotoxin. The clinical features of *Shigella shigae* dysentery may include severe diarrhoea, dehydration and prostration and there is a high mortality rate in untreated cases. This disease is only rarely imported into Britain from tropical countries.

Epidemiology

The disease has an incubation period of about two days and has a peak incidence in winter and spring.

In Britain, outbreaks of bacillary dysentery are most frequent in infant nurseries and kindergarten, primary schools, geriatric and mental handicap institutions. The spread of the organisms occurs by direct contact. The dose of organisms required to cause infection is low (less than 10^3 organisms) and the organisms survive in the dark moist areas associated with lavatories. These factors facilitate the spread of the organism by the faecal-oral route, and by contaminated fomites. Outbreaks are particularly prone to occur when there is poor washing and drying of hands after defaecation, as is often the situation with the very young, the old and the mentally ill patients. Within a home, it is frequent for all the members of a family to be infected but the adults may have no symptoms.

In warm climates and underdeveloped countries, flies may spread the infection and polluted water used for drinking or washing is an important source of infection.

Microbiological investigations

Microscopic examination of a fleck of mucus, collected from the faeces of a patient, characteristically shows a different type of exudate with bacillary dysentery as compared with amoebic dysentery:

	Bacillary exudate	*Amoebic exudate*
Smell	+	+ + + (offensive)
Polymorphs	+ + +	±
Red cells	+ + (scattered)	+ + (agglutinated)
Other cells	Few monocytes (non-motile)	*Entamoeba histolytica* (motile amoebae with red cells inside) or *E. histolytica cysts*

Culture of faeces yields growth of *Shigella* species in most cases of bacillary dysentery. However, there are occasionally technical difficulties with isolation of the organism and, when in doubt, a further one or two faeces samples for culture may be desirable if the first culture is negative.

Antibiotic treatment

Antibiotic therapy is not indicated for patients with mild or moderate bacillary dysentery.

Severely affected cases, especially when the organism is *Shigella dysenteriae*, require urgent antibiotic therapy together with rehydration. Some *Shigella* strains are multiple antibiotic resistant but a choice, later helped by the sensitivity test results, can be made between ampicillin, cotrimoxazole, tetracycline and chloramphenicol. Many *Shigella* strains are resistant to sulphonamides.

Prevention

Dysentery is notifiable. In hospital, a patient with suspected dysentery or gastro-enteritis must be isolated and barrier nursed.

Outbreaks of bacillary dysentery in institutions and mental hospitals may be difficult to control and the closest collaboration between the clinicians, the environmental health department and the consultant microbiologist is essential.

Amoebic Dysentery

The causative organism, *Entamoeba histolytica*, invades the colonic mucosa to form shallow ulcers with undermined edges. It causes dysentery predominantly in tropical regions such as Africa, India, Pakistan and Bangladesh. The organism has a worldwide distribution. In some people, *E. histolytica* colonizes the colon without causing disease and this may be due to variations between strains of *E. histolytica* as well as host factors. Inflammation of the colon in diseased patients is mainly due to secondary bacterial infection of the amoebic mucosal ulcers.

Incubation period

From 5 days to several weeks.

Clinical features

Clinically there is a wide range of symptoms associated with intestinal amoebiasis varying from no symptoms to fulminating colitis. Most patients are only mildly or moderately severely affected and consititutional upset is uncommon.

With severe infection, the faeces consist predominantly of blood and mucus. Subacute diarrhoea cases may have loose stools, up to 12 a day, mixed with much mucus, and the attack usually resolves clinically within a few weeks. Chronic amoebic dysentery cases may have no or only mild symptoms and apparently normal faeces mixed possibly with a little mucus.

Complications

a. Intestinal

i. Very rarely fulminating infection can lead to toxaemia, a severe colitis that is clinically similar to ulcerative colitis, perforation, peritonitis and death. Amoebiasis should always be considered in any patient with 'ulcerative colitis', especially before giving steroids or contemplating surgery.
ii. A chronic localized lesion, an 'amoeboma', can rarely occur that may cause intestinal obstruction and be confused with a tumour, an appendix abscess or tuberculosis.

b. Hepatic

Invasion of the capillaries by *E. histolytica* frequently occurs in patients with chronic amoebic dysentery who may have no obvious intestinal symptoms. This leads to acute amoebic hepatitis and later amoebic liver abscess which is common in endemic areas such as Bangladesh. Patients with amoebic liver abscess may have a high swinging pyrexia, an abnormal liver scan or ultrasound and a raised blood white cell count. Rarely other organs, such as the lungs, resulting in 'anchovy sauce sputum', and the brain may become infected as well as the liver.

Epidemiology

Amoebic dysentery is usually acquired in the tropics by swallowing food, such as fruit and vegetables, that is contaminated by the cysts of *E. histolytica*. The cysts usually originate from the faeces of an asymptomatic cyst carrier; 10–25% of the population in endemic areas are cyst carriers. Cysts are relatively resistant to drying and may be transferred to food by the hands of a carrier, or by flies, or the use of human faeces as fertilizer, or through polluted water supplies.

Microbiological investigations

a. Faecal material

Mucus in faeces may show a typical exudate (*above*). Faeces, scrapings from an ulcer seen at sigmoidoscopy, or biopsy material are examined, while still warm, by microscopy for the typical motile *E. histolytica* trophozoites containing ingested red cells. The finding of such trophozoites is highly suggestive of invasive intestinal amoebiasis.

Cysts of *E. histolytica* containing characteristically 1–4 nuclei, are looked for in the faeces of subacute, chronic or asymptomatic cases by microscopy. Three faeces, not necessarily warm, may need to be examined since the cysts can be intermittently excreted, and concentration techniques should be included.

b. Serology

Serology is of great value, especially for the diagnosis of amoebic liver abscess since the serum amoebic immunofluorescent antibody test is nearly always strongly positive with titres of about 1/200 or greater in this condition. The serum cellulose acetate precipitin (CAP) test using amoebic antigens is less sensitive than the immuno-fluorescent test but is also useful since the CAP test is usually only positive when there is invasive disease. The CAP test is also useful in monitoring treatment. Patients who have only intestinal amoebiasis have lower titres of the serum amoebic fluorescent antibody than those with liver abscess, the titres often being about 1/80 when active disease is present. The serum fluorescent amoebic antibody test titre is usually less than 1/80 when the patient is a cyst passer without active disease.

Antimicrobial treatment

a. *Intestinal amoebiasis* is best treated by metronidazole, 800 mg three times a day for 5–10 days. However, this treatment does not always eradicate the infection although the symptoms are relieved. The faeces should be re-examined, $\times 3$, a few weeks later after stopping the treatment. If cysts are seen, a 10-day course of diloxanide furoate, 500 mg three times a day can be given to eradicate the infection. Severe intestinal amoebiasis can be treated by a combination of tetracycline, 500 mg twice a day, and metronidazole.

b. *Hepatic amoebiasis* responds promptly to metronidazole, 400 mg three times a day, which is given for 5 days. (This cannot be regarded as a convincing 'therapeutic trial' for the diagnosis of amoebic liver abscess when microbiological results are negative since anaerobic bacteria, also sensitive to metronidazole, are an important cause of pyogenic liver abscess.)

Prevention

Adequate cleaning of vegetables, fruit and other foods and use of boiled water for drinking in endemic areas; careful hand hygiene, provision of modern sewage disposal, separate drinking water facilities and limiting the access of flies to food are also desirable measures in underdeveloped countries where the disease is most common.

CHOLERA

Clinically cholera is characterized by the sudden onset of profuse diarrhoea and vomiting. At first the diarrhoea is faeculent but rapidly becomes effortless and watery; typically the faeces are like colourless water with mucous flecks known as 'rice water stools'. In severe cases, there is rapid and severe dehydration, prostration, and electrolyte imbalance, leading to peripheral circulatory failure, renal damage and often death. The severe forms of cholera are particularly associated with the 'classical' biotype of *Vibrio cholerae*. Milder forms of cholera, clinically similar to gastro-enteritis, are commonly associated with the 'El Tor' biotype although this biotype can occasionally also cause fatal cholera.

Causative Organisms

There are only two biotypes of *Vibrio cholerae*—the 'classical' and 'El Tor' biotypes—and these can be distinguished in the laboratory by their different sensitivities to polymyxin and specific phages.

Marked differences in the epidemiology of cholera are associated with the two biotypes (*see below*).

Incubation Period

The incubation period is usually about 24 hours. It can be up to a few days.

Pathogenesis

The *Vibrio cholerae* organisms multiply in the small intestine without causing any macroscopic or microscopic damage or invasion of the epithelium. Enterotoxin is produced by the vibrios which becomes attached to the epithelium and through its active 'peptide A' component, the enterotoxin stimulates the enzyme adenylate cyclase in the mucosa. This results in an increase in the adenosine cyclic 3′:5′-monophosphate (cyclic AMP) concentrations which leads to an outpouring of almost isotonic fluids and electrolytes into the lumen of the bowel.

Epidemiology

Man is the only host for *Vibrio cholerae*. Cholera pandemics due to the 'classical' biotype occurred several times during the 19th and 20th centuries, often originating in Asia, particularly the Indian Subcontinent. Endemic foci of 'classical' cholera continued in Asia between pandemics. The importance of water as a vehicle of infection was clearly shown by Dr John Snow during a cholera outbreak in London that was stopped by removing the handle of the Broad Street pump in 1832. In 1961, a new cholera pandemic, due for the first time to the 'El Tor' biotype, originated from the Celebes in Indonesia.

During the 1960s and 1970s, 'El Tor' cholera spread to S.E. Asia, the Indian Subcontinent, the Middle East, Australia, Russia, Africa and eventually Europe.

Table 14.3. Factors affecting the spread of the two biotypes of *Vibrio cholerae*

	Vibrio cholerae biotype	
Factors affecting spread of organism	*El Tor*	*Classic*
1. Most patients have mild or asymptomatic infection?	Yes	No
2. Duration of faecal carriage of vibrios during convalescence	Weeks or months (or years)	Days (up to a few weeks rarely)
3. Duration of survival of vibrios in water	Weeks	Days
4. Transmission by case-to-case spread (poor hygiene)?	Yes	No
5. Transmission by		
a. Infected water	Yes	Yes
b. Infected vegetables, seafood and other non-acid foods	Yes	No

Some cases were imported into Britain during the 1970s. There was a large outbreak in Italy, associated with contaminated seafoods (mainly mussels) that had been harvested from polluted tidal waters near Naples.

The 'El Tor' biotype has now virtually replaced the 'classical' biotypes and persists in many parts of the world today. In Bangladesh and some other parts of the Indian subcontinent, the 'classic' biotype also continues to be endemic.

Factors that facilitate the spread of the 'El Tor' biotype rather than the 'classical' biotype are included in *Table 14.3*. Where there is poor hygiene in an underdeveloped region, the 'El Tor' *Vibrio cholerae* often persists after its introduction to the region. The higher infectivity of the 'El Tor' biotype is a particular problem when infected people travel rapidly about the world by land, sea and air.

Microbiological Investigations

Cholera should be suspected whenever a person with diarrhoea has recently travelled abroad and particularly if there has been a visit to an endemic area during the previous week.

Microscopy and culture of the faeces or rectal swab on suitable selective (TCBS) and enrichment media (alkaline peptone water) is urgently necessary before the start of any antibiotic therapy. The results of microscopic examination by Gram-stain or dark-ground illumination can strongly suggest the diagnosis when vibrios are seen, especially if the specimen is a 'rice water stool'. However, the definitive diagnosis must await the results of culture and the local laboratory will send the isolate for confirmatory tests to a recognized reference laboratory.

After treatment, six faecal samples should be examined and negative results obtained before the patient is declared 'free' of carriage of the vibrios.

Antimicrobial Treatment

Antimicrobial treatment has second place to the urgent need to rehydrate the patient, with intravenous fluids in severely affected cases and by the oral route using modern glucose salt solution methods for less severely affected cases.

Tetracycline, 500 mg four times a day, for 3 days, in an adult is given as soon as practicable since this is very active against the 'El Tor' vibrio, reduces the duration of symptoms and the excretion of the organism and allows less fluids to be used for rehydration. However, there have been recent reports of tetracycline resistance emerging in 'El Tor' strains of *V. cholerae* and the results of antibiotic sensitivity tests may need to be taken into account.

Prevention

The most important measures to prevent the spread of cholera in a country include:

1. Sewage disposal—separate from
   i. drinking or washing water
   ii. sea where sea foods are harvested
   iii. farming—human faeces not to be used as fertilizer.
2. Modern filtered and chlorinated water supplies.

When a case of cholera is imported into a developed country the following measures are necessary:

1. Immediate notification of the medical environmental health authorities.
2. Isolation and barrier nursing of the case until at least three negative faeces are obtained after stopping antibiotic treatment.
3. Tetracycline should be administered to the patient as this reduces the duration of excretion of vibrios (*see* Treatment *above*).
4. Contacts need to observe strict hygiene—isolate if diarrhoea develops. (No secondary spread of cholera has been reported in Britain in recent years.)
5. Close contacts may be given prophylactic tetracycline (not vaccination).

For travellers to endemic areas a killed cholera vaccine, preferably administered as two doses one month apart, will give some protection against clinically severe disease. However, the protection is for a few months only (up to 6 months) and the vaccine does not prevent infection by *Vibrio cholerae*. Travellers should try to drink heat-treated water and foods in such areas whenever possible and follow high standards of hygiene.

GIARDIASIS

Giardia lamblia is a flagellate pear-shaped protozoon which is a common bowel pathogen in countries throughout the world including Britain. Cysts of giardia are swallowed in contaminated food or water and develop into trophozoites in the duodenum. The trophozoites become attached to the villi of the small intestine and cause mucosal damage in some patients which results in abdominal discomfort, flatulence and diarrhoea. Symptoms usually start within a couple of weeks of ingesting the organism. Occasionally steatorrhoea and malabsorption can develop in chronically infected patients. Sometimes there is a history of intermittent attacks of diarrhoea. Children and adults are commonly infected.

Certain cities, including Leningrad, appear to have a higher incidence of infection due to *Giardia* than other cities and this is probably related to the persistence of giardia cysts in the chlorinated drinking water supplies.

Microbiological Investigations

Faeces collected from a patient with acute diarrhoea may show the trophozoite of *Giardia* on microscopy. When the patient has subacute or chronic giardiasis with formed faeces, microscopy usually reveals the typical giardia cysts. Three faecal samples collected on different days, and examined by concentration methods,are necessary to obtain a positive result in some patients.

Duodenal aspiration or examination of a villous biopsy specimen is necessary to establish the diagnosis in a minority of patients who have negative results of faeces examination.

Antimicrobial Treatment

Metronidazole, 200 mg, three times a day for 8 days is recommended. Occasionally it is necessary to repeat this course of treatment after one week.

Mepacrine, 100 mg, three times a day for 8 days can be used for, metronidazole-failed treatment cases.

WINTER VOMITING DISEASE

Outbreaks of illness characteristically nausea and vomiting and diarrhoea, lasting for 1–2 days affecting adults or children has been recently shown due to a virus, the 'Norwalk Agent'. This infection may be spread by the respiratory route.

TRAVELLER'S DIARRHOEA

Visitors to places abroad such as Mexico, the Middle East, Southern Europe and the Far East, may develop diarrhoea which is not due to the known bacterial, viral or protozoon bowel pathogens mentioned above. It is probable that various strains of *E. coli*, particularly 'LT' enterotoxin producers, are implicated. Doxycycline has been shown to be effective for prophylaxis of infection by tetracycline-sensitive enterotoxin-producing strains of *E. coli*. There are no reports of effective treatment of traveller's diarrhoea with antibiotics once symptoms have started.

TROPICAL SPRUE

The exact aetiology of this chronic diarrhoea or steatorrhoea condition, sometimes accompanied by malabsorption, is unknown but secondary bacterial infection of the small intestine probably occurs in many cases.

Tetracycline appears to relieve the symptoms in some patients.

BLIND LOOP SYNDROME

Patients with a 'blind loop' of small intestine after gastric surgery may develop diarrhoea, steatorrhoea and malabsorption. This is due to the overgrowth of normal flora bowel organisms, such as *Bacteroides fragilis*, which may split bile salts and cause disturbances of the small bowel mechanisms for fat absorption.

A [^{14}C]glycolic acid breath test has been used to detect bacterial overgrowth but the definitive demonstration of overgrowth depends on anaerobic and aerobic quantitative cultures of aspirated duodenal/jejunal fluid.

Antibiotic sensitivity results of the bacteria isolated from the intestinal fluid will help the choice of an antibiotic to suppress the overgrowth which may then relieve symptoms. Surgical shortening or elimination of the loop may be possible in some cases.

ANTIBIOTIC-INDUCED DIARRHOEA

Many antibiotics, including ampicillin, tetracycline and lincomycin may cause diarrhoea side effects, probably by upsetting the normal bowel flora. When the drug is stopped, the symptoms usually quickly disappear.

PSEUDO-MEMBRANOUS COLITIS

Pseudo-membranous colitis is a serious, occasionally fatal, complication of antibiotic therapy that may occur during or shortly after a course of antibiotic therapy. Clinically the disease is characterized by severe diarrhoea, often bloodstained, dehydration and toxaemia with typical colonic changes apparent on sigmoidoscopy.

Several antibiotics have been implicated, but especially clindamycin or lincomycin, when given to elderly patients or those with previous known bowel disease. Clindamycin and lincomycin should be avoided in the latter circumstances, and only used when essential.

The condition has recently been shown to be due to a superinfection of the bowel by antibiotic-resistant strains of *Clostridium difficile* which produces a toxin in the faeces and gut that damages the colonic mucosa. The toxin (neutralized by *C. sordelii* anti-serum) is demonstrated in the faeces of patients using tissue culture techniques by reference laboratories.

Most strains of *Clostridium difficile* are sensitive to vancomycin and this drug has proved useful for treating pseudo-membranous colitis (*see also* Chapter 9, p.165).

Further Reading

CIBA Foundation (1976) *Acute Diarrhoea in Childhood.* Amsterdam, Elsevier.

*Geddes A. M. (1973) Enteric fever, salmonellosis and food poisoning. *Br. Med. J.* **1**, 98–100.

Hobbs Betty C. and Gilbert R. J. (1978) *Food Poisoning and Food Hygiene,* 4th ed. London, Edward Arnold.

Leading Article (1976) Is the cholera pandemic waning? *Br. Med. J.* **2**, 390.

*Skirrow M. B. (1977) Campylobacter enteritis, a 'new' disease. *Br. Med. J.* **3**, 9.

* Particularly recommended for further study by undergraduates.

Chapter 15

Hepatic infections

VIRAL HEPATITIS

Viruses that cause hepatitis include hepatitis A virus, hepatitis B virus, hepatitis non-A, non-B virus, yellow fever virus, cytomegalovirus, Epstein-Barr virus and herpes simplex. All of these viruses may cause subclinical hepatitis infections as well as illness associated with hepatitis. The great majority of clinically significant hepatitis infections are due to the first three hepatitis viruses mentioned above (*see Table 15.1*).

Table 15.1. Differences between three types of viral hepatitis

	Hepatitis A	*Hepatitis B*	*Hepatitis non-A, non-B*
Causative virus	Hepatitis A virus (22 nm diameter)	Hepatitis B virus (in the 42 nm Dane particle)	Unknown
Incubation period	2–6 weeks	6 weeks to 6 months	1–3 months
Mode of transmission	Faecal-oral mainly	Parenteral; close personal contact	Parenteral
Epidemic spread	Frequent	Rare	?
Clinical course	Short, generally mild	Prolonged, more severe than hepatitis A	Generally mild but fatal cases have occurred
Ages	Schoolchildren mainly	Young adults; infants of affected mothers	Adults
Post-transfusion hepatitis?	Yes	Yes	Yes
Carrier state?	No	Yes	Yes
Chronic liver disease?	No	Yes	Yes
Microbiological diagnosis	Serum anti-HAV, IgM positive or rising titres soon after infection	Serum HBsAg positive or 'e' positive, or rising titres of serum anti-HBcAg or anti-HBsAg	Exclusion of recent hepatitis A or hepatitis B

Hepatitis A ('Infectious Hepatitis')

Epidemiology

Hepatitis A particularly occurs in parts of the world where there are inadequate sewage disposal measures or poor standards of food hygiene. Countries where the disease is very common include those in the Middle East, Indian sub-continent, Africa, S.E. Asia, Latin America and Mediterranean areas. Sporadic cases, as well as cases involved in outbreaks, do still frequently occur in Britain and other developed countries although these are much less common than 40 years ago.

Spread of infection is mainly by the faecal-oral route and via contaminated food and water. Children and young people are most often infected in endemic areas. Foods that have been incriminated as sources in outbreaks in Britain in recent years include contaminated shellfish and oysters, and contaminated soft fruit such as frozen raspberries.

Incubation period

Two–six weeks.

Period of infectivity

During the 10 days before to only a few days after the onset of symptoms.

Clinical features

Recent serological studies have indicated that the great majority of hepatitis A infections are either subclinical or associated with only a relatively mild illness without jaundice (known as 'anicteric hepatitis'). The most common clinical presentation is malaise and anorexia, sometimes accompanied by fever, and this is followed in some patients by jaundice. Most patients develop an enlarged liver and the serum aminotransferases (transaminases) are usually markedly elevated in the acute stage of the disease. Pale stools and dark urine are often noticed in the early stage of jaundice. The jaundice is not usually severe and gradually disappears within one or two weeks. Most patients recover completely within a few weeks of the onset of symptoms although the serum aminotransferases may take up to two or three months to return to normal levels. A few patients suffer from more severe clinical infection lasting for up to several weeks and a relapse may occasionally occur following an initial clinical recovery. Very rarely death may result from fulminating hepatitis A infection.

Microbiological diagnosis

Serological tests for the specific diagnosis of recent hepatitis A infection are carried out only in a reference laboratory and are mainly useful when the clinical diagnosis of 'infectious hepatitis' is in doubt and there is not serological evidence of recent hepatitis B infection. These tests are also valuable for investigating outbreaks of hepatitis.

The serological tests depend on the recent discovery of hepatitis A virus particles (HAV) in the faeces of patients with acute hepatitis A, during the week before the onset of symptoms, as seen by electron microscopy. The HAV particles rapidly disappear from the faeces during the week after the onset of symptoms. These particles are agglutinated by antibody present in convalescent serum. Antigens from the particles are used for performing various antibody tests on samples of serum including a radio-immunoassay test.

When serum is collected from a patient with hepatitis A during the first week of illness and compared with a later serum sample during the subsequent several weeks, a rising titre of anti-HAV antibody is demonstrated. A single serum sample may also show conclusive evidence of recent hepatitis A infection; a sample collected between 1 and 6 weeks following clinical illness nearly always shows a high titre of specific anti-HAV, IgM antibody. Anti-HAV, IgG antibodies characteristically persist for a long time after the original infection, possibly for many years, and this correlates with the fact that there appears to be life-long immunity following an attack of hepatitis A. If only IgG anti-HAV antibodies are demonstrated in a serum sample this is suggestive of past rather than recent hepatitis A infection.

Specific prophylaxis

A single injection of pooled normal human immunoglobulin provides effective specific prophylaxis against hepatitis A for up to about 3 months after the injection and is recommended for travellers to highly endemic areas. The immunoglobulin contains a high titre of anti-HAV antibodies and these help to attenuate the course of the illness if the injection is given before or during the early incubation period.

Hepatitis B ('Serum Hepatitis')

Incubation period

Six weeks to six months.

Period of infectivity

During the 6 weeks before the onset of symptoms and for an indefinite period after the acute attack of hepatitis, possibly for life in a minority of persistent carriers.

Epidemiology

Hepatitis B virus is characteristically spread by the parenteral route rather than the faecal-oral route. There are several major differences between hepatitis due to the hepatitis A virus and the hepatitis B virus (*Table 15.1*). Epidemic spread of hepatitis B in the general community is relatively rare but occurs commonly with hepatitis A.

The incidence of hepatitis B varies greatly between different parts of the world. The disease is very common in many countries in Asia including China, the Philippines and other S.E. Asian countries, the Middle East and Africa. Up to 20% of the population in these highly endemic areas may be asymptomatic HBsAg positive chronic carriers. Vertical transmission of the hepatitis B virus (i.e. from one generation to the next generation) is probably a major reason for the high incidence of hepatitis B infection in the above developing countries, infants acquiring the virus from infected mothers *in utero*, at birth or shortly after birth. In Britain and other developed countries in Europe and North

America, there is a low incidence of hepatitis B; only about 1 in 1000 of the indigenous population are healthy chronic HBsAg carriers.

In developed countries, the risks of exposure to hepatitis B appear to be greatest in certain groups of people including:

a. *Drug addicts*
Spread of hepatitis B is associated with the sharing of contaminated needles and syringes used for intravenous injections of drugs. As these patients are debilitated there may sometimes also be impaired immunity with an increased risk of persistent carriage.

b. *Homosexual males*
There is a high incidence of hepatitis B in promiscuous homosexual males. Heterosexual spread of hepatitis B is also possible but at a lower rate than that associated with male homosexual spread.

c. *Renal dialysis patients*
In the past, hepatitis B spread between patients and from patients to staff via shared contaminated haemodialysis machines and the spillage of infected blood. The immunity of the patients was probably impaired and high titres of infective hepatitis B virus could circulate persistently without clinical signs of infection; handling of these patients by hospital staff was extremely hazardous, and in several outbreaks in the 1960s there were fatalities in medical, nursing and technical staff. Following the implementations of the Rosenheim Report (1972) to exclude hepatitis B from renal units, there have been no further reported outbreaks in these units in Britain.

d. *Individuals undergoing tattooing or acupuncture*
Inadequate sterilization of shared needles used for these techniques has occasionally been associated with outbreaks of hepatitis B in the past. The risks have probably decreased during the last few years in Britain as the hygienic precautions taken by the performers of these techniques have improved. The individuals do not have any obvious reason for impaired immunity and persistent hepatitis B carriage following an attack of hepatitis occurs infrequently.

e. *Infants born to HBsAg positive mothers*
As in the third world, there is a risk that a baby born to an asymptomatic hepatitis B mother will acquire the virus from the mother. However, the risk is much greater when a pregnant mother develops acute hepatitis B near the time of delivery of the neonate. The most frequent route of transmission of the virus is probably via inoculation of highly infected blood into the freshly abraded skin or conjunctivae of the infant during delivery and possibly also by the baby swallowing the blood. The immunity of the baby is impaired compared with later life and the infant is then at increased risk of developing persistent hepatitis B carriage with possible associated chronic liver disease.

f. *Patients receiving transfusion of blood or injection of blood products*
Patients who are given multiple transfusions and those with bleeding disorders, such as haemophilia, requiring injections of appropriate human blood products are at increased risk of acquiring hepatitis B. However, this risk has become much reduced in Britain and other countries since blood donors are serologically screened for evidence of hepatitis B carriage.

g. Hospital staff (other than those in renal units)
Hepatitis B is an occupational risk of those hospital staff who regularly have contact with the blood or body fluids of patients. Accidents involving needles or 'sharps' and inoculation injuries, including splashing of the eye with fluid from a patient, occasionally occur as well as contamination of fresh cuts in the skin of the hand, etc. Sporadic cases of hospital-acquired hepatitis B occur but outbreaks of hepatitis B arising from contact with a patient are fortunately rare (*see* Shanson, 1980). The incidence of hepatitis B in laboratory workers has decreased greatly, possibly associated with increased awareness of safety precautions, and it is now a very rare disease in laboratory staff in Britain (*see also* Chapter 24).

Clinical features and complications of hepatitis B

The clinical features in the early stages of hepatitis B are similar to those described for hepatitis A except that the onset may be more insidious and in the prodromal period, polyarthralgia and a transient urticarial type rash may also appear. The attack of hepatitis is frequently more severe than that seen with hepatitis A with jaundice or greatly disturbed liver function tests lasting for several weeks. In a significant proportion of patients, complications such as acute fulminating hepatitis or persistent infection leading to chronic active hepatitis may occur (*Fig. 15.1*). In parts of Asia and Africa, it is probable that hepatitis B is an important aetiological factor in the pathogenesis of primary liver cancer. Healthy carriage of hepatitis B associated antigens or of the hepatitis B virus or both is another major possible consequence of hepatitis B infection (*Fig. 15.1*).

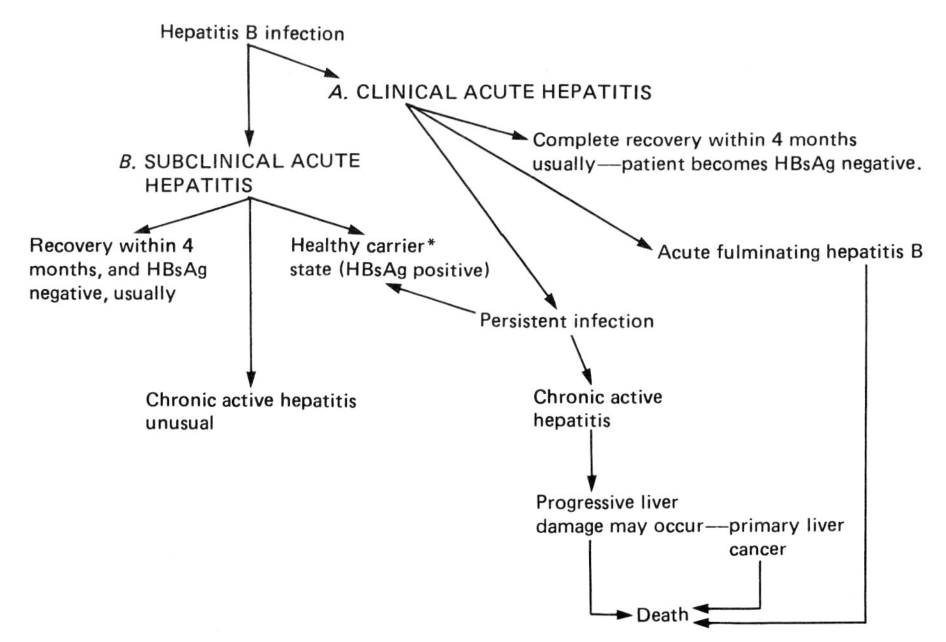

Fig. 15.1. Consequences of hepatitis B infection. * Not usually infectious to contacts; depends on whether 'e' antigen positive and other factors.

Microbiological diagnosis and features associated with hepatitis B infection

a. *HBsAg and the Dane particle*
Hepatitis B surface antigen, HBsAg ('Australian Antigen' component), characteristically appears in the serum of the majority of patients with acute hepatitis B during the first few days of the illness and tests to recognize this antigen are valuable diagnostically (*Table 15.2*). Serum samples for testing for HBsAg must be collected with care and transported to the laboratory clearly marked with 'hepatitis risk' labels.

Table 15.2. Some tests available to detect evidence of hepatitis B infection

Hepatitis B associated antigen or antibody	*Serological tests available and their relative sensitivity*			
	Passive haemagglutination	*Countercurrent immunoelectro-phoresis*	*Ouchterlony gel-diffusion*	*Solid-phase radio-immunoassay*
HBsAg	+++*	++	+	++++
'e' antigen			+	
Anti-HBcAg		+		++++
Anti-HBsAg	+++	++	+	++++

* A useful rapid 'screening' test is commercially available for routine laboratories but occasional 'false positives' occur

The titre of HBsAg in the serum rapidly declines during the first 6 weeks after the onset of illness; it is even possible for a patient with acute hepatitis B to have a negative serum HBsAg test result after only a few days of jaundice due to the rapid clearing of the antigen from the blood. The great majority of patients are serum HBsAg negative, by the most sensitive immunological tests, by 3–4 months after the onset of symptoms. The HBsAg is associated with the Dane particle which can frequently be seen together with other spherical or tubular particles (of 22-nm diameter) during electron microscopy of serum collected during the most acute stages of hepatitis B (*Fig. 15.2*). The Dane particle is a 42-nm diameter double-shelled particle and the surface component contains the HBsAg. The inner core of the Dane particle contains the hepatitis B core antigen (HBcAg). Dane particles probably contain the infective hepatitis B virus which includes single-stranded DNA and DNA-dependent DNA polymerase. Following hepatitis B infection antibodies develop first to the core antigen and later to the HBsAg; tests for these antibodies may help to show past or recent hepatitis B infection.

b. *Anti-HBc antibody*
Rising titres of antibody to the core antigen are usually demonstrable in the serum during the first few months following the onset of symptoms. This antibody may sometimes be detectable some years after an attack of hepatitis B.

c. *Anti-HBsAg antibody*
This antibody characteristically appears in high titre in the serum between 3–6 months after the onset of symptoms.

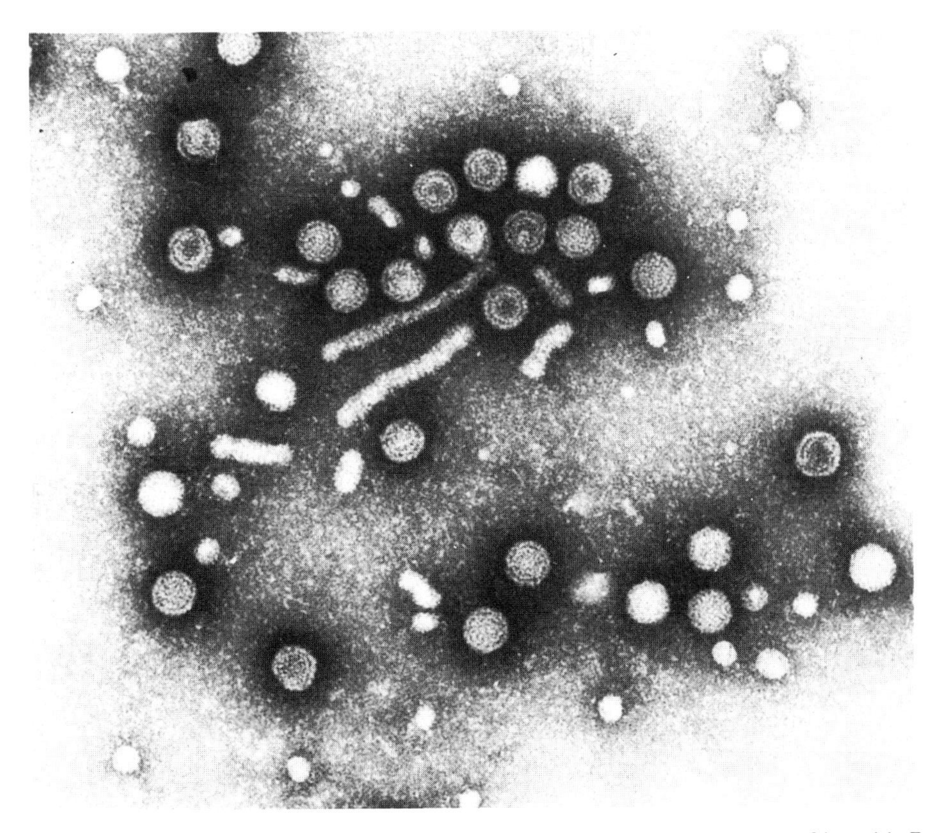

Fig 15.2. Electron micrograph (× 160 000) showing the three morphological forms of hepatitis B antigen (*see text* on p. 297).

d. 'e' antigen

This antigen is distinct from HBsAg and HBcAg and is characteristically present in the serum in high titre during the last 5 weeks of the incubation period and during the acute attack of hepatitis B. Its presence is closely associated with the infectivity of the patient. Only 0·0001 ml of serum which is HBsAg positive and 'e' antigen positive may be required to transmit hepatitis B to another patient. Patients who have persistent carriage of HBsAg probably have a higher risk of chronic liver disease when 'e' antigen is detected in the serum as well. Unfortunately tests for 'e' antigen are not as routinely available at present as the other tests for hepatitis-B-associated antigens and antibodies, but the test can be performed in a reference centre on selected cases.

Prevention of hepatitis B

General measures to educate those at risk about sensible hygienic precautions: including the use of separate sterile needles and syringes (helped greatly in hospitals by disposable plastic syringes and needles), avoiding close contact with blood and body fluids, reporting of all mishaps to an appointed safety officer or other appropriate senior member of staff and implementing of hospital policies to reduce the spread of hepatitis B (*see* Chapter 24). *Specific hyperimmune anti-hepatitis B immunoglobulin* should be given to persons exposed to hepatitis B because of an inoculation injury, preferably within 24–48 hours of the injury. In a few cases, administration of the immunoglobulin can also be considered for up to 10 days following the injury. A second dose of this immunoglobulin is normally recommended at about 1 month after the first dose. Babies born to HBsAg positive mothers may also need to be protected within 48 hours of birth by this immunoglobulin. Hepatitis B vaccines are under evaluation and probably will be available for selected groups of people at high risk in the near future. They may have an important use in reducing the incidence of the disease in Asia and Africa.

Hepatitis, Non-A, Non-B

In the last few years many cases of hepatitis, non-A, non-B have been recognized and this type of hepatitis is the most common cause of post-transfusion hepatitis in U.S.A. today. The diagnosis is normally made by excluding hepatitis A or B and other types of viral hepatitis.

Other Types of Viral Hepatitis

Yellow fever is discussed in Chapter 22. Jaundice due to hepatitis caused by the Epstein-Barr virus, cytomegalovirus or herpes simplex virus is uncommon.

OTHER INFECTIVE CAUSES OF JAUNDICE

Viral hepatitis is by far the most common infective problem associated with jaundice. Jaundice may also occur occasionally with other infections including:

a. Liver abscess—pyogenic or amoebic.
Clinical jaundice is rare but disturbed liver function tests are common, sometimes involving raised serum bilirubin.

b. Leptospirosis—jaundice is an occasional feature of Weil's disease (*L. icterohaemorrhagiae* infection).

c. Legionnaires' disease—hepatitis is occasionally severe in this infection.

d. Atypical pneumonia due to *Mycoplasma pneumoniae*—occasionally jaundice occurs in severe cold agglutinin positive cases in children.

e. Clostridial toxaemia associated with septic abortion or gas gangrene due to *Cl. welchii*—here jaundice is frequently a terminal feature.

f. Biliary tract obstruction due to worms—*Ascaris lumbricoides*, *Fasciola hepatica* or *Clonorchis sinensis*.

g. Cholangitis—possibly with empyema of gall bladder. Secondary bacterial infection usually associated with gall stones—resulting in jaundice and fever, and sometimes accompanying Gram-negative bacteraemia.

h. Hepato-renal syndrome associated with a few cases of Gram-negative sepsis.

i. Rare syphilitic hepatitis.

j. Jaundice may be a non-specific presentation of severe infection at any site in an infant—including urinary tract infection and septicaemia.

LIVER ABSCESS

Amoebic Liver Abcess

Amoebic liver abscess has been described elsewhere (*see* Chapters 4, 14, 22); it can be confused clinically with pyogenic liver abscess occasionally as both conditions may initially respond to metronidazole treatment. However, whereas amoebic liver abscess may be cured by a course of metronidazole alone, pyogenic liver abscess often will not be (*see below*).

Pyogenic Liver Abscess

Liver abscess may follow portal pyaemia associated with abdominal sepsis or it may occur in association with spreading infection from the biliary tract. A hydatid may become secondarily infected. Haematogenous spread from a focus elsewhere in the body, such as osteomyelitis, can also occur. In many cases, no obvious predisposing cause is found. The right lobe of the liver is more frequently affected than the left lobe.

Organisms

The most common bacteria causing pyogenic liver abscesses are:

a. Non-sporing anaerobes, such as *Bacteroides fragilis*, or anaerobic cocci.
b. Coliforms, such as *E. coli*, often mixed with a non-sporing anaerobe.
c. Streptococcal species, especially *Streptococcus milleri*, which may also be associated with collections of pus elsewhere in either the abdomen or chest.

Clinical features

There is often an insidious onset, and the patients may present with PUO. Eventually swinging pyrexia, malaise and pain in the right hypochondrium are characteristic features. Chest manifestations are frequent including cough and right basal pleural effusion. The blood usually shows a neutrophil leucocytosis.

Special investigations

Liver scans or ultrasound investigations usually reveal a hepatic filling defect.

Microbiology investigations

Blood cultures, at least three sets, just as the temperature is beginning to rise, should be collected. Isolation of *Bacteroides fragilis* (possibly mixed with *E. coli*) or *Strep. milleri* would suggest the presence of a collection of pus probably in the abdomen or liver.

Pus itself may be occasionally collected by fine needle aspiration but it is usually not available until after open surgical drainage of an abscess. Gas-liquid chromatography examination of the pus may reveal the presence of an anaerobe. Microscopy, prolonged culture and antibiotic sensitivity testing of any isolated organism will help greatly in the rational choice of an antibiotic for the patient. A search for amoebae should also be carried out.

Serum fluorescent amoebic antibody tests should be routinely carried out—a negative test helps to make a diagnosis of amoebic liver abscess less likely (*see* Amoebiasis, in Chapter 22 and in p. 286).

Treatment

Surgical drainage and antibiotic therapy are required. Initially a combination of ampicillin plus gentamicin plus metronidazole is necessary to cover *Strep. milleri*, coliform or anaerobic infections, respectively. The treatment can be modified once the results of culture and sensitivities are known.

Further Reading

Coleman J. C., Waugh M. and Dayton R. (1977) Hepatitis B antigen and antibody in a male homosexual population. *Br. J. Vener. Dis.* **53**, 132.

Cossart Y. E. (1977) *Virus Hepatitis and Its Control.* London, Baillière Tindall.

Farrow L. J., Stewart J. S., Stern H. et al. (1981) Non-A, non-B hepatitis in West London. *Lancet* **1**, 982–984.

Leading Article (1980) Immunisation against Hepatitis B. *Br. Med. J.* **2**, 1585.

Rosenheim Advisory Group (1972) *Hepatitis and the Treatment of Chronic Renal Failure.* D.H.S.S. London, H.M.S.O.

Shanson D. C. (1980) Outbreak of hepatitis B affecting operating theatre and intensive care unit staff. *Lancet* **2**, 596.

Zuckerman A. J. and Howard C. R. (1980) *Hepatitis Viruses of Man.* London, Academic Press.

Chapter 16

Skin infections and infestations

NORMAL FLORA OF SKIN

There are two types of skin flora, resident and transient:

1. *The resident flora* represents the organisms that are always present on the whole skin surface including those in the deeper parts of the skin such as the ducts of sebaceous and sweat gland follicles. This flora consists predominantly of *Staph. epidermidis,* micrococci and diphtheroids. Small numbers of anaerobic cocci and propionibacteria also may be present.

2. *The transient flora* consists of a wider range of organisms than the resident flora and may come in contact with the superficial aspects of the skin from the environment, another person or from the person's own alimentary tract. Limitation of the survival and growth of these organisms occurs as a result of:

a. cleaning and washing;

b. presence of an intact mechanical barrier of normal skin; however, when there are cuts or other lesions in the skin, the transient flora can multiply in these lesions causing either colonization or infection;

c. drying of some intruding bacteria on the skin;

d. fatty acids on the skin inhibit many bacteria;

e. antimicrobial substances produced by the resident skin flora.

Frequent examples of organisms that may transiently occur on the skin, especially of the hands, include *Staph. aureus, E. coli, Klebsiella* and other enterobacteria. Unless effective washing and drying of the skin follows the introduction of these organisms they may survive on the skin for several hours. This fact has particular importance for the control of cross-infection in hospitals (*see* Chapter 24). Less frequent examples include other bacteria, viruses and fungi.

Carriage of Staph aureus

A minority of individuals may carry *Staph. aureus* asymptomatically on moist areas of skin especially in the anterior nares. Outside of hospitals, 10–30% of healthy adults are nasal carriers. There is a higher nasal carriage rate in hospital staff varying between 20 and 60%. For the treatment of staphylococcal carriage *see* Chapter 24 and p. 485.

CAUSATIVE ORGANISMS

Organisms causing skin infections are included in *Table 16.1. Staph. aureus* and *Strep. pyogenes* are by far the most frequent causes of skin infections. Enterobacteria rarely cause skin infections unless there is a wound or devitalized tissue present (*see* Wound infections). *Candida albicans* infections of the skin are most likely to occur when the skin is subjected to excessive moisture.

Staph. aureus

Most strains of *Staph. aureus* do not invade and establish themselves in healthy skin tissues unless the dose of the organisms is high; however, if there is a skin lesion including skin disease, such as eczema, or foreign body present, the dose required is considerably less. The virulence of the organism varies greatly between different strains, and may depend partially on the protein A in the cell wall. Enzymes, such as coagulase and lipase, and toxins, such as alpha-toxin and leucocidin, may help the organism to establish itself in the tissues in spite of the host defence mechanisms that include phagocytosis, humoral antibody production and the activation of complement. In some patients, chronic and recurrent staphylococcal infections may occur, particularly if there is a congenital deficiency of phagocytic white cell function or of humoral antibody.

Strep. pyogenes

Strep. pyogenes often establishes itself easily in the skin tissues and the dose of organism required to initiate infections is much less than for *Staph. aureus*. The enzymes produced such as streptokinase and hyaluronidase may help the organism to lyse fibrin and spread rapidly through the tissues. The antigenic M protein in the cell wall is related to virulence and is anti-phagocytic. DNAase and leucocidin produced by the organism destroy white cells.

Organisms Associated with Vesicles/Pustules

Staph. aureus
Strep. pyogenes } *See* Impetigo, Pyoderma and Acne, *below*
Corynebacterium acnes

Neisseria—crops of vesicles/pustules, particularly occuring on the hands, may be associated with chronic gonococcal or meningococcal bacteraemia.

Viruses frequently cause vesicular lesions of the skin. These may become secondarily infected and pustules result. The most frequent viral causes include:

a. Herpes simplex (cold sores/lesions—particularly at mucocutaneous junctions)
b. Varicella-zoster, causing vesicles in one or more dermatomes in herpes zoster (shingles) and more generalized in chickenpox
c. Enteroviruses—especially Coxsackie A. Coxsackie A16 is sometimes associated with hand, foot and mouth disease
d. Vaccinia is a less frequent viral cause. Smallpox has now been eradicated—Orf and Molluscum contagiosum are mentioned later in this section.

Organisms Associated with Ulcers

Secondary infection of ulcers

This is a common problem in pressure sores, and varicose ulcers and is due to a mixture of organisms often including staphylococci, streptococci, Gram-negative bacilli, anaerobes and yeasts.

Table 16.1. Some causative organisms of skin infections (or infestations)

Bacteria		
1. *Gram-stainable*:	*Gram-positive*	*Gram-negative*
	Staph. aureus	Coliforms
	Strep. pyogenes	*Pseudomonas aeruginosa*
	Other haemolytic streptococci	*Neisseria gonorrhoeae*
	Anaerobic cocci	*Neisseria meningitidis*
	Clostridium sp.	*Pasteurella multocida*
	Corynebacterium diphtheriae	*Francisella tuluraemia*
	Actinomyces israelii	*Bacteroides* and fusiforms
	Nocardia asteroides	*Pseudomonas pseudomallei*
	Streptomyces	*Pseudomonas cepacia*
	Erysipelothrix rhusiopathiae	
	Bacillus anthracis	
	Corynebacterium minutissimum	
2. *Acid-fast bacilli*:	*Mycobacterium tuberculosis, M. ulcerans, M. chelonei, M. balnei* *Mycobacterium leprae*	
3. *Spirochaetes*:	*Treponema pallidum, pertenue, carateum* *Borrelia vincenti*	
Viruses	*DNA viruses*	*RNA viruses*
	Smallpox and vaccinia, Molluscum contagiosum, Orf } Pox viruses	Coxsackie A, Echo } enteroviruses
	Herpes simplex, Varicella-zoster } herpes viruses	
	Papovavirus	
Fungi	*Yeasts*	*Filamentous*
	Candida albicans	*Microsporum* species, *Trichophyton* species, *Epidermophyton floccosum* } dermatophytes
	Malassezia furfur	*Sporothrix schenckii*, *Histoplasma capsulatum*, *Coccidioides immitis*, *Blastomyces dermatidis* } dimorphic fungi
	Cryptococcus neoformans	*Madurella*, *Allescheria*, *Phialophora* } fungal causes of mycetoma

Primary microbial causes of ulcers

These include:

a. Bacteria

i. *Pseudomonas aeruginosa*—causes black necrotic ulcers—'ecthyma gangrenosum'—in patients with impaired host defences or receiving immunosuppressive therapy, who develop pseudomonas bacteraemia.

Table 16.1 continued

Protozoa	*Middle East, Africa and Asia*	*S. America*
	Leishmania tropica *Leishmania aethiopica*	*Leishmania brasiliensis* *Leishmania mexicana* *Leishmania peruana*
Helminths	*Filarial*	*Other*
	Onchocercus volvulus *Loa loa*	*Dracunculus medinensis* *Strongyloides stercoralis* Dog and cat hook worm
Arthropod	*Britain and other countries*	*Endemic only outside Britain*
	Sarcoptes scabei *Pulex irritans* and other fleas *Pediculus humanus* *Pediculus capitis* *Phthirus pubis* *Cimex lectularius*	*Tunga penetrans* *Cordylobia anthropophaga*

ii. *Treponema pallidum*—'hard chancre' in primary syphilis, which sometimes is extra-genital, and 'gumma' in tertiary syphilis which typically has a 'wash leather' base.
Treponema pertenue—(*see* Yaws *below*).

iii. *Mycobacterim tuberculosis*—'lupus vulgaris'—can present as tuberculous ulceration of the skin or as warty lesions.

iv. *Mycobacterium ulcerans*—'Buruli ulcer' due to *M. ulcerans* occurs in Central Africa and is associated with spreading chronic infection of the subcutaneous fat at flexure sites such as the elbow and forearm. Unless treated by surgery and anti-mycobacterial drugs, extensive fibrosis may result and cause severe disability.

v. *Mycobacterium balnei*—can cause superficial skin granulomas and ulcers in tropical fish tank enthusiasts and in those using swimming pools.

vi. *BCG vaccination*—usually causes a papule but as a complication either cheloid formation or ulceration may occasionally result especially if the immunization has inadvertently been given subcutaneously instead of intradermally or to an immunodeficient patient.

vii. *Anaerobes*—can cause acute ulceration in Meleney's synergic gangrene, particularly at an abdominal site when necrotizing fasciitis occurs, due to a combination of anaerobic streptococci and pyogenic cocci (*see* p. 314 for treatment). Fournier's gangrene presents similarly, usually at a perineal or scrotal site.

viii. *Bacillus anthracis*—'malignant pustule' (*see below*).

ix. *Corynebacterium diphtheriae*—in the tropics (*see below*).

x. '*Tropical ulcer*'—usually due to fusiforms and *Borrelia vincenti* following minor trauma, especially in malnourished young people in the tropics (*see* p. 314 for treatment).

xi. *Francisella tularensis*—tuluraemia—following bites or scratches from dogs, cats and wild animals in the U.S.A., Norway and other endemic areas outside Britain (*see* p. 315 for treatment).

b. Viruses/Mycoplasma

Serious vaccinial ulceration may follow smallpox vaccination when complications occur, especially in immunodeficient patients.

Orf can be associated with an ulcer on the hand or arm.

'Stevens-Johnson syndrome' involving skin and mucous membrane ulceration is occasionally associated with *Mycoplasma pneumoniae* infection.

c. Fungi

Certain deep fungal infections may result in skin ulceration including sporotrichosis and histoplasmosis.

d. Protozoa

Cutaneous leishmaniasis affecting the face or limbs is often associated with chronic skin ulceration and is usually due to *Leishmania tropica* and *Leishmania aethiopica* in Africa and Asia, respectively, and often *Leishmania brasiliensis* (cause of 'Espundia') in Latin America. Characteristically the ulcerated nodule has satellite papules. Serious destructive lesions are particularly associated with *L. brasiliensis*. The disease is spread by a sandfly with the reservoir of infection including dogs and rodents.

e. Worms

Guinea worm (*Dracunculus medinensis*) may cause an ulcer usually on the leg or foot in endemic parts of Africa and Asia and Latin America (*see* Chapter 23).

f. Insects

Tunga penetrans, the chiggoe or jigger flea, can penetrate the skin usually of the foot from the soil in tropical countries including Latin America, West Indies and Africa. Each early symptomless lesion appears as a black dot but the painful or itchy lesion enlarges and ulcerates. Tetanus can occur as a complication.

South African Tick vector of typhus and the Mite vector of scrub typhus often cause an 'eschar' at the site of the bite of the vector (*see* Chapter 22).

SKIN LESIONS ASSOCIATED WITH BACTERIAL INFECTION

Boils and Carbuncles

Boils (furuncles) result from *Staph. aureus* invasion of hair follicles or sebaceous glands. As with many other types of staphylococcal infection, there is a fibrous walling off of the suppurative lesion. Carbuncles are larger and deeper than boils and result from *Staph. aureus* infection of more than one hair follicle. They often appear on the back of the neck. If a patient complains of recurrent boils, microbiological investigations for carriage of *Staph. aureus* in the nose and other sites may be indicated and antiseptic (such as hexachlorophane) treatment of the carriage sites might help prevent future recurrences when the patient reinfects his skin from these sites. Also any patient with recurrent boils or carbuncles should have the urine tested for glucose in cases diabetes mellitus has predisposed to re-infection.

Cellulitis and Erysipelas

Spreading marked erythema, often accompanied by pain and brawny thickening of the skin and swelling of subcutaneous tissues, is indicative of cellulitis. When cellulitis spreads across the face the patient has 'erysipelas' which is rare today. Sometimes there is a history of an accidental wound or a discharging lesion may be evident, but with many cellulitis cases there is no history of an accident. When there is severe cellulitis, the patient shows marked constitutional upset, is febrile and may have septicaemia. Unless the patient receives rapid and effective treatment, death may occur.

Strep. pyogenes (β-haemolytic streptococcus, Lancefield group A) may invade the skin after a minor abrasion; it is nearly always the cause of spreading cellulitis. Haemolytic streptococci of other Lancefield groups, such as C and G, can also occasionally cause cellulitis. Rarely anaerobic streptococci may also be a cause. Lymphangitis and painful enlargement of lymph glands is also characteristic of streptococcal cellulitis.

Staph. aureus, alone, is an infrequent cause of cellulitis and the spreading erythema is less marked. More frequently, *Staph. aureus* occurs together with *Strep. pyogenes* and this is particularly important with regard to treatment (*see below*).

Impetigo

Impetigo is a superficial infection of the epidermidis which occurs in children and is characterized by vesicles that become golden crusted in the usual type of impetigo which is caused by *Strep. pyogenes*. The vesicular lesions usually occur on the limb extremities or on the face. Serous fluid from a vesicle infects adjacent skin areas and large extended lesions up to 10 cm in diameter may result. Secondary infection of the vesicles by *Staph. aureus* often develops causing pustular lesions. There is usually little constitutional upset, and fortunately scarring of the skin rarely occurs as a complication as deep skin tissues are not affected. The infection may spread from child to child by direct contact.

Another less common type of impetigo, characterized by persistent bullous lesions, with only transient thin white crusts, is due to *Staph. aureus* of a group II phage type, such as phage type 71. This type can occur in epidemic form in hospitals amongst neonates when it is then known as Impetigo Neonatorum (Pemphigus Neonatorum).

Ritter's Disease

Toxic epidermal necrolysis, also known as Ritter's disease, Lyell's syndrome, 'Scalded Child' syndrome, is characterized by the sudden appearance of toxaemia, fever and erythematous tender skin lesions over the face or other parts of the body of neonates and children up to 10 years old. Occasionally adults are affected. The skin lesions are due to a toxin secreted by certain phage group II strains of *Staph. aureus*, often phage type 71, that causes the epidermidis to be split by fluid. The *Staph. aureus* strain may cause infection in the upper respiratory tract, skin or other parts of the body and bacteraemia may occur. Outbreaks of the disease may occur in nurseries and deaths can follow rapidly (*see* Chapters 7 and 24).

Pyoderma

Impetigo is a form of pyoderma, but the term 'pyoderma' includes many other skin lesions which are secondarily infected by *Strep. pyogenes* or *Staph. aureus*. These skin lesions include minor trauma such as may follow a game of rugby and so-called 'scrum pox', usually an outbreak of streptococcal impetigo, can then occur. Other lesions include insect bites, scabies, eczema and herpes. In overcrowded circumstances in warm countries, such as the West Indies, outbreaks of streptococcal pyoderma are particularly liable to occur. Sometimes these outbreaks are followed by outbreaks of acute glomerulonephritis when *Strep. pyogenes* of certain nephritogenic types such as M types 49 or 55 have caused the pyoderma. Indirect skin complications of streptococcal infections such as erythema nodosum do not appear to follow the pyoderma.

'Sycosis barbae' is a superficial skin infection over the beard area of the face and, when pustular, is usually due to *Staph. aureus*.

Abscesses

Subcutaneous abscesses may arise especially in the axillae, groin, perineum and post-partum breast as well as at injection sites (particularly in drug addicts and diabetics). *Staph. aureus* is by far the most frequent causative organism at these sites followed by *Strep. pyogenes*.

When a foreign body is present in the subcutaneous tissues, such as suture material, a cardiac pacemaker, haemodialysis shunt or a drain, *Staph. aureus* is again the most frequent causative organism of infection; however, many other organisms may also cause infection including some strains of streptococci, Gram-negative bacilli and *Staph. epidermidis*.

Other causes of subcutaneous abscesses include:

Anaerobes—Bacteroides or anaerobic cocci—may cause infections of the sweat glands—especially in the axilla, breast and sebaceous cysts.

Bacteroides fragilis, frequently mixed with coliforms, often cause the suppuration in ischio-rectal and peri-anal regions and in the Bartholin's glands.

NB Lesions which discharge and are accompanied by a foul smell are often due to anaerobes.

Mycobacterium tuberculosis—especially in immigrants; atypical presentations can occur with 'cold abcesses' subcutaneously; also in immunosuppressed patients.

Mycobacterium chelonei and other environmental bacteria, particularly at injection or foreign body sites.

Pseudomonas pseudomallei—cause of melioidosis—'glanders' occurring in Indo-China, India and Malaysia.

Nocardia asteroides—particularly in immunosuppressed patients receiving steroids.

Actinomyces israelii—actinomycosis of skin can occur as a metastatic complication of actinomycosis eslewhere.

Paronychia

Infection of the subcutaneous tissues around the nails—paronychia—can present as an acute or chronic lesion.

The pyogenic cocci, *Staph. aureus* and *Strep. pyogenes*, are the main causes of acute paronychia. Herpes simplex virus can also cause paronychia (*see* Herpes simplex, p. 315.)

Chronic paronychia, involving the loss of the cuticle, mainly occurs when there is a predisposing factor present such as chronic moist conditions and devitalized tissues around the nails. This occurs where there is a lot of wet work and mechanical trauma—as with 'washerwoman's hands'. Gram-negative bacilli, such as *E. coli*, *Pseudomonas aeruginosa*, *Proteus mirabilis*, *Bacteroides fragilis* and yeasts, especially *Candida albicans*, are the usual causative organisms, although *Staph. aureus* and streptococci can also occasionally cause chronic infections.

Cat and Dog Bites and Scratches

Pasteurella multocida is an important cause of subcutaneous infection which often follows bites or scratches from cats and dogs. Characteristically, there is some suppuration at the site of the injury, regional enlargement of the lymph glands and possibly some cellulitis.

Other organisms may cause infection alone or mixed in with *Pasteurella multocida* following these injuries, particularly non-sporing anaerobes such as *Bacteroides* species, *Clostridium tetani*, *Clostridium perfringens* and streptococci. Tetanus prophylaxis is advisable. Cat scratch fever, after cat scratches, has very rarely been described. When the injury occurs in an endemic area, the possibility of rabies developing should also be considered and prophylaxis started if necessary. In endemic areas outside Britain the possible development of tuluraemia should be considered (*see* Chapter 21).

Erysipeloid

Erysipeloid, due to *Erysipelothrix rhusiopathiae*, should be suspected in meat or fish handlers who develop pain followed by the appearance of a blue–red discoloration of the skin with a well-demarcated edge on the hands or forearms.

Erythrasma

Erythema spreading in moist folds of the skin, particularly the axillae, may be 'erythrasma' which is caused by *Corynebacterium minutissimum*. The skin lesion fluoresces under ultraviolet light.

Intertrigo

Intertrigo consists of a weeping dermatitis at the site of moist skin folds where the skin surfaces rub one another occurring particularly under the breasts and in the crutch area. *Candida albicans* is the most common infecting organism but secondary infection due to streptococci or staphylococci may also occur. Nappy rash in babies may be associated with *Candida albicans* infection.

Acne vulgaris

The unsightly pimples of acne on the face and upper trunk are due to blockage of pilo-sebaceous openings by the 'blackhead' and hormonal imbalance during adolescence. Bacteria, including *Corynebacterium acnes* and coagulase-negative staphylococci, may invade the blocked sebaceous glands and cause pustules. Exacerbation of the acne lesions due to bacteria may be due to the local production of free fatty acids due to the action of bacterial lipases. The low doses of tetracycline that are sometimes useful in treatment might help through reducing this lipase activity but the pathogenesis of acne and the mode of action of antibiotics remains unclear.

Infected Burns

Infection of burns is extremely common and continues to cause significant mortality in many centres. Mild superficial infection or colonization by *Staph. aureus* and Gram-negative bacilli including *E. coli* and *Klebsiella* is often seen without serious complications developing. However, occasionally these organisms can infect deeper tissues and cause septicaemia. Infrequently infection occurs due to *Strep. pyogenes* and is always potentially serious as this organism can delay healing, prevent grafts from taking and can rapidly cause fatal septicaemia. *Pseudomonas aeruginosa* frequently infects burns unless appropriate preventive measures are taken possibly including the use of topical silver compounds. This organism can reduce the chances of a graft taking successfully and pseudomonas septicaemia in burned patients is associated with a particularly high mortality. Patients with severe burns are particularly liable to infection by *Pseudomonas* and a further preventive measure under investigation involves immunization against *Pseudomonas*.

All patients with burns need management with much attention to aseptic technique and should preferably by nursed in protective or protective plus source isolation, since cross-infection is very liable to occur (*see* Chapter 24). A policy involving the restriction of antibiotics is essential to reduce the development of organisms with multiple antibiotic resistance.

Cutaneous Diphtheria

Corynebacterium diphtheriae can secondarily infect skin lesions, mainly in the tropics, causing a small ulcer. Only very rarely are the classic toxic complications of diphtheria produced.

Anthrax

Cutaneous anthrax (malignant pustule) follows contact with infected animals, hides and other animal products including bone meal. The disease is rare in

Britain and most often occurs in gardeners, farmers, vets and dock and tannery workers. The lesion starts as a small 'pimple' which becomes pustular within 48–72 hours and is surrounded by inflammation. The centre of the lesion becomes necrotic resulting in a dark 'eschar'. An area of induration and some vesicles may develop around the eschar. Early treatment is necessary; if the patient develops widespread oedema, toxic signs or septicaemia, the prognosis is poor. (*See also Bacillus anthracis* p. 521, and Chapter 21.)

Leprosy

The two main types of skin lesions due to *Mycobacterium leprae* are (i) depigmented anaesthetic skin patches of 'tuberculoid leprosy' and (ii) nodular 'lepromatous leprosy' (*see* Chapter 13).

Yaws (Framboesia)

Yaws occurs in humid tropical parts of Latin America, West Indies, Africa and Asia, due to *Treponema pertenue*. The chronic infection is usually spread by direct contact and possibly by gnats, and affects mainly the skin and later bone. The initial skin lesion is papular, extra-genital and subsequently ulcerates. Generalized exuberant lesions may occur several weeks later on the limbs, face and genitalia.

Pinta

Pinta may affect the natives of Central and South America and the West Indies and is caused by *Treponema carateum*. The primary lesion appears as a small scaly patch, extra-genitally. Generalized hyperkeratotic lesions may follow several months later. The disease is spread by direct contact and by gnats. Cardiovascular and central nervous system complications can occur later.

BACTERIOLOGICAL INVESTIGATIONS

Specimens that are representative of the site of infection are collected whenever possible before the start of antimicrobial chemotherapy as with infections at other sites.

1. Collection of specimens

Pus

Pus is always preferable to a swab and, when there is a subcutaneous abscess or a superficial closed lesion, aspiration of the contents using a syringe and needle is usually possible, even if surgical drainage is not performed. The pus needs to be put in a sterile dry container, which is then transported promptly to the laboratory. When there are only small quantities of pus in a lesion, a swab may have to suffice. Ideally two swabs should be collected—one 'dry' swab for making a smear for microscopy for cells and organisms and another 'wet' swab broken off into Stuart's transport medium for culture of all bacteria including those that might otherwise die during transport on a dry swab such as delicate anaerobes and neisseria organisms. The swabs are also transported in less than 2–3 hours to the laboratory. If only one swab is collected it should be the 'wet' swab.

When there is an open discharging lesion, or a deep infected ulcer, the results obtained from a superficial swab taken from an uncleaned lesion may reflect superficial colonization only. A swab of a lesion that has first been carefully cleaned using a sterile gauze may yield more representative results reflecting the organisms present at the site of the infection.

When *actinomycosis* is suspected, pus that has been collected from a sinus including that on the most recent dressing should also be examined for 'sulphur granules'.

Foul-smelling pus may be examined by a gas–liquid chromatography method for a rapid indication of whether anaerobes are present. *Proteus* and *Pseudomonas* can also be associated with unpleasant smelling pus and occasionally *Pseudomonas*-induced pus has a greenish colour. Ultraviolet light directed at septic lesions which fluoresces red may indicate *Bacteroides melaninogenicum* infection.

Blood cultures

Blood cultures should always be collected from patients with cellulitis and severe or unusual sepsis.

Biopsies

When unusual infections, such as erysipeloid and mycobacterial infection, are suspected, a *biopsy* of the skin lesion is sometimes necessary for microscopy and culture, and a sample is sent also to histopathology. Good clinical collaboration between the clinician and clinical microbiologist is always desirable especially when unusual infections are suspected. A split-skin biopsy is collected from possible leprosy skin lesions as well as from the ear lobes, and perhaps nasal septum, for a search for acid-fast bacilli (*see* Chapter 13).

Serous exudate

Primary or secondary syphilitic lesions may need *serous exudate* collecting for dark-ground illumination or fluorescent antibody microscopy for spirochaetes.

2. Microscopy

The Gram-stain is a frequently useful rapid indicator of the causative organisms present and is routinely performed. Acid-fast and fluorescent stains and dark-ground illumination microscopy are only performed when clinically indicated.

3. Cultures and antibiotic sensitivities

Pus, swabs and biopsy material should always be cultured on fresh blood agar aerobically and anaerobically, and the anaerobic atmospheres should include added CO_2 to culture carboxyphilic organisms. Cultures are incubated for at least 48 hours and for up to 5 days when organisms apparent in the Gram-stain or suggested clinically (such as actinomycosis) are not cultured by 48 hours. The microbiologist may wish to include other media, such as MacConkey agar, when infections with coliforms or *Proteus* are possible and 'Lowenstein-Jensen' media at various temperatures when mycobacteria are suspected. Skin commensals are normally disregarded but suspected pathogens would have antibiotic sensitivity tests performed.

4. Serology

Patients with suspected syphilis, yaws or pinta should have treponemal serological investigations performed (*see* Chapter 20).

TREATMENT

Many minor common skin infections, such as boils, will resolve spontaneously and require no treatment. The need for and choice of treatment will mainly depend on the severity and type of skin infection or infestation encountered.

Examples of bacterial infections where surgical drainage of pus or débridement of tissues is usually necessary include abscesses, septic wounds following animal bites, badly infected burns, paronychia, Buruli ulcer, anaerobic skin infections and some mycetoma. Systemic antibiotics may be necessary as an adjunct to the surgery and in most instances the final choice of antimicrobial drug depends on the results of the microbiological investigations including antibiotic sensitivity tests.

Antibiotics often need to be given without surgery.

Some principles of therapy include:

a. No treatment necessary or topical therapy only

Systemic antibiotics are not helpful for minor to moderate degrees of secondary infection of ulcers or eczema and for most boils and mild impetigo.

Antiseptics such as chlorhexidine, hexachlorophene and topical hypochlorite (e.g. Eusol) may help when topically applied together with local toilet and removal of crusts where applicable. Also, depending on the results of cultures and sensitivity, topical treatment with antibiotics that are seldom used systemically such as bacitracin, polymyxin or chloramphenicol may occasionally help. Gentamicin should never by applied topically as gentamicin-resistant strains of *Staph. aureus* and Gram-negative bacilli may rapidly emerge following such therapy.

b. Systemic antibiotic therapy necessary

Closed spreading cellulitis is nearly always due to *Strep. pyogenes* which is always sensitive to benzylpenicillin. Benzylpenicillin alone, 1 MU 4-hourly, usually will start to control the infection within 24–48 hours. In addition, flucloxacillin, 500 mg–1 g 6-hourly, is recommended to cover a possible coexistent penicillinase-producing *Staph. aureus.* Flucloxacillin by itself is active against both *Strep. pyogenes* and *Staph. aureus* infection, but in all but very very mild cases it is best to treat with benzylpenicillin as well, as this is the drug of first choice for a *Strep. pyogenes* infection.

For pyoderma, impetigo and other bacterial soft tissue infections where *Staph. aureus* and *Strep. pyogenes* are likely pathogens, a combination of high-dose cloxacillin plus benzylpenicillin is again the safest therapy.

Tetracycline should not be used 'blind' as tetracycline resistance is frequently seen amongst both *Strep. pyogenes* and *Staph. aureus* strains.

Chronic infections—it is best to wait for the results of investigations and antibiotic sensitivity tests before selecting antimicrobial drugs.

Allergy to penicillin

For patients allergic to penicillin: erythromycin is active against nearly all *Strep. pyogenes* strains and the majority of *Staph. aureus* strains and is effective clinically when used instead of penicillin and flucloxacillin. (Erythromycin stearate, 500 mg–1 g 6-hourly, orally.)

Cephalosporins can also be used instead of erythromycin again when the penicillin allergy history is only doubtful.

Fusidic acid is active against most strains of *Staph. aureus* and may be useful when given systemically for severe staphylococcal infection in combination with flucloxacillin or erythromycin. It should not normally be used alone or topically because of the risk of developing fusidic acid resistance.

Burns

Antibiotics are not required systemically for most mildly infected burns except when there is *Strep. pyogenes* infection when cloxacillin is usually indicated (this drug is resistant to the penicillinases produced by other organisms which may also be present in the infected burn).

The closest collaboration between the clinician and microbiologist is necessary to discuss treatment of each severely infected case. An attempt at treating *Pseudomonas aeruginosa* infections can be made using a combination of tobramycin or gentamicin and carbenicillin when the strain is sensitive to carbenicillin.

Outlines of Treatments for Specific Bacterial Infections Include:

Acne—low dose tetracycline therapy may be beneficial
Neisseria infections—penicillin
Nocardiosis—surgical drainage and cotrimoxazole often helpful
Actinomycosis—penicillin
Tropical ulcers—penicillin therapy or metronidazole and skin grafting
Syphilis, yaws, pinta—penicillin therapy
Erysipeloid—penicillin
Erythrasma—erythromycin
Anthrax—penicillin
Buruli ulcer—surgery and rifampicin
Pasteurella multocida infection—penicillin or tetracycline
Meleney's synergic gangrene—metronidazole plus benzylpenicillin plus cloxacillin

Leprosy—dapsone for tuberculoid leprosy
dapsone, rifampicin and clofazimine for lepromatous leprosy
Tularaemia—streptomycin

SKIN LESIONS ASSOCIATED WITH VIRAL INFECTION

Herpetic Vesicles and Herpetic Whitlow

Herpes simplex may cause recurrent cold sores and genital lesions (*see* Chapter 20). Herpetic whitlow may be an occupational disease of nursing staff. Kaposi's varicelliform eruptions may result from herpes simplex superinfection of disseminated eczema.

Other Viruses Associated with Vesicular Lesions

See above Organisms associated with vesicles or pustules—varicella-zoster, vaccinia, enteroviruses, etc. (p. 303).

Warts

A papovavirus is the cause of the common wart. Plantar warts often cause discomfort and may require treatment. Genital warts may also be caused by a virus and these are transmitted venereally. Viral-induced warts frequently regress spontaneously. The more flat Condylomata lata occurs in the genital or perianal regions and is syphilitic. Chronic trichomonal infections in women also can be associated with genital warts.

Molluscum contagiosum

A pox virus causes molluscum contagiosum which is most often seen in children. Fleshy papules, up to 4 mm diameter, appear which may become umbilicated. The lesions usually spontaneously disappear within a few months but occasionally treatment may be necessary by squeezing the waxy contents out of a pierced lesion.

Orf (Contagious Pustular Dermatitis)

A pox virus, with a characteristic criss-crossed basket-like structure apparent on electron microscopy, is the causative organism of Orf which is most frequently seen in shepherds or other people in contact with infected sheep and goats. The skin lesion in Orf usually consists of a solitary papulovesicular lesion on the hand or forearm which may ulcerate. Orf is less common than in the past, since the introduction of an effective sheep vaccine against the disease.

Milker's Nodule

Milker's nodule is similar to the lesion of Orf and is caused by a morphologically identical virus to the virus of Orf. The reservoir of the disease is in cows (vesicles on teats of udders) and it affects the hands of people working with infected cattle.

Virological Investigations

1. Collection of specimens

Fluid from vesicular lesions is collected into sealed capillary glass tubes for subsequent microscopy and culture, and also directly at the bedside into viral transport medium. A swab of the base of the lesion should also be broken off into viral transport medium and sent to the laboratory. Biopsy material of the nodules, ulcer or papules of Orf, Milker's nodule or Molluscum contagiosum may also be collected to confirm the diagnosis, but microbiological investigations of the common wart or plantar wart are not usually necessary.

2. Microscopy

Characteristic inclusion bodies are seen in epithelial cells infected by Molluscum contagiosum on light microscopy. Electron microscopy is often used to provide rapid evidence of herpesvirus infections (herpes simplex, varicella-zoster) when vesicular fluid is examined on the carbon-coated grid by negative-staining methods and also characteristic pox viruses when material from vaccinial lesions or Orf is examined. Historically, electron microscopy was of enormous importance for the rapid investigation of suspected smallpox.

3. Culture

Tissue cultures and culture in chick embryos are used to identify the causative viruses.

Treatment of Virus Infections

a. Herpes

Varicella-zoster (shingles) and herpes simplex lesions can be treated topically with idoxuridine in dimethyl sulphoxide provided treatment is given in the early stages of the disease. Acycloguanosine may be useful for treating severe lesions in immunodeficient patients (*see* Genital herpes, in Chapter 20).

b. Vaccinia

Ectopic vaccinial lesions can be treated by methisazone and hyperimmune antivaccinial globulin should be given to immunodeficient patients who have inadvertently received vaccination.

SKIN LESIONS ASSOCIATED WITH FUNGAL INFECTIONS

Tinea Infections (Ringworm)

Many different dermatophyte fungal species may invade the keratinized layers of the skin, the nails or hair to cause tinea infections. The three genera of dermatophytes are *Trichophyton, Microsporum* and *Epidermophyton.* Some dermatophyte infections are zoonoses (*see* Chapter 21, p. 419). Ringworm is particularly common in the hands and feet.

Tinea capitis (Scalp Ringworm)

Microsporum audouini affects pre-pubertal schoolchildren and is sometimes associated with an epidemic form of tinea capitis (*see Fig. 16.1*). Invasion of the hair shafts deep to the scalp results in circumscribed patches of alopecia with grey lustreless hairs broken just above the scalp. When a Wood's ultraviolet light is used the affected scalp fluoresces.

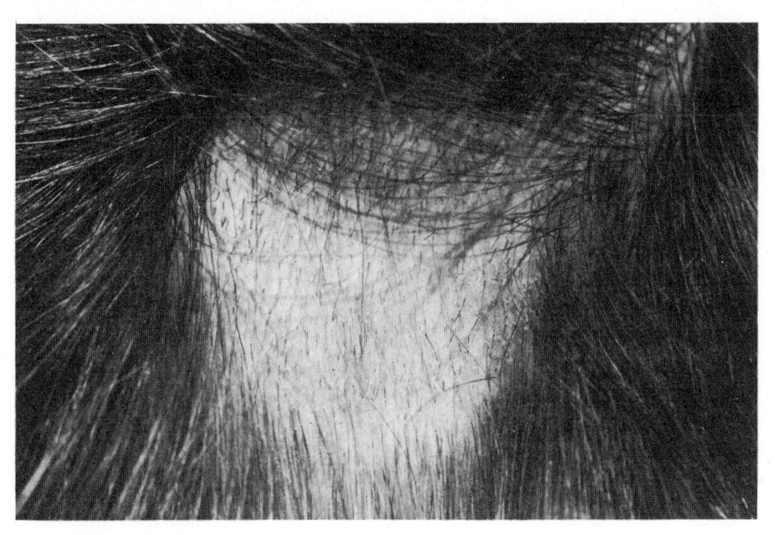

Fig. 16.1. Tinea capitis lesion.

Microsporum canis causes tinea capitis which is associated with inflammatory lesions unlike *Microsporum audouini*. The organism is acquired by children from cats or dogs.

Favus

Trichophyton schoenleinii causes a variety of scalp ringworm seen more commonly amongst Asians than Europeans.

Tinea pedis (Athlete's Foot)

Peeling, maceration and the development of fissures between the toe clefts due to dermatophytes is extremely common. The three main causative organisms are *Trichophyton rubrum*, *Trichophyton mentagrophytes* var. *interdigitalis* and *Epidermophyton floccosum*. The infection is spread by person to person especially when there are shared shower or bathing facilities.

Tinea corporis (Body Ringworm)

Characteristically, dermatophytes, mainly *Trichophyton* species, affecting glabrous skin cause rounded lesions which spread centrifugally and heal in the centre (*Fig. 16.2*).

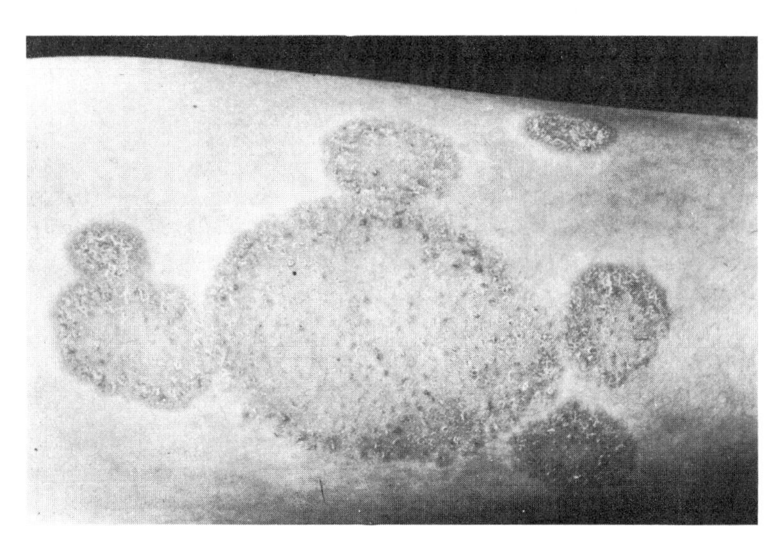

Fig. 16.2. Tinea corporis.

Tinea barbae (Ringworm of the Beard)

A pustular eruption, associated with much inflammation, is associated with tinea barbae due to *Trichophyton verrucosum* which is acquired from cattle.

Tinea cruris

Trichophyton rubrum or *Epidermophyton floccosum* are the main organisms causing tinea in the intertrigous areas of the groin in men.

Tinea unguium (Ringworm of the Nails) ***Onchomycosis***

Trichophyton rubrum is the commonest cause of ringworm of the nails and Man is the main source of the organism. Affected nails usually show yellow discoloration at the side of the nail and the nails become brittle and thickened.

Pityriasis versicolor

Clinically the lesions in Pityriasis versicolor usually appear as a macular rash on the trunk of a young adult with brownish lesions on a white skin and depigmented lesions on a skin that is otherwise tanned by sunlight. The disease is more common in tropical countries and is caused by a yeast, *Malassezia furfur*. The lesions fluoresce golden-brown colour under Wood's ultraviolet light.

Chronic Mucocutaneous Candidiasis

Chronic infection of the skin and mucous membranes by *Candida albicans*, to form severe and widespread granulomatous lesions, may occur in some children or adults with impaired phagocytic or T lymphocyte immunity, or hypoparathyroidism, or iron deficiency. Correction of the underlying predisposing factor may help in the treatment of the infection.

Sporotrichosis

A skin ulcer forms at the site of a wound which has been in contact with either soil or part of a plant contaminated with the causative organism of sporotrichosis, *Sporotrichium schenckii*. The wound is often penetrating and is commonly caused by a thorn.

Mycetoma

Deep destructive suppurative or granulomatous lesions affecting the subcutaneous tissues and occasionally bone, often localized in the foot, and frequently associated with sinuses, may be caused by a variety of fungi or bacterial species belonging to the genera *Actinomycetes*, *Streptomyces* and *Nocardia*. *Madurella mycetoma* is an important example of a fungal causative organism. These infections are more common in countries with warm or tropical climates, and occur especially in people who walk barefoot; the organisms frequently are acquired by people in rural areas from contaminated soil.

Mycological Investigations

1. Collection of specimens

Skin scrapings taken from the edge of the lesion using a blunt 'banana' scalpel, nail clippings and broken hairs taken from the follicles in the scalp are collected from suspect ringworm lesions and transported in envelopes or plastic containers, preferably in the folds of black paper. Biopsy material is usually preferable when mycetoma or sporotrichosis is suspected. Skin scrapings are collected from the suspected lesions of Pityriasis versicolor.

2. Microscopy

The specimens are first examined under direct microscopy after 'clearing' the tissue in warm potassium hydroxide so that fungal hyphae and spores can be seen. A wet mount in lactophenol blue may help better visualization of the hyphae and characteristic spores such as macroconidia of dermatophytes (*see Fig. 16.3*). *Malassezia furfur* is diagnosed by a characteristic microscopic appearance (*see Fig. 16.4*). Biopsy material is also examined using PAS staining techniques. *Candida* species are obvious on bacteriological Gram-stain when a pseudomycelium and Gram-positive candida buds are seen.

3. Culture

Sabouraud's medium is usually used for fungal isolations either in Petri dishes or as a slide culture which is particularly useful for showing the typical morphology of colonies. The medium is incubated for a prolonged period at 22–26 °C in a moist atmosphere, and sometimes also at 35 °C. Pigmentation on the reverse side of dermatophyte colonies often aids identification of the fungus (such as the red–violet colour of *Trichophyton rubrum*).

Blood agar also supports the growth of most fungi including *Candida albicans*.

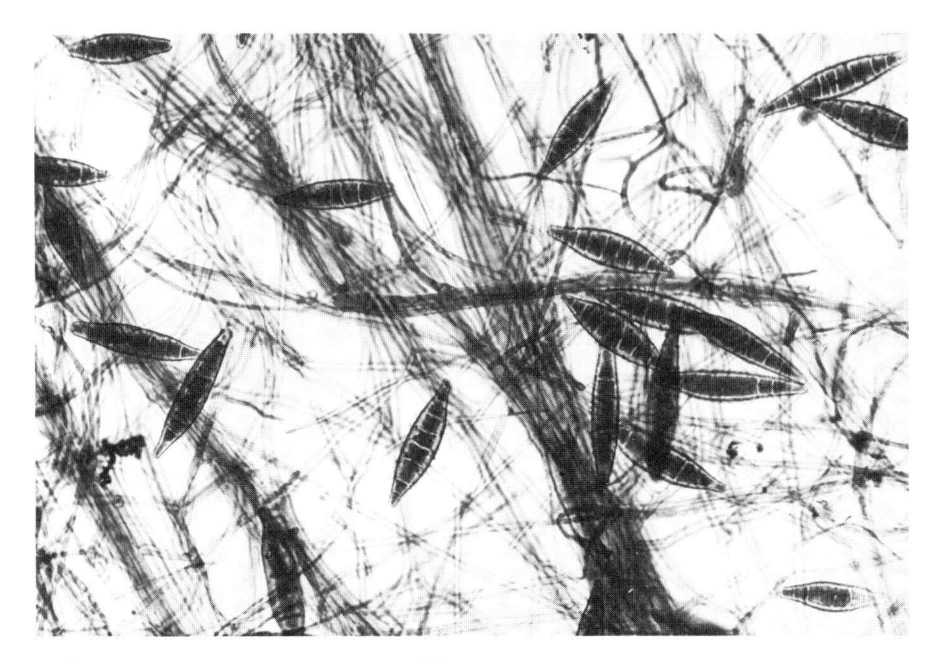

Fig. 16.3. Microsporum canis macroconidia.

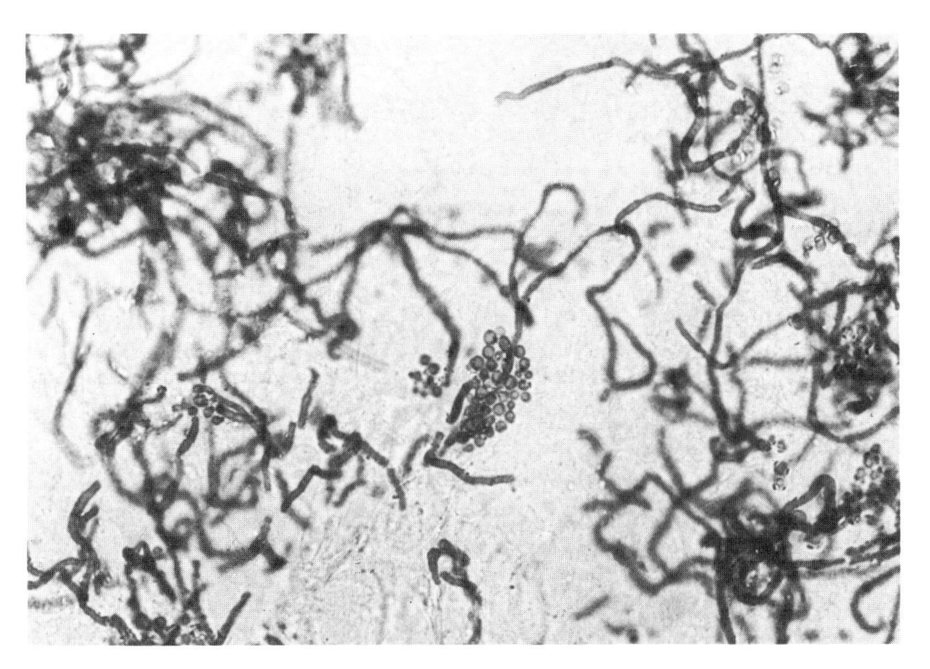

Fig. 16.4. Malassezia furfur in a skin scraping.

4. Antimicrobial sensitivities

Sensitivity tests to antifungal agents are only carried out on a few selected pathogens in special circumstances in reference laboratories. The sensitivities to agents such as amphotericin B, nystatin, clotrimazole and griseofulvin is usually predictable without having to do sensitivity tests.

Treatment of Fungal Infections

a. Ringworm

Tinea pedis, cruris, corporis and barbae are usually successfully treated with a topical anti-fungal agent, active against dermatophytes; Whitfield's ointment or local clotrimazole are usually successful.

Hair ringworm and nail ringworm usually respond to systematic treatment with griseofulvin. This drug becomes incorporated into the newly formed keratin layers and prevents further infection. It usually needs to be given for 2–6 months.

b. Candida albicans lesions

Intertrigo associated with *Candida* responds to topical nystatin or amphotericin B, gentian violet or miconazole.

Systemic agents such as 5-fluorocytosine, clotrimazole or amphotericin B are necessary for treating chronic muco-cutaneous candidiasis.

c. Pityriasis versicolor

Local treatment with Whitfield's ointment, selenium sulphide shampoo or clotrimazole is often successful but relapses are common.

d. Sporotrichosis

Oral potassium iodide solution continued for about 1 month after the skin lesion has disappeared. For iodine-resistant cases, amphotericin B is given.

e. Madura foot

Severe deep subcutaneous mycoses may require extensive surgery, possibly even amputation of the foot or leg, in addition to systemic amphotericin B.

SKIN LESIONS ASSOCIATED WITH PROTOZOA

See Ulcers, p. 303.

Investigations for Protozoa

Suspected cutaneous leishmaniasis lesions should have material collected by either a split-skin smear of the edge of the lesion or a biopsy from the deepest parts of the ulcer, avoiding contamination by blood.

Microscopy of the material smeared on a slide is examined after staining by Leishman's stain. A search for typical oval forms of the organism is made.

Culture of the leishmania organisms can also be attempted from the collected material using NNN medium.

The leishmania skin test is useful in people who are not natives in the endemic areas, a positive test developing about 4 months after infection.

Treatment of Protozoal Infections

Cutaneous leishmaniasis can be successfully treated with pentavalent antimony given locally into the lesion or systemically.

SKIN LESIONS ASSOCIATED WITH WORM INFECTIONS

a. Loiasis

The adult filarial worm *Loa loa* is rarely observed as it moves in the subcutaneous tissues where it resides. Calabar swellings (fugitive swellings) can appear in the skin as transient erythematous swellings on the upper limbs and face resulting from an allergic inflammatory reaction to the worm. This disease, which is spread by the *Chrysops* gnat, occurs in West Africa only (*see* Chapter 23, p. 456, and Chapter 11, p. 211.

b. Onchocerciasis

The adult filarial worm *Onchocerca volvulus* resides in the subcutaneous tissues and is associated with the development of much more obvious skin symptoms and signs than *Loa loa*. The disease occurs in Africa, from approximately 15 °N to 15 °S and in parts of Latin America. Onchocerciasis affects large numbers of people in Africa, particularly near fast-flowing rivers where the black fly vector, *Simulium,* breeds. Both the adult worms and the microfiliariae which also occur in the subcutaneous tissues excite an inflammatory response so that itchy papules and oedematous lesions develop. Thickened skin and depigmented patches may also occur in long-standing cases. The skin lesions are particularly common about the waist and over the iliac crests, thighs, skull and chest.

The main complication of the disease is involvement of the eye—'river blindness' which is regrettably common in endemic areas (*see* Chapters 11 and 23).

c. Strongyloidiasis and Cutaneous Larva migrans

The larvae of *Strongyloides stercoralis* penetrate the skin and may cause a weal and flare serpentine reaction as they migrate several centimetres across the skin. This cutaneous larva migrans reaction may recur although each line of irritating eruption may last for a few hours only. Strongyloidiasis is prevalent in many tropical areas of the world including the Far East, West Indies and Latin America. There are other worms that may cause cutaneous larva migrans including hook worms of the cat and dog.

d. Schistosomiasis (Bilharzia)

Papular eruptions can result from the penetration of the cercariae of *Schistosoma* species following bathing in contaminated fresh water (*see* Chapter 23).

e. Guinea Worm

See Ulcer *and* Investigations *below.*

Investigation for Worms

Eosinophilia is nearly always present when the skin is infested by worms. A heparinized blood sample is collected during the day and after filtration and staining by Leishman stain the characteristic microfiliariae of *Loa loa* can be demonstrated in patients with loiasis.

Skin strips are collected at the site of the nodular lesions of patients with suspected onchocerca infection and immersed in saline. After 30 minutes or after 24 hours the microfiliariae of *Onchocerca volvulus* may be seen during microscopic examination of the saline.

When strongyloidiasis is suspected, the rhabtidiform larvae of *Strongyloides stercoralis* are looked for during the wet microscopy of faeces. The adult guinea worm *Dracunculus medinensis* is seen during extraction through the skin ulcer associated with it. The guinea worm embryos may be detected in the affected joint fluid or in the fluid from the vesicular skin ulcer.

Treatment of Worm Infestations

Loiasis and onchocerciasis are treated by diethylcarbamazine in specialized centres; this drug kills the microfilariae but can also cause toxic complications. The same drug is useful for treating guinea worm infestation since it prevents the maturation of the larvae.

Cutaneous larva migrans is treated locally with ethyl chloride freeze spraying and thiabendazole.

SKIN LESIONS ASSOCIATED WITH INSECT INFESTATIONS

a. Scabies

The mite *Sarcoptes scabiei* is the cause of scabies which is common throughout the world, and is spread by direct contact and infected clothes. It is particularly prevalent in immigrants who may have the chronic form of the disease and in travellers returning to Britain who usually have the acute disease. The female mite burrows into the skin to lay eggs in the clefts most often between the fingers and in the skin of the hands, wrists, forearms, perineal and genital (especially penile) regions. Generalized papular urticaria may result as an allergic reaction. Genital scabies is frequently a sexually transmitted disease. Punctate erythematous papules, itching which is worse at night, and the pathognomonic burrows are characteristic in the acute disease, but these features may be absent in the chronic form of the disease when there is often only thickened skin apparent. Norwegian crusted scabies is a rare severe chronic form of the disease occasionally seen in neglected mental or geriatric patients.

b. Fleas

Papular urticaria and irritating erythematous macules, particularly on the lower limbs of young adults, may be due to flea bites. Common fleas in Britain include

Pulex irritans (human flea), *Ctenocephalides felis* (cat flea) and *Ctenocephalides canis* (dog flea). Fleas from other animals, often kept as pets such as rabbits and guinea-pigs, can also cause skin lesions. The rat flea *Xenopsylla cheopsis* has great historic significance as it is the vector of bubonic plague which rarely occurs today (mainly in the Far East).

c. *Lice* (Pediculosis)

The three types of lice that may infest man are *Pediculus capitis* ('head louse'), *Pediculus corporis* (or *humanus*) ('body louse') and the *Pythirus pubis* (pubic or 'crab' louse). These insect infestations frequently cause itching and red papular lesions. The presence of nits (eggs) attached to hairs is often obvious. The lice are spread by direct contact and are common in vagrants. In some urban areas, as many as 10% of school children are infested by head lice. The crab louse is often seen in patients attending genito-urinary medicine clinics who have a reasonable standard of hygiene; it is commonly spread venereally and may affect the eyelashes, eyebrows, axillary hair as well as the pubic hair region in some patients.

The pediculus lice can act as vectors for louse borne and epidemic typhus fever (caused by *Rickettsia prowazeki*) and for relapsing fever, caused by *Borrelia recurrentis*.

d. Bed Bugs

The bed bug of temperate climates is *Cimex lectularius*, which is predominantly a human parasite. The flat triangular insect has stink glands, in adults, and this gives a charactistic odour. During the day, the insect hides in inaccessible places in furniture and under carpets. At night, it bites humans to suck blood causing minor skin lesions. The parasite can survive for many months between 'meals'. No disease is transmitted by bed bugs.

e. Cutaneous Myiasis

Patients arriving from Africa and India may complain of itchy boil-like skin lesions particularly on the trunk, which are due to the deposition in the skin of the larvae of the fly *Cordylobia anthropophaga*. This fly may lay its eggs on clothes left out to dry and the eggs develop into larvae when the clothes are worn because of the warmth of the body. The lesions may become secondarily infected by bacteria.

f. Chiggoe

See Insect cause of ulcer *above*.

g. Investigations for Insects

Scabies is diagnosed by inserting a needle under a mite at the anterior end of a characteristic burrow hooking it out on to a slide and observing the features of *Sarcoptes scabei* under direct microscopy.

The capture of a suspected flea, louse or crab louse or bed bug, and its examination under low power microscopy, will lead to a definitive diagnosis. The demonstration of nits, i.e. eggs, in the hairs indicates lice infestation and a special fine-toothed comb can be used to search for the nits of the head louse in children.

Liquid paraffin applied over the punctum of a suspected swelling of cutaneous myiasis may cause the larva to appear and it can then be extracted from the lesion and its identity is thereby confirmed.

A needle is used to widen the punctum of a suspected chiggoe lesion in the foot and the jigger flea *Tunga penetrans* is removed.

Treatment of Insect Infestations

a. Scabies

Benzylbenzoate (25%) applied to the whole of the body surface from the chin to the soles is the traditional and effective treatment for scabies. Alternatively, gamma-benzene hexachloride or crotamiton can be used.

b. Lice

Bathing, clean clothing and malathion or gamma-benzene hexachloride are effective for treating pediculosis.

c. Cutaneous myiasis and chiggoes

Insects extracted at the time of diagnosis—*see* Microbiological investigations *above*.

Secondary staphylococcal infection in the lesions may need treatment with flucloxacillin.

Further Reading

*Bryceson A. (1978) Imported skin infections. *Medicine*, 3rd series, **4**, 171.

Garrod L. P., Lambert H. P. and O'Grady F. (1981) Infections of skin, soft tissues and bones. In: *Antibiotics and Chemotherapy*, 5th ed., p. 306. London, Churchill Livingstone.

Hewitt M., Walton G. S. and Waterhouse M. (1971) Pet animal infestations and human skin lesions. *Br. J. Dermatol.* **85**, 215.

*Pembroke A. and Howard A. (1978) Fungal infections. *Medicine*, 3rd series, **5**, 219.

Rook A. (1968) Skin diseases caused by arthropods. In: Rook A., Wilkinson D. S. and Ebling F. G. J. (ed.) *Textbook of Dermatology*, p. 979. Oxford, Blackwell Scientific Publications.

Tyrell D. A. J., Phillips, I., Stewart Goodwin C. et al. (1979) Subcutaneous and deep mycoses. In: *Microbial Disease. The Use of the Laboratory in Diagnosis, Therapy and Control*, p. 270. London, Edward Arnold.

Youmans G. P., Paterson P. Y. and Sommers H. M. (1975) Cutaneous infections. In: *Biological and Clinical Basis of Infectious Diseases*. Philadelphia, U.S.A., W. B. Saunders Company.

* Particularly recommended for further study by undergraduates.

Chapter 17

Bone and joint infections

PATHOGENESIS

Bones and joints may become infected either by the haematogenous or by direct routes.

In acute infections, the causative organism, usually *Staph. aureus*, most often reaches the bones or joints via the bloodstream. Other examples of organisms that usually infect the skeletal system via the blood include *Haemophilus influenzae, Strep. pyogenes, Neisseria gonorrhoeae, Brucella melitensis* and *Salmonella typhi*. When the acute infections are not recognized and treated promptly, chronic infection may result.

Direct infection from a skin site to bones or joints may follow trauma or surgery resulting in acute or chronic infections. In this situation, the most common causative organism is *Staph. aureus* but infection by Gram-negative bacilli, including coliforms and *Pseudomonas*, is also frequent. The risk of direct infection is great when there is a compound fracture or an open deep wound overlying a bone or joint.

The metaphysis of a long bone is affected by osteomyelitis and, when the infection spreads, it may also involve an adjacent joint.

Joints are very susceptible to infection. The joint fluid is, of course, normally clear and sterile and devoid of phagocytic cells. The articular cartilage is also avascular. Therefore only a few organisms are required to initiate a joint infection which may ultimately cause serious destruction, if not treated quickly. The susceptibility of the joint to infection is further increased when there is previous damage to the joint, as occurs in rheumatoid arthritis, and when the patient's general host defences are impaired by steroid therapy.

A prosthesis inserted into a joint or bone increases the susceptibility of infection and the range of possible infecting organisms is extended by the presence of the prosthesis. Low-grade pathogens, such as *Staph. epidermidis*, have frequently infected prostheses in hip joints many weeks or months after hip joint replacement operations.

Joints may become inflamed as a result of infection at a distant site—'reactive' arthritis. Although not true infections of joints, these are also briefly mentioned below. The joint may become involved as a result of an immunological response to the organism, because of a possible antigenic cross-reaction between synovial membrane and the cell wall of the organism, such as *Strep. pyogenes*, or because of the deposition of immune complexes at the joint site (e.g. HBsAg complexes). Alternatively, inflammation of the bowel could, by itself, cause a reactive arthritis following some shigella, salmonella, campylobacter or other intestinal infections. The genetic constitution of an individual may predispose to the development of a reactive arthritis. Patients with HLAB27 histocompatibility antigen on their lymphocytes appear more likely to develop reactive arthritis following *Yersinia enterocolitica* bowel infections than other patients lacking this antigen. A similar genetic predisposition may apply to some patients with reactive arthritis associated with previous chlamydia genital tract infection or campylobacter intestinal infection.

BONE INFECTIONS

Acute osteomyelitis is suggested clinically by the presence of a painful tender bone lesion of acute onset and general systemic upset. The infection occurs most commonly in children.

Chronic osteomyelitis frequently occurs in adults as well as children and is characterized by chronic pain in the back or other bone sites. There is usually radiological evidence of osteomyelitis.

Causative Organisms of Bone Infections

a. Staphylococcus aureus

Staph. aureus is by far the most common causative organism of both acute and chronic osteomyelitis (*Table 17.1*). Sometimes the original source of the infection is obvious as a septic focus in the skin but often no source is apparent.

Table 17.1. Some causative organisms of osteomyelitis

Group of organisms	*Acute osteomyelitis*	*Chronic osteomyelitis*
1. *Bacteria*		
a. Gram-positive bacteria	*Staph. aureus* (>90% cases)	*Staph. aureus* (>60% cases)
	Strep. pyogenes	*Strep. milleri*
	Strep. pneumoniae	*Strep. pneumoniae*
	Clostridium welchii	*Actinomyces israelii*
		Propionibacteria
b. Gram-negative bacteria	*Haemophilus influenzae*	Coliforms
		Pseudomonas aeruginosa
		Bacteroides species
		Haemophilus species
		Salmonella species
		Brucella species
c. Acid-fast bacilli		*Mycobacterium tuberculosis*
d. Spirochaetes		*Treponema pallidum**
		Treponema pertenue
2. *Fungi*		*Madurella mycetoma*
		Cryptococcus neoformans
		Histoplasma duboisii
3. *Protozoa*		*Entamoeba histolytica*
		Leishmania braziliensis

* Cause of congenital syphilitic bone lesions in children and a gumma in adults.

b. Haemophilus influenzae

Haemophilus influenzae, capsulated type b strains, invade the bloodstream from the respiratory tract and causes acute bone or joint infections in young children less than 5 years old, particularly in infants up to 2 years old.

c. Streptococcus pyogenes and Strep. pneumoniae

Strep. pyogenes occasionally causes acute osteomyelitis in infants. It is also an infrequent cause at other ages. *Strep. pneumoniae* is a rare cause, sometimes associated with direct spread of infection from an ear or sinus infection.

d. Clostridium welchii

Clostridial bone infection is rare and usually post-traumatic (*see* Chapter 9).

e. Other organisms

The range of other organisms is much wider with chronic than with acute osteomyelitis as is shown in *Table 17.1*. These other organisms cause chronic osteomyelitis less frequently than *Staph. aureus*.

i. *Mycobacterium tuberculosis*
   Myco. tuberculosis is an important cause of chronic osteomyelitis (*see* TB of bone and joints *below*).
ii. *Pseudomonas aeruginosa*
   Pseudomonas often directly superinfects established bone infections when previous antibiotic therapy has been given and particularly when there is a sinus or open wound linking the skin surface and bone.
iii. *Salmonella* species
   Salmonella typhi, *Salmonella choleraesuis* and many 'food-poisoning' *Salmonella* species may infect bones via the bloodstream, particularly in patients with sickle cell disease. Salmonella osteomyelitis is rare in Britain but frequently occurs in Africa. 'Typhoid spine' is a recognized complication of typhoid. Many patients with salmonella bone infections give no previous history of gastro-intestinal symptoms.
iv. *Brucella* species
   Brucella melitensis and *Brucella abortus* can cause chronic osteomyelitis in various bony sites including the sacro-iliac region and spine. Brucellosis is rare in Britain.
v. Coliforms and *Bacteroides*
   Gram-negative bacilli from the faecal flora often infect bones directly when there is an open fracture, bullet wound or other trauma or surgery. Gangrenous toes of diabetics may particularly become infected by *Bacteroides fragilis*.

   E. coli or other coliforms sometimes reach the spine, or other skeletal sites, by the bloodstream from a urinary tract or prostatic infection in elderly male patients.

   Gram-negative bacilli from the faecal flora (and *Pseudomonas*, above) are frequent causes of chronic osteomyelitis in Britain.

vi. *Actinomycetes israelii*
Actinomycosis of the jaw may particularly follow trauma or surgery to the mandible.

Microbiological Investigations of Bone Infections

Blood cultures

Blood cultures, ideally collected just as the temperature of the patient starts to rise, are the mainstay of the microbial diagnosis of acute osteomyelitis. Two or three sets should be collected before the start of antibiotic therapy. *Staph. aureus* is isolated from the blood of the great majority of patients with acute osteomyelitis. *Haemophilus influenzae* is isolated from the blood cultures of some infants.

The numbers of positive blood cultures in chronic osteomyelitis are much less than with acute osteomyelitis but are, nevertheless, worthwhile sometimes yielding growth of organisms such as *Staph. aureus*, salmonellae and *Brucella melitensis*.

Pus from infected bone biopsy

Whenever possible pus, rather than a swab of pus, is collected and transported promptly to the laboratory for microscopy and culture. This type of specimen is not available from patients with acute osteomyelitis who have closed lesions, unless a surgeon exceptionally decides to perform a bone biopsy or drainage of the infected bone lesion. However, when there is an open lesion or surgery on a patient with chronic osteomyelitis, it is usually possible to collect a sample of pus. Microscopy and culture for acid-fast bacilli, as well as pyogenic bacteria, is especially indicated in samples from immigrant patients.

Faeces and urine

Culture of faeces and urine for salmonellae should be carried out in chronic osteomyelitis patients who have no microbial diagnosis.

Serology

Serological tests may be useful when blood cultures are negative in patients with chronic osteomyelitis.

i. *Staphylococcal antibodies*
Raised serum antibody titres of staphylococcal anti-alpha haemolysin, anti-gamma haemolysin, anti-leucocidin and anti-nuclease may suggest *Staph. aureus* infection. These tests, which are carried out by a reference laboratory, are sometimes difficult to interpret as false negatives and false positives may occur. Advice from the reference centre is often desirable.

ii. *Brucella antibodies*
Tests for chronic brucella infection include serum direct (saline) and indirect (Coombs test) agglutinins and the complement fixation test (*see* Brucellosis, in Chapter 21, p. 404).

iii. *Salmonella antibodies*
The Widal test may help indicate *Sal. typhi* infection but the results need to be interpreted with caution (*see* Widal test in Chapter 14, p. 263).

Treatment of Bone Infections

See below.

JOINT INFECTIONS (SEPTIC ARTHRITIS) AND 'REACTIVE' ARTHRITIS

Mono-articular arthritis is most common with septic arthritis whereas poly-articular arthritis frequently occurs with 'reactive' arthritis. Charcot's joints, a rare painless arthropathy, is a neuropathic disorder of the joints, due to neurosyphilis.

Infective Causes of Arthritis

Staphylococci and other infective causes of arthritis are included in *Table 17.2*. In Britain, the three most frequent causes of septic arthritis are *Staph. aureus*,

Table 17.2. Some microbial causes of arthritis

Organism	*Septic arthritis*	*'Reactive' arthritis*
1. *Bacteria*		
a. Gram-positive	*Staph. aureus* (>80% cases) *Staph. epidermidis** *Strep. pyogenes* *Strep. pneumoniae*	*Strep. pyogenes*
b. Gram-negative	*Haemophilus influenzae* *Neisseria gonorrhoeae* *Neisseria meningitidis* Coliforms *Pseudomonas aeruginosa* *Bacteroides fragilis* Fusiforms *Salmonella* species *Brucella* species *Pasteurella multocida*	*Neisseria meningitidis* *Neisseria gonorrhoeae* *Yersinia enterocolitica* *Shigella* (not *sonnei*) *Salmonella* species *Campylobacter jejuni* ? *Klebsiella*
c. Acid-fast bacilli	*Mycobacterium tuberculosis*	
d. Spirochaetes	*Treponema pallidum* *Leptospira icterohaemorrhagiae*	
2. *Mycoplasma*		*Mycoplasma pneumoniae*
3. *Chlamydiae*		*Chlamydia trachomatis*
4. *Viruses*	Rubella Arbo (e.g. Onyong-nyong fever) Enterovirus Mumps	Hepatitis B Epstein-Barr (glandular fever)

* Mainly in prosthetic hip joints.

Haemophilus influenzae and *Neisseria gonorrhoeae*. Important causes of reactive arthritis include *Neisseria gonorrhoeae*, *Neisseria meningitidis*, *Chlamydia trachomatis*, *Campylobacter jejuni* and *Strep. pyogenes*.

Staphylococcus aureus

Staph. aureus causes more than 80% of cases of acute septic arthritis. Clinically, the affected joint appears painful, tender, hot and swollen, and the patient is usually febrile. Children are most often affected and common sites of infection include the knee or hip joints. These features may become less obvious when the patient is an adult with rheumatoid arthritis who is receiving steroids since steroids may mask the infection.

Haemophilus influenzae

Pittman capsulated type b strains of *H. influenzae* are important causes of septic arthritis in infants and young children (*see* Haemophilus bone infections *above*).

Neisseria gonorrhoeae

Gonococcal arthritis occasionally occurs in young adults, affecting a large joint, such as the knee, or a number of small joints, such as in the hand. Some patients may also have vesicular gonococcal skin lesions.

Staphylococcus epidermidis

Chronic low-grade infection of prosthetic hip joints by *Staph. epidermidis* may follow hip joint replacement.

Streptococcus pyogenes

Haemolytic streptococcal infection of joints is uncommon. Rheumatic fever often affects joints (fleeting arthralgia) about 2 weeks after a streptococcal sore throat; in the past the disease was much more common.

Pseudomonas aeruginosa

In 'mainlining' drug addicts, *Pseudomonas* may enter the bloodstream. It characteristically infects the sterno-clavicular joint.

Yersinia enterocolitica

The sacroiliac, lower limb and other joints may become affected by a reactive arthritis 2–3 weeks after yersinia gastro-enteritis, especially in Scandinavia (*see* Pathogenesis *above*).

Chlamydia trachomatis

Many cases of non-specific urethritis are caused by *Chlamydia trachomatis* and, occasionally, these patients develop a reactive arthritis that may be associated with this organism (sometimes together with uveitis as part of Reiter's syndrome).

Microbiological Investigations of Septic and Reactive Arthritis

Joint fluid

When acute septic arthritis is suspected, it is nearly always possible to aspirate fluid from the affected joint under scrupulous aseptic and antiseptic conditions. The fluid from septic joints is usually pus with greater than 10^8 polymorphs per litre of fluid. However, other non-septic causes of inflammatory joint disease, such as rheumatoid arthritis, may also result in turbid joint fluids with many polymorphs present. A Gram-stain of a centrifuged deposit of pus from a joint may quickly show the presence of a causative organism—Gram-positive cocci in clusters suggesting staphylococcal infection. Cultures and direct antibiotic sensitivities, when available on the following day, help the optimal management of the patient. The isolation of some organisms may take 2 days or longer and antibiotics usually must be given without waiting for the results of culture.

Surgery is occasionally necessary to aspirate material from deeper joints, such as the hip joint and in chronic infections involving such sites as the spine. Cultures for acid-fast bacilli are included when there has been chronic infection.

Blood cultures

Although pus is usually available for culture, blood cultures should always be collected also. Occasionally blood cultures are positive when joint fluid culture results are negative, particularly when the causative bacteria are *Neisseria*, *Haemophilus* or *Brucella* species.

Throat swab

A throat swab is collected for streptococcal culture when rheumatic fever is suspected.

Faeces culture

Cultures for shigellae, campylobacter and yersinia organisms may indicate a bowel pathogen that is implicated in 'reactive' arthritis. The isolation of *Salmonella* suggests the possibility of a salmonella joint infection or a salmonella reactive arthritis.

Urethral, cervical and rectal swabs

Swabs, transported in Stuart's transport media, or direct cultures from these sites, may indicate a possible gonococcal aetiology of arthritis, particularly in a young person.

Urethral and cervical cultures for Chlamydia trachomatis

There are only a few reference centres with facilities for the isolation of chlamydiae. Urethral and cervical secretions should be sent in appropriate chlamydial transport media from selected patients following discussion with the medical microbiologist.

Serology

a. Streptococcal antibody tests
Serum antistreptolysin O (ASO) titres and anti-streptococcal DNAase antibody estimations can indicate a recent streptococcal infection in patients with a suspect reactive arthritis.

b. Brucella antibodies
c. Salmonella antibodies } *See* p. 329

d. Gonococcal complement fixation test (GCFT)
This test is of limited value as the antigen used is often unsatisfactory. A positive result may indicate past gonococcal infection which may be unrelated, and false negatives occur. Nevertheless, a rising or very high GCFT titre may occasionally suggest that the arthritis is gonococcal in origin when the cultures are negative.

e. WR (or VDRL, TPHA, etc.) and FTA
Syphilis serology (*see* p. 379) will be positive in patients with arthritis due to secondary or tertiary syphilis.

f. Mycoplasma pneumoniae CFT
When there has been a recent or current respiratory infection, paired sera to look for a rising *Mycoplasma pneumoniae* CFT titre should be collected.

g. Yersinia serology
The presence of agglutinins to *Yersinia enterocolitica* and *Yersinia pseudotuberculosis* should be looked for in patients who have had bowel symptoms, particularly if there has been a recent visit to Scandinavia, Belgium or South Africa. Yersinia arthritis only rarely occurs in British patients who have not travelled abroad.

h. Leptospiral CFT
Leptospiral antibody tests may be indicated when there is a relevant animal contact, occupational history or clinical features suggesting leptospirosis.

i. Rubella
Rubella HAI and CFT should be carried out if there has been recent contact or a rubella-like rash.

j. Chlamydiae antibodies
There is no 'routine' chlamydia antibody test available yet for investigating patients with reactive arthritis who have had recent non-specific urethritis but discussion with chlamydiae reference centres may be worthwhile for particular cases.

TREATMENT OF BONE AND JOINT INFECTIONS (NON-TUBERCULOUS)

1. *Acute Infections*

Acute osteomyelitis and acute septic arthritis can usually be effectively treated by antibiotics without the need for surgical intervention. However, it is essential that systemic antibiotics are given early in the disease and that the correct choice and dosages of drugs are used for effective therapy.

'Blind' systemic antibiotic therapy

As soon as the samples for microbiology have been collected 'blind' antibiotic therapy is given mainly on the basis that the most likely causative organism is a penicillinase-producing *Staph. aureus*—cloxacillin 1 g 4-hourly, intramuscularly in adults and 25 mg per kg 4-hourly in children:

a. For patients older than 5 years, benzylpenicillin 1 MU 6-hourly, can be added to the cloxacillin regimen to treat possible penicillin-sensitive staphylococci and other less frequent coccal causes.

b. For children less than 5 years old, ampicillin, 25 mg per kg 4-hourly, should be added instead of penicillin to the cloxacillin regimen to treat possible *Haemophilus influenzae* infections also.

When the *Gram-stain* result of pus suggests a particular microbial cause the 'blind therapy' should always include antibiotics that would be expected to treat that cause.

Local instillation of antibiotics

When a septic joint is aspirated, local instillation of cloxacillin into the joint can be considered. Once the culture and sensitivity results are known, further regular injections of the appropriate antibiotic into the joint can be considered, but there is a risk of superinfection with repeated taps. Another potential disadvantage of local instillation of an antibiotic into a joint may be that chemical irritation results, especially if inappropriate doses are used.

Surgical drainage

For patients with severe subacute osteomyelitis or suspected acute infection of the hip joint, surgical drainage under a general anaesthetic is sometimes indicated. Aspirated material is sent for microbiological investigation, and systemic antibiotics are given as soon as the cultures have been obtained (repeated surgical aspirations of a septic hip joint may be necessary).

Modification of treatment once the culture and antibiotic sensitivity results are available

Staph. aureus

The minority of patients who have penicillin-sensitive *Staph. aureus* infections are best treated with high doses of benzylpenicillin. When the strain is resistant to penicillin but sensitive to fucidic acid and cloxacillin, this combination should normally be given.

When there is resistance to cloxacillin (methicillin), a combination of fucidic acid and erythromycin or lincomycin can be considered if the strain is sensitive to these antibiotics. Occasional patients have developed pseudo-membranous colitis due to lincomycin and any patient who develops diarrhoea during therapy should be warned to stop taking the drug immediately. Fusidic acid penetrates bone well and is an excellent anti-staphylococcal drug but should never by used alone otherwise resistant mutants may emerge. Gentamicin can beneficially be added to cloxacillin when there is *Staph. aureus* infection of bone or joints in association with a serious septicaemic illness (*see* Chapter 5).

Streptococci, pneumococci, gonococci and Pasteurella multocida

Infections due to these organisms usually respond best to high doses of benzylpenicillin.

Haemophilus influenzae

Capsulated Pittman type b strains of *H. influenzae* are usually sensitive to ampicillin. Ampicillin-resistant strains (due to beta-lactamase production) can usually be effectively treated by cortimoxazole, cefuroxime or chloramphenicol.

Penicillin-allergic patients

When there is a doubtful history of penicillin allergy, a cephalosporin can be used in place of cloxacillin and penicillin. Alternatively, and when there is a definite history of penicillin allergy, a combination of fucidic acid and erythromycin or lincomycin can usually be given in place of cloxacillin for treating staphylococcal infections.

Duration of therapy

In all cases antibiotics should be continued for at least 10 days. Some patients may need to have therapy continued for up to 4 weeks depending on the clinical and radiological findings.

2. *Chronic Infections*

Since the range of organisms causing chronic infections is much wider than with acute infections, there is a greater need to obtain an exact microbial diagnosis before starting treatment than with acute infections. Therefore surgical intervention in order to obtain suitable material for microbiology as well as to effect debridement and drainage is often necessary.

Blind therapy

Blind therapy is needed when an exact microbial diagnosis cannot be obtained, as may happen when it is not feasible to perform surgery. The main difficulty is often to differentiate chronic staphylococcal or Gram-negative infection from tuberculosis infection (*see below*). If non-tuberculous infection is suspected, a prolonged course of anti-staphylococcal treatment (cloxacillin and fucidic acid) should be tried in the first instance. When this approach fails, drugs that treat Gram-negative causes, such as cotrimoxazole, can be considered. With all such difficult cases, there should be the closest collaboration between the clinician and clinical microbiologist to discuss the best management of the individual patient.

Prosthesis

Infections of prosthetic joints occasionally can be effectively treated by antibiotics and surgical drainage when the microbial diagnosis is known, but often removal of the infected prosthesis is necessary. This removal is particularly necessary at an early stage when the infection is due to multi-antibiotic-resistant organisms, such as many strains of *Staph. epidermidis*.

Modification of treatment once the culture and sensitivity results are known

Staph. aureus

The principles for *Staph. aureus* are similar to those above for acute infections, but the duration of treatment may need to be prolonged for up to 6 weeks or longer (*see below*). Some authorities recommend the repeat estimation of anti-staphylolysin titres for monitoring response to therapy.

Coliforms and Pseudomonas

The choice of antibiotic is based on the sensitivity results. *Pseudomonas aeruginosa* infections are often best treated by a combination of gentamicin or tobramycin and carbenicillin. Repeat cultures are indicated, when possible, during treatment to check that the causative Gram-negative bacillus cannot be reisolated and regular serum antibiotic assays are essential when aminoglycosides are given.

Bacteroides

Metronidazole is a very effective antibiotic for treating *B. fragilis* infections.

Salmonellae

Chloramphenicol (for typhoid), cotrimoxazole or a combination of mecillinam with ampicillin are useful treatments for some salmonella infections.

Brucella

Tetracycline, initially combined with streptomycin, is usually effective for treating brucellosis of bone and joints. Cotrimoxazole is an alternative.

Duration of treatment

At least 6 weeks and often up to 6 months or longer is necessary depending on the organism, the site and severity of the chronic infection.

Prophylaxis of Bone and Joint Infections

Bone and joint infections can often be avoided following orthopaedic surgery or aspirations of joints by the use of scrupulous aseptic and antiseptic techniques. Skin preparation with 1·5% iodine in 70% ethyl alcohol for joint aspirations is recommended.

Antibiotic prophylaxis with an anti-staphylococcal drug is desirable for hip joint replacement operations and cloxacillin is usually suitable for this purpose.

Prophylactic gentamicin incorporated in the bone cement is especially recommended when revision of an infected hip joint replacement operation is carried out. This type of local prophylaxis is still under evaluation. Prophylaxis against gas gangrene using iodophor skin disinfection and benzylpenicillin is necessary for amputations in patients with ischaemic arterial disease and hip surgery (*see also* Antibiotic prophylaxis, in Chapter 3).

Recent trials have shown that a laminar air flow system in the operating theatre may reduce the sepsis rates in patients who have hip joint replacement operations.

TUBERCULOSIS OF BONES AND JOINTS

Tuberculosis affecting non-pulmonary sites including bones and joints is about ten times more common in immigrants than in the native population in Britain.

Many different bone sites may become infected by *Mycobacterium tuberculosis* (human type) including the spine and the bones of the hands and feet. Tuberculosis of the spine usually affects two vertebral bodies, most often T10 and T11, and the intervertebral disc between them becomes narrowed. A 'cold' tuberculosis abscess from a spinal site may track down via the psoas sheath to present as a psoas abscess in the groin. Paraplegia is an important complication resulting from pressure on the spinal cord. Constitutional upset with fever and loss of weight is infrequent.

Joint tuberculosis most often affects a large joint such as the hip or knee. The presenting clinical features include pain and stiffness in the swollen joint and muscle wasting.

Microbiological Investigations

Bone, pus and joint fluid

Fluid aspirated from an affected joint, and pus and bone tissues from sites subjected to needle biopsy or explorative surgery, are examined for acid-fast bacilli by microscopy and culture. Microscopic methods include the fluorescent auramine-phenol method and Ziehl-Neelsen stains.

Material for culture is inoculated onto Lowenstein-Jensen media and, where possible, into guinea-pigs. Histological examination of material removed at surgery or biopsy may also provide evidence of tuberculosis.

Culture of other sites

A few patients may also have clinical or radiological evidence of tuberculosis at other sites such as the genito-urinary system and when this is suspected appropriate specimens, such as early morning specimens of urine, are also examined for acid-fast bacilli.

Skin testing

The tuberculin (Mantoux) intradermal skin test starting at 1 in 10 000 dilution should be performed. Nearly all patients with bone or joint tuberculosis are strongly Mantoux positive but a strongly positive Mantoux does not by itself indicate active tuberculosis.

Treatment

Conservative measures rather than extensive surgery are usually indicated and often include immobilization of the affected site. Antituberculous chemotherapy is always necessary. The modern 9 month recommended combination of drugs for treating pulmonary tuberculosis has not formally been evaluated for treating bone and joint TB. Nevertheless, the recommended treatment consists of rifampicin, isoniazid and ethambutol for 8 weeks followed by daily rifampicin and isoniazid for a total period of 9 months (*see* Pulmonary tuberculosis, Chapter 13, p. 250).

Further Reading

Garrod L. P., Lambert A. P. and O'Grady F. (1981). *Antibiotic and Chemotherapy*, 5th ed. London, Churchill Livingstone.

Horney N. (1978) Non-pulmonary tuberculosis. *Medicine,* 3rd series, **6**, 306–312.

Keat A. C., Thomas B. J., Taylor-Robinson D. et al. (1980) Evidence of *Chlamydia trachomatis* infection in sexually acquired reactive arthritis. *Ann. Rheum. Dis.* **39**, 431–437.

McAlister T. A. (1974) Treatment of osteomyelitis. *Br. J. Hosp. Med.* **12**, 534–545.

Taylor A. G., Cook J., Fincham W. J. et al. (1975) Serological tests in the differentiation of staphylococci and tuberculous bone disease. *J. Clin. Pathol.* **28**, 284.

Chapter 18

Infections of the heart

INFECTIVE ENDOCARDITIS

Incidence and Clinical Features

The incidence of infective endocarditis today, about 1500 cases each year in Britain, is similar to that observed over 30 years ago. The disease is still serious and in spite of antibiotic therapy the overall mortality rate is 15–30%.

The mode of clinical presentation has changed because many more patients over 50 years are seen than formerly. The onset of symptoms is often insidious, particularly in the older patients, and the main clinical features include tiredness, anaemia, worsening heart failure, pyrexia and changing heart murmurs. In recent years echocardiograms have often proved useful diagnostically in patients where the clinical diagnosis is uncertain, as they may reveal vegetations or other cardiac abnormalities compatible with infective endocarditis.

Predisposing Factors

Predisposing factors include previous rheumatic heart disease (less common than in the past) congenital heart disease, atherosclerotic aortic valve disease, homograft or prosthetic valve heart surgery and drug addiction. Infective vegetations are most likely to develop on the damaged endothelium of the aortic or mitral valves. Congenital lesions that may become infected include patent ductus arteriosus and ventricular septal defect.

Pathogenesis

Damage to the endothelium occurs when there is a high pressure gradient and turbulence around a valve or septal defect. The roughened endothelium that results becomes the site of deposition of fibrin and platelets. Organisms may enter the blood from a number of sites including the gums and teeth or directly during open-heart surgery to reach the fibrin-platelet layer. Invasion and colonization of the fibrin-platelet layer of organisms leads to microbial vegetations (*see Fig. 18.1*).

The factors that determine whether a microbial vegetation is formed or not include:

i. the type of organism and the number of organisms reaching the endothelium;
ii. the site and type of heart defect;
iii. the host defence mechanisms.

Some organisms may infect the endocardium of patients who have no previous evidence of heart damage, such as *Staph. aureus* or, rarely, *Strep. pyogenes* or *Strep. pneumoniae*.

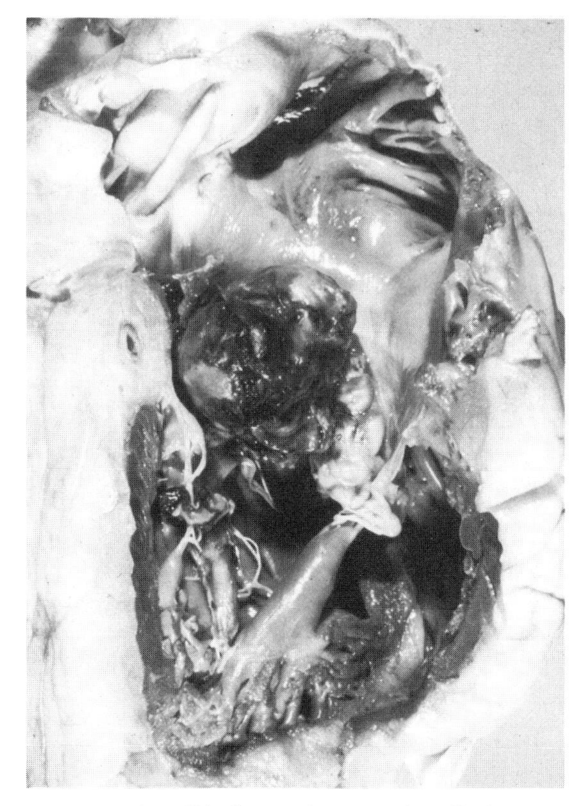

Fig. 18.1. Staph. aureus endocarditis: heart valve vegetation affecting tricuspid valve.

High titres of antibodies against the infecting organism usually develop during the disease and many of the clinical features, such as nephritis and Osler's nodes, probably result from immunological mechanisms, particularly the deposition of immune complexes. A few patients die from immunologically induced renal failure.

Emboli from an infected heart lesion, both 'septic' and non-bacterial, frequently reach many different organs, including the skin and central nervous system and may cause fatal complications.

When there has been substantial damage to the heart from infective endocarditis, such as severe aortic incompetence, the patient can die from cardiac insufficiency even though the infection may have been cured by antibiotics.

Causative Organisms

Scores of different bacterial species, *Coxiella burnetii*, chlamydiae and fungi can cause infective endocarditis.

The pattern of causative agents varies according to whether the patient has had previous heart surgery, and some important causes of endocarditis are included in *Tables 18.1* and *18.2*. The great majority of cases of endocarditis occur in

Table 18.1. Causative organisms of endocarditis in patients who have not had heart surgery

Organism	*Approx. percentage of positive blood culture cases*
'*Streptococcus viridans*'	65
Streptococcus faecalis	7
Microaerophilic streptococci	7
Anaerobic streptococci	1
Staphylococcus aureus	11
Staphylococcus epidermidis	1
Haemophilus species	3
Other bacteria	5

Table 18.2. Some organisms causing endocarditis in patients who have undergone heart valve surgery

	Approx. percentage of blood culture positive cases	
Organism	*Early onset*	*Late onset**
'*Streptococcus viridans*'	2	41
Streptococcus faecalis	1	3
Staphylococcus aureus	39	13
Staphylococcus epidermidis	28	24
Diphtheroids	8	3
Gram-negative bacilli	18	13
Fungi	4	3

* Late onset: more than 2 months after cardiac surgery.
Late onset cases occur more frequently than early onset cases.

patients who have not had previous heart surgery. However between 1 and 5% of heart valve or septal defect patients undergoing surgery develop infective endocarditis as a complication and the numbers of patients receiving homograft or prosthetic heart valves is increasing.

Bacterial causes

Streptococci

A. 'STREPTOCOCCUS VIRIDANS'

'*Streptococcus viridans*' was responsible for about 90% of endocarditis cases 35 years ago when most patients were less than 40 years of age and had rheumatic heart disease. Although the patients seen today are often older than in the past and the proportion of cases due to '*Streptococcus viridans*' has fallen, this type of organism is still the most frequent cause of endocarditis (*see Table 18.1*).

Most cases of prosthetic valve endocarditis occur more than 2 months after cardiac surgery and '*Streptococcus viridans*' is the most frequent cause of late onset endocarditis (*see Table 18.2*).

'*Streptococcus viridans*' is not one species but a heterogeneous group of different alpha-haemolytic and non-haemolytic streptococcal species that are included in the normal mouth flora. These species include *Streptococcus sanguis*,

Streptococcus mitior, *Streptococcus mutans* and *Streptococcus milleri*. The two species most often isolated from endocarditis patients are *Streptococcus sanguis* and *Streptococcus mitior*. *Streptococcus bovis* is not strictly a viridans streptococcus as it is a Lancefield group D streptococcus, but this species is usually fully sensitive to penicillin, like most strains of '*Streptococcus viridans*', and can conveniently be grouped together with those viridans streptococci that are closely associated with endocarditis.

The viridans streptococci can enter the blood from the gums after dental extraction and the asymptomatic bacteraemia lasts from about 2 to 20 minutes after extraction. Any procedure that causes gingival bleeding can cause a streptococcal bacteraemia. Occasional cases of '*Streptococcus viridans*' endocarditis have been reported in edentulous patients.

Characteristically the clinical features of endocarditis due to viridans streptococci have an insidious onset and a patient can develop an illness lasting many weeks before death occurs, in the absence of chemotherapy; this disease was previously known as subacute bacterial endocarditis (SBE). A few patients have a more rapidly progressive course of the disease. Nearly all patients with '*Streptococcus viridans*' endocarditis have a previous heart lesion and about a quarter give a history of a recent dental procedure as a precipitating cause.

B. STREPTOCOCCUS FAECALIS

Streptococcus faecalis is important because of its reduced sensitivity to penicillin. It is more common among older male patients who have genito-urinary disease.

The organism can enter the blood following manipulations of the genito-urinary tract or gut and after dental procedures in patients who have received recent penicillin therapy.

Staphylococci

Staphylococci are the most frequent causes of endocarditis after streptococci (*Tables 18.1* and *18.2*).

A. STAPHYLOCOCCUS AUREUS

Staph. aureus endocarditis usually runs an acute course. The clinical features often include those of staphylococcal septicaemia, such as disseminated intravascular coagulation and metastatic abscesses in the lungs, brain and kidney. This organism often attacks a previously healthy heart valve, particularly the aortic valve. The organism may enter the bloodstream originally from a septic skin focus or from infected lungs. Endocarditis can occur as a complication in any patient with *Staph. aureus* septicaemia.

Drug addicts are particularly at risk of developing *Staph. aureus* septicaemia and endocarditis. The tricuspid valve may be infected in 'mainliners'. Occasionally drug addicts develop polymicrobial endocarditis when the *Staph. aureus* is mixed with other organisms such as coagulase-negative staphylococci, Gram-negative bacilli or *Candida* species.

B. STAPHYLOCOCCUS EPIDERMIDIS

Staphylococcus epidermidis (*Staph. albus*) is an important cause of endocarditis following cardiac surgery and may enter the patient's heart either from the patient's skin or from the skin of the surgeon.

Staphylococcus epidermidis, together with *Staph. aureus*, have been responsible for the great majority of early onset endocarditis cases after cardiac surgery (*Table 18.2*). In the late onset endocarditis case group *Staph. epidermidis* is the second most frequent causative organism after '*Streptococcus viridans*'. Rarely, *Staph. epidermidis* can also cause endocarditis in susceptible infants with infected Spitz-Holter valves.

C. HAEMOPHILUS SPECIES

Haemophilus parainfluenzae, *H. influenzae* and *H. aphrophilus* are uncommon but well-recognized causes of endocarditis (*Table 18.1*), often affecting younger patients than streptococci and originally entering the bloodstream from the respiratory tract.

D. DIPHTHEROIDS

Diphtheroids infrequently cause prosthetic valve endocarditis (*Table 18.2*).

E. GRAM-NEGATIVE BACILLI

Coliforms, such as *E. coli* and *Klebsiella aerogenes*, *Pseudomonas* species, *Serratia* species, anaerobic Gram-negative bacilli, such as fusiforms or *Bacteroides fragilis*, may enter the bloodstream from the gut or genito-urinary tract or an infected wound and cause endocarditis after cardiac surgery, mainly during the first few post-operative months, or in drug addicts. In both these situations, the organisms can cause endocarditis singly or in various mixtures. The mortality of endocarditis caused by Gram-negative bacilli is very high.

Non-bacterial causes

a. Coxiella burnetii

Coxiella burnetii, a rickettsia-like organism, can cause Q fever in patients who live in urban as well as rural areas (*see* Chapter 21). It is a rare but important cause of endocarditis that requires different management from bacterial endocarditis (*see below*).

b. Chlamydiae

Chlamydia psittaci, the cause of psittacosis, and *Chlamydia trachomatis*, the cause of many cases of non-specific urethritis, can very rarely cause infective endocarditis.

c. Fungi

Candida species, particularly *Candida albicans* and less often *Aspergillus* species, can rarely cause infective endocarditis. However, unlike the other non-bacterial causes of endocarditis these fungi are of most importance after open-heart surgery. They can reach the heart during the post-operative period from infected intravenous drip-sites or, less often, during surgery itself.

Microbiological Investigations

The mortality rate is less in those endocarditis patients who have a definite microbiological diagnosis than in those where the infecting organism is unknown. The rational selection of optimal antimicrobial therapy is only possible when an exact diagnosis has been obtained.

a. Blood cultures

Blood cultures remain the most important investigation. It is essential to collect at least two sets of blood cultures *before* the start of antibiotic therapy, in a scrupulous aseptic manner, from a well-cleaned venepuncture site. These two sets are collected over a 1–2-hour period from an acutely ill patient who clinically appears to need urgent chemotherapy. When the patient is less severely ill, three sets of cultures are collected over a 24-hour period irrespective of the patient's temperature. Characteristically in endocarditis there is a low-grade persistent bacteraemia. If recent antibiotics have been administered for any reason then it is usually best to stop the antibiotics and collect several sets of blood culture spaced out over a 10-day period.

Each blood culture set should always consist of aerobic and anaerobic bottles. Many organisms, such as some streptococci and *Haemophilus*, require added carbon dioxide during incubation of the broths and subculture plates for their successful isolation.

When the initial routine blood cultures are negative, sometimes additional special laboratory methods for fastidious organisms such as pyridoxal dependant streptococci may be helpful (*see* Further reading list on blood culture techniques).

Interpretation of results

Generally any organism which is isolated from at least two different blood culture sets should be considered as significant. *Staph. epidermidis* and diphtheroids are common skin contaminants that usually only grow in one or two bottles. Further tests including antibiotic sensitivity testing and phage typing of staphylococci may help to differentiate some strains and help demonstrate contamination rather than infection. In every suspected case, the clinical and microbiological facts need careful consideration; any organism can cause endocarditis in a patient with a prosthetic valve. Certain 'diphtheroid-like' organisms on further investigation may prove to be viridans streptococci.

Occasionally a viridans streptococcus is isolated from only one or two bottles and its significance is uncertain. A fluorescent serum antibody test using the patient's own serum against the organism may help to show a very high antibody titre ($>1/400$) which is characteristic of streptococcal endocarditis. Fortunately, the majority of endocarditis cases have easy-to-interpret blood culture results, with the same organism isolated within a few days of incubation from most of the bottles of the first two or three sets, in more than 90% of blood culture positive cases.

Blood culture negative endocarditis

About 25% of suspected endocarditis cases have negative blood cultures due to:

i. previous antibiotic therapy,
ii. fastidious bacteria,
iii. non-bacterial causes.

In some patients the clinical diagnosis may be incorrect.

b. Serology

Paired sera are collected from all cases of blood culture negative endocarditis and, when cultures are yielding growth of uncertain clinical significance for the following tests:

i. *Coxiella burnetii*, CFT phase 1 and 2
ii. *Chlamydia psittaci*, CFT
iii. *Brucella* CFT

} Necessary in all blood culture negative cases

iv. Fungal serology Candida precipitins (20% of normal people may have low titres of these)
Aspergillus precipitins

Fungal serology is necessary in patients who have undergone heart surgery.

v. Immunofluorescent test for antibodies against viridans streptococci may be particularly helpful when only an occasional bottle yields growth of a streptococcus and its significance is uncertain—using the patient's isolate as the antigen.

c. Other investigations

Only rarely do other investigations help the management of an individual patient:

i. Heart valves removed at surgery—microscopy and culture of vegetations can occasionally reveal an aetiological agent which is not otherwise demonstrated.
ii. Emboli, lodged in a blood vessel and removed by surgery, or rarely large emboli lodged in the skin—microscopy and culture can reveal the causative organism—particularly when this is a fungus.

Antimicrobial Treatment

It is vital to provide complete bactericidal therapy so that all the organisms in the endocardial vegetations are eradicated. With good antimicrobial treatment, which is dependent on previously obtaining a microbiological diagnosis, the mortality rate of the disease is reduced from 100% to 10–15%. In all cases, close collaboration between the clinician and microbiologist is essential.

Blind therapy

Many acutely ill patients need to start immediate blind treatment as soon as the two or three blood culture sets have been collected.

With the majority of patients, who have not had previous heart surgery, a combination of benzylpenicillin and gentamicin will cover streptococcal causes of endocarditis. The gentamicin is also active against *Staph. aureus*, but if clinical clues suggest staphylococcal infection such as skin sepsis, disseminated intravascular coagulation or a history of 'mainline' drug addiction, then cloxacillin should also be added to the penicillin plus gentamicin regimen. This will give more effective treatment for possible penicillinase-producing *Staph. aureus* strains. Details of suggested blind antibiotic regimens are included in *Table 18.3*. The doses of antibiotics mentioned below and in *Table 18.3* are for adults with normal renal function. The doses of aminoglycoside drugs and vancomycin may need adjustment according to the results of repeated serum antibiotic assays (*see* Antibiotic assays, in Chapter 3 and Notes on antibiotics, in Appendix, p. 548).

Blind antibiotic treatment of prosthetic valve endocarditis varies according to whether the endocarditis is of early or late onset. Staphylococci are the most frequent causes in early onset endocarditis followed by Gram-negative bacilli and diphtheroids (*Table 18.2*). Streptococci and staphylococci are the main causes of late onset endocarditis. Some *Staph. epidermidis* strains are resistant to penicillin or methicillin (and cloxacillin) but sensitive to gentamicin. Gentamicin is therefore included in the blind therapy of both early and late onset prosthetic valve endocarditis (*Table 18.3*).

Therapy based on a microbial diagnosis

Antibiotic sensitivity tests on the blood culture isolate must always include an estimation of the minimum bactericidal concentration (MBC) as well as the minimum inhibitory concentration (MIC). Tests of combinations of antibiotics are sometimes necessary to select an optimal combination that gives the best synergic bactericidal effect when single antibiotics give an incomplete bactericidal effect against the isolate (*see Fig. 18.2*). Suggestions for therapy for different types of organism isolated follow:

a. 'Streptococcus viridans' fully sensitive to pencillin

The MBC of penicillin for most strains of viridans streptococci is equal or less than 0·12 mg/l. Endocarditis in such patients without previous heart surgery is effectively treated by benzylpenicillin, given alone, 4 MU every 6 hours by the intravenous bolus administration for 2 weeks followed by oral antibiotics for a further 3–4 weeks. The oral regimens used are either pencillin V, 1 g 6-hourly, plus probenicid or amoxycillin, 500 mg 6-hourly, plus probenecid, 500 mg 6-hourly. The serum bactericidal activity against the patient's own blood culture isolate should be estimated during both parenteral and oral therapy, to check that a serum bactericidal titre of preferably at least 1 in 4 is achieved shortly before the next dose of antibiotic is due.

Recently, there has been controversy over whether an aminoglycoside should be combined with penicillin to treat endocarditis due to penicillin-sensitive streptococci (*see* Shanson, 1981).

Table 18.3. Initial blind antibiotic treatment of suspected bacterial endocarditis

Situation	*Likely organisms*	*Antibiotics*	*Suggested dosage*
1. No previous heart surgery	'*Streptococcus viridans*' *Streptococcus faecalis*	Benzylpenicillin	5 MU, i.v. bolus route every 6 hours
		plus	
		Gentamicin	80 mg, i.v. bolus or i.m. route every 8 hours
2. Prosthetic or homograft valve endocarditis			
a. Early onset	*Staphylococcus aureus* *Staphylococcus epidermidis* Gram-negative bacilli Diphtheroids	Cloxacillin	2 g, i.v. bolus route every 4 hours
		plus	
		Gentamicin	80 mg, i.v. bolus route every 6 hours
		plus	
		Benzylpenicillin	2 MU, i.v. bolus route every 6 hours
b. Late onset	'*Streptococcus viridans*' *Staphylococcus epidermidis* *Staphylococcus aureus*	Benzylpenicillin	4 MU, i.v. bolus route every 6 hours
		plus	
		Gentamicin	80 mg, i.v. bolus route every 6 hours
		plus	
		Cloxacillin	2 g, i.v. bolus route every 6 hours

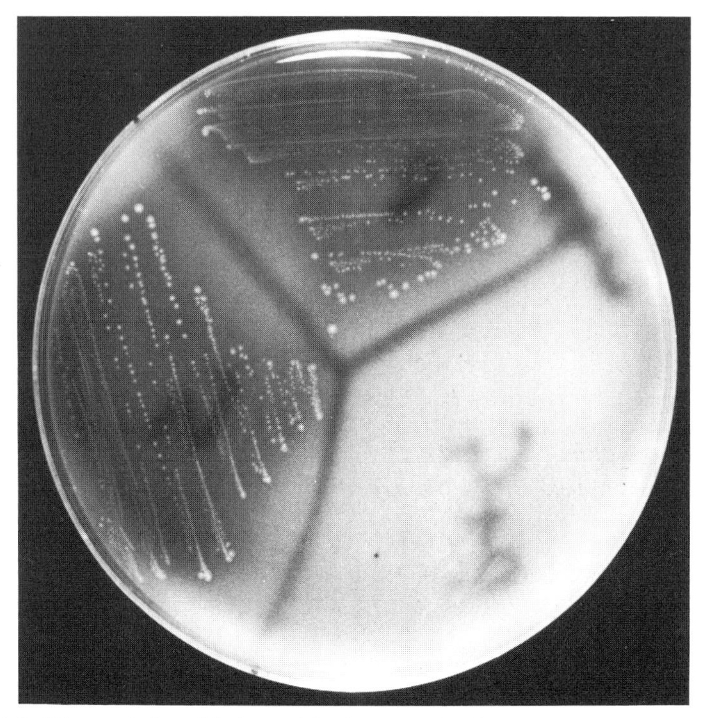

Fig. 18.2. 'Three-tube' antibiotic combination test, showing bactericidal synergy between penicillin and gentamicin against a 'penicillin-resistant' streptococcal strain from a patient with bacterial endocarditis.

b. 'Streptococcus viridans' and Streptococcus faecalis strains with reduced sensitivity to pencillin

The MBC to penicillin is greater than 0·12 mg/l for a minority of strains of viridans streptococci and the majority of *Streptococcus faecalis* strains and frequently the MBC to penicillin is greater than 6 mg/l for *Streptococcus faecalis* strains.

Laboratory guidance is essential in these cases and therapy may depend on the results of antibiotic combination tests for synergy between various aminoglycosides and penicillin or ampicillin (or amoxycillin). Often suitable therapy is provided by a combination of benzylpenicillin, 5 MU every 6 hours intravenously plus gentamicin, 80 mg, every 6 hours intravenously.

c. Staphylococcus aureus

Staphylococcal endocarditis is often rapidly fatal unless urgently treated with large doses of appropriate bactericidal antibiotics.

Most strains of *Staph. aureus* are resistant to penicillin but sensitive to cloxacillin and gentamicin. Cloxacillin, 2 g intravenously by bolus administration every 4 hours, should be given together with gentamicin, 80 mg 8-hourly, intravenously or intra-muscularly. For the few cases of endocarditis due to *Staph. aureus* sensitive to penicillin, benzylpenicillin, 4 MU every 6 hours, should be given intravenously instead of the cloxacillin, as penicillin is much more active than cloxacillin against these strains.

d. Gram-negative bacilli
A combination of ampicillin and gentamicin is often suitable, but the choice must depend on the results of antibiotic sensitivity tests.

e. Coxiella burnetii
Q fever endocarditis needs treatment by tetracycline drugs for many months and surgical excision of the infected valve is sometimes necessary. Following the insertion of the new valve treatment may need to be continued for at least 1 year. Rifampicin has been used successfully in one patient in whom tetracycline therapy failed.

f. Fungal causes
Amphotericin B together with surgical treatment is usually necessary.

Prosthetic valve endocarditis

Antibiotics are selected on the same principles as for patients without prosthetic valves. However, when penicillin-sensitive streptococci are isolated it is always preferable to add an aminoglycoside to the benzylpenicillin parenteral therapy to obtain a more rapid bactericidal effect.

The duration of therapy in endocarditis in patients who have not had heart surgery is usually for 4–6 weeks but in prosthetic valve endocarditis therapy should be continued for at least 6 months.

Many patients with prosthetic valve endocarditis are not curable by antibiotic therapy alone and excision of the infected valve during appropriate antibiotic treatment is often necessary.

Allergy to penicillin

When only a doubtful history of penicillin allergy is obtained it is often best to give penicillin under anti-histamine and steroid cover. Alternatively, cephaloridine or cephazolin has been effective for treating endocarditis due to '*Streptococcus viridans*' fully sensitive to penicillin. This is best given in combination with an aminoglycoside, such as streptomycin, depending on the results of laboratory combination tests. Cephalosporins should never be used for treating streptococci with reduced sensitivity to penicillin, such as *Streptococcus faecalis*, because the results of treatment are often unsatisfactory.

When a clear-cut penicillin allergy situation occurs, treatment of *Strep. viridans* with vancomycin alone or with an aminoglycoside should be considered. Rifampicin may also be useful, in combination with either gentamicin, vancomycin or erythromycin, under laboratory guidance.

Laboratory monitoring of treatment

The serum bactericidal titre against the patient's blood culture isolate is the most useful test during treatment and post-dose titres of 1/8 or greater and pre-dose titres of 1/4 or greater are preferable. Serum antibiotic assays of gentamicin or other aminoglycosides, and of vancomycin, have already been mentioned.

Pyrexia during treatment

Although the patient generally feels much better after 1–2 days of appropriate treatment, the temperature may continue to be raised above normal for 3–14 days after the start of treatment. If pyrexia worsens or persists, the following possibilities are considered:

i. drug reaction;
ii. superinfection—especially from a contaminated intravenous line or drip-site infection;
iii. lack of control of the original infection—? mixture of organisms or ineffective antimicrobial therapy against the single organism.

Further blood cultures and culture of the intravenous line are indicated if the pyrexia persists.

Prevention of endocarditis

A high standard of oral hygiene is vital in susceptible patients to reduce the chances of dental bacteraemia. This is probably of greater importance than chemoprophylaxis. For hospital inpatients great care should be taken over aseptic and antiseptic techniques for intravenous therapy and any invasive procedures.

Chemoprophylaxis

Basic principles for effective chemoprophylaxis include:

i. Select bactericidal rather than bacteriostatic antibiotics.
ii. Arrange for timing of the first dose just before the expected bacteraemia. (If chemoprophylaxis is started too soon, antibiotic-resistant bacteria strains may rapidly appear and cause subsequent infection.)
iii. Continue chemoprophylaxis for the critical 'at risk' period following bacteraemia—rarely more than 24–48 hours.
vi. Use adequate dosage of antibiotics.
v. Use different prophylaxis if patients are already receiving a penicillin drug or have done so recently.

The scientific basis for most of these principles has recently been demonstrated in a rabbit model for experimental endocarditis.

Chemoprophylaxis for dental procedures

The risk of endocarditis developing after a dental extraction in a susceptible patient without any antibiotic prophylaxis is low—about 1 in 500. Nevertheless, about 25% of patients presenting with '*Strep. viridans*' endocarditis give a recent history of dental procedure and, as the disease is potentially fatal, adequate chemoprophylaxis should always be arranged to cover dental procedures. Dental extraction is the main procedure, but any other procedure that causes gingival bleeding also requires prophylaxis.

Suggested antibiotic prophylactic regimens for dental procedures are included in *Table 18.4*. Most patients who require prophylaxis visit a dentist outside hospital and in this situation high dose oral amoxycillin is recommended.

Table 18.4. Prophylaxis of endocarditis in susceptible adult patients undergoing 'at risk' dental procedures

Regimen	If allergic to penicillin
1. *Parenteral prophylaxis for hospital patients or those receiving general anaesthesia* I.m. injection of Fortified Benzathine penicillin, BPC (Penidural All purpose, Wyeth, I vial) containing a mixture of Benzylpenicillin 190 mg Procaine penicillin 300 mg Benzathine penicillin 450 mg Administered 15–30 minutes before the procedure	*If allergic to penicillin* i. Erythromycin lactobionate, 1 g, intravenously, just before procedure, followed by oral erythromycin, 500 mg 6-hourly for 24 hours or ii. Vancomycin, 1 g intravenously, over 20 minutes, starting 30 minutes before the procedure
2. *Oral prophylaxis for patients outside hospital receiving local anaesthesia* Single 3-g oral dose of amoxycillin, given under supervision, 1 hour before the procedure Second dose of 3 g taken 6–8 hours after the procedure	*If allergic to penicillin* Erythromycin, 1·5 g orally, 1–2 hours before the procedure followed by 500 mg 6-hourly for 24 hours
3. *Patients with prosthetic heart valves*—parenteral prophylaxis* I.m. injection of Fortified Benzathine penicillin, BPC (*see* (1) *above*) plus i.m. injection of streptomycin 1 g Both injections given 15–30 minutes before the procedure	*If allergic to penicillin* Vancomycin, 1 g intravenously by slow infusion, 30 minutes before the procedure plus Gentamicin, 80 mg i.m. or i.v., 15–30 minutes before the procedure

* Also patients receiving penicillin prophylaxis for rheumatic fever and patients who have had a previous episode of endocarditis.
N.B. Paediatric dosage: up to 12 years use half adult dose.

Combined antibiotic prophylaxis with injections of penicillins plus an aminoglycoside is recommended for patients who have recently received penicillin or who have a prosthetic heart valve.

Chemoprophylaxis for manipulations or surgery on the genito-urinary or intestinal tract

The main organism that can cause endocarditis following such procedures as cystoscopy of the bladder, complicated vaginal delivery of a baby or surgery on the large bowel is *Streptococcus faecalis*.

Ampicillin, 1 g parenterally, is suggested, 15–30 minutes before the procedure plus gentamicin, 80 mg by a separate injection, at the same time. Repeat doses of these antibiotics are given 6 and 12 hours after the procedure.

Chemoprophylaxis for open-heart surgery

Staphylococcus aureus and *Staphylococcus epidermidis* are the two most important organisms that may cause endocarditis during the early post-operative period in patients undergoing prosthetic or homograft valve surgery. Parenteral prophylaxis should start with the pre-medication, consisting of a combination of cloxacillin, penicillin and gentamicin, and continue for 24–48 hours after surgery.

INFECTIVE MYOCARDITIS AND PERICARDITIS

Clinical Features

Infections of the myocardium and pericardium often present clinically in young people as an acute illness with breathlessness or pain in the chest. In severely affected patients there may be clinical confusion with a myocardial infarction. The electrocardiogram (ECG), as well as microbiological investigations, may help to differentiate these different pathologies.

Both the myocardium and pericardium are usually infected but occasionally separate infections of these heart tissues may occur. Many patients have no symptoms of infection.

Chronic infections are more common in underdeveloped countries, especially in the tropics, than in Britain or the U.S.A.

Causative Organisms

Acute infections

Viruses cause the majority of acute infections and the most frequent viral causes in Britain are Coxsackie B1–B6 and influenza A viruses (*Table 18.5*). Arboviruses are important in some tropical countries.

Bacteria infrequently cause infections of the pericardium or myocardium in Britain. *Strep. pyogenes* commonly affected the heart in the past by an immunological mechanism when rheumatic fever was common (*see* Chapter 11, p. 204). *Neisseria* species and *Staph. aureus* rarely cause a pyogenic pericarditis. *Corynebacterium diphtheriae* exotoxin can cause myocarditis.

Non-bacterial agents that can cause acute pericarditis or myocarditis include *Mycoplasma pneumoniae*, *Chlamydia psittaci* and *Coxiella burnetii*.

Table 18.5. Causative organisms of myocarditis and pericarditis

Organism	*Comment*
Viruses	
Coxsackie B1–B6 } Influenza A }	Most frequent known causes of acute infections in Britain
Arboviruses	
Rubella	Cause of foetal myocarditis and congenital lesions
Bacteria	
Strep. pyogenes	Indirect effect on heart in rheumatic fever
Staph. aureus	
Strep. pneumoniae	
Neisseria meningitidis	
Neisseria gonorrhoeae	
Corynebacterium diphtheriae	Toxic effect on heart
Mycobacterium tuberculosis	
Treponema pallidum	
Leptospira	
Mycoplasma, chlamydiae and Coxiella	
Mycoplasma pneumoniae	
Chlamydia psittaci	
Coxiella burnetii	Acute or chronic myocarditis possible in Q fever
Protozoa	
Toxoplasma gondii	Acute or chronic myocarditis may occur in toxoplasmosis
Trypanosoma cruzi	Chagas' disease
Entamoeba histolytica	
Fungus	
Cryptococcus	

Chronic infections

Tuberculous pericarditis is particularly important and may cause a chronic constrictive fibrinous pericarditis. Chagas disease caused by *Trypanosoma cruzi* is often associated with a chronic myocarditis and occurs in poorer parts of South America (*see* Chapter 21, p. 422).

Toxoplasma can cause an acute or chronic myocarditis and this infection of the heart is occasionally reported in Britain.

Fungi, amoebae and worms can very rarely cause chronic pericarditis.

Microbiological Investigations

a. Viral studies

i. Throat swab collected and immediately put in viral transport medium—for Coxsackie B and influenza virus isolation attempt.
ii. Faeces specimen sent for Coxsackie B virus isolation.
iii. Acute serum early on in the illness and a convalescent serum 10–14 days later, to demonstrate rising neutralizing antibody titre against any

Coxsackie B virus isolated and also for influenza CFT's. In some centres paired sera can be tested against Coxsackie B viruses. Paired sera above can also be tested for mycoplasma, Q fever and psittacosis CFT's.

b. Bacteriology and parasitology

i. Blood cultures—for isolation of *Neisseria* or *Staphylococcus* or other possible bacterial causes.
ii. Pericardial fluid—for microscopy, culture and sensitivity including a search for acid-fast bacilli in chronic cases.
iii. Paired sera—for leptospiral CFT, ASO titre, Toxoplasma Dye test.

Antimicrobial Treatment

Tetracycline is given when mycoplasma, coxiella or chlamydia infections are suspected.

Benzylpenicillin is appropriate for treating neisseria and leptospiral infections. When other bacteria are isolated the antibiotics are selected in accordance with results of culture and sensitivities.

Pyrimethamine and sulphonamides are given when toxoplasma mycocarditis is suspected.

Further Reading

Editorial (1979) Preventing endocarditis. *Br. Med. J.* **1**, 290.

Hamer J. and O'Grady F. W. (1977) In: Hamer J. (ed.) *Recent Advances in Cardiology*, 7th ed. London, Churchill Livingstone.

Lerner A. M. (1979) Myocarditis and pericarditis. In: Mandell G. L., Douglas R. G. and Bennett J. E. (ed.) *Infectious Diseases*, pp. 711–723.

Oakley C. M. and Darrell J. H. (1980) Treatment of infective endocarditis. *Prescribers Journal* **20**, 98.

Oakley C. M. and Somerville W. (1981) Prevention of infective endocarditis. *Br. Heart J.* **45**, 233–235.

Shanson D. C. (1978) Blood culture techniques. In: Williams J. D. (ed.) *Modern Topics in Infection*. London, Heinemann.

Shanson D. C. (1980) The chemotherapy of infective endocarditis. In: Grüneberg R. N. (ed.) *Antibiotics and Chemotherapy. Current Topics*. London, MTP Press.

Shanson D. C. (1981) Prophylaxis and treatment of infective endocarditis. *J. R. Coll. Physicians Lond.* **15**, 169–172.

Shanson D. C., Ashford R. F. U. and Singh J. (1980) High dose oral amoxycyllin for preventing endocarditis. *Br. Med. J.* **280**, 446.

Chapter 19

Infections of the urinary tract

Urinary tract infections are common and cause significant morbidity and mortality.

NORMAL FLORA OF THE URINARY TRACT

The bladder urine is normally sterile, as is the entire urinary tract.*

DEFINITION OF URINARY TRACT INFECTION

This is the presence of micro-organisms in the urinary tract (Medical Research Council Report, 1979).

SIGNIFICANT BACTERIURIA

'Significant bacteriuria'—greater than 10^8 bacteria per litre ($>10^5$ bacteria per ml) in a suitably collected and well-transported mid-stream sample of urine (MSU)—is the usual diagnostic criterion for a urinary tract infection. Originally, this term was used by Kass to distinguish between infected and contaminated urine specimens in patients without symptoms, but it has also become widely used to define the presence of urinary infection in symptomatic patients. However, occasionally in symptomatic patients, the count may fall to 10^7 bacteria per litre (10^4 bacteria per ml), or even lower, in the absence of antibiotics. This is taken into account in the 1979 revised terminology.

CLINICAL PATHOLOGICAL CATEGORIES

The terminology has been recently revised (M.R.C. Report, 1979).

1. *Frequency and Dysuria Syndrome*

Dysuria and frequency of micturition, sometimes accompanied by supra-pubic pain. This may be due to:

a. Bacterial cystitis
Characterized by 'significant bacteriuria' and often pyuria and haematuria also occur.

b. Abacterial cystitis
Previously known as 'urethral syndrome' when no bacteria are demonstrable in the bladder urine. The cause is usually unknown.

* The distal anterior urethra is lightly colonized with skin or faecal flora.

2. *Acute Bacterial Pyelonephritis*

Syndrome consisting of loin pain, tenderness and pyrexia accompanied by bacteriuria and pyuria. In this syndrome particularly, 'significant bacteriuria' may not occur. Bacteraemia is often detected.

3. *Chronic Interstitial Nephritis*

The renal interstitium and tubules are affected by a chronic inflammatory disease which may lead to a progressive shrinkage of a kidney due to fibrosis. Tubular function in particular may become impaired.

Bacterial infection, usually associated with structural abnormalities of the urinary tract, is an important cause but there are numerous other causes, including analgesic abuse, methicillin nephropathy, and irradiation. In many patients, no aetiological agent is found.

4. *Covert bacteriuria*

Previously known as 'asymptomatic bacteriuria'. Significant bacteriuria is found during the screening of apparently healthy people.

PATHOGENESIS

Organisms from the faecal flora usually enter the urinary tract by the ascending route starting at the perineum and peri-urethral sites. The organisms then ascend up the urethra to the bladder and sometimes further on to the kidneys. In females the short urethra facilitates this route of infection.

During micturition, a few organisms may enter the neck of the bladder in females, occasionally, and with normal defence mechanisms these may be quickly eradicated. However, the chances of trans-urethral passage of organisms into the bladder is increased in some women after coitus and in all people by instrumentation. Sometimes there is no clear history of a 'sub-umbilical event' that precipitates infection and the pathogenesis of urinary tract infection is unclear.

The normal defence mechanisms include:

a. Hydrodynamic factors—flushing out infected urine and replacement by sterile urine.
b. Phagocytosis by polymorphs.
c. Humoral antibody—IgA especially.
d. Non-specific antibacterial substances in prostatic, urethral and bladder mucosa secretions.

Colonization of the Vaginal Introitus, 'O' Serotypes of E. coli. Bacterial Adhesion and 'K' Antigen

The vaginal introitus or peri-urethral area typically becomes colonized by the causative organism from the faecal flora before infection of the urinary tract. Relatively few 'O' serotypes of *E. coli* (such as O2, O4, O6) cause the majority of *E. coli* urinary tract infections and this mainly reflects the prevalence of these serotypes in the faeces. However, recent work has suggested that certain strains of *E. coli*, within a particular 'O' serogroup, may vary in their ability to adhere to uroepithelial cells and strains which show great adhesiveness may be more likely to cause urinary tract infections than others. The bacterial adhesion to epithelial cell surfaces may be due to bacterial fimbriae becoming attached to specific epithelial cell 'receptors'. Research to elucidate the mechanisms of bacterial adhesion and, incidentally, to develop possible drugs or chemical agents which might interfere with this adhesion is in progress.

Once bacteria have invaded the urinary tract, the organisms can ascend to cause infection of the upper urinary tract although this probably occurs in only a minority of patients. Predisposing factors, such as vesico-ureteric reflux in infants or renal calculi in adults, often determine whether upper urinary tract infection will occur but organism-related factors may sometimes be relevant also. The amount and type of polysaccharide 'K' antigen present in the 'capsular' surface of an infecting *E. coli* strain may be related to the likelihood of certain strains causing acute bacterial pyelonephritis.

E. coli strains with K1 antigen are more often associated with pyelonephritis than cystitis (although these strains also frequently cause cystitis) and strains with abundant K1 antigen are relatively resistant to the bactericidal effects of fresh human serum. Similarly, *E. coli* O6 strains with K2a or K2c capsular antigens frequently cause pyelonephritis but are infrequently found in the normal faecal flora.

Residual Urine

In the healthy urinary tract, the bladder is virtually completely empty after micturition. When there is some structural abnormality or a neurogenic bladder the residual urine may constitute more than 2 or 3 ml and then the chances of infection developing and persisting are greatly increased.

Haematogenous Infection

In a few cases, the kidney can become infected by the haematogenous route, particularly after a *Staph. aureus* bacteraemia. The peri-nephric tissues can also become infected by this route and a peri-nephric abscess may develop—one cause of 'PUO'.

PRE-DISPOSING FACTORS

Age

The incidence of urinary tract infection increases greatly with age (*see Fig. 19.1*).

Sex

The short female urethra greatly pre-disposes to infection of the urinary tract by the ascending route and the great majority of symptomatic infections are in females up to the age of 50 years. Urinary infections are much more common in women who have sexual intercourse than in those who abstain from sex.

A significant number of infections occur in men only after the age of 50 years when prostatic hypertrophy or other urinary tract abnormalities may occur.

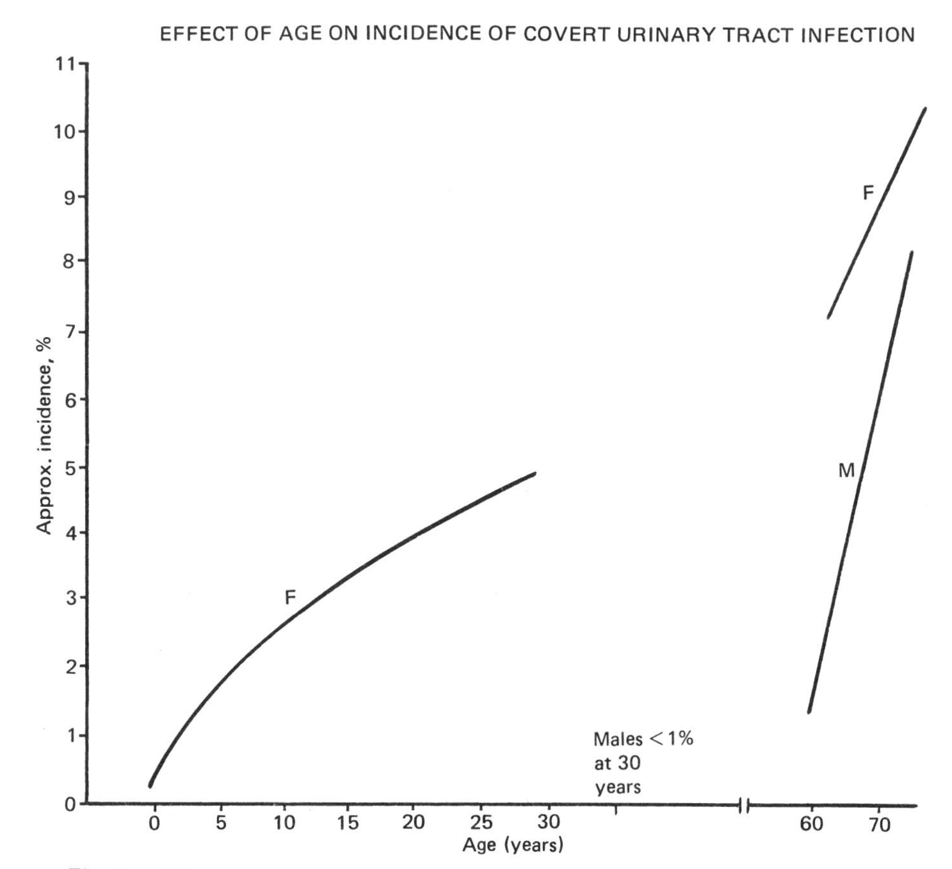

Fig. 19.1. Effect of age on incidence of covert urinary tract infection. M = males. F = females.

Urinary tract infection in a young man is unusual and requires further investigation.

Structural/Neurological Abnormalities of the Urinary Tract

There are numerous possible abnormalities of the urinary tract that are associated with a 'residual urine' which increase the chances of infection occurring and which may become associated with repeated attacks of urinary tract infection. Some of these are included in *Table 19.1*. Paraplegic patients and patients with multiple sclerosis who have a neurogenic bladder may need long-term urinary catheterization.

Instrumentation and Surgery

Indwelling urinary catheters are probably the most frequent pre-disposing cause of urinary infections in hospital patients. Re-infection with successively more

Table 19.1. Some abnormalities of the urinary tract pre-disposing to urinary tract infections

Abnormality	*Comment*
Vesico-ureteric reflux	Mild to moderate degrees of reflux usually resolve spontaneously as child grows older Severe degrees of reflux may cause intra-renal lesions associated with 'back pressure' as well as infection—surgery usually indicated
Ureterocoele Urethral valves Urethral stricture	Occasional congenital causes that require surgical correction
Calculus formation Prostatic hypertrophy	Common causes of obstruction often requiring surgery
Bladder diverticulum	
Genital prolapse	
Neurogenic bladder	Permanent indwelling catheterization associated with recurrent UTI

UTI, urinary tract infections.

antibiotic-resistant strains of bacteria frequently occurs. This subject is further discussed under Hospital-acquired urinary infections, in Chapter 24.

Any instrumentation or surgery on the urinary tract increases the chances of hospital-acquired infection.

Other Host Factors

a. Diabetes mellitus—increases the risk of severe bacterial pyelonephritis developing with acute papillary necrosis.

b. Immunosuppression—steroids or cytotoxic drugs, as given to renal transplant patients, greatly increase the chances of recurrent urinary tract infections and infection of the kidney by unusual organisms, such as *Salmonella, Serratia, Candida* and *Nocardia.*

EFFECTS OF URINARY TRACT INFECTIONS

a. Symptoms

Most symptomatic patients complain of frequency and dysuria. In some patients with bacterial cystitis there is also supra-pubic pain.

Loin pain or tenderness suggests acute pyelonephritis and this condition is often accompanied by fever and some vomiting. Jaundice is sometimes the presenting feature of urinary tract infection in neonates. Bed wetting in a child or increasing 'stress incontinence' in an elderly person are amongst the many alternative possible presenting features of urinary tract infection.

b. Gram-negative Septicaemia

This may particularly occur when there is any obstruction to the upper urinary tract and also when there is pre-existing kidney infection. Instrumentation or surgery on an infected urinary tract is frequently followed by septicaemia (*see* Chapter 5).

c. Renal Damage

Chronic urinary tract infection, both symptomatic and asymptomatic, in young children can lead to scarring of the kidney and damage to growing nephrons, often in association with vesico-ureteric reflux. This can result in chronic pyelonephritis in young adulthood and renal failure. For these reasons, urinary infections in childhood must be fully investigated and treated effectively together with long-term follow up.

In a small number of adults, especially those with abnormal urinary tracts, chronic urinary tract infection may also contribute to the impairment of renal function.

d. Prolonged Hospital Stay

Urinary infection in hospital in-patients, especially post-operative patients, may lead to a prolonged hospital admission until the infection responds satisfactorily to therapy.

CAUSATIVE ORGANISMS

Bacteria (and fungi) are the main organisms that infect the urinary tract.

Bacterial Causes

Bacteria are by far the most frequent group of organisms causing urinary infection, but the pattern of bacterial agents depends to a large extent on whether the infections are acute or recurrent and whether they are occurring outside or inside of hospital. Scores of different bacterial species have, at one time or another, caused urinary tract infections. The main bacteria causing urinary infections in hospital and in general practice in 1979 are included in *Table 19.2*.

Table 19.2. Bacterial causes of urinary tract infection

	UTI (%) in	
Organism	*General practice*	*Hospital practice*
Escherichia coli	82	55
Staphylococcus albus or *saprophyticus*	9	4
Proteus species	3	12
Strep. faecalis	1	3
Klebsiella aerogenes	2	13
Other 'coliforms'	2	5
Pseudomonas aeruginosa	1	7
Serratia marcescens	0	1

Figures from 500 infections in each practice from the Microbiology Laboratory at St Stephen's Hospital, Fulham Road, London.
UTI, urinary tract infections.

Escherichia coli (E. coli)

Most infections in both general and hospital practice are due to *E. coli*, but the percentage in hospital is much less than that in general practice as is shown in *Table 19.2*. The most frequent serotypes of *E. coli* causing urinary tract infections include O1, O2, O4, O6, O7, O25 and O50, and this probably reflects the prevalence in the faecal flora rather than differences in virulence between serotypes. The percentage of urinary tract infections, due to *E. coli* in patients with single attacks of infection, is greater than in patients who have repeated attacks of infection. Also the strains of *E. coli* from patients with recurrent urinary tract infections are often more resistant to antibiotics than those from patients who have only suffered one or two attacks of infection.

Staphylococcus saprophyticus and Staphylococcus albus (epidermidis)

The causative organisms of bacterial cystitis in young women patients seen in general practice is usually *E. coli* but the next most common cause is *Staph. saprophyticus* (previously known as novobiocin-resistant micrococcus subgroup 3).

Staph. albus is also an occasional cause of urinary infection in hospital, sometimes associated with catheterization.

Staph. aureus is only rarely a cause of urinary tract infection, but gives severe symptoms and sequelae as a post-operative infection.

Proteus Species

Proteus mirabilis (indole negative) is the most frequent *Proteus* species associated with urinary tract infections, but indole-positive *Proteus* species like *Pr. vulgaris*, which are more often resistant to ampicillin, may also cause urinary tract infections.

These species are often associated with an alkaline urine. The organisms split urea through their enzyme urease to form ammonia and this helps to encourage the growth of calculi. *Proteus* species are often associated with large staghorn calculi in the renal pelvis, acute pyelonephritis and septicaemia.

Although infection of the urinary tract in boys aged 2–12 years is uncommon, *Proteus* is one of the most frequent causes in this age group and is often associated with isolation of the same organism from the prepuce.

Klebsiella Species

These bacteria are increasingly found to cause urinary tract infections in hospital patients and may be involved in outbreaks of hospital infection. They are common in patients with repeated attacks of urinary tract infections who have received previous antibiotics.

Klebsiella aerogenes strains are nearly always resistant to ampicillin and the widespread use of ampicillin in hospitals encourages the spread of these organisms. Many *Klebsiella* strains are resistant to several antibiotics and the multiple antibiotic resistance is often plasmid mediated. In recent years, there have been outbreaks of gentamicin-resistant klebsiella infections mainly in male hospital patients with urinary catheters (*see* Urinary tract infections, in Chapter 24).

Pseudomonas and Serratia Species

These species are usually resistant to many antibiotics and are particularly associated with recurrent urinary tract infections in hospital patients.

Streptococcus faecalis

This organism appears to have a low-grade pathogenicity compared with Gram-negative bacilli and staphylococci. No antibiotic treatment is indicated for some *Strep. faecalis* urinary tract infections although ampicillin may be necessary when there are associated symptoms.

Other Bacteria

i. *Mycobacterium tuberculosis* must always be considered as a possible cause of chronic urinary tract infection (*see* Chapter 13).
ii. *Anaerobes*, such as *Bacteroides fragilis* or anaerobic cocci, rarely cause urinary tract infections, but may need to be looked for in selected cases where pyuria has occurred without a previously demonstrable bacterial cause.
iii. *Neisseria gonorrhoeae* is an infrequent cause of pyuria but this is due to urethritis rather than to urinary tract infections.

Fungi

Candida albicans causes bladder infections, predominantly in diabetics and in patients who have had repeated courses of antibiotics, or who have their general host defences impaired. Candida infections of the kidney may also occur in immunosuppressed patients, including recipients of renal transplants.

INVESTIGATION OF URINARY TRACT INFECTIONS

Microbiological Investigation of Urine

Specimens of urine are frequently contaminated with normal flora from the perineum or genitalia. This contamination is reduced although it sometimes cannot be entirely prevented, when efforts are made to explain to the patient exactly how the mid-stream specimen of urine (MSU) should be collected. It is particularly necessary to explain the importance of adequate cleansing with tap water and drying of the genitalia before micturition. However, this may not be a practical procedure in children, but should be attempted if the perineum is obviously faecally soiled.

In infants and the elderly, excessive contamination of urine specimens is a particularly great problem.

Methods of urine collection

Whichever method is used, urine samples should be collected before the start of antibiotic therapy.

a. *MSU*—main method

b. i. *Adhesive bags*—infants
ii. *Clean-catch specimen*—infants
Preferable to an adhesive bag when possible to arrange.

(*a* and *b*:) Collect two specimens rather than one where possible, since the percentage confidence of detecting a bona fide urinary tract infection is increased if the same organism is isolated in significant numbers from two specimens.

c. *Supra-pubic aspiration*—occasionally necessary in infants; rarely necessary in pregnancy.

d. *Catheterization of urethra*
i. Should *never* occur just to obtain a urine specimen for microbiology because of the danger of introducing infection.
ii. If the patient is already catheterized, this is a valid method provided that urine is collected from the catheter into a syringe and needle before it enters the drainage bag and not from the bag itself.

e. *Ureteric catheterization* in the operating theatre during urological examination may provide valuable information concerning the localization of the infection (*see below*).

Transport to laboratory

The urine sample, in its sterile container, should reach the microbiology laboratory for culture within 2 hours of collection to avoid undue multiplication of possible contaminants.

When delay in transport is inevitable, one of the following methods can be used:

i. *Refrigeration at 4 °C*
The urine will be suitable for culture for 24–48 hours if kept at 4 °C. However, the cellular elements may deteriorate during storage.

ii. *Dip-slide technique*
There is a commercially available slide, covered on each side with culture medium. This is immersed in freshly voided urine, drained and then sent to the laboratory through the post for incubation at 36 °C.
The dip-slide culture method is semi-quantitative and is mainly suitable for general practices that are situated some distance from a laboratory.

iii. *Boric acid*
A few practitioners use urine containers with boric acid so that when the urine sample is added, there is a final concentration of 1·8% boric acid in the urine. This preserves the bacterial count of most urinary bacterial pathogens and also the white cells. A few bacterial strains are inhibited by boric acid.

Microscopic examination of urine

The white cells are routinely counted in a well-mixed urine sample by a counting chamber method. An abnormal white cell count is indicated by any count greater than 10 per mm^3. Pyuria of higher numbers than this is usually present in acute urinary tract infections but urinary infection may occur without pyuria.

Casts and red cells are best looked for in a gently centrifuged deposit of a fresh sample of urine, from selected patients with suspected renal disease (or infective endocarditis), numerous granular, leucocyte or epithelial casts suggesting renal involvement in an infected patient.

Culture of urine and determination of bacterial counts

a. *Surface viable count*

Measured volumes of urine are diluted in sterile water and spread on the surface of a dried solid medium such as cysteine lactose electrolyte deficient medium (CLED). After incubation, each colony represents at least one bacterium in the original urine and the approximate number of bacteria per litre of urine can then be estimated. In practice, this method is time consuming and is only used for selected urines.

b. *Semi-quantitative*

i. *Filter paper screening method of Leigh and Williams*

A commercially available strip of absorbent paper is folded so that a foot is formed and this is dipped into the urine sample. The foot has a measured standardized area and the urine inoculated foot is pressed against the surface of a CLED agar plate. Each plate is inoculated with up to eight tests each in duplicate. After incubation, the number of colonies in the impression area is counted and if over 25 colonies are present the original urine sample is known to have contained greater than 10^8 organisms per litre.

This method is reliable and inexpensive and is widely used. Urines that are positive on the screening test may be further investigated by the surface viable count method if there is a possibility of a mixed culture, provided the urine under investigation has been kept in the refrigerator in the meantime.

ii. *Standard loop method*

A standard loop is dipped vertically into the urine and inoculated onto a CLED agar plate. This method is relatively inaccurate.

iii. *Dip-slide method*

Particularly suitable for use in some general practices (*see* Transport *above*).

c. *Chemical screening methods*

Chemical screening tests which depend on the active metabolism of bacteria have been used when there is a lack of bacteriological facilities. A colour change in each method used indicates the presence of 'significant bacteriuria', but unfortunately each method is associated with a significant number of false positive or false negative results. The tests include the triphenyl tetrazolium chloride test, the Griess test for nitrite and the estimation of urinary glucose.

Interpretation of the Results of Microscopy and Culture

The culture results are far more important than the results of microscopy. Interpretation of the culture results depends on the type of urine specimen collected, whether antibiotics have recently been given (negative results are then of limited value), and on knowledge of the circumstances of transport of the specimen. Ideally, the time of collection should be recorded on the specimen container and the time noted when the specimen arrives in the laboratory; 'positive' results obtained from specimens that have been at room temperature for more than 2 hours should be interpreted with caution. Urine is a good culture medium in which contaminants may multiply and 'significant bacteriuria' applies only to well-collected urine specimens that have been suitably transported or refrigerated soon after collection.

Mid-stream, clean-catch and adhesive bag urine samples:

Significant bacteriuria	—greater than 10^8 bacteria per litre —usually a pure growth of one organism when indicative of urinary tract infection —indicative of urinary tract infection with 80% confidence when present in one urine sample —confidence of urinary tract infection is further increased in one urine sample when characteristic symptoms and pyuria also occur —confidence of urinary tract infection increases to 95% when the same organism is isolated in significant numbers from two different MSU samples.
No evidence of infection	—less than 10^7 bacteria/litre and patient not receiving antibiotics
Equivocal results	—10^7–10^8 bacteria/litre—may indicate infection, especially if *Proteus* or staphylococci are present, or patient extremely well hydrated —suggest repeat cultures
Probable contamination	—mixed growths in MSU sample —count less than 10^7 bacteria/litre —epithelial cells in microscopy suggesting vaginal contamination

Catheter or supra-pubic urine samples:

Evidence of infection	—counts usually greater than 10^8 bacteria/litre when infected urine —two organisms common when indwelling catheter —counts less than 10^7–10^8 per litre may still be significant

Interpretation of sterile pyuria:

Possible tuberculosis	—consider early morning specimen of urine (EMSU) × 3 for acid-fast bacilli culture, especially if persistent pyuria
Treatment/Non-infective causes	—antibiotic therapy; tumours or foreign bodies in genito-urinary tract including catheters; recent surgery; analgesic nephropathy
Urethuritis/abacterial cystitis	—pus cells from 'urethritis' and 'abacterial cystitis' if low to moderately high counts of white cells
Vaginal discharge	—pus cells from vaginal contamination from a patient with a discharge—suggested by presence of epithelial cells and also by long Gram-positive bacilli (probable lactobacilli) in a Gram-stained smear of urine deposit
Other possible causes	—urinary infection due to a fastidious organism such as *Mycoplasma* or L form—consider prolonged cultures
	—look at Gram-stain of urine deposit for evidence of bacterial infection when cultures are negative and the patient is not receiving antibiotics—if numerous short bacilli are present infection due to diphtheroids, *Haemophilus vaginalis* or anaerobes is a possibility
	—if patient has had recent cotrimoxazole, consider possibility of thymidine-dependent coliform strains that would require prolonged incubation to grow

Urines from patients with sterile pyuria should be incubated in an aerobic plus CO_2 atmosphere and also anaerobically plus CO_2 for at least 3 days and a repeat urine sample requested (i.e. when patients are not receiving antibiotics).

Antibiotic sensitivity tests

Antibiotic sensitivity tests are carried out on all significant bacterial isolates using about six 'routine' different antibiotics. Patients who have large numbers of pus cells present in the urine or who have severe symptoms, may have their urine selected for direct antibiotic sensitivity tests using the original urine as the test inoculum, so that the results of antibiotic sensitivity tests are available the day after receipt of the specimen.

Screening for Asymptomatic Urinary Tract Infections

a. Pregnant women

About 5% of women attending the ante-natal clinics have covert (asymptomatic) bacteriuria of pregnancy. An MSU for microscopy, culture and sensitivity should be routinely collected early in pregnancy and, if infection is demonstrated, appropriate antibiotics are necessary. If no antibiotic therapy is given to this group of patients, 20–30% of the patients will develop acute pyelitis of pregnancy. This complication can be prevented by effectively treating the covert bacteriuria.

b. Other adults

Elderly people have a high incidence of asymptomatic urinary tract infections (*Fig. 19.1*) and treatment is not usually indicated. It is not worthwhile screening these and other adults for covert bacteriuria.

c. Infants and children

Studies are in progress to see if it is worthwhile routinely screening infants under 5 years old in the community for the presence of covert bacteriuria. This is the age group in which kidney growth is at its maximum and it is necessary to detect possible abnormalities of the urinary tract in order to avoid subsequent impairment of renal function. It is generally considered that it is not worthwhile arranging routine screening of infants over 5 years old at present.

Children with Symptomatic Urinary Tract Infections and their Investigation

Urinary tract infections are about two to three times more common in girls than boys. About 12% of all children with symptomatic urinary tract infection have renal scarring or reflux nephropathy on initial radiological investigation, and this incidence is highest in those with recurrent urinary tract infections. There is about a 50% chance of infection recurring within 1 year of treatment of a urinary tract infection in girls. The investigation, long-term follow up and appropriate treatment of urinary infections in children is of the greatest importance to reduce the chances of serious hypertension or renal failure occurring in later childhood or young adult life. These latter complications may otherwise result from progressive kidney damage to growing kidneys by renal infection.

The clinical features of urinary tract infection may be confused with those of infection of the gastro-intestinal tract or respiratory tract as well as of other illnesses, especially in young infants. Urine samples should be collected for culture from these infants, especially when fever occurs, before the start of antibiotics whenever possible. Other symptoms, such as enuresis or vomiting, as well as 'conventional' urinary tract infection symptoms, such as frequency, dysuria, loin or abdominal pain, should also alert the clinician for the need to collect urine samples for culture. In an acutely unwell child, it may not be possible to collect more than two 'clean-catch' or other urine samples before the start of treatment but at least three samples should be collected whenever possible. Dip-slides are often useful to overcome problems of transportation of urine samples.

Radiological investigations are necessary in all children who present with a bacteriologically proven urinary tract infection to identify possible structural abnormalities of the urinary tract, such as vesico-ureteric reflux, stones or ureterocele (including the child who presents with a first urinary tract infection). This involves an intravenous pyelogram (IVP) in the first instance and micturating cysto-urethrography (MCU) in selected infants. The latter is especially considered in those with recurrent urinary tract infections. Surgical correction of the underlying abnormality is necessary in an important minority of the children especially those who have severe vesico-ureteric reflux with some element of renal involvement. Lesser degrees of vesico-ureteric reflux often show spontaneous resolution as the child grows older.

Long-term low dose antibiotic prophylaxis is given to infants with a structural abnormality of the urinary tract and is considered for all children with recurrent urinary tract infections. Regular long-term bacteriological monitoring of the urine of all children who present with a urinary tract infection is essential.

Investigation of Recurrent Urinary Tract Infections in Adults

An abnormality of the urinary tract associated with residual urine is often present when there is relapse of infection, and radiological investigations including an IVP are usually indicated when there are more than two or three infections in one year in an adult. Sometimes surgical correction of an abnormality revealed by X-rays is possible under appropriate antibiotic cover.

Renal function tests including blood urea and creatinine clearance are necessary. Localization tests, referred to below, may help in a small proportion of cases; the problem is more serious if recurrent renal infection occurs. Generally relapses of infection are often associated with renal abnormalities and re-infection is most often seen with bladder abnormalities.

When *E. coli* is the pathogen, 'O' serotyping may help to distinguish relapse from re-infection although it is unlikely to alter the management of an individual patient.

Localization of the Site of Infection

Clinical features of acute bacterial pyelonephritis, such as fever and loin pain, combined with the finding of significant bacteriuria on culturing the urine, would be sufficient to indicate that kidney infection has occurred. In general practice, patients presenting with the frequency and dysuria syndrome, the finding of significant bacteriuria would suggest acute bacterial cystitis but it is difficult to exclude the possibility that infection of the upper urinary tract has also occurred. Some patients have atypical or no symptoms and may still have pyelonephritis. In adult men with significant bacteriuria, acute prostatitis, especially due to *E. coli*, may be suggested by perineal pain after sitting, a tender prostate and fever. Many symptomatic patients without significant bacteriuria may be suffering from urethritis and a few of these patients may suffer from sub-acute or chronic bacterial prostatitis. Localization tests have been developed to help to determine the site of urinary tract infection since clinical features alone are unreliable. These tests may be worth considering in patients with recurrent urinary tract infections but, in practice, they are usually unhelpful in the management of an individual patient. Radiological investigations, such as intravenous pyelograms and micturating cystograms, are of much more practical value than localization tests. However, localization tests performed mainly as a research procedure yield particularly valuable information about urinary tract infections in general.

Bacterial urethritis might be present if bacteria are only isolated in the first 2–3 ml urine passed and if this urine sample contains more numerous pus cells than subsequent urine samples that are collected immediately afterwards. However, in practice, this kind of localization test is rarely possible and the results are difficult to interpret.

Localization tests that are well established include direct and indirect tests (*see below*). Most of these tests have been developed to distinguish upper urinary tract infection from lower urinary tract infection. (Some patients suffer of course from simultaneous upper and lower urinary tract infections.) Only rarely can tests distinguish between the different sites of upper urinary tract infection—the upper ureter, renal pelvis (pyelitis) and kidney tissue (pyelonephritis). Histological study of nephrectomy specimens are of particular value in this respect. Of course, such specimens are rarely available.

Direct localization tests include:

1. *Ureteric catheterization*
   Bilateral ureteric catheterization gives accurate information about the presence of unilateral or bilateral upper urinary tract infection.
2. *Neomycin bladder wash-out test (Fairley's)*
   In this test:
   a. the patient empties the bladder and an MSU sample is collected
   b. a catheter is introduced
   c. neomycin is instilled locally into the bladder
   d. sterile water is used to wash out the bladder repeatedly
   e. serial urine samples are collected at 10 minute intervals for culture over a period of about 30 minutes. These samples represent ureteric urine and if obviously infected indicate upper urinary tract infection
3. *Prostatic massage to detect chronic prostatitis*
   This has been recommended by certain North American authorities but is rarely carried out in Britain.
   Three urine samples are collected:
   a. at the start of micturition
   b. MSU sample and
   c. a sample (about 10 ml) which is first passed after prostatic massage
   Highest counts of bacteria demonstrable in the third sample may suggest the presence of sub-acute prostatitis in a symptomatic patient who does not have 'significant bacteriuria' in the MSU sample. In practice, this test rarely demonstrates convincing sub-acute or chronic bacterial prostatitis.
4. *Nephrectomy*
   Surgery on the kidney can incidentally provide samples of kidney tissue which can be examined both histologically and microbiologically to provide accurate evidence about the presence of renal infection.

Indirect localization tests

These indirect tests often provide less conclusive evidence about the site of infection than the direct tests, but have the advantage of not requiring instrumentation or manipulations on the patient's urinary tract. These tests include:

1. *Renal concentration test*
   Deprivation of water may be followed by the failure to concentrate urine normally and this then indicates possible renal tubular damage associated

with renal infection. In practice, there are many potential pitfalls in the interpretation of this test.

2. *Antibodies to the infecting organism*
   Serum antibodies to the 'O' antigen of the infecting Gram-negative bacillus can be detected by a direct agglutination technique. Generally higher titres of antibody are found in patients with pyelonephritis compared to those with bladder infection. This test is most reliable in young children who may produce an IgM antibody response to the organism causing renal infection.
3. *Antibody-coated bacteria test*
   Bacteria which are coated with antibody are detected in the urine by an immunofluorescent antibody test. The presence of antibody-coated bacteria is suggestive of tissue infection in the kidney (or prostate), since antibodies are most likely to be produced and coat bacteria when the bacteria have invaded the tissues. However, some recent work has shown that IgA immunoglobulins, possibly produced in the lower urinary tract, may coat the bacteria and this test does not necessarily distinguish between upper and lower urinary tract infection in an individual patient.
4. *Analysis of the results of short-term treatment*
   In non-pregnant, non-catheterized symptomatic patients with lower urinary tract infection the results of short-term treatment, such as with a single dose of antibiotic, are usually good. When the results of single-dose treatment are retrospectively analysed, there is a lower cure rate in patients with infections of the upper urinary tract. However, the response to short-term treatment is an unreliable guide to the localization of the site of infection in an individual patient.

Abacterial Cystitis (Urethral Syndrome)

About 50% of women presenting to a general practitioner with symptoms of frequency and dysuria will not have a urinary tract infection and their symptoms are not expected to improve with antibiotic therapy. However, a few authorities recommend a short course of an antibiotic, such as cotrimoxazole. The causes of 'abacterial cystitis' are usually not apparent in an individual patient but possible causes include urethritis due to trauma or organisms such as chlamydiae, *Mycoplasma* and *Trichomonas*. Genital tract infection due to the gonococcus, *Candida albicans*, herpes simplex virus and *Haemophilus vaginalis* (*Gardnerella*) may also need consideration.

TREATMENT OF URINARY TRACT INFECTIONS

General Comments

The majority of symptomatic patients are women with bacterial cystitis and these patients need encouragement to drink large quantities of fluids so that flushing out of the infected urine occurs. Urine samples should be collected before the start of antibiotic therapy, but the decision as to whether to wait for the results or not before giving an antibiotic depends on the clinical severity of the infection. In practice, the laboratory can often give 'direct' antibiotic sensitivities the day after the receipt of the urine sample and in hospital practice it is particularly important that rational antibiotic therapy should only be given after the results of the sensitivity tests are known whenever possible.

In general practice, the great majority of urinary tract infections are due to *E. coli* strains that are sensitive to most antibiotics. Bacteriological investigations should be awaited to distinguish bacterial cystitis from abacterial cystitis otherwise antibiotics are given unnecessarily to about half the patients with frequency and dysuria. An incubator in the surgery can help give a clear result overnight if the dip-slide screening method is used for those surgeries far away from a laboratory. (A medical microbiologist should always see all possible positives and carry out further investigations as necessary.)

The patient is advised to empty the bladder last thing at night before going to sleep and also to take the last dose of antibiotic at this time to achieve a high concentration of antibiotic in the urine during sleep when the bladder is not emptied. During the day, frequent micturition and double micturition is encouraged to help eliminate residual infected urine.

Catheterized patients with asymptomatic urinary tract infection should not usually receive systemic antimicrobial agents. However, when the patient has symptoms or gross pyuria, a week's course of chemotherapy is often necessary and treatment would also be essential to cover any operation that is to be performed.

Antimicrobial agents that are available for treating urinary tract infections are included in *Table 19.3*. It is preferable that agents are selected routinely on the basis of antibiotic sensitivity test results but there are situations in practice where 'blind' chemotherapy is occasionally necessary.

A first or second attack of bacterial cystitis in a general practice adult patient usually responds to sulphonamides, ampicillin, cotrimoxazole, nalidixic acid or nitrofurantoin. Any general practice patient with recurrent cystitis must be fully investigated and treatment based on sensitivity test results.

Sulphonamides, usually excellent for treating domiciliary urinary tract infections, are cheap and excreted in high concentration in the urine, but the incidence of *E. coli* strains resistant to sulphonamides is about 20% in many areas. Cotrimoxazole, or trimethoprim, is active against greater than 90% of general practice bacterial isolates from urine. Trimethoprim alone has recently been recommended, instead of cotrimoxazole, for treating uncomplicated urinary tract infections in adults in general practice. It is probably as effective as cotrimoxazole but is associated with a lower incidence of unwanted effects such as skin rashes or blood dyscrasias.

Tetracyclines are frequently not effective and in any case should not be given to young children, pregnant women or any patient with renal impairment.

A child with a suspected urinary tract infection, presenting for the first time, should usually be given cotrimoxazole after urine samples have been collected for microbiology (*see above*). Occasionally, ampicillin, or, when infection is due to antibiotic-resistant bacteria, cephalexin, may be indicated. Ampicillin, pivmecillinam and cephalosporins are also reasonably safe drugs to give to a pregnant woman with a proven urinary tract infection, provided the pathogens are sensitive to these agents.

Nalidixic acid and nitrofurantoin are sometimes referred to as 'urinary antiseptics'. They are not suitable for treating systemic infections as adequate concentrations of these agents are not achieved in the blood. They should not

Table 19.3. Some antimicrobial drugs for urinary tract infections (UTI)

Drug	*Dosage (adult)*	*Comment*
Sulphadimidine	1 g 6-hourly orally	Main use in general practice
Trimethoprim	100 mg 12-hourly orally (full dosage)	Should probably not be used alone for treatment of acute infections in hospital as resistant strains may become more common if widely used. Useful for long-term low-dosage antibiotic prophylaxis in selected patients
Cotrimoxazole	2 tabs 12-hourly (full dosage)	Particularly valuable for long-term low-dose therapy for chronic urinary tract infections. Emergence of trimethoprim-resistant strains is rare during therapy
Ampicillin or Amoxycillin	500 mg 6-hourly orally/parenterally; 250 mg 8-hourly orally	Many *E. coli* strains resistant to ampicillin in hospital practice
Nalidixic acid	1 g 6-hourly orally	Resistance can develop during therapy. Inactive against staphylococci causing UTI in general practice. Only for use in treating bladder infections
Nitrofurantoin	100 mg 8-hourly orally	For bladder infections only. Not effective for most proteus infections
Pivmecillinam; Cephalexin	200–400 mg 6-hourly orally; 500 mg 6-hourly orally	Useful for treating some ampicillin-resistant *E. coli* urinary infections
Gentamicin or Tobramycin	80 mg 8-hourly i.m./i.v.*	Treatment of serious infections due to multiple antibiotic-resistant strains of coliforms and *Pseudomonas*
Polymyxin; Kanamycin	100 mg per 100 ml; 40 mg per 100 ml	For local instillation into bladder when indwelling catheter for some patients

* Dosage may need modification according to state of renal function.

therefore be used for treating suspected kidney infection or septicaemia. These two 'urinary antiseptics' may cause nausea, and psychiatric or neurological side effects, respectively, if given to patients with renal impairment. Nitrofurantoin is usually ineffective for treating proteus urinary tract infections. However, this drug may be useful in prophylaxis (*see below*).

Nalidixic acid is not suitable for treating young women who present with the frequency and dysuria syndrome caused by *Staph. saprophyticus* infection, as the organism is almost always resistant to this drug. However, most strains of this *Staphylococcus* are sensitive to nitrofurantoin. Resistance to nalidixic acid often emerges in a Gram-negative bacillus strain during a course of treatment of a complicated urinary tract infection (as when a patient has an enlarged prostate or an indwelling catheter).

Hospital patients with urinary tract infections are frequently infected with *E. coli* strains resistant to sulphonamides (greater than 30%) or ampicillin (between 30–60%) or *Klebsiella* strains which are always resistant to ampicillin. *Proteus* strains are usually sensitive to ampicillin. The sensitivity pattern expected of each pathogen will vary from hospital to hospital and the bacteriologist can advise about the expected current sensitivity patterns in each hospital. This advice can be followed when blind treatment is necessary. For a very severe urinary tract infection in hospital, accompanied possibly by septicaemia, a blind combination of ampicillin and gentamicin is usually effective until the results of investigations are available.

It is usually possible to wait for the results of antibiotic sensitivity tests before giving antibiotic treatment to hospital patients. When coliform strains resistant to ampicillin, sulphonamides and trimethoprim are encountered, new agents including pivmecillinam and cephalosporins can sometimes be useful. Gentamicin or tobramycin should only be used when absolutely necessary. When there is impairment of renal function, antibiotic assays, particularly of aminoglycosides, are often necessary to avoid accumulation of the drug and toxic effects. *Pseudomonas aeruginosa* infections can sometimes be treated by tobramycin in combination with carbenicillin. An ester of carbenicillin is commercially available which is broken down to form carbenicillin which is suitably concentrated in the urine for treatment of certain pseudomonas infections on an outpatient basis, but this is only rarely necessary.

Local instillations of polymyxin or kanamycin, or a disinfectant such as chlorhexidine, may be useful for treating persistent urinary infections due to antibiotic-resistant bacteria, especially in paraplegic patients.

Duration of Antimicrobial Treatment

In general practice, where the great majority of non-pregnant adult patients present with simple acute bacterial cystitis, short courses of 3-day ampicillin treatment give as good results as 10 day ampicillin treatment. Single dose treatment is under investigation, but it is clear that it is often effective in patients who have no complications.

A child with a first symptomatic urinary tract infection requires treatment, with a drug such as cotrimoxazole, for at least 1 week. Long-term low-dose prophylaxis may subsequently become necessary (*see above*).

In hospital practice when many more patients with complicated urinary tract infections are seen, therapy is usually necessary for at least a week.

At least 10 days' treatment is desirable for any patient who presents with acute bacterial pyelonephritis and for the treatment of asymptomatic bacteriuria of pregnancy.

Tests of cure

Although symptoms may disappear within a few days of starting suitable antibiotic treatment, the infection may persist asymptomatically when the treatment is stopped. Urine samples for tests of cure are collected:

a. between 3 and 5 days after stopping antibiotics

b. between 4 and 6 weeks after stopping antibiotics.

When the original infecting organism is not re-isolated from either (*a*) or (*b*), the patient is regarded as bacteriologically cured.

Treatment of Recurrent Urinary Tract Infections

Some patients with recurrent urinary tract infections should undergo surgery to remove an obstruction or correct another structural abnormality of the urinary tract that pre-disposes to recurrent infection. However, many patients have to receive medical treatment only.

When there are relatively few attacks of re-infection, each infection is treated separately in an adult according to the sensitivity of the pathogen each time. However, when there are more frequent attacks or a serious complicated chronic urinary infection that is not amenable to surgical correction, long courses, for many months or years, of antibiotics such as cotrimoxazole or nitrofurantoin are often necessary. The dosage of cotrimoxazole is reduced to the minimum which controls the symptoms and also suppresses the infection during treatment. There is a high success rate with long-term low-dose cotrimoxazole prophylactic (against re-infection) or suppressive (against relapse) therapy and this is particularly valuable in children. Recently trimethoprim alone has also proved effective for the long-term prophylaxis of urinary tract infections.

PREVENTION OF URINARY TRACT INFECTIONS

Prevention of Urinary Tract Infections in Sexually Active Women

In a substantial minority of women there is a suggestive association between sexual intercourse and the onset of urinary tract infections. When this history is obtained, advice about micturating immediately after intercourse is advised. In a few selected cases, it might be advisable also to take a prophylactic tablet of nitrofurantoin.

Cross-infection and Prevention of Urinary Tract Infections

Many patients acquire urinary tract infections in hospital either from their own faecal flora or through various cross-infection routes from other patients or from contaminated hospital environmental sources such as contaminated urinals. The most frequent procedure associated with hospital-acquired urinary tract infection is catheterization. Many incidents of cross-infection are associated with contamination of nurses' hands by organisms, such as *Klebsiella*, and spread of infection between patients who have indwelling catheters. The overuse of broadspectrum antibiotics in recent years in hospitals has been associated with outbreaks of infection due to multiple antibiotic-resistant strains of Gram-negative bacilli which carry R factors for antibiotic resistance. Of particular concern is the recent increase of outbreaks of infection due to gentamicin-resistant strains of *Klebsiella* in catheterized patients.

Prevention of catheter-associated infection depends on:

a. Aseptic catheter techniques.
b. Antiseptic lubricant containing chlorhexidine and local instillation of 1% chlorhexidine into the bladder.
c. Closed drainage catheter technique.
d. Excellent hand washing techniques, using chlorhexidine detergent and good drying of hands.
e. Use of gloves and isolation of patients with infections due to multiple antibiotic-resistant strains.

Some patients will acquire urinary tract infections in spite of these measures when there is prolonged indwelling catheterization. Every effort should be taken to remove a catheter as early as possible in each patient.

Catheter-associated and other hospital-acquired urinary tract infections are further discussed in Chapter 24 (*see also* Kunin, 1979).

Further Reading

Asscher A. W. (1975) Urinary tract infection in women In: Jones N. F. (ed.) *Recent Advances in Renal Disease.* London, Churchill Livingstone.

Asscher A. W. (ed) (1980) *The Management of Urinary Tract Infection, an International Symposium.* Oxford, The Medicine Publishing Foundation.

Brumfitt W., Percival A. and Williams J. D. (1975) Estimation of bacteria and white cells in the urine. *Association of Clinical Pathologists Broadsheet No. 80.*

Garrod L. P., Lambert H. P. and O'Grady F. (1981) *Antibiotics and Chemotherapy,* 5th ed. London, Churchill Livingstone.

Grob P. (1978) Urinary tract infection in general practice. Practical problems. *The Practitioner* **221**, 237–241.

Kunin C. M. (1979) *Detection, Prevention and Management of Urinary Tract Infections.* Philadelphia, Lea and Febiger.

Leading Article (1981) Acute urethral syndrome in women. *Br. Med. J.* **282**, 3.

Medical Research Council Report (1979) Recommended terminology of urinary tract infection. *Br. Med. J.* **278**, 717–719.

Smellie J. M., Grüneberg R. N., Leakey A. et al. (1976) Long term low dose cotrimoxazole in prophylaxis of childhood urinary tract infection. *Br. Med. J.* **2**, 203–206.

(*See also* Further reading on Catheter-associated urinary tract infections, in Chapter 24.)

Chapter 20

Sexually transmitted diseases

CAUSATIVE ORGANISMS

Bacteria, chlamydiae, mycoplasma, viruses, fungi, protozoa and arthropods may cause sexually transmitted diseases (*Table 20.1*).

INCIDENCE OF SOME SEXUALLY TRANSMITTED DISEASES

The incidence of both gonorrhoea and non-specific urethritis has increased dramatically during the last two decades in many countries in the Western

Table 20.1. Causative organisms of sexually transmitted disease

Organism	*Associated disease or syndrome*
1. *Bacteria*	
Treponema pallidum	Syphilis
Neisseria gonorrhoeae	Gonorrhoea
Donovania granulomatis	Granuloma inguinale
Haemophilus ducreyi	Chancroid
Gardnerella vaginalis	Gardnerella vaginitis ('non-specific' vaginitis)
2. *Chlamydiae*	
Chlamydia trachomatis	Non-specific urethritis (NSU)
Chlamydia A	Lymphogranuloma venereum (LGV)
3. *Mycoplasma*	
Mycoplasma urealyticum (T-strains)	? non-specific urethritis
4. *Viruses*	
Herpes simplex (type II and type I)	Genital herpes
Papova	Genital warts
Pox virus of Molluscum contagiosum	Molluscum contagiosum
Hepatitis B	HBsAg +ve hepatitis
5. *Fungi*	
Candida albicans	Vaginal thrush, balanitis
6. *Protozoa*	
Trichomonas vaginalis	Trichomonas vaginitis, urethritis, balanoposthitis
7. *Arthropods*	
Sarcoptes scabei	Genital scabies
Phthirus pubis	Pediculosis pubis

Hemisphere, Africa and Asia. During the last few years, the incidence of gonorrhoea in England and Wales has been approximately 70 000 new cases each year. The incidence of non-specific urethritis is continuing to increase greatly each year and in England and Wales there are over 80 000 new cases diagnosed each year.

Genital herpes has become increasingly recognized during the last 15 years and is now a common sexually transmitted disease amongst young adults with several thousand new cases diagnosed each year in England and Wales.

Syphilis is fortunately uncommon in Britain today with only about 3000 new cases diagnosed each year in England and Wales. The majority of cases occur amongst promiscuous homosexuals. New cases of late syphilis are very rare.

Granuloma inguinale, chancroid and lymphogranuloma venereum are exceedingly rare in Britain—these diseases occur mainly in the tropics.

BACTERIAL INFECTIONS

Syphilis

Syphilis is still an important disease which is most often recognized in homosexuals in Britain today.

Organism

Treponema pallidum. This spirochaete has 6–14 fine spirals, is the length of a red blood cell, has a characteristic motility, cannot be cultured in vitro and requires special stains (silver, immunofluorescent) or dark-ground illumination microscopy to visualize it. The organism can be cultivated in testes of immunosuppressed rabbits.

Incubation period

Ten to ninety days, but usually about 3 weeks.

Stages of untreated disease

Primary stage

A primary chancre develops on the genitalia or peri-anal or rectal sites. Rarely it may occur at other extra-genital sites. At first the chancre is a papule but this breaks down to form an indurated painless ulcer ('hard' chancre). The chancre may be evident for up to about 6 weeks. Regional lymph nodes become enlarged.

Secondary stage

Occurs 6–8 weeks after the primary stage. Generalized symptoms of an infection including malaise, fever, headache and sore throat may be present. Characteristically a widespread, non-itchy maculo-papular rash occurs and there is often generalized lymphadenopathy. Some patients develop mucosal ulcers in the mouth which may be serpigenous—'snail-track ulcer'.

Condylomata lata, exuberant warty-like lesions, may occur in moist warm sites such as the peri-anal regions, the vulvae or scrotum.

A few patients may develop patchy alopecia, iritis or evidence of infection in the central nervous system.

The patient is potentially infectious during the primary and secondary stages.

Latent stage

When the features of secondary syphilis have gradually resolved, the patient may appear clinically well but continues to have a syphilitic infection which is 'controlled' by immunological factors.

Some patients may have latent syphilis for 3–30 years before tertiary syphilis becomes evident. Other cases may never develop any of the late complications of syphilis.

Late syphilis stages

a. TERTIARY SYPHILIS

The first complications of late syphilis, occurring 3–30 years or more after the original infection, usually involve one or more of the following sites:

Skin, subcutaneous tissues
Mucous membranes of the upper respiratory tract
Bones—especially affecting subperiosteal sites of long bones
Joints—Charcot's joints

The lesion at these sites is characteristically a gumma which may be single or else many gummatous lesions may occur together. The gumma varies greatly in size and consists of a granuloma with ultimately 'ghost cell necrosis'.

A 'gummatous' skin ulcer characteristically has a 'wash-leather base'.

b. QUATERNARY SYPHILIS

May occur 5–30 years after the original infection. Serious complications affecting the cardiovascular system or the central nervous system (CNS) may occur with or without the above features of tertiary syphilis. These serious complications are more common in men than women. Occasionally cardiovascular system or CNS late syphilis has been referred to as quaternary syphilis as the lesions may appear after those outlined in (*a*) above.

Cardiovascular syphilitic complications include:

Aortic valve incompetence
Ascending aortitis and coronary ostial stenosis
Aortic aneurysm
} may lead to a fatal outcome

CNS syphilitic complications include:

Asymptomatic neurosyphilis—CSF syphilis tests, positive, clinically normal—may progress to the other types
Meningovascular syphilis (low grade meningitis)
Tabes dorsalis (Argyll-Robertson pupils, lightning pains, paraesthesia—posterior columns of spinal cord affected)
General paralysis of the insane (GPI) (cerebral cortex affected)

New cases of late syphilis only rarely occur in Britain today as syphilis is much less common in the penicillin era and every attempt is made to recognize and treat the disease in the early stages.

Congenital syphilis

Since the advent of routine ante-natal serological screening for syphilis this disease has become extremely rare (*see* Congenital syphilis, in Chapter 7).

Microbiological investigations for suspected syphilis

Serological tests for syphilis

At every stage of suspected syphilis serological investigations for syphilis are used for diagnosis and they are also used for monitoring treatment. There are two main groups of tests:

1. Cardiolipin (or reagin) antibody tests which are relatively non-specific.
2. Treponemal antibody tests which specifically indicate the presence of spirochaetal antibodies.

   One cardiolipin and one treponemal test should always be used for the initial serological investigation of syphilis (e.g. VDRL and TPHA, *see below*).

CARDIOLIPIN ANTIBODY TESTS

The *Wassermann Reaction* (WR) depended on a mixture of cardiolipin, lecithin and cholesterol as a lipoidal antigen for this complement fixation test which was used for many years for the diagnosis of syphilis. The *Kahn test* was a flocculation test using lipoidal antigen. These tests have largely become superseded by other cardiolipin flocculation antibody tests which include:

Venereal Disease Reference Laboratory (VDRL) Slide Test
Rapid Plasma Reagin (RPR) Test

These cardiolipin antibody tests are positive in the serum of the great majority of untreated secondary, latent and tertiary syphilis cases. They are sometimes falsely positive (*see* Biological false positive reactions *below*).

During the successful treatment of early active syphilis, the cardiolipin antibody test titres fall and the test gradually becomes negative, thus making the tests particularly useful for monitoring treatment.

TREPONEMAL ANTIBODY TESTS

Treponemal antigens are used for these tests which are generally more specific and more sensitive than cardiolipin antibody tests for detecting syphilis. These tests include:

a. *Reiter Protein Complement Fixation Test (RPCFT)*
   This test uses an antigen from culturable Reiter treponemes and detects 'group' specific treponemal antibodies. Rarely false positives may occur as this test is not as specific as tests (*b*), (*c*) and (*d*) below which use *Tr. pallidum* antigens.

b. Treponema pallidum Haemagglutination Test (TPHA)
In this test the antigens of *Tr. pallidum* are attached to tanned red cells which are agglutinated by treponemal antibodies in the serum. It is almost as sensitive as the fluorescent antibody test (*c*), mentioned below. This test has now largely superseded the RPCFT and is used as the main treponemal antibody screening test by many laboratories.

c. Fluorescent Treponemal Antibody Test–Absorbed (FTA–Abs)
Indirect immunofluorescent antibody test using killed whole *Tr. pallidum* spirochaetes as the antigen (*see Table 20.2*). This test is more specific still than the other *Treponema pallidum* antibody test (*b*) above and is mainly used as a 'verification test' in selected cases. The FTA–Abs test is nearly always positive in cases of current (except in the very early primary stage) old or treated syphilis.

Table 20.2. Principle of serum fluorescent treponemal antibody test–absorbed (FTA–Abs)

1. Patient's serum first reacted with 'sorbent' to absorb out non-specific group treponemal antibodies while leaving unabsorbed any specific antibodies present against *Tr. pallidum*.
2. Absorbed patient's serum applied to slide covered with killed *Tr. pallidum* suspension as the antigen.
3. Fluorescein conjugated anti-human immunoglobulin serum applied to slide in the final stages of this indirect fluorescent antibody test.
4. Slides examined under ultraviolet microscope fitted with dark-ground condenser:

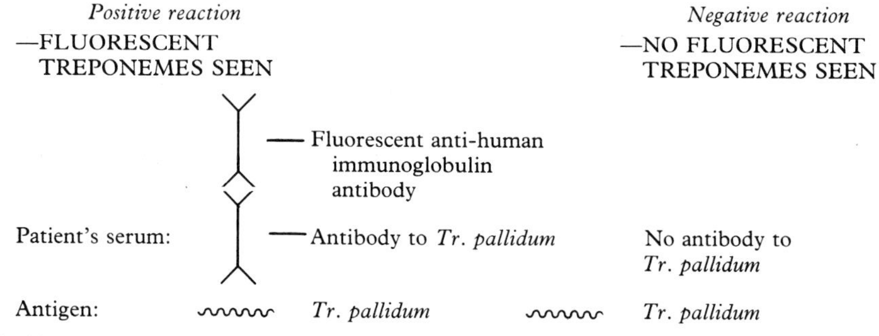

5. Positive reaction expected in nearly all patients with treponemal infections—syphilis, yaws and pinta.

d. Treponema pallidum Immobilization Test (TPI)
Live motile *Tr. pallidum* becomes immobile by the action of treponemal antibody—this test is extremely specific, in the absence of antibiotics, but is rarely necessary since the advent of the highly specific FTA–Abs test. It is a dangerous test to perform and is available only at a reference centre.

Interpretation of results

See Table 20.3.

Table 20.3. Interpretation of some results of serological tests for syphilis

Cardiolipin test *VDRL*	*Treponemal test* *TPHA*	*Interpretation*
+	+	Almost certainly indicates treponemal infection (syphilis or yaws)—other tests rarely necessary
+	–	Probably indicates a biological false positive reaction—verification treponemal test indicated (e.g. FTA–Abs)
–	+	Probably indicates treated or old treponemal infection—verification test (FTA–Abs) necessary. False positive TPHA in $<2\%$ cases (FTA–Abs will be negative)
–	–	Syphilis unlikely (do FTA if this is suspected). Rarely—late syphilis (FTA). Occasionally—early primary syphilis

Investigations for each suspected stage of syphilis

Primary stage

A. DARK-GROUND AND IMMUNOFLUORESCENT MICROSCOPY OF EXUDATE FROM A CHANCRE

Any suspected penile or female genital syphilitic lesion should be squeezed using the gloved hand, to obtain serous exudate. A drop of exudate is examined under dark-ground microscopy to look for spirochaetes with the characteristic appearance and motility of *Treponema pallidum*. Scanty spirochaetes in late lesions may also be examined by direct immunofluorescent microscopy using fluorescein-tagged antibodies to *Tr. pallidum*.

Microscopy is of greater importance than serology for the diagnosis of primary syphilis.

B. SEROLOGY

Cardiolipin (reagin) antibodies may be negative in early primary syphilis. The fluorescent treponemal antibody (FTA) test may be positive (*see Table 20.4*).

Secondary stage

A. DARK-GROUND AND IMMUNOFLUORESCENT MICROSCOPY

Exudate from skin lesions, mucous ulcers or condylomata lata should be examined for the presence of *Treponema pallidum* in a similar way to that described above from the diagnosis of primary syphilis.

B. SEROLOGY

Both groups of antibody tests, cardiolipin and treponemal, usually show strongly positive results in secondary syphilis (*see Table 20.4*).

Table 20.4. Characteristic results of serological tests for syphilis

Clinical condition	*Sample*	*Test* — *VDRL* (cardiolipin antigen)	*TPHA* (treponemal antigen)	*FTA–Abs*
1. *Early syphilis*:				
Primary syphilis	Serum	− or +	− or +	+ usually
Secondary syphilis	Serum	+ (strongly)	+	+
2. *Latent syphilis*	Serum	+ usually	+	+
3. *Late syphilis*	Serum	− or +	+	+
4. *Neurosyphilis*	CSF	+ usually	+	+
5. *Recently treated syphilis*	Serum	− or + (weakly)	+	+

Latent syphilis

SERUM SAMPLES

Serological tests for syphilis are characteristically positive although the patient appears well.

CSF

It may be necessary to perform a lumbar puncture on some patients who may have had latent syphilis for a long time to see if there is any evidence of asymptomatic neurosyphilis in which case the FTA and possibly other tests would be positive in the CSF.

Late syphilis

SERUM SAMPLES

Serological tests for syphilis are nearly always positive. The cardiolipin antibody tests may be negative in patients with old syphilis or partially treated syphilis, while the treponemal antibody tests are positive (*see Table 20.4*).

CSF

The cardiolipin and treponemal antibody tests for syphilis are usually both positive in the CSF in patients with active neurosyphilis, although some patients may only have treponemal antibody tests positive.

Congenital syphilis

Microscopy of exudate for *Treponema pallidum* from congenital mucosal lesions and syphilis serology are used for the microbiological diagnosis of congenital syphilis. Characteristically the affected infant's serum will show a high IgM FTA+ titre (*see* Chapter 7).

Recurrent syphilis

Certain promiscuous homosexual patients may suffer many repeated attacks of syphilis and their serum always show positive treponemal antibody test results. Clinically it may be difficult to differentiate a new infection from a previous one. A high titre of cardiolipin antibody, e.g. VDRL strongly positive, would indicate a recent infection which needs fresh treatment. Also a positive IgM FTA may also suggest recent treponemal infection.

Biological false positive (BFP) reactions

BFP: no clinical evidence of syphilis and treponemal antibody tests are negative.

Clerical and laboratory errors should first be excluded and repeat serum samples are usually indicated.

A 'false' positive cardiolipin antibody test (VDRL pos and Treponemal test neg.) may be present for up to 6 months—an acute BFP—or for more than 6 months—a chronic BFP.

Acute BFP causes include:

Recent immunization, e.g. smallpox vaccination
Pneumonitis—bacterial or viral pneumonia
Malaria attack

Chronic BFP causes include:

Autoimmune disease	Associated with raised IgM antibody sometimes
	SLE—in presymptomatic stage sometimes and other collagen diseases
	Acquired haemolytic anaemia
Chronic infection	Leprosy especially
Drug addiction	

Treatment of syphilis

Primary, secondary or latent syphilis

Procaine pencillin, 600 000 units, intra-muscularly daily for 10 days. If penicillin allergy present, tetracycline or erythromycin can be given instead, 500 mg 6-hourly orally for 2 weeks. The results of treatment are not as good as with penicillin.

Follow-up with regular clinical and serological examinations are necessary for at least 2 years. In the majority of cases the cardiolipin antibody tests become negative or only weakly positive (*see Table 20.4*), although in some cases the treponemal antibody tests may remain positive for many years. Adequate treatment and follow up is essential to avoid the serious complications of late syphilis.

Jarisch–Herxheimer reaction

Many patients with active syphilis develop a transient acute worsening in their general condition shortly after the start of penicillin treatment, the Herxheimer reaction, probably resulting from an inflammatory response due to the increased release of treponemal antigens from antibiotic-damaged spirochaetes. Local lesions may also become temporarily more inflamed during this reaction and this may be particularly important during the start of treatment of cardiovascular or neurosyphilis. In the latter situations, it may be desirable to reduce the effects of this reaction by covering the start of treatment with steroids.

Cardiovascular and neurosyphilis

Procaine penicillin, 600 000 units, intra-muscularly, daily for 21 days. Care is necessary to reduce the risk of complications from a Herxheimer reaction at the start of treatment (*see above*).

The treatment may stop further damage to cardiovascular or central nervous system tissues from the spirochaetes. However, the previous tissue damage and its effects will remain and may still get worse. In many cases of advanced cardiovascular syphilis or tabes dorsalis the prognosis is poor in spite of adequate penicillin treatment.

Control of syphilis

Contact tracing is essential. Health education programmes.

Yaws and pinta

Yaws due to *Treponema pertenue* and pinta due to *Treponema carateum* are non-venereal treponemal diseases (*see* Chapters 16 and 17). The serological tests for syphilis give similar results in these diseases as for syphilis and there are no satisfactory tests to distinguish serologically between these different treponemal infections.

Patients from Jamaica especially may have a positive FTA–Abs test which can be due to a previous yaws infection acquired in childhood in Jamaica.

Gonorrhoea

Organism

Neisseria gonorrhoeae, Gram-negative intracellular diplococcus. Pili of the organism probably a virulence factor, helping the coccus to become attached to mucosal surfaces.

Incubation period

Usually about 2 days, but can be 1–10 days. The great majority of male cases with gonorrhoea have symptoms of infection, but most of the female cases are asymptomatic. Females constitute the main 'reservoir' of the disease.

Clinical features and complications in the male

a. Urethritis—the gonococcus causes an acute anterior urethritis in men which results in an obvious purulent urethral discharge and dysuria in most cases.

b. Rectal gonorrhoea occurs particularly in homosexuals and symptoms of a discharge or tenesmus may be present. Many patients have no symptoms but some proctitis may be evident during proctoscopy.

c. Pharyngeal gonorrhoea is increasingly recognized amongst those participating in oral-genital sexual practices and is often asymptomatic or else a sore throat may be present. Pharyngitis or tonsillitis is sometimes seen on examination.

Other sites in the male urogenital tract may also occasionally become infected causing possible complications:

i. *Posterior urethritis* may occur at the same time as anterior urethritis and in a few cases which are not promptly treated chronic posterior urethritis resulting in a urethral stricture might occur.
ii. *Prostatitis* which can become chronic may occur causing an intermittent low backache and occasional urethral discharge.
iii. *Acute epididymo-orchitis.*
iv. *Bacteraemia—skin and joint infection.* A few patients may develop bacteraemic complications including gonococcal arthritis (*see* Chapters 16 and 17).

Clinical features and complications in the female

a. Asymptomatic cases of gonorrhoea most often occur in spite of active gonococcal infection of the endocervix in nearly all cases. Other sites that are asymptomatically infected in most females with gonorrhoea are the urethra and rectum. These patients are seen mainly because of a history of possible contact with a man with gonorrhoea.

b. Vaginal discharge or dysuria may be present in a small number of patients with gonorrhoea. These symptoms are much more often due to non-gonococcal causes.

c. Symptomatic rectal or pharyngeal gonorrhoea occasionally occurs but is less frequent in women than in male homosexuals. Proctitis is clinically more likely to occur following anal intercourse.

Other sites may also become infected causing possible complications:

i. *Bartholinitis*—following infection of one or both Bartholin's glands.
ii. *Pelvic inflammatory diseases* may occur after the gonococcus has ascended up the female genital tract from the infected endocervix to affect the salpinges. Clinically the patient may present with acute abdominal pain, fever and severe constitutional upset. Urgent surgery is sometimes required. In some patients the infection may spread to involve pelvic peritoneum and the ovaries, and cause severe widespread inflammation of the pelvic tissues.

   The long term sequelae of pelvic inflammatory disease include extensive fibrosis which distorts the salpinges and uterus so that infertility or ectopic pregnancy may eventually result.
iii. *Bacteraemia* may occur at the same time as pelvic inflammatory disease or in association with chronic infection and skin manifestations (*see* Chapter 16).
iv. *Arthritis* can occasionally complicate bacteraemia. (*See* Chapter 17.)
v. *Ophthalmia neonatorum* may occur in a 1–2-day-old neonate born to a mother who has gonorrhoea.

Childhood gonococcal vulvo-vaginitis

Gonococcal inflammation of the vulvae and vagina may occur in young female infants who have close contact with an adult with gonorrhoea. Sexual assault may need to be ruled out. The usual means of acquiring the infection is by poor hygiene because of contact between the child's genitalia and the contaminated hands of an adult with gonorrhoea or contaminated towels or bedclothes.

Microbiological investigations

Investigation of the male patient

Gram-stains of smears of material collected from the urethral discharge usually shows numerous Gram-negative intracellular diplococci in pus cells. In this situation, an immediate presumptive diagnosis of gonorrhoea can be made but confirmation of the diagnosis must await the results of culture.

CULTURE OF URETHRAL DISCHARGE

Direct culture of the urethral discharge material in the clinic, on to gonococcal selective medium, gives the best results. The selective medium generally used is a VCT (vancomycin, colistin and trimethoprim medium) lysed blood agar. The inoculated plates are incubated in moist conditions in an incubator with added CO_2.

Alternatively a charcoal-coated swab is inserted into the anterior urethra and broken off into Stuart's transport medium for transport to the laboratory. Unless a suitable transport medium is used the gonococci rapidly die on the swab.

The culture is confirmed as gonococcal by sugar fermentation tests and specific fluorescent antibody tests.

CULTURE OF PHARYNGEAL OR RECTAL SITES

In selected cases who have recently practised oral sex or homosexuality, or where there is evidence of inflammation present, swabs of the pharynx or rectum should also be cultured for gonococci using direct selective media or Stuart's transport medium.

BLOOD CULTURES

Blood cultures should be collected, as well as urethral cultures, from suspected cases of gonococcal epididymo-orchitis or skin or joint infections.

ANTIBIOTIC SENSITIVITIES

The sensitivity to penicillin of gonococci isolated is determined using a '3 disc test'. The MIC to penicillin is determined on selected strains showing reduced zones and β-lactamase tested for also in these strains.

Investigation of the female patient

Smears of the cervical, urethral or rectal sites for Gram-staining are not generally worthwhile. *Cervical, urethral and rectal site* swabs (or loopfuls of exudate from the endocervix) for culture are always necessary and should be collected under direct visualization by using a speculum. Culture of the urethral as well as cervical sites is the minimum routine requirement but the highest yield of positive gonococcal cultures is obtained when the rectal site is also cultured. Swabs of the rectum are positive for gonococci in between 40 and 60% of patients with gonorrhoea.

CULTURE OF THE PHARYNX

This is indicated in patients who have practised oral sex and who have a sore throat or signs of pharyngitis or tonsillitis.

MICROSCOPY AND CULTURE OF PUS

When a Bartholin's gland abscess is drained or a patient with an acute abdomen is found to have pelvic inflammatory disease and has pus collected at operation, the pus is cultured immediately for gonococci on selective media and chocolate agar.

BLOOD CULTURES

Blood should be cultured from all patients with possible pelvic inflammatory disease or arthritis or possible skin manifestations of disseminated gonococcal disease.

SEROLOGY

The Gonococcal Complement Fixation Test (GCFT) is associated with so many false negative results that it is of little routine value. Also a positive test can result from a previous attack of gonorrhoea.

Other simultaneous investigations for candida, trichomonas and syphilis infections

In a woman a high vaginal swab (HVS) for candida and trichomonas investigation is usually generally desirable (*see below*).

In all patients, a serum sample should be collected for syphilis serological tests in case there is also incubating early syphilis, before penicillin treatment is given which may otherwise mask syphilis. A further serum sample, 3 months later, is also desirable for syphilis serology.

Antimicrobial treatment of gonorrhoea

Gonococcal strains have gradually shown a slight reduction in penicillin sensitivity over the last 20 years but the overwhelming majority of uncomplicated infections in Britain can still be effectively treated by a single intramuscular injection of 1·2MU of procaine penicillin when given in conjunction with 2 g oral probenecid to delay excretion of the drug. For infections due to non-β-lactamase-producing penicillin 'resistant' organisms an injection of 4·8 MU procaine penicillin combined with 5 MU benzylpenicillin, divided between two sites, and given with 1 g oral probenecid is an effective treatment.

An effective alternative single oral dose treatment consists of 2 g ampicillin given with 1 g probenecid. The highest cure rates with uncomplicated infections are achieved with a single oral dose of 3 g amoxycillin. In complicated severe gonococcal infections, such as gonococcal pelvic inflammatory disease, a course of high dose penicillin injections is usually desirable. Alternatively a 10-day course of ampicillin 500 mg 6-hourly following the loading dose of 2 g ampicillin given with 1 g probenecid.

Infections due to β-lactamase-producing gonococci are usually treated effectively by spectinomycin, 4 g, intra-muscular injection (once only). (Most of the infections due to penicillinase-producing strains of gonococci have been imported into Britain from the Far East, Middle East or Africa.)

Patients who are allergic to penicillin can be treated by cotrimoxazole, 4 tablets b.d. for 2 days, or by spectinomycin.

Follow-up treatment

This is desirable in all patients but particularly necessary in female patients since gonococcal infection is more difficult to eradicate from women than men.

The patients should be seen 1–2 days after treatment and twice during the next 2 weeks. Repeat cultures are arranged, particularly if there is any discharge. Evidence of urethritis should also be looked for by the two glass urine test; when mucous strands or pus cells are seen in the first glass but not in the second glass the persistence of anterior urethritis is suspected.

Contact tracing

Efficient contact tracing, with the help of trained social workers, is essential for the adequate control of the spread of the disease.

Prophylaxis

High-risk groups of men, such as those in the armed services visiting foreign countries, can be given some protection against contracting the disease if sheaths are worn. The use of certain antibiotics has also had some success prophylactically, but there is no generally agreed prophylactic regimen which will prevent the acquisition of both gonorrhoea and syphilis.

Granuloma Inguinale

Granuloma inguinale occurs mainly as an uncommon sexually transmitted disease in the tropics and is characterized by the development of papules on the genitalia or groins. These papules subsequently form large ulcers and these become secondarily infected. The causative organism is *Donovania granulomatis*.

Diagnosis is made by biopsy of the lesion and seeing intracellular capsulated short bacilli (Donovan bodies) in macrophages.

Treatment with tetracycline, 500 mg four times a day for 2–3 weeks, may be effective.

Chancroid

The causative organism is *Haemophilus ducreyi*. Chancroid occurs in tropical countries as a sexually transmitted disease where the 'soft chancre' is the typical lesion which may occur singly or as multiple papules on the genitalia. These papules ulcerate but are different from the syphilitic 'hard chancre' as there is a lack of induration.

The inguinal lymph nodes become enlarged and may break down to form an abscess. Subsequently discharging sinuses may develop in the groin.

A microbial diagnosis is sometimes difficult but can be attempted by taking scrapings of the lesion and looking for the short Gram-negative bacilli in smears. Culture of the *Haemophilus ducreyi* organisms is occasionally successful using media containing defibrinated rabbit blood.

Treatment, with tetracycline, is similar to that outlined for treating granuloma inguinale.

Gardnerella vaginalis Infection

Gardnerella vaginalis (otherwise known as *Corynebacterium vaginale* or *Haemophilus vaginalis*) has been implicated as a possible cause of non-specific vaginitis and is thought to be a sexually transmissible organism. Characteristically, the patient has a malodorous thin vaginal discharge. It has been suggested that the symptoms are produced by the combined activity of *Gardnerella vaginalis* together with anaerobic organisms. Treatment with metronidazole, 400–500 mg twice daily for a week, preferably for both partners, appears to be effective.

LYMPHOGRANULOMA VENEREUM (LGV)

This disease, like granuloma inguinale and chancroid, mainly occurs in tropical countries. However, the two latter diseases are caused by bacteria and LGV is caused by a group A chlamydia organism.

The initial genital lesion is usually a small ulcer that passes unnoticed and the patient may present with painful enlarged inguinal lymph nodes. These nodes may become involved in multiple abscess formation. Sometimes the overlying skin is discoloured. Eventually the abscess may rupture to discharge thick pus and the infection can spread to the genitalia to cause extensive ulceration or to the pelvic tissues to cause rectal stricture.

The diagnosis is confirmed either serologically, by finding raised antibodies against chlamydiae in the serum LGV complement fixation test, or by observing a positive intradermal skin tests using Frei's lymphogranuloma venereum antigen. A positive Frei test does not necessarily indicate current or recent infection, since it may remain positive for years after the original infection.

The antimicrobial treatment usually recommended is tetracycline, given in a similar regimen as that suggested for treating granuloma inguinale.

NON-SPECIFIC URETHRITIS

Non-specific urethritis is now the commonest sexually transmitted disease in Britain. It is also known as 'non-gonococcal urethritis' (NGU).

Most male patients with urethritis due to the gonococcus alone have a urethral discharge containing thick creamy pus whereas the majority of men with 'non-specific urethritis' (NSU) where no gonococcal cause can be found, have a thinner, more mucoid purulent urethral discharge. However in an individual male patient it is clinically impossible to distinguish between gonorrhoea and NSU. Also some patients may suffer from a simultaneous mixed infection due to the gonococcus and one of the causes of NSU, characteristically *Chlamydia trachomatis*. This double infection sometimes becomes apparent after a male patient apparently relapses with post-gonococcal urethritis, following the successful penicillin treatment of gonorrhoea and is found to have persistent chlamydial infection. The chlamydial urethritis does not respond to penicillin therapy.

Female patients with 'NSU' usually have no symptoms but may have either urethritis or, much more frequently, cervicitis. The cervicitis may be accompanied by a vaginal discharge but usually is only apparent during direct examination of a female contact of a male case of NSU.

Causative Organisms of NSU

Possible causes of NSU include:

a. *Chlamydia trachomatis*
b. *Ureaplasma urealyticum* ('T' strains of *Mycoplasma*)
c. *Trichomonas vaginalis*
d. Secondary bacterial infective causes, such as coliforms, group B streptococci, anaerobes, *Gardnerella vaginalis* and yeasts possibly following trauma to the genitalia.

Chlamydia trachomatis is almost certainly the predominant cause of 'NSU' infections; this organism can be seen on microscopy or isolated from 30 to 60% of patients with NSU. The organism multiplies intracellularly in epithelial cells to cause characteristic large intracytoplasmic inclusions which stain with iodine stains or by a specific fluorescent antibody technique. The incubation period of chlamydial urethritis is usually 1–3 weeks. *Chlamydia* often causes chronic infection and recurrent clinical attacks of urethritis.

T strains of Mycoplasma are found in the genital tract of a high proportion of sexually active individuals without any clinical evidence of infection. However, these *Mycoplasma* strains have occasionally undoubtedly caused clinically evident urethritis and they are probably responsible for a minority of 'NSU' infections.

Trichomonas vaginalis occasionally colonizes the male urethra without symptoms or else causes urethritis in a few patients.

The role of other organisms in 'NSU' is largely speculative.

Complications of NSU due to Chlamydia trachomatis

The possible complications of chlamydia genital tract infections include:

a. Pelvic inflammatory disease.
b. Trachoma inclusion conjunctivitis (TRIC)
c. Prostatitis or epididymitis; Bartholinitis
d. Reiter's syndrome

Pelvic inflammatory disease is frequently due to chlamydial infection ascending from the cervix to affect the salpinges and pelvic tissues. There may be long-term complications of infertility and other gynaecological disorders, as with fibrotic damage due to gonococcal pelvic inflammatory disease.

Chlamydial cervicitis in a mother may result in a neonate acquiring a TRIC eye infection during birth. A purulent discharge of the eye, accompanied by a follicular conjunctivitis, may start between the second and fifth day of life (*see* Chapter 11).

Prostatitis or epididymitis in a young person where no gonococcal cause is found is often due to *Chlamydia* following an attack of NSU. In the female, Bartholinitis may occasionally be caused by *Chlamydia*.

Reiter's Syndrome may complicate NSU in up to 5% of patients and possible symptoms include arthritis, conjunctivitis, uveitis, pustular hyperkeratosis of the skin on the feet (keratodermia blenorrhagica) and circinate balanitis. This complication is much more likely to occur in individuals who have the HLAB-27 histocompatibility antigen—80% of patients with Reiter's syndrome have this antigen.

Microbiological Investigations of NSU

The two glass urine tests will show some mucous threads and leucocytes in the first urine sample.

In every patient the investigations for gonococci, previously described, are essential and investigations for *Trichomonas* are also necessary. An incidental but necessary investigation is syphilis serology in case coincidental syphilis is present.

Specific chlamydial or mycoplasma investigations are not routinely available and the possible presence of these agents must be presumed when gonococcal investigations are negative.

In a few institutions with special facilities, urethral or cervical scrapings can be collected for microscopy onto glass slides. For culture of urethral or cervical material it is necessary to use appropriate buffered transport media which lack any antibiotics (even penicillin may inhibit the organism in vitro) which may cause false negatives. The chlamydia organism can be relatively easily cultured using irradiated McCoy tissue culture cells or certain lines of HeLa cells.

Antimicrobial Treatment of NSU

Treatment started early in the disease is more likely to be successful than when started many months or years after recurrent attacks of NSU. The treatment of chlamydia and mycoplasma urethritis is fortunately similar.

Tetracyclines given for 3 weeks may effectively treat the disease in about three-quarters of patients who present early. Either oxytetracycline, 250 mg q.d.s., or a long-acting tetracycline such as triple tetracycline (Deteclo), 1 tablet b.d., can be given. Abstinence from sexual intercourse during treatment is essential.

Erythromycin is an alternative to tetracycline for patients who have relapsed after tetracycline treatment or for treating a pregnant mother just before delivery to prevent chlamydial neonatal eye infection. Pelvic inflammatory disease due to *Chlamydia* can also be treated initially by intravenous erythromycin lactobionate.

Follow-up of treated cases is necessary for at least 3 months.

Contact Tracing

The sexual contacts of the patient should be investigated and female patients are usually only diagnosed by a contact history.

Prophylaxis

It is possible that the contraceptive sheath affords some protection against acquiring NSU although the degree of protection is probably less than that given against acquiring gonorrhoea.

PELVIC INFLAMMATORY DISEASE

Clinical features of pelvic inflammatory disease in a woman include lower abdominal pain, backache, malaise, dyspareunia and altered periods. The incidence of acute pelvic inflammatory disease in sexually active young women is increasing and these patients may be seriously ill on admission to hospital with acute abdominal pain. Physical signs include lower abdominal tenderness, fever, signs of peritonism, tenderness in the fornices and sometimes a tender mass can be felt *per vaginam*. Frequently surgery is necessary to differentiate the condition from acute appendicitis or to drain a tubo-ovarian abcess.

Causative Organisms

The main organisms that have been implicated in the aetiology of salpingitis, tubo-ovarian abscess and pelvic peritonitis include:

Neisseria gonorrhoeae
Chlamydia trachomatis
Coliforms and streptococci
Anaerobes—*Bacteroides* and anaerobic cocci

The gonococcus can cause pelvic inflammatory disease alone or, after an initial gonococcal cervical infection, other organisms from the lower genital tract may ascend to cause a mixed infection. The gonococcus is probably more frequently implicated in the aetiology of pelvic inflammatory disease than any other organism.

Chlamydia trachomatis may cause infection alone or mixed with the gonococcus or other organisms and is probably a frequent cause of pelvic inflammatory disease.

Many cases of pelvic inflammatory disease cannot be attributed to either the gonococcus or chlamydiae. In these cases mixtures of aerobes and anaerobes that originally ascended the genital tract from the vagina contribute to the polymicrobial aetiology of pelvic infection. Aerobic organisms would include *E. coli* or other coliforms, group B streptococci, and rarely staphylococci. Anaerobic organisms would include *Bacteroides melaninogenicum* or *Bacteroides fragilis*, fusiforms, peptococci or peptostreptococci.

Microbiological Investigations

1. Investigations for gonorrhoea including cervical, urethral and rectal cultures (*see* Gonorrhoea).

2. High vaginal swab for anaerobes and aerobes, transported in Stuart's transport medium.
3. If pus or peritoneal fluid is available at operation, this is immediately cultured for gonococci, other aerobes and anaerobes.
4. Blood cultures should always be collected.
5. Syphilis serology is always incidentally necessary.

In the U.S.A., some centres have performed culdocentesis and cultured the pelvic fluid from the pouch of Douglas aerobically and anaerobically. More relevant culture results have been claimed for this technique than those obtained by cervical culture.

In special centres chlamydia culture of cervical or operative specimens can also be performed. Also the demonstration of a rising antibody titre against *Chlamydia trachomatis* using a micro-immunofluorescence technique may retrospectively indicate *Chlamydia* as the cause of the pelvic inflammatory disease.

Antimicrobial Treatment

As soon as the cultures have been collected, antibiotic therapy should be started usually consisting of (*a*) plus (*b*):

a. *Ampicillin*, given as a 2-g loading dose parenterally, followed by 500 mg 6-hourly parenterally at first, followed by oral administration for up to 10 days, should effectively treat most of the cases where gonococci or other aerobic bacteria or penicillin-sensitive anaerobes like anaerobic cocci are the causative organisms.

b. *Metronidazole*, 500 mg intravenously or 400 mg orally 3–4 times daily for 5–7 days should be given to treat anaerobes such as *Bacteroides* and anaerobic cocci, in addition to the ampicillin mentioned in (*a*).

c. If the patient gives a doubtful history of allergy to penicillins, *cefuroxime*, 750 mg intra-muscularly, can be given four times a day for 7–10 days instead of the ampicillin.

d. *Erythromycin* lactobionate, 600 mg intravenously g.d.s., followed by erythromycin stearate, 500 mg 6-hourly orally, can be given together with ampicillin and metronidazole if *Chlamydia* is suspected because of a contact history. In severe cases of pelvic inflammatory disease all the main causative organisms should be covered by the ampicillin plus metronidazole plus erythromycin combination.

VIRAL INFECTIONS

Genital Herpes

Genital herpes is caused by herpes simplex type II virus usually, although occasionally it can also be caused by herpes simplex type I, the type usually responsible for 'cold sores' around the mouth. The genital herpes virus probably persists in a latent form in the peripheral nerve fibres supplying the affected muco-cutaneous sites.

Clinical lesions on the genitalia first appear in a primary infection, in a more florid form than in later recurrent infections. The lesions consist of clusters of vesicles which break down to form shallow painful ulcers which often become secondarily infected. The primary infection occurs after an incubation period of

3–7 days. Constitutional upset may accompany the primary infection and the patient can be febrile and have severe malaise. The primary infection is generally more severe in females.

Recurrent crops of vesicles may appear on any part of the penis or vulvae and occasionally the urethra may be affected causing dysuria. Before the vesicles appear there is sometimes irritation lasting a day or two. Recurrent herpetic cervicitis is present in some women as a symptomless infection but occasionally severe ulcers may appear on the cervix.

Complications of herpes infection include:

a. Central nervous system—aseptic meningitis or encephalitis may rarely follow a severe primary attack of genital herpes.
b. Hepatitis—another, very rare, complication of systemic herpetic infection.
c. Neonatal disseminated herpes or herpetic encephalitis—these infections carry a high mortality and may occur when the mother has primary herpes near the time of delivery of the baby. In the latter situation, delivery of the baby by Caesarian section may be advisable as a prophylactic measure.
d. Carcinoma of the cervix—possibly—there is an association between herpes simplex type II cervicitis and carcinoma of the cervix.

Investigations

Fluid from a vesicle and material collected from the base of the ulcers are put into viral transport medium for culture of herpes simplex. (A rapid diagnosis is possible using electron microscopy, but this technique is not generally available or strictly necessary in most cases.)

The main differential diagnosis is with primary syphilis which can also occur coincidentally so that dark-ground illumination microscopy and syphilis serology, repeated 3 months later, is necessary.

Treatment

Cleanliness is essential to avoid secondary bacterial infection of the lesions. The lesions spontaneously heal in 8–15 days. For severe local lesions preferably seen at an early stage, specific anti-viral therapy may be advisable using idoxuridine in 5% dimethylsulphoxide. When there are systemic complications it may be necessary to use parenteral anti-herpes drugs, such as parenteral acycloguanosine.

Hepatitis B

HBsAg-positive hepatitis can be transmitted by both hetero- and homosexual practices but there is a particularly high risk of transmission of hepatitis B amongst homosexuals. The risk of acquiring hepatitis B is greatest in 'passive' homosexuals and in those with many sexual partners.

Serum, suitably labelled with 'hepatitis risk' labels and transported to the laboratory in a plastic bag, is collected from patients with possible symptoms of hepatitis and from close contacts of these patients. The tests indicated include

HBsAg. 'e' antigen may be looked for in HBsAg positive cases as carriage of 'e' antigen is associated with a higher infectivity. (*See* Chapter 15.)

There is no specific treatment but liver function tests are indicated in HBsAg positive cases. A referral to a physician for possible liver biopsy is occasionally necessary. When the patient is an asymptomatic HBsAg positive carrier, it is difficult to do more than monitor his close contacts. Ideally some restraint should be exercised by promiscuous homosexuals who are 'e' antigen positive to reduce the number of possible new cases of hepatitis B.

Genital Warts (Condylomata Acuminata)

Warts can appear on the vulvae, lower vagina, perianal regions and penis and be transmitted sexually. They are caused by a papovavirus and the incubation period varies between 1 and 6 months.

The diagnosis is clinical and condylomata acuminata must be differentiated from the syphilitic condylomata lata. Viral genital warts may persist for many months when untreated and can be very unsightly, particularly when they spread.

Treatment consists of keeping the affected skin areas cool and dry and local applications of podophyllin. If the lesions are extensive and resistant to treatment with podophyllin, electric cautery under anaesthesia may be required.

Molluscum Contagiosum

Small pink or white papules may appear in the genital region and be sexually transmitted. The lesions spontaneously disappear. Occasionally electrocautery may be indicated (*see* Chapter 16).

FUNGAL INFECTION

Candida Vaginitis

Candida albicans vulvo-vaginitis is very common. The yeast is often sexually transmitted and male patients may complain of balanitis (*see below*) or else have asymptomatic colonization of the penis. The organism may also cause endogenous infections which may be recurrent when it colonizes the gastro-intestinal tract. *Candida* in the faecal flora may colonize the female genital tract.

Predisposing factors

The yeast thrives in a warm moist environment and infection is more likely when there is poor hygiene in the genital areas.

Many patients have no obvious predisposing factors present but often one or more of the following additional factors are relevant:

- Diabetes mellitus
- Oral contraceptives
- Pregnancy
- Broad spectrum antibiotics
- Steroid therapy

Microbiological investigations

A vaginal swab of the white exudate on the vaginal mucosa, or a high vaginal swab, should be collected. The swab should be plated onto Sabouraud's selective medium for fungi. A smear for wet microscopy or a Gram-stain will show budding yeasts and a pseudo-mycelium in most cases of vaginal thrush. If a delay in culture is anticipated, the swab should be broken off into Stuart's transport medium for culture on Sabouraud's medium. Rectal swabs for *Candida* may be relevant in a few cases of recurrent candida vaginitis.

Antimicrobial treatment

Local anti-yeast drugs are advisable together with good hygiene. Nystatin pessaries inserted into the vagina each night for 2 weeks and nystatin cream may help to relieve symptoms. Other drugs that can be used instead of nystatin include clotrimazole, miconazole or econazole.

Recurrent attacks of candida vaginitis may be difficult to treat successfully using various local antifungal creams or pessaries gently applied to the vagina. When there is evidence of intestinal colonization with *Candida*, an oral suspension of nystatin, 500 000 units t.d.s. for 2 weeks, may be given in an attempt to reduce the chances of persistent recolonization of the genital tract from the faecal flora. Also when there is a known predisposing factor present, this may sometimes be removed, such as substitution of other methods of contraception for oral contraception. Finally, investigation and treatment of sexual partners who may be colonized or infected with *Candida* are advisable.

PROTOZOAL INFECTION

Trichomonas Vaginitis

Trichomonas vaginalis is a common cause of vaginal discharge which is typically thin, frothy and yellow in appearance with an offensive smell. Other symptoms may include vulval pruritis, dysuria and dyspareunia. Some patients have no symptoms. Occasionally the organism causes urethritis in both sexes.

On examination the mucosa of the vagina is usually reddened and abundant frothy discharge is typically evident. In severe long-standing cases, there may also be extensive genital warts present.

Microbiological investigations

Fluid should be aspirated from the posterior vaginal fornix and placed onto a slide for immediate wet microscopy. Characteristic motile, pear-shaped trichomonas organisms, larger than leucocytes, are often easily seen under the microscope in the clinic. The protozoal organism is flagellated but the flagella are not always apparent. Some fluid should also be put into a trichomonas liquid culture medium (such as Feinberg's medium).

Alternatively, and slightly less satisfactory than the above, a high vaginal swab broken off into Stuart's transport medium is sent to the laboratory for wet microscopy and culture of *Trichomonas*.

A cervical smear, stained by the Papanicoloau method, occasionally detects trichomonas genital tract infection when other methods have failed to show this.

Coincident gonococcal infection sometimes occurs with trichomonas infection and cervical and urethral swab for gonococcal culture should also be collected.

In the male patient with possible asymptomatic or symptomatic urethritis, *Trichomonas* may be difficult to detect by microscopy of a urethral swab and liquid culture of the swab in trichomonas medium is advisable.

Antimicrobial treatment

Metronidazole, 400 mg orally b.d. for 5 days, is usually very effective treatment.

Follow-up of the patient with repeat microscopy and culture for *Trichomonas* is desirable.

The sexual partner may need a simultaneous course of metronidazole treatment, especially when there is a recurrence of trichomonas vaginitis.

'Gay Bowel Syndrome'

Recently it has become recognized that enteric protozoal pathogens, such as *Giardia lamblia* and *E. histolytica*, can be sexually transmitted between male homosexual patients.

BALANITIS

Poor hygiene, diabetes mellitus or a tight prepuce predisposes to this infection of the glans penis and subpreputial space.

The main causative organisms are *Candida albicans* or, in Negroes, *Trichomonas vaginalis*, both of which may be sexually transmitted.

Investigations

Wet microscopy, Gram-stain and culture of swabs from the penis will show evidence of *Candida* or *Trichomonas* when these are the causative organisms.

Treatment

Cleaning of the lesion is always necessary.

Candida infections should be treated by nystatin cream and trichomonas infection by oral metronidazole. The sexual partner will also need specific investigation and treatment.

Correction of a tight prepuce, by circumcision, may be necessary. Strict attention to hygiene should help to prevent a relapse of infection.

ARTHROPOD INFESTATIONS

Genital Scabies

Sarcoptes scabiei, the 'itch mite', can cause generalized skin infestations, rashes or eczema (*see* Chapter 16) or it may cause more localized infestations on the genitalia. Genital scabies is usually sexually transmitted and is frequently seen in special clinics. The clinical features include itching, worse at night, with the formation of discrete erythematous papular lesions. Occasionally the mite can be

Table 20.5. Summary of the main investigations required for a new patient attending with suspected sexually transmitted disease

	Female patient	
Gonococcal cultures: When history of contact with gonorrhoea or vaginal discharge—cervical, urethral and rectal sites Pharyngeal site cultured also when history of oral sex and a sore throat or signs of pharyngeal inflammation	*Vaginal discharge*: HVS for microscopy and culture for *Candida* and *Trichomonas* *Vesicles/ulcers on genitalia or oral site* DGI microscopy for spirochaetes Herpes simplex cultures	*Always syphilis serology* (and consider repeat in 3 months)
	Male patient	
Gonococcal microscopy and cultures: When history of urethral discharge or contact history—urethral site Rectal or pharyngeal sites also cultured if relevant history or signs of inflammation	*Close contact hepatitis B*: Serum HBsAg tests *Vesicles/ulcers on penis/pharyngeal/peri-anal/rectal sites* DGI microscopy for spirochaetes Herpes simplex cultures	*Always syphilis serology* and consider repeat in 3 months

seen in a burrow or a papule in the genital region but often the diagnosis is a clinical one. A few patients may have evidence of scabies elsewhere with burrows between the fingers or toes.

Antiscabies treatment consists of whole body (below neck) applications of benzyl benzoate, 10%, or gamma-benzene hexachloride, 1%.

Pediculosis Pubis

Phthirus pubis, the 'crab louse', is a commonly seen sexually transmitted cause of infestation of the pubic hair. The patient complains of itching and on examination the eggs of the insect, called 'nits', are seen attached to pubic hairs or the crab louse is seen on the pubic skin. Occasionally other hairy sites also become affected, such as eyebrows or axillae. The itching is caused by the bites of the crab louse. The typical 'crab-like' features of the louse are easily seen under the low power lens of a microscope or under a hand lens.

Treatment to all affected hairy sites with malathion is recommended.

SUMMARY OF DIAGNOSTIC MICROBIOLOGICAL INVESTIGATIONS FOR PATIENTS ATTENDING WITH SUSPECTED SEXUALLY TRANSMITTED DISEASE

More than one sexually transmitted disease is often present in an individual patient presenting with suspected sexually transmitted disease. *Table 20.5* summarizes the main investigations that are required which include tests to detect diseases incidental to the one with which the patient presents, such as syphilis.

Further Reading

Catterall R. D. and Nicol C. J. (1976) *Sexually Transmitted Diseases*, 2nd ed. London, Academic Press.

Clay J. (1981) Non-specific vaginitis: its diagnosis and treatment. *J. Antimicrob. Chemother.* 7, 501–502.

Epidemiology (1981) Sexually transmitted disease surveillance 1979. *Br. Med. J.* **282**, 155–156.

Johnston N. A., Kolator B. and Seth A. D. (1981) A survey of lactamase-producing gonococcal isolates reported in the United Kingdom 1979–80. The present trend. *Lancet* **1**, 263–264.

King A. and Nicol C. (1975) *Venereal Diseases*, 3rd ed. London, Baillière-Tindall.

Leading Article (1980) Genital herpes. *Br. Med. J.* **1**, 1335–1336.

Leading Article (1981) Recalcitrant gonococci, plasmids and antibiotics. *Lancet* **1**, 816–817.

Lim K. S., Taan Wong V., Fulford K. W. M. et al. (1977) Role of sexual and non-sexual practices in the transmission of hepatitis B. *Br. J. Ven. Dis.* **53**, 190–192.

Morton R. J. and Harris J. R. W. (1975) *Recent Advances in Sexually Transmitted Diseases*. Edinburgh, Churchill-Livingstone.

Ridgway G. (1979) Chlamydia infection of the genital tract. In: Reeves D. S. and Geddes A. M. (ed.), *Advances in Infection*. Edinburgh, Churchill-Livingstone.

*Wisdom A. (1973) *A Colour Atlas of Venereology*. London, Wolfe Medical Books.

* Particularly recommended for further study by undergraduates.

Chapter 21

Zoonoses

DEFINITION

Zoonoses are diseases mainly of vertebrate animals that can also be transmitted to man.

In many instances the animals may not have obvious illness but may still be infective for man. Domesticated animals and pets are usually the reservoirs of disease in Britain whereas wild animals are often the main reservoirs of disease in tropical countries.

MODES OF TRANSMISSION

Once the modes of transmissions of a zoonoses are known, it becomes possible to consider preventive measures to effectively break the cycle of transmission and reduce the incidence of the disease in man. There are numerous modes of transmission (*Fig. 21.1*) which include:

1. Direct contact

The occupation of a person may result in direct contact with an infected animal or its products. A farmer or vet may acquire brucellosis by handling the infected

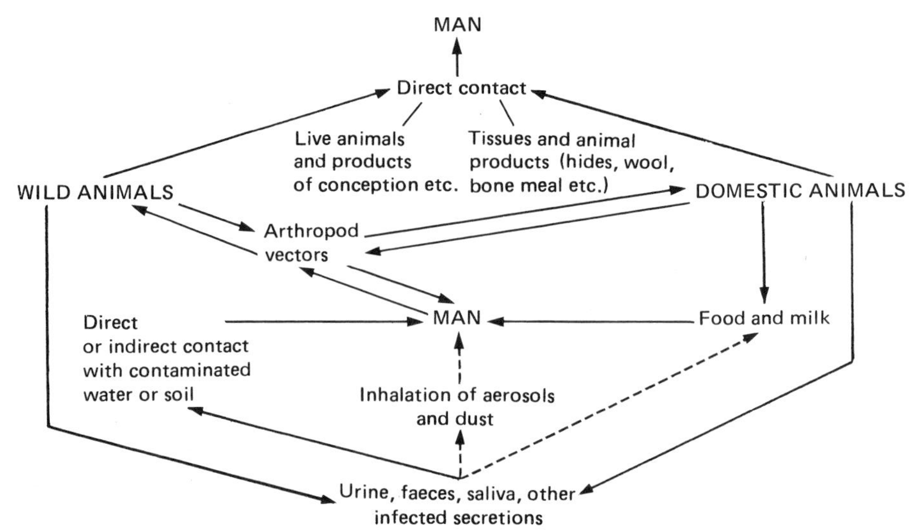

Fig. 21.1. Modes of transmission of zoonoses to man.

genital tract of a cow during calving or by touching the products of conception. A shepherd may contract orf from an infected lamb. A gardener or tannery worker could acquire anthrax from handling infected bone meal or hides, respectively. An abattoir worker could acquire Q fever or toxoplasmosis and a fish handler erysipeloid by handling infected flesh. There are scores of other examples.

2. Inhalation

Inhalation of aerosols of infected animal excreta, secretions or other products may occur as in psittacosis (droppings), Q fever (infected excreta in dust), brucellosis (infected secretions) or pulmonary anthrax (spores in wool).

3. Food and milk products

Ingestion of infected meat, fish, eggs, milk or dairy products often results in diseases of humans such as salmonellosis, campylobacter infections, brucellosis, Q fever, toxoplasmosis and trichinosis. Unpasteurized milk is the potential source of several zoonoses (*Table 21.1*).

Table 21.1. Unpasteurized milk as a source of zoonoses

Disease	*Organism*
Tuberculosis (bovine)	*Mycobacterium tuberculosis*
Brucellosis	*Brucella abortus* (cattle) *Brucella melitensis* (sheep and goats)
Salmonellosis	*Salmonella typhimurium* *Salmonella dublin* Other *Salmonella* species
Q fever	*Coxiella burnetii*
Listeriosis	*Listeria monocytogenes*
Campylobacter infections	*Campylobacter jejuni*

4. Saliva

Bites or licks from infected animals may result in transfer of the causative organism of disease from the saliva of the animal to man, as occurs in rabies, rat bite fever and *Pasteurella multocida* infections.

5. Faeces

Infected faeces from animals may contaminate foods, soil or surfaces handled by man, or be inhaled in droplet or dust form by man. As a result diseases, such as salmonellosis, hydatid, tetanus, toxocara infection, or ornithosis, may occur in man.

6. Urine

Urine from infected animals with leptospirosis may infect man directly while handling animals or indirectly while swimming in or having an occupational reason for exposure to contaminated water.

7. Blood and live tissues

Animal house attendants, zoo and laboratory workers may rarely become exposed to serious disease by direct handling or by inhaling aerosols from infected blood or tissues of monkeys. Monkeys may have several dangerous infections that can be transmitted to man, including Marburg virus disease, Herpes Simian 'B' virus disease and Yellow Fever.

8. Arthropod vectors

Scores of zoonoses may be spread to man by arthropod vectors and these are summarized below. (*See also* Chapter 22.)

BACTERIAL ZOONOSES

Tuberculosis

Bovine tuberculosis has been eradicated in Britain and other developed countries by various control measures, including the tuberculin testing of cattle, the slaughter of infected animals and the pasteurization of milk. However, the disease is still common in many underdeveloped countries throughout the world. The bovine type of *Mycobacterium tuberculosis* mainly infects the lungs of cattle but the mammary glands of cows may become infected during the chronic disease and the organism may then be present in the milk. Humans acquire the infection by drinking the infected unpasteurized milk. This may result in infection involving the cervical glands or abdomen (*see* Chapter 13).

Salmonellosis

Hundreds of different *Salmonella* species may infect the intestines of a wide range of animals including poultry, cattle, pigs, rodents and terrapins. Chickens and turkeys are particularly important reservoirs of the disease. (*See* Salmonella food poisoning, Gastro-enteritis and Septicaemia, in Chapter 14.)

Brucellosis

Causative organisms and epidemiology

The causative organisms are *Brucella abortus* from cattle, *Brucella melitensis* from goats and sheep, and *Brucella suis* from pigs. Brucellosis occurs in many European, African, Asian and American countries.

Brucella abortus causes contagious abortion in cows and the organism is spread between cattle largely by contact with infected vaginal secretions or infected semen. The organism has a particular predilection for a sugar compound, erythritol, which is present in significant concentrations in bovine but not human placenta. The brucella organisms also localize in the mammary glands of infected cows which is important in the spread of the infection to man as well as other cattle.

Man, especially farmers and vets, usually acquire *B. abortus* by direct contact with infected vaginal secretions or the infected products of conception of cattle. The other main method of acquiring the infection is by drinking unpasteurized milk from infected cows. Occasionally vets vaccinating calves with the S19 attenuated vaccine strain of *B. abortus* have accidentally inoculated themselves through the skin or conjunctiva with the vaccine and have acquired a mild form of brucellosis. Laboratory accidents have rarely occurred when microbiology staff have had contact with or inhaled the organism and then developed brucellosis. The brucella organisms can infect man through the abraded skin, conjunctival or alimentary tract mucosa or by inhalation.

Brucellosis is mainly an occupational disease of vets, farmers and abattoir workers acquired by contact with cattle or drinking raw milk. In Scotland, England and Wales, the number of human cases of brucellosis and the number of herds of cattle not accredited as brucellosis free declined greatly between 1971 and 1979. The campaign in Britain to slaughter brucella-infected cattle and to obtain the maximum number of accredited brucella-free herds has progressed well. Vaccination of calves with the S19 vaccine was used in the past but will probably become completely unnecessary. Within a short time, it is likely that few further cases of brucellosis due to *B. abortus* will be acquired in Britain.

Brucella melitensis is the cause of Mediterranean or Malta fever and is frequently present in unpasteurized milk or cheese products from goats and sheep in Mediterranean or Middle East countries. Patients either enter Britain with brucellosis due to *B. melitensis* acquired abroad or become infected by consumption of imported infected goats cheese.

Brucella suis is the most important cause of brucellosis in the U.S.A. Humans may become infected while handling the pig carcasses particularly in slaughter houses, and occasionally from eating infected ham.

Pathogenesis

Brucella organisms become intracellular parasites of cells of the reticulo-endothelial system, in bone marrow, liver, spleen, lymph nodes and other sites so that they subsequently become relatively inaccessible to circulatory phagocytes; infection then often becomes chronic, especially with *B. abortus* or *B. suis* and is frequently subclinical. No man-to-man spread of the disease occurs.

Clinical features of brucellosis ('Undulant fever', 'Mediterranean fever')

Brucellosis can occur clinically as an acute, subacute, chronic or subclinical disease. In addition, those with repeated exposures to the disease with high antibody titres to *Brucella*, particularly vets, may develop a hypersensitivity state often marked by rashes on the arms after examining cows.

Acute brucellosis may occur after an incubation period of 2–3 weeks, and occurs with many cases of *B. melitensis* infection and a minority of cases of *B. abortus* infection. The predominant symptoms include high fever, headache, drenching sweats, fatigue and joint pains. Occasionally there is splenomegaly and slight liver enlargement.

Subacute brucellosis may occur when infection with *B. abortus* persists for more than a month and is mainly characterized by recurrent attacks and extreme lassitude in an apparently well-looking patient. The joints may be painful and possibly swollen.

Chronic brucellosis lasting for many months or years may occur characterized by recurrent episodes of headache, flu-like illnesses, lassitude, backache, anxiety and depression. Death by suicide may very rarely result. Other rare serious complications of brucellosis may occur including endocarditis, thrombophlebitis, meningo-encephalitis and chronic arthritis which can affect the spine (*see* Chapter 17). Granulomata may appear in the liver, marrow or spleen in chronic brucellosis which occasionally can be histologically confused with sarcoidosis.

Subclinical—no active brucellosis but patients may have raised antibody titres—common in vets and farmers.

Haematological investigations

The blood count in acute brucellosis is usually low or normal. Characteristically there is a neutropenia and a lymphocytosis.

Microbiological investigations

Blood cultures are positive in up to 20% of cases of brucellosis, usually during the acute phase of the illness, and are more likely to become positive when the brucellosis is due to *B. melitensis* than *B. abortus*. The latter organism in particular has a requirement for a high CO_2 concentration and at least one bottle of the routine blood culture sets should be incubated in an aerobic atmosphere containing 10% CO_2. When brucellosis is suspected clinically a few additional sets of blood cultures using diphasic (Castenada) media may be collected as the temperature of the patient rises and these should be incubated in a CO_2 atmosphere for up to 6 weeks.

Liver biopsy for isolation of the organism and histology may be helpful in blood culture negative cases where the diagnosis is suspected.

Serology

1. *Standard agglutination test*

During the acute phase of the illness, repeated serum samples should be collected and simultaneous serological tests are performed on paired sera to demonstrate a rising (greater than four-fold) titre of brucella agglutinins in the standard phenol-saline agglutination tests. High titres are usually encountered by the second or third week of illness, over 1/80, and may be in the thousands—a prozone phenomenon may occur.

In the subacute or chronic phase of brucellosis, the standard agglutination test may be particularly difficult to interpret or may be negative and other tests need also to be done including:

—the 2-mercaptoethanol test
—brucella complement fixation test (CFT)
—anti-human globulin test (AHG or Coombs' test)

2. *The mercaptoethanol test*

When the brucella agglutinin titre is lower in the mercaptoethanol test than in a simultaneous standard saline agglutination test, the difference may be explained due to the presence of IgM antibodies which suggest active disease in the acute or subacute phase rather than subclinical infection.

3. *The brucella CFT*

This test detects IgG antibodies against *Brucella* and is especially useful in chronic brucellosis as the CFT may then be positive while the agglutination tests are negative. The CFT is also useful in the acute or subacute phases when the results of the agglutination tests are equivocal; the titres are often strongly positive, between 1/32 and 1/1024 during these phases. In practice, many laboratories routinely use the CFT and standard agglutination tests together as the two main screening tests for the serological diagnosis of brucellosis. The patient is unlikely to have brucellosis if the CFT is negative.

4. *The anti-human globulin test*

This type of agglutination test is mainly useful for detecting 'incomplete' antibodies in cases of chronic brucellosis. In these circumstances the information gained is similar to that found with the complement fixation test.

Two antigens are usually used in these tests and because of antigenic cross-reactions, antibodies to all the various types of *B. abortus* or *B. melitensis* may be detected. It is nearly always possible to differentiate active brucellosis from subclinical brucellosis in a patient with occupational exposure to the disease when the clinical circumstances and results of a combination of these tests are considered together.

Antimicrobial therapy

Tetracycline, administered in a well-absorbed oral form such as clomocycline, for 3 months, together with daily streptomycin for the first month is the best treatment for acute brucellosis. Occasionally it is necessary to repeat this treatment after a few months. Relapses may occur due to the intracellular location of the brucella organism which makes it relatively inaccessible to antibiotics.

Cotrimoxazole is satisfactory alternative treatment for acute brucellosis given in high dosage until the patient is better and treatment should be continued for two to three months.

It is doubtful that tetracycline is effective in the management of chronic brucellosis although cotrimoxazole has occasionally proved useful for treating this condition.

Prevention

The pasteurization of milk, the vaccination of female calves, the monitoring of cattle for infection (using tests such as the milk-ring test with a methylene blue stained antigen to detect antibody in the milk) and the eradication of brucella-infected cattle are important control measures used in Britain. In some countries including the U.S.A., protective clothing and goggles are also recommended for vets and farmers for high risk exposure situations.

Campylobacter Infections

Campylobacter vibrios have been isolated from the faeces of a wide range of farm animals, especially poultry, and pets including dogs. These organisms are a common cause of febrile illness and gastro-enteritis in humans who acquire the infection by eating contaminated meat or occasionally by handling raw meat or close contact with the animal (*see* Chapter 14). There have been some recent raw milk-borne outbreaks of campylobacter infections.

Leptospirosis

Epidemiology, causative organisms and main clinical characteristics

Leptospires can survive for long periods in stagnant water and wet soil, especially when the pH is alkaline and the various wet sources may become contaminated by the infected urine of many different animals. There are two main groups of animal reservoirs of infection, small wild animals such as rodents, voles and hedgehogs and larger farm or domestic animals such as pigs, cattle and puppies. The cycle of infection may involve more than one animal species in a given location and the leptospira spirochaetes in a wet source can penetrate the abraded or intact skin, conjunctiva or mucous membranes of new animal hosts or man. The leptospires then invade the blood and localize in various sites, including the kidneys, so that leptospiruria results which perpetuates the cycle of infection. The majority of infections are asymptomatic or associated with only mild disease.

Humans throughout the world may become infected because of a 'wet' occupation such as working in rice fields (e.g. in Italy, Spain or the Far East), wet sugar cane fields or on farms (in Britain—especially with pigs or cattle in rodent-infested areas), mines or sewers. Alternatively, leptospirosis can result from a leisure pursuit such as swimming in contaminated fresh water or playing with an infected pet dog. The incubation period varies between 5 and 14 days. There are three main serogroups of *Leptospira*:

1. *Leptospira canicola serogroup*—the animal host is often canine and children playing with puppies can develop 'Canicola fever' which may be associated with aseptic meningitis (*see* Chapter 10). Pigs are often the animal reservoir which subsequently cause infection in farm workers while rodents may also become infected and help perpetuate the cycle of infection on farms.
2. *Leptospira icterohaemorrhagiae serogroup*—rats are the most well-known reservoir for this serogroup but other animals may also become infected. Humans infected by this serogroup may develop Weil's disease which is classically characterized by fever, jaundice, subconjunctival haemorrhages and proteinuria. Rarely, severe hepatorenal failure and death may occur.

Many patients suffer milder forms of the disease and may not have jaundice at all.

3. *Leptospira hebdomadis serogroup*—cattle, fieldmice and voles are the main animal reservoirs of infection with this serogroup.

Microbiological investigations

Blood dark-ground microscopy and cultures

Leptospira can sometimes be seen in the blood by DGI or isolated during the first weeks of the illness from the blood using special culture media (e.g. Fletcher's or Korthoff's) or guinea-pig innoculation.

Urine dark-ground microscopy and cultures

The urine should be alkalinized before collection and then examined by DGI and guinea-pig inoculation—positive results may be obtained during the second week of illness.

Serology

Leptospiral CFT and micro-agglutinins may become positive during the second week of illness and repeated serum samples should be collected to demonstrate a rising titre of antibody.

Treatment

Benzylpenicillin (or tetracycline in penicillin-allergic patients) is effective only if given at the start of the illness and, in severely ill cases, high initial doses such as 10 MU parenterally a day may be necessary. Deaths rarely occur although a few patients may require management of renal failure by haemodialysis.

Prevention

Protective clothing for those at occupational risk, such as sewer or abattoir workers, rodent control and disinfection of infected premises, are important public health measures. People who develop cuts or abrasions while at risk may require prophylactic penicillin. For selected high risk situations, vaccination against relevant serogroups of *Leptospira* may be considered. The incidence of the clinical disease in Britain is now low with only about 40–70 cases of leptospirosis diagnosed each year.

Anthrax

Bacillus anthracis is an aerobic Gram-positive spore-forming bacillus which causes anthrax, a disease primarily of sheep and cattle. Preventive measures have helped to make this disease almost unknown in Britain and many developed countries today. It still occurs in Asia and parts of Africa.

Spores of the anthrax bacillus may survive for many years in contaminated soil and herbivore animals become infected by ingesting the spores. A terminal septicaemia occurs and many organs of the body become infected. Anthrax in man is mainly an occupational disease since infection occurs in workers handling contaminated hides, hair or other products of cattle, the wool of sheep and bone meal. In Britain, infected imported bone meal has been the main source of infection in the few gardeners and others who have acquired the disease in recent years.

Cutaneous anthrax is the main clinical type of disease seen. It is acquired by direct contact with a contaminated animal product and characterized by the 'malignant pustule' (*see* Chapter 16). Swabs of the lesion cultured onto blood agar confirm the diagnosis and parenteral penicillin treatment, if given early in the disease, is usually effective treatment. The patient should be isolated and the Medical Officer for Environmental Health informed.

Pulmonary anthrax is exceedingly rare and associated with a high mortality. In the past, it occurred in workers who inhaled anthrax spores from contaminated wool—'woolsorters disease'.

Prevention

All imports of wool, hides and hair into Britain are decontaminated at special disinfectant facilities near Liverpool docks. Workers at high risk who handle the above products and bone meal are vaccinated against anthrax. The disease no longer occurs in British animals partly because of vaccination in the past. If anthrax appears in an animal there are stringent regulations that include notification and burying it in quick lime.

Listeriosis

Although listeriosis in man is rare, it has become increasingly recognized in Britain in recent years.

Listeria monocytogenes, a Gram-positive bacillus that is sometimes confused in the laboratory with streptococci or diphtheroids, causes infection in scores of different animal species including cattle, pigs, rodents, birds and fish and occasionally in man. The organism may be a cause of abortion in cows. It is present in the faeces of infected animals and can be found sometimes in soil. Man probably becomes infected by direct contact with the live animal or by handling raw meat or drinking infected milk. The organism may also be spread sexually.

Clinical syndromes associated with listeria infection include:

1. *Perinatal listeriosis*
   An influenza-like illness due to *Listeria* acquired during pregnancy may rarely cause stillbirth. More frequently a live neonate is born prematurely with granulomatous pneumonia, respiratory distress and septicaemia occurring within the first 2 days of life, following intra-uterine infection. A predominantly meningitic illness may develop after the fifth day in other infants who might also acquire the organism from other babies or the attendants in hospital instead of the mother (*see* Chapters 7 and 10).
2. *Febrile illness in vets, abattoir workers, butchers, poultry workers or other farm workers*
   A febrile illness due to listeriosis may be confused with influenza. The illness may be accompanied by pharyngitis, diarrhoea, generalized pains

or symptoms of genital tract infection. The occupation of the person may suggest the diagnosis.

3. *PUO, pneumonia or meningo/encephalitis in immunocompromised adults* Children or adults who have had a splenectomy or have a lymphoma, or are immunosuppressed, may develop serious listeria infections. These infections include septicaemia and infections of lungs or central nervous system.

Microbiological investigations

Blood cultures in adults and neonates. Culture of the CSF and of skin lesions in neonates, and high vaginal swabs in the mother usually yield growth of *Listeria monocytogenes* on blood agar from suspected sporadic cases (*see also* Chapter 10).

If there is an epidemic, which is a rare event, faeces and swabs from other babies in the nursery and possibly from other mothers and hospital staff may also be required for culture.

Antimicrobial treatment

Ampicillin is the drug of choice which should be given parenterally. Some authorities suggest a combination of ampicillin and gentamicin for treatment of febrile mothers suspected of having listeriosis and a combination of ampicillin and chloramphenicol for treating listeria meningitis.

If treatment is given early on in the disease, in neonates, the prognosis is reasonably good but, if treatment is delayed, there is a high mortality rate.

Plague

Plague is caused by the *Yersinia pestis*, a short Gram-negative bacillus. Rodents, particularly rats, are the usual animal reservoirs for plague which is spread from rat to rat and from rat to man by the rat flea *Xenopsylla cheopsis*. The black rat, *Rattus rattus*, is the most important rat reservoir. Following an incubation period in man of 2–6 days, the inguinal or other lymph glands become tender and the patient febrile in sporadic cases of bubonic plague. Unless treatment is quickly given the yersinia organisms invade the blood and death usually follows a haemorrhagic illness ('the Black Death'). When the organism causes lung infection, the patient develops pneumonic plague which may spread from person to person in epidemic plague by respiratory droplets.

Plague is extremely rare in Europe but a few cases have occurred in America and small epidemics during the 1970s have occurred in the Far East, usually at times of war.

Microbiological investigations

Lymph node aspiration can give a rapid indication of the disease when characteristic Gram-negative bipolar staining coco-bacilli are seen in the smear. Cultures of the aspirate and blood and sputum cultures may yield growth of *Yersinia pestis* after prolonged culture.

Antimicrobial treatment

Streptomycin is the recommended drug and alternatives include chloramphenicol or tetracycline.

Prevention

Quarantine measures have long been used to prevent the spread of plague. Rodent control measures in ports and on ships are enforced in many countries. The eradication of plague-infested rats and rat fleas may be more difficult in some underdeveloped warm countries with poor public hygiene.

When a patient is diagnosed as having plague, strict isolation measures are essential and immediate notification of the Medical Officer for Environmental Health is necessary. Contacts of a case of pneumonic plague may need chemoprophylaxis with tetracycline. For certain workers in endemic areas of the world, repeated administration of a vaccine against *Y. pestis* may be desirable.

Tularaemia

The causative organism of tularaemia, *Francisella tularensis*, may infect rabbits, ground squirrels and many rodents, wild mammals, dogs and cats as well as the ticks that may parasitize these animals, particularly in North America and Scandinavia, but not in Britain.

The disease is mainly seen in hunters and butchers in endemic regions who usually acquire francisella infection through the skin while handling infected animals. The infection can also be acquired from animal bites or scratches, tick bites or inhaling infected aerosols or by ingesting contaminated food or water.

Clinically the usual form of the disease is ulceration of the skin followed by regional lymphadenopathy, fever, headache and hepato-splenomegaly.

Microbiological investigations

Culture of a skin biopsy of the ulcerated skin lesion may yield growth of *Francisella tularensis* on glucose–cysteine enriched media or a guinea-pig inoculation.

A rising titre of specific agglutinins may be demonstrated during the second week of the illness (there are weak cross-reactions with *Brucella*).

Antimicrobial treatment

Streptomycin is the drug of choice.

Prevention

Protective clothing against ticks and the wearing of gloves when handling rabbits or other animals in endemic parts of North America or Scandinavia reduces the risks of infection.

Erysipeloid

Erysipelothrix rhusiopathiae causes zoonotic infection in pigs, fish and other animals and man may develop the skin infection erysipeloid following handling of the meat or fish, especially if there is abraded skin. Butchers, fish handlers and others with occupational exposure, acquire the disease. Rarely septicaemia and endocarditis result (*see* Chapter 16).

Glanders

Horses are the main animals infected by *Pseudomonas mallei* which causes skin, subcutaneous or respiratory infections. Man very rarely becomes infected following contact with an infected horse or accidentally in the laboratory. This disease is virtually unknown in Britain.

Rat-bite Fever

Rats can, after biting man, produce skin ulcers or wound abscess, local lymphadenopathy and fever, but there are two different causative organisms of 'rat-bite fever' disease in man, *Spirillum minus* or *Streptobacillus moniliformis*. The spirillum type of rat-bite fever occurs mainly in the Far East, especially in Japan where it is called Soduku. Penicillin is effective treatment. *Spirillum minus* can be seen on dark-ground illumination or by Leishman stains of blood or aspirate from infected glands. It cannot be cultured on an artificial media but it can sometimes be isolated using guinea-pig inoculation.

Streptobacillus moniliformis causes rat-bite fever in America and the illness may include polyarthritis. In addition to acquiring the disease by rat bites, the infection may follow drinking of contaminated milk, as occurred in an outbreak in Haverhill (Haverhill fever). The organism, which may occur as L forms, can be isolated using special media or guinea-pig inoculation from the blood or joint fluids. The infection responds to tetracycline therapy.

Pasteurella multocida Infections

Pasteurella multocida (*P. septica*) is found in the upper respiratory tract of many animal species including cats, dogs, cattle and poultry. Bites or scratches from these animals can result in human wound infections due to *P. multocida*. Alternatively, spread can occur by the respiratory route. Sometimes bacteriuria, respiratory tract infection or meningitis can occur in man due to this organism.

Microbiological investigations

P. multocida, a short Gram-negative bacillus with bipolar staining, can be easily isolated from wound swabs on blood agar or from blood cultures, sputum or CSF.

Antimicrobial treatment

Benzylpenicillin is effective treatment for *P. multocida* infections. Tetracyclines are also usually effective but the results of antibiotic sensitivity tests should be checked to ensure that the organism is sensitive to the antibiotic selected.

Tetanus

Clostridium tetani is frequently found in the intestines of many animals, including horses and cattle but only occasionally in the intestine of man. Man is infected when spores from an animal source germinate under anaerobic conditions (*see* Chapter 9).

Relapsing Fever

There are two types of relapsing fever, louse-borne and tick-borne due to *Borrelia recurrentis* or *Borrelia duttoni*, respectively. The main differences between the two types of disease are summarized in *Table 21.2*. Only the tick-borne variety is strictly a zoonosis since the main vertebrate reservoir of louse-borne relapsing fever is man.

Table 21.2. The two types of relapsing fever

	Tick borne	*Louse borne*
Other name	African relapsing fever	'European'* relapsing fever
Organism	*Borrelia duttoni*	*Borrelia recurrentis*
Arthropod vector	Soft tick infective for life after biting mammal and transovarial vertical transmission occurs	Body louse—body contents infect man when crushed against skin
Reservoir of disease	Wild rodents mainly pigs and armadillos	Man
Geographical distribution today	Africa, Asia and Latin America	Ethiopia
Patterns of disease	Sporadic cases	Epidemics may occur in overcrowded and insanitary circumstances

* Misnomer today.

The main clinical features of relapsing fever include fevers lasting 2–4 days, headache and an enlarged spleen; characteristically, relapses of fever occur after an afebrile period of about a week in patients who survive the first attack. The relapses are probably due to new antigenic variants of *Borrelia recurrentis* occurring, particularly in louse-borne relapsing fever.

Microbiological investigations

Thick and thin blood films should be collected during the febrile stage for Giemsa or Leishman staining and the borrelia spirochaetes can then be demonstrated; alternatively the motile spirochaetes can be seen during dark-ground illumination examination of the blood.

The organisms can also be isolated by inoculation of the patient's blood into rats which show the spirochaetes in the blood in large numbers after a couple of days.

Antimicrobial treatment

Tetracyclines provide effective treatment.

Prevention

Vector control is the most important method of avoiding infection and rodents should be kept out of dwelling places.

RICKETTSIAL ZOONOSES

Q Fever ('Query Fever')

Q fever is caused by a rickettsia-like organism, *Coxiella burnetii*. The disease is relatively rare in Britain.

Domestic sheep and cattle are the main animal reservoirs of infection in countries throughout the world and ticks play a part in the cycle of infection amongst animals.

Man may become infected during occupational exposure by handling infected animals or animal products, particularly infected placentae or infected meat, by inhaling contaminated dust or by drinking infected unpasteurized milk. Men are more commonly infected than women.

Clinical features

Fever, severe headache, anorexia and general aches and pains are later followed by features of primary atypical pneumonia in about 50% of cases. Hepato-splenomegaly may also occur. Within a few weeks, most patients completely recover but infective endocarditis is an important though rare complication which carries a worse prognosis (*see* Chapter 18).

Microbiological investigations

Paired sera should be collected to show a rising titre of antibodies in the Q fever complement fixation test (CFT). This test uses two antigens of *Coxiella burnetii*:

1. Phase 1 antigen prepared from freshly isolated strains of *Coxiella* which reacts with sera from patients with chronic infections such as Q fever endocarditis
2. Phase 2 antigen, prepared from passaged strains of *Coxiella*, which reacts with sera from patients in both the acute and chronic stages of infection

Material from infected heart valves can be stained by Macchiavello's stain, or specific immunofluorescence, to show the cocco-bacillary form of *Coxiella*. The organism may be isolated by guinea-pig inoculation. Subsequently, antibodies may be demonstrated in the sera of infected guinea-pigs using the Q fever CFT.

Antimicrobial treatment

Tetracycline or chloramphenicol is effective treatment for Q fever. Long courses of tetracycline and surgical removal of the infected heart lesion is usually necessary for cases of Q fever endocarditis (*see* Chapter 18).

Typhus

Rickettsia species cause typhus fevers (*see Table 21.3*).

Murine typhus, scrub typhus (Tsutsugamushi fever), Rocky Mountain spotted fever and other tick-borne rickettsial fevers are all zoonoses but epidemic louse-borne typhus is not a zoonoses as man is the only vertebrate reservoir of this disease (*Table 21.3*).

Table 21.3. Causative organisms, animal or human reservoirs, vectors and serological diagnosis of typhus diseases

				Weil–Felix serology: Agglutinins against		
Typhus diseases	*Rickettsial organism*	*Main reservoirs of disease*	*Vector*	*Proteus OX 19*	*Proteus OX K*	*Proteus OX 2*
Epidemic typhus (Brill's disease when relapse occurs)	*R. prowazeki*	Humans*	Body louse	+ +	–	+
Murine typhus	*R. mooseri* (*typhi*)	Rats	Rat flea	+	–	±
Scrub typhus (Tsutsuga-mushi fever)	*R. orientalis* (*tsutsuga-mushi*)	Mongooses Birds	Mite (trans-ovarial)	–	+	–
Spotted fever (SF)	*R. rickettsi* (Rocky mountain SF) *R. conori* (African tick typhus)	Dogs Rodents Rabbits	Ticks (trans-ovarial)	Variable results		

* Debilitated—as in Ethiopia today.

In most typhus diseases there is fever, severe prostration and a maculo-papular rash which may become haemorrhagic. In severe cases of epidemic or murine typhus, coma and death may result. One of the commonest but less severe forms of typhus seen today is tick-borne typhus in tourists who go on safaris to countries in Eastern or Southern Africa; occasionally an eschar can be seen at the site of the initial tick bite.

The Weil–Felix test is a useful serological test for diagnosing some forms of typhus (*Table 21.3*) provided paired sera are collected to show rising titres of antibody. Other serological tests are available in reference laboratories.

Tetracycline or chloramphenicol started in the early stages of the disease may provide effective treatment.

Prevention of the disease depends mainly on arthropod vector control.

VIRAL ZOONOSES

Rabies

A bullet-shaped rhabdo RNA virus is the causative organism of rabies. This virus can penetrate skin abrasions or wounds and intact mucous membranes of dogs and man, spreading subsequently via the nerves to the central nervous system. The virus is present in the saliva of infected animals from a few days before the start of signs of disease in the animal. When an apparently healthy dog bites man and is still healthy 10 days afterwards, it is extremely unlikely that the animal had rabies on the day of the bite.

The disease is worldwide with only Britain and Scandinavia free of rabies. The range of animals that may develop rabies is very wide including dogs, foxes, cats, skunks, mongooses, cattle, monkeys and vampire bats. In Europe, rabies is endemic amongst the wild animals of many areas and is especially spread by fox epizootics. Foxes are responsible for the spread of rabies, during the 1960s and 1970s from Germany and Belgium to wide areas of Northern and Eastern France, up to the Channel ports. Dogs on the Continent can become infected and are the usual animals that cause rabies in man following bites. The threat of spread of rabies by importing an infected dog or other pet from the Continent to Britain has greatly increased during the last ten years. Rabies was eradicated from Britain by 1921 and imported animals must satisfy the quarantine regulations; vigilance has to be exercised against the smuggling in of potentially infected animals. In Latin America, the vampire bat is the main wild animal reservoir of rabies. After a bite from an infected bat, man can develop 'paralytic rabies' with flaccid paralysis due to ascending myelitis because of spinal cord lesions.

Man is mainly infected following a bite from an infected animal but occasionally acquires the disease after an animal has licked his skin or mucosa or from scratches from the animals.

Incubation period and pathogenesis

From 4–13 weeks, but occasionally up to 6 months following contact with a rabid animal. Rabies is especially likely to develop and the incubation period is shorter when a person is bitten on the head, neck or fingers, rather than the trunk or lower limbs. The virus penetrates peripheral nerves and is carried to the central nervous system where it causes an encephalomyelitis. Other organs also may become infected including skeletal muscle, myocardium and salivary glands. Within the neurones, the virus causes characteristic intracytoplasmic inclusions—Negri bodies.

Clinical features of 'furious' rabies

'Furious' rabies is the usual clinical presentation when the disease follows contact with a rabid dog. Initial symptoms include sore throat, headache, irritability, fever and discomfort at the site of a wound.

The characteristic features of rabies develop including excitement, muscle spasms and convulsions, particularly affecting the muscles of swallowing when attempting to drink water which gave rise to the alternative name for rabies, 'hydrophobia'. Opisthotonus and other convulsions almost invariably finally result in death following cardiac or respiratory arrest. Treatment in an intensive care unit may delay death for a few days and is rarely curative.

Microbiological investigations

a. Of patients

Rapid diagnosis of rabies in patients is possible by immunofluorescence of skin biopsy (showing rabies antigen in nerve fibres of hair follicles), corneal impression smear or brain biopsy.

Isolation of the virus is possible by inoculating saliva, urine, CSF or brain tissue from the patient into mice intracerebrally but the results take some days.

b. Of animals

Often the diagnosis of rabies in an animal that has bitten a person is all important in order to assess the risks of rabies developing and to help determine the preventive measures that are necessary. The animal should be observed and the brain normally examined only after disease appears in the animal, so that Negri bodies are then easily seen by immunofluorescence or histological examination of 'Ammon's horn' of the hippocampus.

Preventive measures

As rabies is virtually always fatal once the disease is apparent, the main measures against the disease must be preventive. These measures are (*a*) general, and (*b*) for an individual exposed to potential risk of rabies—post-exposure prophylaxis.

a. General preventive measures

In Britain, which is rabies free, the exclusion of possibly infected imported animals is the main preventive general measure.

In France and other countries where rabies is endemic, domestic animals require animal vaccination and stray animals are killed. People at occupational risk, such as veterinary surgeons, are given pre-exposure vaccination with intradermal injections of human diploid cell strain vaccine with regular boosters.

b. Post-exposure prophylaxis

Any person who is bitten, scratched or licked by a possibly rabid animal in an endemic area should be encouraged to seek immediate medical help to:

i. Ascertain the degree of risk by trying to establish whether the animal indeed is rabid or incubating rabies.
ii. Give prompt local toilet to the wound using alcoholic iodine solutions and *prompt passive immunization* using human rabies immunoglobulin (HRIG) when there is any possibility of a rabies risk. Half the dose of HRIG is given intra-muscularly and half locally into the site of the wound.
iii. Start *active rabies immunization* as soon as possible in all those at definite risk. The chances of successful prevention of rabies are improved when the person is vaccinated in the early part of the long incubation period of rabies. The wild rabies virus is known as 'street' virus and the attenuated virus used in the first rabies vaccine developed by Pasteur using rabbit spinal cords was known as 'fixed' virus. The early preventive vaccines (such as Semple vaccine) were associated with an unacceptably high

chance of neuroparalytic reactions and had to be given by a course of numerous abdominal subcutaneous injections.

Duck-embryo killed virus vaccine administered subcutaneously is recommended in the U.S.A. and is much safer than the previous nerve tissue vaccines. However doubts have been raised about its effectiveness in preventing the development of rabies and, in Europe, the human diploid cell strain vaccine is preferred.

The human diploid cell strain (HDCSV) live attenuated strain of rabies vaccine is the vaccine of choice for both active pre- and post-exposure vaccination. It is associated with very few side effects and produces a good antibody response against rabies; it still has to be given early in the incubation period since wild rabies virus in nerve tissue is relatively inaccessible to humoral antibody. The HDCSV vaccine is administered as 1·0-ml intra-muscular injections on five different days over a month with a sixth dose at 90 days after exposure.

Lymphocytic Choriomeningitis

Mice are the animal reservoirs of this arenavirus which causes a rare type of aseptic meningitis in man. Human infection may follow inhalation of dust contaminated by infected mouse excretions.

Lassa Fever and Marburg Virus Disease

Lassa fever is endemic in certain rural areas of West or Central Africa and is caused by an arenavirus. The main reservoir of the disease appears to be the rat *Mastomys natalensis*. Man may become infected through contact with the urine or saliva of an infected rat and occasionally family members and hospital staff looking after patients with Lassa fever have become infected.

Marburg virus disease first became recognized in persons who were in contact with infected African green monkeys.

These rare viral haemorrhagic fevers from Africa are further outlined in Chapter 22.

Arbovirus Diseases Associated with Animal Reservoirs of Disease

Arboviruses are spread by arthropod vectors from animals, mainly small mammals such as rodents, birds and monkeys, to man and cause many different viral zoonoses in Africa, the Far East, America, Eastern Europe and Australia. Other arboviruses are associated with human reservoirs of disease only such as urban yellow fever or dengue. Most infections due to arboviruses cause no symptoms or only mild disease.

Arboviruses are classified as togaviruses, consisting of alphaviruses and flaviviruses, and are associated with zoonoses that are spread by mosquitoes or tick vectors from animal reservoirs to cause encephalitis in man (*see* Chapter 10), such as Equine Encephalitis or Murray Valley Encephalitis. In Britain a flavivirus, louping-ill, spread by ticks from infected sheep or cattle can rarely cause encephalitis in man.

Other arboviruses may cause fevers, sometimes with haemorrhagic rashes or other haemorrhagic manifestations. The flavivirus of yellow fever in jungle regions of equatorial Africa or South America causes sylvan yellow fever with a reservoir of the disease in tree-dwelling monkeys. The disease is spread from monkey to monkey and from monkey to man by mosquitoes (*see also* Urban yellow fever in Chapter 22).

Herpes Simiae 'B' Virus

Herpetic ulcers in the mouth or on the lips of old world monkeys such as Rhesus or cynomolgus monkeys, due to Simian 'B' herpes virus, can cause fatal encephalomyelitis in man after spread by bites, scratches or aerosols. Laboratory or animal house workers have been mainly affected in the past.

Prevention by avoiding contact with unwell monkeys is most important and the use of protective clothing and gloves as well as quarantining imported monkeys.

Newcastle Disease

Newcastle disease, due to a myxovirus, mainly affects chickens and is spread by respiratory or intestinal secretions. Rarely, man is infected by close contact with infected poultry or by laboratory accidents and the virus causes an acute conjunctivitis, usually unilateral.

Orf

Orf is a viral disease primarily affecting sheep, especially lambs at spring time which may develop vesicles in the mouth. Shepherds or vets are occasionally infected on their hands or forearms following direct contact while handling the sheep. A maco-papular lesion develops at the site of trauma which becomes a multiloculated vesicle accompanied by some fever and regional lymphadenopathy. Within a few weeks the lesion heals completely spontaneously and there is good immunity preventing any further infections. The diagnosis can be confirmed by seeing the characteristic pox virus on electron microscopy of material from the skin lesion (*see* Chapter 16).

CHLAMYDIAL ZOONOSES

Ornithosis and Psittacosis

Chlamydiae B are intracellular organisms which may infect the respiratory tract, alimentary tract, liver and spleen of birds. Ornithosis refers to generalized chlamydial infection in birds, such as pigeons or turkeys, and psittacosis refers to a chlamydial disease of psittacine birds, in particular, which includes parrots and budgerigars.

Man may become infected by inhaling dust from faecal or other discharges from infected birds or by direct contact. The birds may not have obvious illness but some birds, especially if under stress in captivity, fall ill with diarrhoea, weakness or purulent nasal discharge. Occasionally, birds die of the disease and the carcasses are highly infectious. Infection in birds is widespread across the world but man is only infrequently infected.

Occupational exposure to infected birds is closely associated with disease in man, amongst poultry farm workers, bird keepers and pet shop owners. Also those who keep pet budgerigars or parrots are at risk of acquiring the disease, especially if the birds have recently been imported. Rarely man can become infected in the laboratory by handling sputum from a patient with psittacosis under unsafe conditions.

In Britain, there are between 150 and 250 new cases of ornithosis or psittacosis diagnosed each year. The main sources of infection are budgerigars, parrots and pigeons.

Clinical features

Headache, a flu-like febrile illness, joint pains or PUO are common presentations of psittacosis and respiratory symptoms are often not marked. The patient may have a dry cough or expectorate some mucoid or muco-purulent sputum. The chest radiograph often shows more marked patchy signs of consolidation than would be expected from examination of the chest, which is usually the situation in atypical pneumonia due to either psittacosis or *Mycoplasma*. The radiological features may persist for many weeks, while clinically the patient usually greatly improves after 1–2 weeks. A few cases develop serious 'septicaemic' type infections with widespread consolidation of the lungs and rarely death can occur.

Complications of infection infrequently occur and include myocarditis, pericarditis and, rarely, infective endocarditis which may be fatal (*see* Chapter 18).

Microbiological investigations

Isolation of the organism from sputum or blood is possible using egg yolk sac inoculation, but is dangerous.

Serological investigations using paired sera are the mainstay of diagnosis. A rising antibody titre or a single high titre can be demonstrated against chlamydial B antigens using a psittacosis CFT.

Antimicrobial treatment

Treatment in the early stages of the disease with tetracyclines is effective.

Prevention

Care to avoid buying or handling birds that are ill or have been recently imported is necessary to avoid infection.

FUNGAL ZOONOSES

Many dermatophytes throughout the world may cause ringworm in man following contact between man and an infected animal. Up to 50% of human ringworm is acquired from animals, particularly in rural areas. Examples include *Trichophyton verrucosum* from infected cattle causing pustular tinea barbae lesions in man, *Microsporum canis* from infected dogs and cats causing tinea capitis, and *Trichophyton mentagrophytes* from infected horses, hedgehogs and other animals causing tinea corporis in man. Children are more liable to become infected than adults and the dermatophyte may be acquired following direct contact with the animal or by indirect contact via a surface such as a farm gate (*see* Chapter 16).

PROTOZOAL ZOONOSES

Toxoplasmosis

Epidemiology and pathogenesis

Toxoplasmosis has a worldwide distribution. *Toxoplasma gondii* multiplies in the ileum of the cat, ultimately sexually to produce gametocytes, which combine to produce zygotes and these develop into oocysts which are excreted in cat faeces. The cat is the main definite animal host and mice are frequent intermediate hosts perpetuating the lifecycle. Humans can acquire toxoplasma infection and become intermediate hosts from contact with cats or soil contaminated by oocysts and also by contact with the raw or undercooked meats of animals that maybe also are intermediate hosts, such as cattle, pigs or horses. The organism is ingested by man but the subsequent development is outside of the alimentary tract, as with other intermediate hosts, and particularly affects the reticulo-endothelial system. The *Toxoplasma* may invade the blood and lymphatics and may be transported to various organs via circulating lymphocytes and macrophages. Almost any organ can become infected but lymph nodes, the eye, the liver and spleen, the central nervous system and the myocardium are some of the most important sites clinically. At each site the trophozoites may form microcysts and rupture of the cysts may result in a hypersensitivity reaction and the development of an inflammatory lesion.

When primary infection occurs in pregnant women, especially during the first trimester, intra-uterine infection of the foetus may occur resulting in a neonate with features of congenital toxoplasmosis. Abortion or stillbirth can also result.

Clinical features of acquired toxoplasmosis

Toxoplasma infection is common in Britain but the great majority of infections are asymptomatic or accompanied by only minor illnesses.

Children and young adults commonly present with either a febrile illness with sore throat, muscle weakness and fatigue or more frequently with painless cervical lymphadenopathy. Clinically the differential diagnosis may include infectious mononucleosis. A few patients may present with complications such as meningo-encephalitis, pneumonitis, myocarditis or choroido-retinitis especially if they are immunosuppressed.

Clinical features of congenital toxoplasmosis

Neonatal features of congenital toxoplasmosis include jaundice, hepato-splenomegaly and purpura. Later in infancy one or more of three classic features of congenital toxoplasmosis may appear: (1) choroido-retinitis resulting in defective vision, (2) hydrocephalus or microcephaly, later associated with mental deficiency or cerebral palsies and (3) cerebral calcification in the basal ganglia and apparent in the ventricular walls.

Microbiological investigations

Serology is the main method of diagnosis—mainly with the Toxoplasma Dye Test. Paired sera to demonstrate a rising titre of antibody to *Toxoplasma* should be collected but sometimes a single high titre in the thousands is strongly suggestive of the diagnosis. In some patients, a positive IgM toxoplasma antibody titre can also be demonstrated by an immunofluorescent antibody technique which indicates recent infection in acquired cases or congenital infection in neonates.

Histological examination of excised lymph nodes can also show changes, such as follicular hyperplasia and the presence of numerous clusters of epithelioid cells in the nodes, suggestive of toxoplasmosis.

Isolation of the organism is possible but hazardous by intra-peritoneal inoculation of mice with lymph-node aspirates or other clinical specimens. After about 2 months, the toxoplasma trophozoites can be seen during histological examination of the brains of the mice.

Antimicrobial treatment

Most cases of toxoplasmosis do not require any specific treatment since the lesions will usually resolve satisfactorily without treatment. However, treatment is indicated in a patient with severe or progressive disease especially in immunosuppressed patients, or in a mother with the disease in pregnancy when it is too late for termination, or in a neonate with signs of congenital toxoplasmosis. Specific anti-toxoplasma treatment can be tried with a combination of sulphonamide and pyrimethamine for 14 days together with folinic acid, since pyrimethamine is a folic acid antagonist. Spiramycin may be a safer alternative to give to pregnant women.

Prevention

Avoidance of close contacts with cats and other animals, as well as care not to handle or eat raw meat (such as 'steak tartare') or undercooked meat, especially during pregnancy, may help to reduce the chances of acquiring toxoplasmosis.

Babesiosis

Babesiae are protozoa that infect various animal species, including cattle, and extremely rarely cause disease in people who have been splenectomized. The affected patients may develop fever, anaemia, jaundice, haemoglobinuria and impaired renal function. Leishman stain examination of the blood films of the patient may reveal the parasite inside the red cells. The antimicrobial treatment of babesiosis is difficult but occasionally chloroquine has appeared effective.

Leishmaniasis

Leishmania donovani, the causative organism of visceral leishmaniasis (kala azar) in Africa, the Middle East, Mediterranean coasts, Asia and South America, *Leishmania tropica,* the causative organism of cutaneous leishmaniasis in the Middle East, and *Leishmania braziliensis,* the causative organism of mucocutaneous leishmaniasis in South America, have many animal hosts including dogs, rodents and other wild animals. Man is infected following the bite or crushing against the skin of the sandfly arthropod vector which spreads the disease from animal to man (*see also* Chapters 4, 16 and 22).

Trypanosomiasis

The Rhodesian form of sleeping sickness is due to *Trypanosoma brucei rhodesiense* and occurs in East and Central Africa. This type rather than the Gambiense form of sleeping sickness is a zoonosis of antelopes, cattle and wild game in these endemic African areas and the disease is spread to man by a tsetse fly, *Glossina morsitans* (*see* Duggan, 1981).

Chagas' disease, due to *Trypanosoma cruzi*, occurs in Central and South America. The main animal reservoirs are wild armadillos and opossums but domestic guinea-pigs, dogs and cats can also become infected. The infection is spread from these animals to man by an arthropod vector, the reduviid triatomid cone-nosed bug (*see Fig. 21.2*), when the infected faeces of the bug are scratched into the skin or settle onto the conjunctiva or mucosae of the patient. Children living in poor homes in rural areas are particularly liable to acquire the infection, especially when houses are made of mud or straw which provide good breeding places for the triatomid bugs (*see* Chapter 18 and Duggan, 1981).

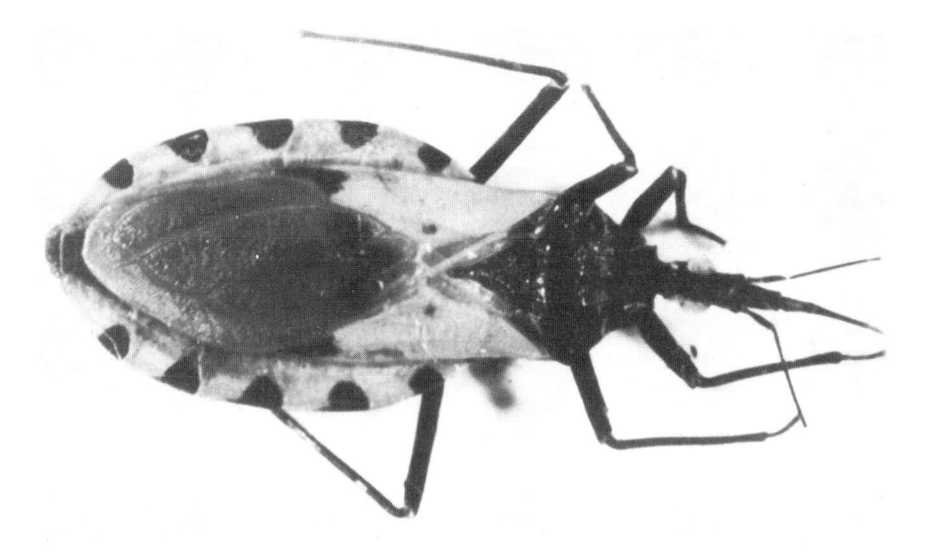

Fig. 21.2. Reduviid cone-nosed triatomid bug.

WORM ZOONOSES

Many worms which cause disease in man have vertebrate animals as the main definitive (sexual and adult stage of the worms life cycle) host and other animals as the intermediate hosts. Man is only incidentally infected. Examples include *Echinococcus granulosus,* the cause of hydatid disease with the adult worm mainly in dogs (*see Fig. 21.3*), *Trichinella spiralis,* the cause of trichinosis with the infected form in old pig meat (as in infected sausages), *Toxocara canis* or *catis* with the adult worm in the intestines of dogs and cats and *Fasciola hepatica* with the adult fluke in the hepato-biliary system of sheep (*see* Chapter 23).

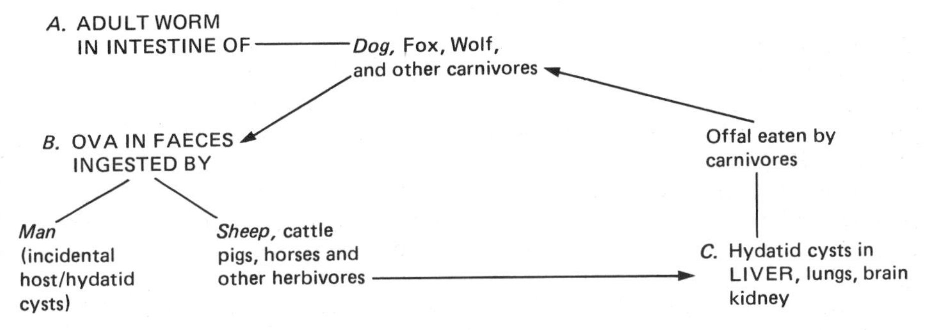

Fig. 21.3. Life cycle of *Echinococcus granulosus.*

Further Reading

Bisseru B. (1967) *Diseases of Man Acquired from His Pets.* London, Heinemann.
*Duggan A. J. (1981) The human trypanosomiases. *Medicine International* **1**, 162–164.
Leading Article (1978) Biological control of arthropods. *Lancet* **i**, 758.
Leading Article (1980) Perinatal Listeriosis. *Lancet* **i**, 911.
Leading Article (1981) Brucellosis. *Br. Med. J.* **282**, 1180.
Leading Article (1981) Toxoplasmosis. *Br. Med. J.* **282**, 249–250.
Vella E. E. (1981) Arbovirus in infections. *Medicine International* **1**, 149–152.
Willmott Sheila (ed.) (1978) *Medical Entomology Centenary.* London, Royal Society for Tropical Medicine and Hygiene.

See Further reading list for Chapters 22 and 23.

* Particularly recommended for further study by undergraduates.

Chapter 22

Arthropod-borne infections and viral haemorrhagic fevers

ARTHROPOD VECTORS OF INFECTIOUS DISEASE

In this section the role of arthropods in spreading both zoonoses and infectious diseases where man is the reservoir of the disease will be summarized.

There are different ways in which arthropod vectors can transmit infectious disease:

1. *Essential biological vectors*
   If the prevention of contact between the vector and man can be expected to totally interrupt the cycle of the spread of the disease to man, the vector role can be stated to be 'essential'. If the life cycle of the causative organism of the disease must continue by multiplication in the arthropod, then the vector is a 'biological' one. An example of an essential biological vector is the female anopheline mosquito which transmits the plasmodial protozoal organisms causing malaria. Another example is the tsetse fly which transmits trypanosomes in African sleeping sickness. There are numerous other examples.

2. *Non-essential biological vectors*
   There are relatively few examples of non-essential biological vectors; ticks which transmit *Coxiella burnetii*, the causative organism of Q fever, play a role in the transmission of organisms between animals but only rarely transmit the disease by biting man. Inhalation of infected dust or drinking infected milk are the usual means by which man acquires Q fever.

3. *Essential mechanical vectors*
   In bubonic plague, the bacillus, *Yersinia pestis*, is transmitted from rats to man by the rat flea *Xenopsylla cheopsis* which acts as an essential mechanical vector in spreading this disease. Another example is the body louse in the spread from man to man of relapsing fever due to the spirochaete *Borrelia recurrentis*. The disease may follow crushing the infected body louse against the skin.

4. *Non-essential mechanical vectors*
   Flies may help to spread enteric diseases such as typhoid and amoebic dysentery, especially in tropical areas with unhygienic circumstances by spreading faecal organisms to food and as there are other means by which these infections are spread by the faecal oral route, the flies are acting as non-essential mechanical vectors.

Horizontal and Vertical Transmission of Disease

The majority of infectious diseases are spread only by horizontal transmission, i.e. from one individual to another individual of a similar generation whether the individual is a person, an animal or an arthropod vector. Arthropod vectors usually contribute to the horizontal transmission of disease. However, a disease can occasionally also be spread by vertical transmission, from one generation to another, examples being hepatitis B in humans and there are several examples in arthropod vectors. In various mites and ticks, rickettsial organisms associated with scrub typhus or spotted fevers and *Borrelia duttoni*, the cause of tick-borne relapsing fever, can be transmitted through the ovaries to the next generation. When vertical transmission occurs, the vector may itself become a reservoir of the disease.

DISEASES TRANSMITTED BY ARTHROPOD VECTORS

A summary of the main diseases that may be spread by each arthropod vector is included in *Table 22.1*. Mosquitoes are particularly responsible for spreading life-threatening or serious debilitating diseases to many millions of people in the world each year and the incidence of many diseases, such as malaria (*see below*), dengue (*see below*) and filariasis (*see* Chapter 23), is increasing in many areas. Many different arbovirus (togavirus) infections and viral haemorrhagic fevers are spread by arthropod vectors and a few examples are discussed below (*see also* Vella, 1981). (*See also* Chapter 21.)

Control of Arthropod-borne Diseases

Elimination of the arthropod vectors, which are essential for the spread of the disease in a given area, would automatically result in the total eradication of the diseases from that area. In spite of early successes, there has been little lasting progress to eradicate important vectors, such as mosquito or tsetse fly, from major endemic tropical areas.

Vectors can often be controlled partially by draining swamps and other wet breeding grounds, and by insecticides. However, it is often politically or administratively impossible to remove all the breeding grounds and the emergence of vectors with resistance to insecticides, such as DDT, has impeded progress. Protection of the individual against arthropod bites by sleeping in mosquito nets and use of insect-repellant creams is often helpful.

ARTHROPOD-BORNE INFECTIONS IMPORTED INTO BRITAIN

The most common arthropod-borne infection imported into Britain is malaria. Visceral leishmaniasis is also occasionally recognized in patients who have travelled abroad. Other imported arthropod-borne infections are rarely seen in Britain (although there has been a small increase in the number of cases of dengue haemorrhagic fever diagnosed following visits to South East Asia). (*See also* Chapter 21.)

Table 22.1. Diseases spread by arthropod vectors

Arthropod vectors	*Diseases transmitted*	*Causative organisms of disease*	*Main reservoirs of diseases*	*Geographical distribution of diseases*
Mosquitoes				
Anopheles species (females transmit disease)	Malaria	*Plasmodia* species	Man	In warm areas of world between 60°N and 40°S in Asia, Africa and S. America
Aedes aegypti	Yellow fever (urban)	Yellow fever flavivirus	Man	Africa and S. America
Forest mosquitoes	Yellow fever (Z) (sylvan)		Monkeys	
Aedes aegypti	Dengue haemorrhagic fever	Dengue flavivirus	Man	Africa and Asia, especially S.E. Asia
Culex fatigans	Filariasis (elephantiasis)	*Wuchereria bancrofti* *Brugia malayi*	Man	Asia and S. America
Various mosquitoes transmitting arboviruses causing encephalitis	1. Eastern, Western and Venezuelan equine encephalitis (Z)	Equine encephalitis alphaviruses	Birds or small mammals (primary) Horses and man (secondary) in epidemics	Americas
	2. Japanese B encephalitis. St Louis encephalitis. Murray Valley encephalitis (Z)	Flaviviruses	Wild birds and small mammals	Japan America Australia
Other mosquitoes (*Aedes/Culex* species)	O'nyong-nyong (break-bone fever) Chikungunya haemorrhagic fever (Z)	Alphaviruses	? Wild birds and mammals	Africa
Sandfly (Phlebotomus)				
Sandfly	Leishmaniasis—visceral, cutaneous and muco-cutaneous (Z)	*Leishmania* species	Dogs, rodents and other wild animals	Mediterranean basin, Africa, Asia and S. America
	Sandfly fever (Z)	Arbovirus	? Rodents	Middle East

Table 22.1. (*Continued*) Diseases spread by arthropod vectors

Arthropod vectors	*Diseases transmitted*	*Causative organisms of disease*	*Main reservoirs of diseases*	*Geographical distribution of diseases*
Ticks				
Soft ticks (Argasidae family, *Ornithodorus* species)	African relapsing fever (Z)	*Borrelia duttoni*	Wild rodents, pigs and armadillos	Africa, Asia and Latin America
Hard ticks (Ixodidae family, *Dermacentor* species)	Tick-borne typhus, e.g. Rocky Mountain spotted fever (Z)	*Rickettsia rickettsii*	Wild rodents, domestic dogs and cats	U.S.A. and Latin America
	Louping-ill	Flavivirus	Sheep and cattle	Britain
	Tick-borne encephalitis	Flavivirus		U.S.A.
	Colorado tick fever	Arbovirus	Rabbits, squirrels, wild mammals (Colorado tick fever and Tularaemia)	North America
	Tularaemia	*Fransicella turalensis*		North America and Scandinavia
	Omsk haemorrhagic fever (Z)	*Flavivirus*	Muskrat	U.S.S.R.
Lice				
Pediculus humanus corporis (body louse)	Epidemic louse-borne typhus (and recrudescent Brill's disease)	*Rickettsia prowazeki*	Man	Africa, especially Ethiopia (historically wartime Europe)
	Louse-borne ('European') relapsing fever	*Borrelia recurrentis*	Man	Africa—today—especially Ethiopia
Fleas				
Rat flea, *Xenopsylla cheopsis*	Flea-borne typhus (murine typhus) (Z)	*Rickettsia mooseri (typhi)*	Rodents especially rats	North Africa and Italy
	Bubonic plague (Z)	*Yersinia pestis*	Rats	Asia—especially S.E. Asia and America
Mites				
Trombiculid mites	Scrub typhus (Z)	*Rickettsia tsutsugamushi*	Rodents	Asia—especially the Far East
	Rickettsial pox (Z)	*Rickettsia akari*	House mice	New York, U.S.A.
Other mites	Korean haemorrhagic fever (Z)	Unclassified arbovirus	Rodents	Asia and Northern Europe

Table 22.1. (Continued) Diseases spread by arthropod vectors

Arthropod vector	*Diseases transmitted*	*Causative organisms of diseases*	*Main reservoirs of diseases*	*Geographical distribution of diseases*
Tsetse fly *Glossina* species	African trypanosomiasis (rhodesiense—Z)	*Trypanosoma brucei rhodesiense*	Antelopes, wild game	Central and Eastern Africa
	(gambiense)	*Trypanosoma brucei gambiense*	Man	Central Africa
Reduviid triatomid bug	American trypanosomiasis (Chagas disease) (Z)	*Trypanosoma cruzi*	Armadillos, opossums, domestic cats and dogs	Central and South America
Simulium black fly	Onchocerciasis	*Onchocerca volvulus* (filarial worm)	Man	Africa and Latin America
Chrysops fly	Loiasis	*Loa loa* (filarial worm)	Man	W. Africa

NB (Z) = Zoonoses.

Malaria

Malaria is a common cause of death thoughout the tropics, especially in children. Adult inhabitants of endemic areas develop immunity to the malaria parasites but immigrants to Britain lose their immunity and may develop severe malaria on re-entering the area. The number of patients seen with malaria in Britain has greatly increased during recent years (mainly due to *P. vivax* and *P. falciparum*).

Causative organisms

Plasmodium vivax is the common cause of benign tertian malaria; *Plasmodium falciparum* causes malignant tertian malaria; *Plasmodium ovale* is an uncommon cause of benign tertian malaria and *Plasmodium malariae* causes quartan malaria.

Geographical distribution

Malaria due to *P. vivax* occurs mainly in the Indian subcontinent, Africa and parts of South East Asia. Malaria due to *P. falciparum* mainly occurs in Africa, South East Asia and Latin America. *P. ovale* malaria occasionally causes malaria in Africa. Quartan malaria is less common than malaria due to *P. vivax* or *P. falciparum*, but occurs throughout the tropical world.

Life cycle

All of the *Plasmodium* species have a sexual multiplication phase, sporogony, in the female anopheline mosquito and an asexual multiplication phase, schizogony, in man (*Fig. 22.1*). *P. vivax*, *P. ovale* and *P. malariae* have subsequent exo-erythrocytic cycles in the liver; relapses up to many months and, occasionally, up to a few years may occur after the initial illness. *P. malariae* may cause relapses of malaria up to 30 years later. The periodicity of schizogony determines the pattern of pyrexia and other symptoms in man.

Incubation period

Eight to sixteen days, although it may be up to 30 days for *P. malariae.*

Main clinical features

Headaches, back and limb aches. Fever is at first often irregular but subsequently with characteristic tertian (every 48 hours) or quartan (every 72 hours) periodicity (*see* p. 76 of Chapter 4). Some patients may never develop the characteristic malaria patterns of fever, especially cases of falciparum malaria. Rigors occurring on every second or third day are typical. Malaria should always be suspected in any person who has a fever who has recently travelled to a malarial area. Gastro-intestinal symptoms, including vomiting, abdominal pain and diarrhoea and mental confusion are frequently present in falciparum malaria. Some patients with chronic malaria have marked splenomegaly.

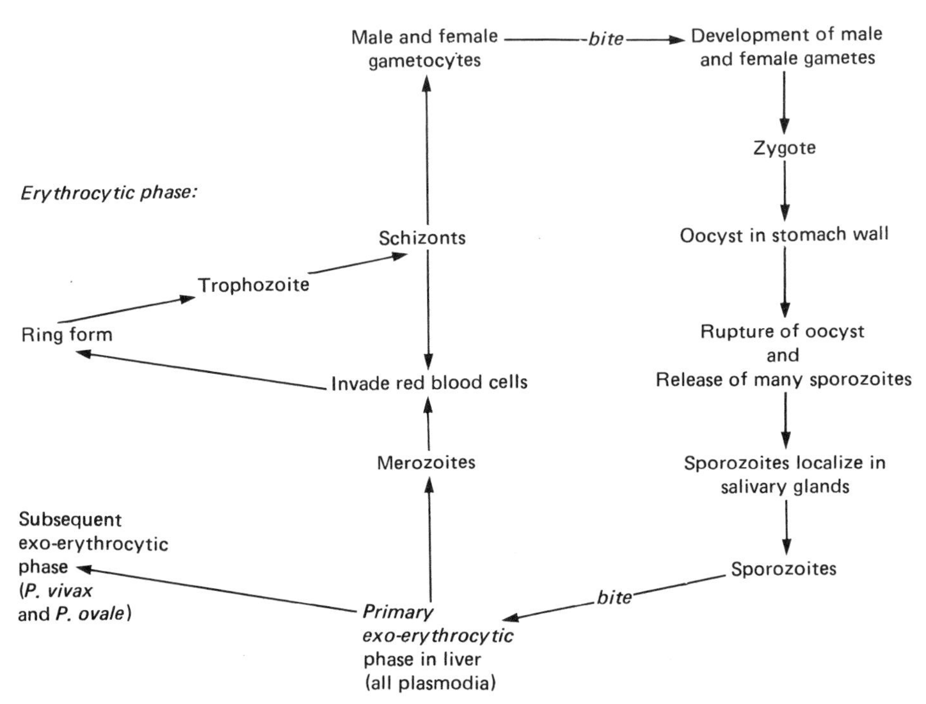

Fig. 22.1. Life cycle of malarial parasite.

Complications

Falciparum malaria can especially cause serious complications and is often rapidly fatal unless recognized and treated promptly. These complications include:

a. Cerebral malaria, manifested by impaired consciousness due to capillary occlusion with many parasitized red cells.

b. Renal failure, sometimes following hypotension.

c. Blackwater fever—haemoglobinuria, following intravascular haemolysis especially after the start of quinine treatment.

d. Disseminated intravascular coagulation has recently been reported.

Falciparum and other forms of malaria may be complicated by the development of severe anaemia and impairment of liver function. An important complication of quartan malaria is the nephrotic syndrome which results from glomerulonephritis associated with the deposition of immune complexes in the basement membrane.

Diagnosis

Thick and thin blood films from blood should be collected as the temperature is rising and stained at pH 7·2 by Giemsa or Leishman stains. The thick films are particularly valuable when relatively few parasites are apparent in the blood. Repeated films may be necessary. The species of *Plasmodium* is usually apparent from examination of the thin blood films (*see Fig. 22.2*). Serology, using a fluorescent antibody test, is usually not useful for an individual ill patient but is valuable in epidemiological surveys. Help in diagnosis and speciation can be obtained from a reference centre such as at the Hospital for Tropical Diseases in London.

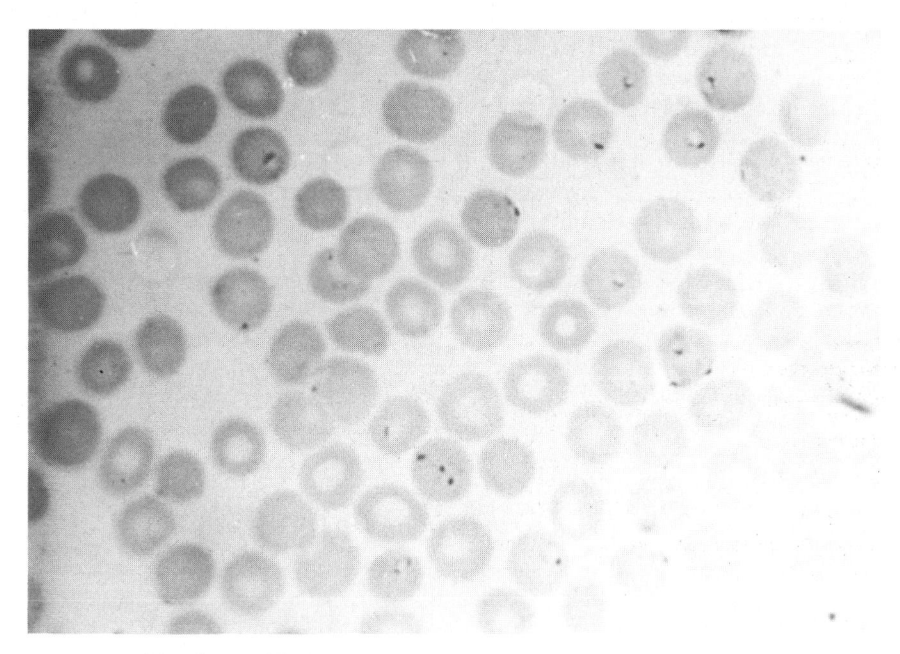

Fig. 22.2. Ring forms of *P. falciparum* malarial parasite in a Leishman stained blood film.

Treatment

Falciparum malaria in patients from Africa, and vivax, ovale and quartan malaria responds to chloroquine in adults. Six hundred mg base orally, followed by 300 mg after 6 hours and further daily doses of 300 mg base on the two subsequent days. Severe cases of malaria, especially when 40% or more of the red cells in the blood film have parasites, require a different dosage of chloroquine given parenterally. Primaquine is required to treat or prevent relapsing vivax malaria by eradicating the exo-erythrocytic phase in the liver but only after glucose-6-phosphate dehydrogenase deficiency has been excluded, otherwise drug-induced haemolytic anaemia may develop. Proguanil may also be used prophylactically to prevent relapse of vivax malaria after treating the first attack with chloroquine.

Chloroquine-resistant strains of *P. falciparum* occur in South East Asia and South America. Patients with falciparum malaria from these areas may need treatment with quinine followed by a combination of sulphadoxine and pyrimethamine (Fansidar). During treatment, repeated blood films are required to check that elimination of the parasites is proceeding satisfactorily. Quinine is also recommended rather than chloroquine for the parenteral treatment of cerebral malaria.

Prevention

Eradication of the anopheline mosquito vectors by draining swamps and other breeding grounds of the mosquito and the use of insecticides has been partially successful in some areas. The avoidance of mosquito bites by sleeping in nets and the use of insect cream repellants may help to prevent the disease, but the only reliable means of prevention for visitors to endemic areas is to take proper chemoprophylaxis. The first two doses of prophylactic drug should be taken before entering the malarial area, with the second dose taken on the day that travel abroad occurs. Therapy should be continued while in the area and for 4 weeks after returning from abroad. A combination of pyrimethamine and dapsone (Maloprim), one tablet weekly, provides suitable prophylaxis against the erythrocytic phase for all the plasmodia except some chloroquine-resistant strains of *P. falciparum* in South America and South East Asia. In the latter situations, prophylaxis with Fansidar, two tablets every 2 weeks, is recommended. Up-to-date expert advice on the best prophylaxis for each area is available at Tropical Disease Hospitals.

Visceral Leishmaniasis (Kala-azar)

Causative organism

Leishmania donovani is a flagellated protozoa in the sandfly and a non-flagellated (amastigote) intracellular organism in the cytoplasm of the reticulo-endothelial cells in man. The oval nucleated amastigotes within the bone marrow, liver, spleen or lymph node cells are known as Leishman-Donovan (LD) bodies.

Geographical distribution

Countries around the Mediterranean including Southern Spain, Southern Italy, Yugoslavia, Greece, Turkey, the Middle Eastern countries, North, East and West Africa, the Sudan, Latin America, India and China.

Life cycle

Dogs are the main reservoir of infection in many Mediterranean countries but man may be the principal reservoir in parts of India. The female sandfly is an essential biological vector transmitting the protozoa to other animals and to man as an incidental host.

Incubation period

Usually 1–3 months, but up to 10 years is possible.

Main clinical features

In many countries, children are particularly affected and adults in endemic areas may have developed considerable immunity to *Leishmania*. Fever is a prominent clinical feature and the patient may often present as a case of PUO (*see* Chapter 4). The illness may have either a gradual or a sudden onset and usually a high intermittent fever develops, sometimes associated with a double notched daily pyrexia on the temperature chart. Within a few weeks hepato-splenomegaly usually develops and occasionally lymphadenopathy also. In chronic cases, the spleen greatly enlarges. Anaemia is present and, characteristically, there is marked neutropenia.

Complications

Severe anaemia, loss of weight and pigmentation of the skin, particularly on the face, may occur. There is a high mortality rate in some areas.

Diagnosis

The serum immunoglobulins are considerably raised when electrophoresis is carried out, especially the IgM fraction. In the past, this was demonstrable by the positive formol-gel test. Direct demonstration of intracellular LD bodies in the macrophages or other reticulo-endothelial cells of a bone marrow biopsy, stained by Leishman or Giemsa stains, is the main method of specific diagnosis. Occasionally the latter biopsy is negative and then liver, lymph node or spleen biopsy may be positive. Splenic biopsy may not be justified in many patients and, if the other biopsies are negative, a serological diagnosis may have to be relied on. In the past, a leishmania CFT test was done but now a serum leishmania immunofluorescent antibody test has replaced this and shows high titres in most patients with kala-azar. Although not often carried out, it is sometimes possible to culture the leishmania protozoa from bone marrow aspirate using NNN medium.

Treatment

Pentavalent antimony compounds, such as sodium stibogluconate, are usually effective given parenterally. Patients from some countries, such as the Sudan, may not respond so well to these compounds and diamidine compounds such as 2-hydroxystilbamidine or pentamidine may be preferred.

Prevention

Infected animal reservoirs and sandflies should be eliminated where possible. Breeding places of sandflies include old buildings and high rocky rural areas where there are shady crevices. Development of modern city areas is associated with a reduction in the breeding places. Insecticide-impregnated mosquito nets will help to prevent contact with sandflies during sleep when the risk is greatest.

VIRAL HAEMORRHAGIC FEVERS

Examples of arthropod-borne viral haemorrhagic fevers include the *mosquito-borne* diseases yellow-fever, dengue haemorrhagic fever and chikungunya

(*Table 22.1*), *tick-borne* diseases such as Omsk haemorrhagic fever (*Table 22.1*) and mite-borne diseases such as Korean haemorrhagic fever (*Table 22.1*). Tick-borne viral haemorrhagic fevers are particularly prevalent in parts of the U.S.S.R. and Eastern Europe, but patients with these diseases are rarely seen in Britain.

Rodent-associated viral haemorrhagic fevers, such as Lassa fever, have gained much publicity in recent years but are exceedingly rarely imported into Britain. Suspected cases must be transferred to an appropriate isolation unit under the supervision of the 'Proper Officer' (*see below*).

Yellow Fever

Yellow fever is notifiable under the International Sanitary Regulations.

Organism

Arbovirus of yellow fever, a flavivirus, is of one major antigenic type only, so that solid immunity occurs after an infection.

Geographical distribution

Yellow fever is particularly endemic in Western and Central Africa and may also occur in the jungles of South America.

Life cycle

In urban areas, man is the main reservoir of infection and *Aedes aegypti* mosquitoes transmit the virus from person to person. Man is also liable to acquire infection when felling trees in jungle areas where monkeys are the main reservoir. Various mosquitoes in the tree tops spread the virus from monkey to monkey but can also incidentally infect man (*see* also Chapter 21). The virus causes lesions mainly in the liver and kidney although many organs may be affected by haemorrhages.

Incubation period

Three to six days.

Main clinical features

In endemic areas, mild infection is frequent with fever, proteinuria, leucopenia and sometimes jaundice, without any complications. Sometimes a severe form of the disease occurs in which there are certain distinct stages. Complications may be fatal. In the initial stages, there is fever of sudden onset which accompanies the maximum period of virus multiplication; this is often manifest by headache, bone pains, backaches and conjunctival injection. The fever is characteristically accompanied by severe bradycardia and proteinuria and lasts for 3–4 days. There then follows a 'calm' second stage for less than a day. Finally, a third 'intoxication' stage starts which is characterized by the development of severe jaundice and haemorrhages into the alimentary tract and skin.

Complications

Severe acute hepatic and renal damage (including acute tubular necrosis) and large haemorrhages from organs contribute to death occurring during the 'intoxication' stage within 2 weeks of the onset of illness. Survivors eventually recover completely from the damage to the various organs.

Diagnosis

Essentially, the diagnosis is a clinical one during the acute stages since virology results are usually of retrospective value. The virus can be isolated from the blood using tissue culture. Post-mortem confirmation of the diagnosis is obtained by histology of a liver biopsy which shows severe mid-zonal degenerative changes and acidophilic 'Councilman bodies' in degenerated parenchymal cells.

Treatment

No specific effective anti-viral treatment is available.

Prevention

Yellow fever vaccine using the live attenuated 17D strain gives lasting immunity for more than 10 years and a valid certificate of vaccination is essential for travellers to endemic areas. Also, great precautions are necessary to prevent spread of the disease to countries which have suitable mosquito vectors but which are free of the disease, especially in Asia. Travellers from endemic areas to these countries must have valid vaccination certificates and rigorous anti-mosquito measures, including the use of insecticides, are enforced at the appropriate airports. Urban yellow fever can be prevented by eradicating moist breeding places for mosquitoes.

Dengue Haemorrhagic Fever

Causative organism

Dengue virus is a flavivirus (with four major antigenic sub-types).

Geographical distribution

Dengue is an increasingly common menace in South East Asia and the Pacific Islands, but is also endemic in parts of India and the Caribbean. Coastal tropical regions, where there are numerous aedes mosquitoes, are particularly affected.

Life cycle

Man is the main reservoir of the infection and the *Aedes aegypti* mosquito is the principal arthropod vector.

Incubation period

Between 4 and 8 days.

Main clinical features

Mild infections where there is malaise followed by a febrile illness lasting for a few days only are common in endemic areas. More severe forms of the disease are characterized by marked fever, generalized aches, especially around joints, painful eye movements and conjunctival injection, nausea and vomiting and mental depression. After about 3 days, a brief afebrile period occurs for 14–48 hours followed by recurrence of fever. During the second bout of pyrexia, a diffuse maculo-papular rash may occur which is particularly prominent on the legs and arms. Prolonged prostration and depression may occur during the convalescent period.

Complications

Death is rare except in young children who may suffer 'dengue haemorrhage shock syndrome'. This syndrome is probably due to a hypersensitivity phenomenon when a child with immunity to one sub-type of dengue virus is infected by another sub-type of the virus and immune complexes are deposited which result in severe haemorrhage and shock.

Treatment

No specific treatment is available.

Prevention

Breeding places for aedes mosquitoes need to be eradicated, especially in South East Asia where repeated epidemics of the disease have occurred in recent years. Sleeping in mosquito nets is recommended in endemic areas.

Lassa Fever, Marburg Disease, Ebola Disease

The possibility of viral haemorrhagic fevers must always be considered in patients with unexplained fevers, who have entered the country from Africa during the previous 3 weeks. However, malaria is a common cause of such fevers, whereas Lassa fever and the other viral haemorrhagic fevers are rare.

Lassa Fever

Lassa fever has been acquired by small numbers of hospital staff attending patients with the disease. There has been much publicity about outbreaks of the disease as there is sometimes a high mortality rate.

Organism

The Lassa fever virus is an arenavirus and is not transmitted by arthropod vectors.

Geographical distribution

The disease was first described in patients from Lassa, in Nigeria, in 1969. Since then it has occurred in patients in various Western and Central African countries including Sierra Leone and Liberia. People living in rural areas are more likely to acquire the disease than those living in towns.

Life cycle

The main reservoir of infection is the multimammate rat, *Mastomys natalensis*. The Lassa fever virus is excreted in the urine and saliva of infected rats and these possibly contaminate water which subsequently may infect man. The virus is present in excreta and blood of infected patients and man-to-man transmission can occur.

Incubation period

Seven to seventeen days.

Main clinical features

In endemic areas, many patients have mild febrile illness only, but, in some outbreaks, there is a high incidence of serious disease with mortality rates of up to 40%. Characteristically, patients with severe disease have persistent fever, pharyngitis with whitish-yellow tonsillar exudates, myalgia, gastro-intestinal symptoms, extreme lethargy and leucopenia during the first week of illness. A maculo-papular rash may also occur. During the second week of illness, complications may occur which can lead rapidly to death.

Complications

Encephalopathy, hypotensive shock leading to oliguria or cardiac failure are frequent complications. Haemorrhages into skin and organs may also occur. Death usually occurs on about the tenth day and is more frequent in pregnant or post-partum women. Visitors from developed countries or from large cities in Africa who have not had any previous contact with the virus are probably more likely to develop serious complications than the local inhabitants of endemic areas.

Diagnosis

The virus can be isolated from blood, throat washings, urine and pleural fluid using vero monkey tissue culture or rat inoculation methods. In Britain, all specimens must be collected with extreme care, under supervision by the Medical Officer for Environmental Health (MOEH) and high security transportation to the Microbiological Research Establishment at Porton Down is necessary where there are special diagnostic facilities. Paired sera for specific Lassa fever antibodies should also be collected. All patients will also need blood films examined for malaria and blood cultures taken for diagnosing a possible bacterial septicaemia, such as typhoid.

Treatment

Most patients should be given antimalarial treatment as death is more likely from *P. falciparum* infection in patients from Africa than from Lassa fever. In suspicious cases, help should always be sought in diagnosis and treatment from recognized reference centres (*see* D.H.S.S. memoranda on Lassa fever, 1976). A convalescent serum from survivors of Lassa fever has probably beneficial effects when administered early enough to patients suffering from Lassa fever.

Prevention

The Medical Officer for Environmental Health should be contacted immediately a case of Lassa fever is clinically suspected. All cases should be strictly isolated until they can be moved to recognized high security isolation hospital units and contacts require careful surveillance.

Marburg Disease

In 1967, laboratory staff in Marburg, Frankfurt and Belgrade acquired a serious viral infection from handling blood or tissues of a contaminated batch of imported African green monkeys and there was a 23% mortality rate. Since then no other outbreaks have occurred, but a tourist who had travelled in Central and Southern Africa died from the disease in 1975. Two contacts of this tourist, including a nurse who attended him in hospital, contracted the disease but survived.

Organism

The causative RNA virus of Marburg disease has a distinctive long filamentous shape with hooked ends.

Geographical distribution

Probably Central and Southern Africa.

Life cycle

Although monkeys were suggested as the reservoir in the original outbreak, it is possible that they contracted their infection from other animals during the journey from Africa. No definite animal reservoir of the disease is known and the life cycle of the organism remains unclear.

Incubation period

Probably between 3 and 10 days.

Main clinical features

There is an initial non-specific febrile illness with malaise, headache, myalgia and leucopenia but the maculo-papular rash with widespread erythema appearing on the fifth or sixth day is characteristic of the disease. Some patients develop marked central nervous system symptoms, gastro-intestinal symptoms and haemorrhagic complications.

Complications

Alimentary tract and urinary tract haemorrhages frequently occur. Shock, hepatitis and renal failure may also develop.

Diagnosis

The virus can be isolated by injecting clinical specimens into guinea-pigs. The same care in the collection and transport of specimens is required as mentioned for Lassa fever.

Treatment and prevention

Similar approach to that described for Lassa fever.

Ebola Disease

Outbreaks of a Marburg-like illness affected hundreds of people in equatorial Sudan and Zaire in 1976 and this illness was due to a virus similar to the Marburg disease virus. The causative virus was sufficiently different from the Marburg disease virus to justify another name—Ebola virus.

Life cycle

Man-to-man transmission occurs in circumstances of close contact.

Incubation period

Usually about a week, but 4–16 days is possible.

Main clinical features

Similar to Marburg disease except that arthralgia and watery diarrhoea accompany the headaches. Fever and lethargy are particularly prominent features. Chest pain and a measles-like rash also develop in most patients.

Complications

Bleeding into the arms, legs, alimentary tract and uro-genital tract commonly occurs. Many patients, especially adults, die of the disease after about 1 week of the illness.

Diagnosis, treatment and prevention

Similar to Lassa fever and Marburg disease.

Further Reading

D.H.S.S. and the Welsh Office (1976) *Memorandum on Lassa Fever*. London, H.M.S.O.

Gillies H. M. (1978) Exotic viral diseases; Marburg virus disease; Ebola virus disease; Lassa fever. *Medicine*, 3rd series, 7, 316.

*Gillies H. M. (1981) Malaria. *Medicine International* **1**, 153–156.

Leading Article (1981) Yellow fever: cause for concern? *Br. Med. J.* **282**, 1735.

*Manson-Bahr P. E. C. (1981) Leishmaniasis. *Medicine International* **1**, 165–169.

Peters W. and Gillies H. M. (1977) *A Colour Atlas of Tropical Medicine and Parasitology*. London, Wolfe Medical Publications.

Vella E. E. (1981) Viral haemorrhagic fever. *Medicine International* **1**, 147–148.

Wilson C. and Manson-Bahr P. E. (1972) *Manson's Tropical Diseases*. London, Ballière Tindall.

*Wright S. G. (1979) Malaria. *Hospital Update* **5**, 309.

* Particularly recommended for further study by undergraduates.

Chapter 23

Worms (helminths)

Many millions of people in the world suffer from serious disease associated with important worm infestations, such as schistosomiasis or hookworm; others have minor symptoms associated with common worm infestations, such as threadworms; many people have asymptomatic infestations due to such worms as whipworms.

The development of disease and its seriousness depends not only on the type of worm, but also on the intensity of infection, the exact sites of infection and the patient's reaction to the infection. Heavy infestations with hookworms, whipworms or onchocerca are more likely to be associated with clinically serious or significant disease than light infestations. *Ascaris lumbricoides* or *Taenia solium* can cause serious disease if biliary tract infection or infection of the brain (cysticercosis) occurs, respectively. Strongyloidiasis can be disseminated and fatal in a patient with an impaired immunological reaction as in an immunosuppressed patient with Hodgkin's disease.

The brief notes that follow summarize the main features of worms which may cause clinical problems in patients living in Britain or arriving from overseas. It should be remembered that simultaneous multiple infestations with different worms often occurs.

CESTODES (TAPEWORMS)

Taenia saginata

The tapeworm *Taenia saginata* is the commonest tapeworm and the adult worm may reach up to 30 feet in length in the small intestine of man. Asymptomatic infestation is common but minor abdominal symptoms including mild discomfort, diarrhoea or vomiting sometimes occurs. Often the passing of a wriggling mature segment through the anus into the toilet is the main complaint.

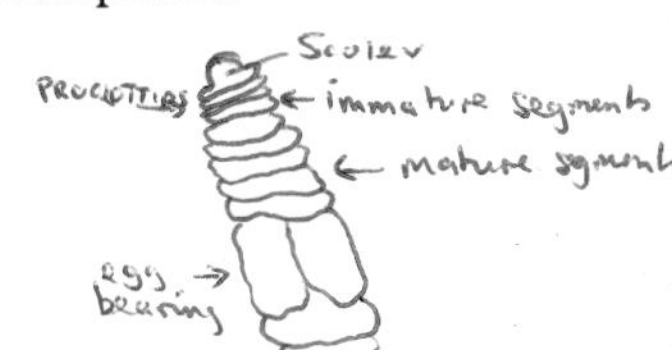

Geographical distribution

Worldwide but especially in Africa and the Middle East.

Life cycle

Man, the definitive host of the worm, eats undercooked beef containing the cysticercus (larval stage). An adult worm develops in the man's intestine and the sexual phase of the life cycle is completed there, ova in the faeces of man are swallowed by the cow which is the worm's intermediate host. The asexual multiplication phase of the life cycle is completed in the cow and the cysticercus is found in its flesh.

Complications
None as a rule.

Diagnosis
Examination of a mature segment (proglottid) shows numerous lateral branches of the uterus which helps to differentiate it from *Taenia solium* which has less uterine branches. Microscopy of a wet preparation of faeces may reveal characteristic cystic ova of *Taenia* species.

Treatment
Niclosamide ('Yomesan'), two 0·5-g tablets on an empty stomach, repeated after 1 hour. Two hours later a saline purge expels the complete worm. See patient again and re-examine faeces 3 months later.

Prevention
Inspection of meat to detect cysts and adequate cooking of beef.

Taenia solium
The *Taenia solium* tapeworm is long, with a multi-segmented ribbon shape similar to *Taenia saginata*, but the scolex (head) of *Taenia solium* is characterized by a ring of hooks which are used for attachment to the intestine. There may be no symptoms or mild clinical problems, as with *Taenia saginata*, including a history of passing segments in the faeces. Infestation by *Taenia solium* is potentially far more serious than that by *Taenia saginata*, because of the possible complication of human cystercercosis. Fever, headache and eosinophilia may occur during human cysticercosis.

Geographical distribution
Similar to *Taenia saginata. Taenia solium* is virtually never acquired in Britain.

Life cycle
Man becomes infected by eating undercooked 'measly pork' containing the cysticercus stage. Life cycle is usually between man as the definitive host, with the adult worm in the intestine, and the pig as the intermediate host, similar otherwise to that of *Taenia saginata*.

Occasionally autoinfection in man may also occur, when the ova are released in the upper intestine during regurgitation, sometimes following treatment, or are ingested, and the cysticercosis stage develops in man.

Complications
Human cysticercosis can result in cysts in the brain, causing epilepsy or fatal encephalopathy, and cysts in muscle, eye, liver, lung or other sites.

Diagnosis

Similar to *Taenia saginata*. Human cysticercosis may be demonstrated by X-rays showing calcified cysts and by radioactive gold scans. A taenia complement fixation test to detect antibodies in the serum may become strongly positive in cysticercosis (performed at the Hospital for Tropical Diseases, London).

Treatment

As for *Taenia saginata* but an anti-emetic is recommended to be given in conjunction with the niclosamide.

Prevention

Inspection of pork and adequate cooking.

Diphyllobothrium latum

Multiple infestation by the adult worms in the jejunum of man may occur unlike the other two long tapeworms affecting man described above.

Geographical distribution

Scandinavia mainly but also the Middle East and Africa.

Life cycle

Man becomes infected by eating undercooked infected fish. The adult worm in man's intestine excretes ova in human faeces which contaminate water. Ova develop into larvae in water which infect the crustacean cyclops (first intermediate host). Cyclops are eaten by fish (second intermediate host) where subsequent development of larvae occurs that finally becomes infective for man.

Complications

Macrocytic anaemia characteristically may occur which disappears on expulsion of the worms and may respond to vitamin B_{12} and folic acid therapy.

Diagnosis

Similar to *Taenia*.

Treatment

Niclosamide, similar to *Taenia saginata*.

Prevention

Adequate cooking of fish.

Hymenolepis nana

Dwarf tapeworm, only 1–3 cm long, in intestine of man. Abdominal symptoms including diarrhoea and pain may occur in children especially when there are heavy multiple infestations.

Geographical distribution

Worldwide.

Life cycle

Ova from faeces of other infected humans or rats pollute water or food which is swallowed by new human host. Ova develop into embryos in internal wall which develop into adult worms in small intestine.

Complications

Convulsions and other neurological complications may occur.

Diagnosis

Microscopy of human faeces may reveal the characteristic ova.

Treatment

Niclosamide, repeated course, is also given 3 weeks later. Heavy or 'resistant' infestations may require treatment with hexylresorcinol. Follow-up 3 months and 1 year later possibly repeating treatment at these times.

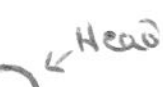

Echinococcus granulosus

Man is incidentally infected when he develops hydatid disease; the infestation is an example of a zoonosis (*see* Chapter 21, and *Fig. 21.3*). The symptoms in man arise from the presence of the hydatid cysts.

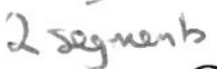

Geographical distribution

Worldwide but particularly in sheep-rearing areas in Mediterranean countries such as Greece, North Africa, Australia and New Zealand. In Britain the infection is more common in Wales.

Life cycle

The adult worm, only a few millimetres long, is present in the intestine of dogs mainly, and the ova excreted in dog faeces are usually swallowed by sheep which become the intermediate host as the larvae emerge and develop into hydatid cysts in the liver and other organs. Offal of the sheep is eaten by dogs. Man is an incidental intermediate host infested by close contact with infected dogs.

When the ovum is ingested by the intermediate host the six-hook embryo develops, penetrates the stomach wall and enters the portal vascular circulation to reach the liver where hydatid cysts form. Hydatid cysts may also develop in any part of the body after the embryos enter the blood but, after the liver, the most common sites are lungs, brain and kidney. Each hydatid cyst has a germinal internal layer from which brood capsules develop into new scolices and daughter cysts.

Complications

Hydatid cysts in the liver, lungs, brain, bone or kidney may cause serious local complications from pressure, inflammation associated with hypersensitivity reactions and secondary infection, occasionally resulting in death. (*See* Liver Abscess in Chapter 15.)

Diagnosis

Radiographs may reveal calcification in cyst walls and scans or ultrasound may also help to reveal the presence of cysts in the liver or other sites. The hydatid CFT may be positive in some patients (carried out at a reference laboratory) and then the Casoni skin test is unnecessary. The fluid contents of a hydatid cyst are normally clear and colourless but 'hydatid sand', consisting of diagnostic scolices with hooklets, is apparent on microscopy.

Treatment

Surgical excision of cysts is occasionally necessary when there are local obstructions or abscess complications. Rupture of a cyst must be guarded against to avoid immediate hypersensitivity reactions including possibly fatal anaphylaxis and also to prevent secondary seeding of daughter cysts. There are no satisfactory drugs.

Prevention

Hot water cleaning of feeding utensils and of floors, possibly contaminated by ova from dogs, and good hand washing and food hygiene may help to reduce infection in an endemic area. Eradication of infected dogs, sheep and other animals may eventually reduce the incidence of hydatid disease in affected areas.

NEMATODES (ROUNDWORMS)

Ascaris lumbricoides

The common roundworm, *Ascaris lumbricoides*, is between 10 and 30 cm long, of cylindrical shape with tapering extremities (*Fig. 23.1*). Patients may have few or no symptoms if the infestation is light except for the passing of the worm in the faeces. Numerous complications may develop when there are large numbers of worms present, especially in children.

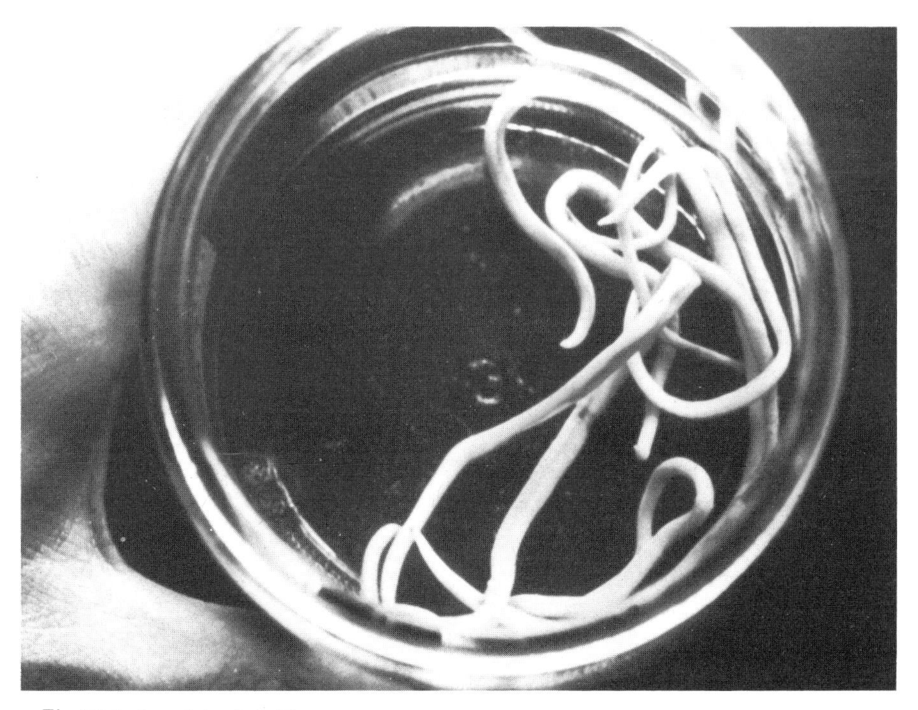

Fig. 23.1. Ascaris lumbricoides.

Geographical distribution

Worldwide, but in the tropics affecting particularly children 3–8 years old.

Life cycle

Man infected by swallowing ova in food or drink or from contaminated hands. Larvae develop from the ova in the small intestine and penetrate blood and lymphatics to reach the lungs where pneumonitis may occur 4–16 days after infection. The larvae then migrate via the bronchioles to the trachea and pharynx and descend the oesophagus to reach the small intestine where they develop into adult worms. The worms excrete ova which are not initially infective in the faeces, but the ova become infective with larvae developing inside while in the soil or other contaminated environmental sites. The faeces may contaminate water or foods, such as vegetables, especially when human faeces have been used for manure.

Complications

1. Pneumonitis during the larval migration stage is characterized by cough, dyspnoea, fever and eosinophilia.
2. Intestinal obstruction caused by a bolus of adult worms may occur, or worms can obstruct the bile duct or pancreatic duct causing cholangitis or pancreatitis when there is heavy infestation. Rarely a worm can

migrate into the gall bladder, liver, eustachian tube, paranasal sinuses or the heart with secondary pyogenic infection possibly occurring at each site.

3. Malnutrition and malabsorption present in some children in the tropics may become worsened when there is a heavy ascaris infestation.

Diagnosis

Microscopy of faeces usually shows the characteristic ascaris ova, either on direct examination or after concentration technique. Three specimens of faeces collected on different days may require examination as with other parasitological investigations of faeces. The adult worm is occasionally passed in faeces or vomit or occurs at an unusual site during surgery. Rarely larvae may be seen in the sputum when pneumonitis occurs.

Treatment

Piperazine salts. Piperazine citrate elixir syrup is effective as a single oral dose given up to a maximum of 4 g with the evening meal. The muscles of the ascaris worms are paralysed and the worms are expelled by peristalsis.

Prevention

Hygienic handling of food and drink, separation of sewage from water supplies in underdeveloped countries and avoidance of use of human faeces for agriculture, and adequate washing and cooking of food.

Enterobius vermicularis (Oxyuris vermicularis)

Infestation by the thread or pin worm *Enterobius vermicularis*, which is only about 1 cm long, is very common, particularly in children. Pruritus is the predominant symptom.

Geographical distribution

Worldwide including Britain.

Life cycle

The complete cycle occurs in man. Ova from contaminated hands, food or drink are swallowed and develop into adult worms in the intestine. The male and female worms mate and the male then dies. The gravid female worms emerge from the anus at night to deposit eggs on the peri-anal skin which causes irritation and insomnia. A cycle of autoinfection may persist when the ova-containing larvae are transferred to the mouth by the fingers. The ova may spread from the contaminated fingers to other children or adults in a family or institution and can occasionally be spread by contaminated bed linen, clothes or dust.

Complications

Secondary infection of peri-anal dermatitis, which results from scratching, may occur.

Diagnosis

Sometimes the patient notices the small white threadworms in the faeces. The most reliable means of diagnosis is to place a strip of Sellotape to the peri-anal skin during the night, remove it the next morning and place it on a glass slide. Microscopy then reveals the characteristic bean-shaped enterobius eggs adherent to the tape (*Fig. 23.2*). Occasionally the worms or ova are seen during microscopy of faeces or of surgical samples of the caecum, appendix or rectum.

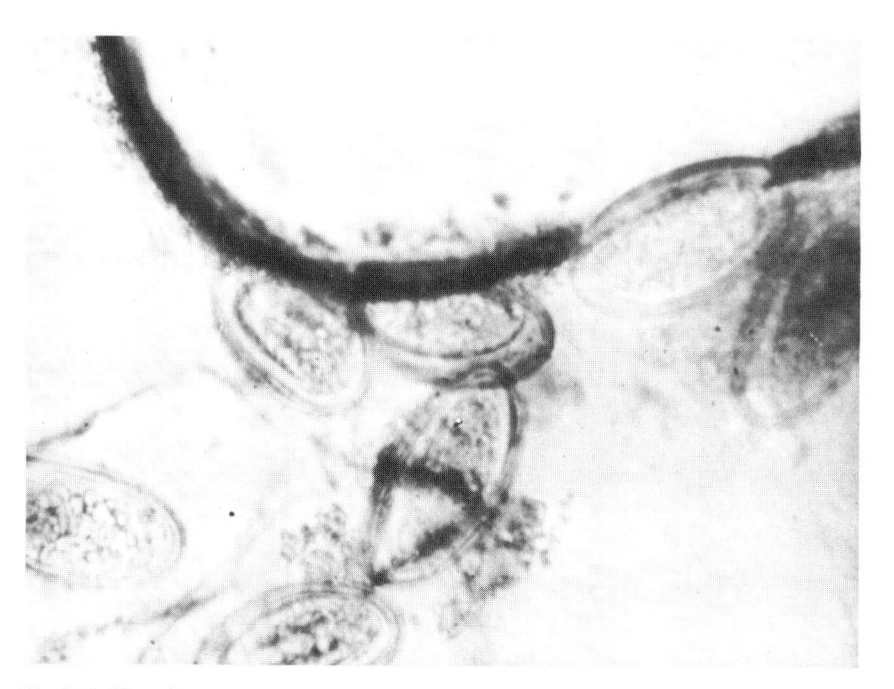

Fig. 23.2. Threadworm ova attached to a Sellotape strip.

Treatment

Piperazine salts. The usual dosage is 2 g daily in divided doses for 1 week but 2 weeks' treatment is occasionally necessary. Treatment of each member of a family at the same time is often indicated. An alternative drug which is also effective is viprynium embonate (Vanquin).

Thorough hand washing after defaecation and before eating, and keeping the nails cut short, are important hygienic measures needed to break the cycle of infection at the same time and following drug treatment.

Prevention

Good personal hygiene and regular laundering of bedlinen, clothes, etc. reduces the chances of acquiring threadworm infestation.

Hookworms—Ancylostoma duodenale and Necator americanus

Hookworm infestation is a common cause of iron deficiency anaemia and oedema in tropical and sub-tropical countries. Each adult hookworm is about 1 cm long and attachment to the small intestine in man may result in the loss of about 0·05 ml blood daily. When there are heavy worm infestations, severe anaemia may result.

Geographical distribution

In the past *Necator americanus* mainly occurred in Latin America and tropical Africa and *Ancylostoma duodenale* was particularly found in India, Ceylon and Africa, but today both types of hookworm are distributed throughout tropical and subtropical countries.

Life cycle

Adult hookworms in small intestine of man. Ova in human faeces develop into infective larvae in soil or contaminated water. Larvae penetrate human skin, usually via the feet, invade the blood, and migrate via lungs and trachea to reach the oesophagus. They then descend to the intestine where they develop into adult worms.

Complications

Chronic anaemia is the main complication which can lead to heart failure. Hypoalbuminaemia as well as iron deficiency may occur in heavy infestations which can cause generalized oedema. When the pulmonary larval stage occurs, some pneumonitis and eosinophilia might occur.

Diagnosis

The diagnosis is confirmed by finding the characteristic ova in the faeces; formol ether concentration techniques may be necessary. Large numbers of ova are usually present when anaemia is due to hookworm infestation.

Treatment

Tetrachlorethylene was widely used in the past and is effective for treating both types of hookworm. However, a disadvantage of this drug is that it may stimulate ascaris worms, which may also be present, to group together and cause intestinal obstruction. If this drug is used, ascaris infestation needs prior treatment. Bephenium hydroxynaphthoate is effective for treating *Ancylostoma duodenale* only. Thiabenzadole is effective for treating both *Ancylostoma duodenale* and *Necator americanus*, and is given orally, 25 mg per kg up to a maximum dose of 3 g on each day for 3 days.

Prevention

Wearing of shoes is desirable when walking on potentially infested soils in warm underdeveloped countries in endemic areas.

Strongyloides stercoralis

Strongyloidiasis affected many troops serving in the Far East during the Second World War. Many ex-Japanese prisoners of war still suffer from recurrent skin lesions and other effects of this disease which exemplifies the persistent nature of this infestation.

Geographical distribution

Tropical countries where there are damp soils contaminated by human faeces. Countries in the Far East, Latin America and West Africa are mainly affected.

Life cycle

Adult worms are in the small intestine of man. Rhabditiform larvae are passed in human faeces and then enter a free-living cycle in the soil. Eventually filariform larvae develop in the soil and penetrate the skin of humans, especially the feet. Larvae migrate via the blood to the lungs and then via the trachea to the intestine where adult worms develop (occasionally the larvae from the adult worms may also ultimately cause autoinfection).

Complications

1. Serpiginous creeping skin eruptions may recur over many years and urticarial lesions also often occur.
2. Pneumonitis, due to the larvae migrating through the lungs with accompanying eosinophilia, may be severe, but is less frequently seen than skin lesions.
3. Gastro-intestinal complications and disseminated disease arising from invasion of larvae from the intestine to mesenteric glands and the bloodstream are rare but important complications. Mucosal lesions due to *Strongyloides* can result in malabsorption or an ulcerative enteritis. The biliary tract may also become inflamed due to the invasion of larvae there. When larvae invade the blood, which is more likely in immunodeficient or immunosuppressed patients, septicaemia, due to *E. coli* or other faecal bacteria, or viraemia, due to enteroviruses such as polio, may result as a further complication with a possible fatal outcome.

Diagnosis

The diagnosis depends on seeing the rhabditiform larvae of *Strongyloides stercoralis* during microscopy of faeces and concentration techniques may be helpful. Occasionally the larvae are seen in duodenal aspirates when microscopy of the faeces gives negative results. A serum strongyloides CFT is sometimes positive when microscopy results are negative.

Treatment
Thiabendazole, which is also active against many other worms, is often effective (*see* Hookworms).

Prevention
Similar measures as for hookworms.

Trichuris trichiura
The whipworm is about 5 cm long in the human colon and light asymptomatic infestation is common. Heavy infestations may be associated with abdominal discomfort, tenesmus and diarrhoea with blood in the faeces, especially in children.

Geographical distribution
Worldwide but most prevalent in moist tropical countries.

Life cycle
Adult whipworm particularly in caecal region. Ova passed in human faeces and develop into infective ova in the soil. Man becomes infected by swallowing the infective ova in contaminated food or water. The infective ova develop into adult worms on reaching the lower small intestine and colon.

Complications
Heavy infestation of adult worms in the caecum or rectum can result in an inflammatory eosinophilic reaction, which causes chronic diarrhoea and, exceptionally, rectal prolapse may occur.

Diagnosis
The characteristic 'tea tray' ova of *Trichuris trichiura* are usually easily recognized during microscopy of faeces. Occasionally adult whipworms are observed during sigmoidoscopy attached to the mucosa.

Treatment
Mebendazole.

Prevention
Similar measures as for *Ascaris*.

Trichinella spiralis
Fever and muscle pains and eosinophilia are the most frequent features of the disease.

Geographical distribution

Trichinosis is rarely seen in patients in Britain. This zoonosis affects man most frequently in underdeveloped countries and outbreaks from a batch of infected food may occur.

Life cycle

The usual cycle is between pigs and rodents. Man eats poorly cooked pork or sausages. Larvae migrate from the intestine via blood to skeletal muscle and other sites.

Complications

1. Myalgia and orbital oedema.
2. Myocarditis.
3. Encephalitis.

The last two complications are infrequent.

Diagnosis

Deltoid muscle biopsy may reveal the spiral larval encysted form of *Trichinella spiralis* in the muscle on histology. Serology may be helpful although the trichinella CFT is not entirely specific.

Treatment

Steroids may help to reduce inflammation during the muscle invasion phase. Thiabendazole may reduce the clinical manifestations of the disease but may not be completely effective against the larvae.

Prevention

Adequate cooking of pork and sausages.

Dracunculus medinensis

The adult 'guinea worm', *Dracunculus medinensis*, 12–120 cm long, infests man as the principal reservoir in many tropical countries where man drinks, washes or bathes in ponds, rivers and wells. The worm lives in the subcutaneous tissues and penetrates the skin often around the joints.

Geographical distribution

Middle Eastern countries, especially Arabia, West and Central Africa, Latin America and the Far East have endemic areas.

Life cycle

Adult guinea worm in subcutaneous tissue or joint penetrates skin when skin in contact with water. Gravid female worm discharges larvae through the skin ulcer so larvae are free in water. Cyclops ingest larvae and the infected cyclops in drinking water are swallowed by man. Larvae migrate from alimentary tract to reach subcutaneous tissues where adult worms develop.

Complications

Secondary pyogenic infection of skin, joints and bone near the site of a skin ulcer where the adult worm has penetrated the skin.

Diagnosis

Adult worm apparent in subcutaneous tissues clinically or obvious if penetrated skin and an ulcer is present. Radiographs may sometimes show calcified worm in subcutaneous tissues.

Treatment

Surgical removal of the worm and debridement.

Prevention

Adequate drinking water supplies are essential where no direct contact with infected humans occurs. When water has to be used which is possibly contaminated by infected cyclops it should be boiled first.

Toxocara canis and Toxocara cati

Toxocara infestation is most likely to occur in children between 3 and 5 years old who play with puppies or kittens, which have not been de-wormed, or who may contaminate their hands with excreta from these animals while playing with soil in gardens or parks. Toxocariasis is a zoonosis.

Geographical distribution

Worldwide including Britain.

Life cycle

The adult roundworm is in the intestine of dogs (*Toxocara canis*) or cats (*Toxocara cati*) and the eggs from the worm passed in the faeces infect other animals including rodents which are eaten by dogs or cats to complete the usual life cycle. Man is incidentally infected when the ova contaminate food or soil which is ingested by man. Larvae develop in the intestine, invade the bloodstream and may migrate to the liver, lungs, brain, eye, heart or other tissues, to cause eosinophilia and local granulomas.

Complications

Many human infestations are asymptomatic or not accompanied by eosinophilia. Asthma can result from the toxocara larvae in the lungs. Epilepsy and other neurological problems can occur from larvae encysting in the brain. A tumour-like mass, that may be confused with malignant retinoblastoma during ophthalmoscopic examination, may occur in the retina when the larvae are encysted in the eye. This ocular lesion may be the only apparent manifestation of the disease.

Diagnosis

A serum fluorescent antibody test using toxocara larvae as the antigen is the main diagnostic method available (at a reference laboratory). The larvae may sometimes be seen in histological examination of biopsy or excised tissues.

Treatment

Diethylcarbamazine is partially effective for treating the migratory larval phase in man but cannot affect fibrosing lesions around larvae which have already been deposited in the tissues. Photocoagulation treatment for a retinal toxocara lesion has been suggested recently.

Prevention

Dogs are more frequently the reservoir of infection for man than cats and measures to ensure that all puppies are de-wormed before becoming pets are important. Control of dogs in shops, parks and other public places is strongly desirable.

FILARIAL NEMATODES

Wuchereria bancrofti and Brugia malayi

Adult filarial worms in the lymphatics of man cause the inflammatory and allergic reactions which ultimately lead to the classical clinical features of elephantiasis and lymphoedema.

Geographical distribution

Tropical or subtropical regions throughout the world may have endemic filariasis. Most frequently affected areas include coastal regions of East Africa, Asia including especially South India, Guyana, Queensland in Australia and the Pacific Islands. The disease affects local inhabitants rather than tourists.

Life cycle

Adult worms up to 10 cm long live in the lymphatics of man. Microfilariae, produced from the worms, emerge in blood at night (*W. bancrofti*) or day (*B. malayi*). The microfilariae are taken up by mosquitoes biting at night or during the day. In the majority of endemic areas, *W. bancrofti* and *Culex fatigans* mosquitoes are involved but *B. malayi* and *Mansonia* mosquitoes are also particularly important in Pacific areas. Once taken up in the mosquito, the microfilariae develop into other forms and become localized in the mouth of the mosquito. The disease is spread to other humans by the bites of the infected mosquitoes. There is an animal reservoir, as well as a human one, for *B. malayi* but not for *W. bancrofti*.

Complications

Lymphatic obstruction due to the adult filarial worms predisposes to recurrent lymphangitis, which ultimately results in fibrosis, lymphoedema and elephantiasis. The lymphangitis may be due to both filarial and secondary bacterial infection. Gross enlargement and deformities of the legs, scrotum, arms and breasts as well as lesions in internal organs and chyluria may result. A hydrocele is almost always present in males with elephantiasis due to *W. bancrofti* infection.

Diagnosis

Blood films stained by Leishman or Giemsa stains show the typical microfilaria in day or night blood during the earlier stages of the disease when there may also be eosinophilia. Serology is also usually positive (e.g. using a filarial CFT) but false positive reactions may occur. However, in the late stages of the disease, when elephantiasis is present, the disease is no longer active and these tests usually give negative results.

Treatment

Diethylcarbamazine, given as a course over 2 weeks, will kill both microfilaria and adult worms. Early elephantiasis lesions may respond to conservative measures, such as elevation of limbs and bandaging. Advanced lesions may sometimes require surgical treatment.

Prevention

Protection from mosquito bites, especially during sleep, is important and, in some areas, monthly doses of diethylcarbamazine is used as a public health measure to reduce carriage of microfilariae.

Tropical Pulmonary Eosinophilia

Asthma, cough, fever and eosinophilia may result from infestation due to filarial species, probably of animal origin. Chronic pulmonary disease accompanied by some radiological changes may occur.

Geographical distribution

Asia mainly, especially the Indian subcontinent.

Diagnosis

The serum filarial CFT is strongly positive.

Treatment
Diethylcarbamazine is effective. The pulmonary symptoms and eosinophilia usually disappear rapidly after the start of treatment.

Loa loa
Inhabitants of West Africa who live near rain forests, which are the breeding places of the biting fly vector *Chrysops*, may complain of seeing 'a worm across their eyes' or from transient oedematous swellings on the hands or arms (Calabar swellings). These clinical features are characteristic of loiasis.

Geographical distribution
West Africa only—Cameroons, Zaire and Nigeria.

Life cycle
Adult worm in man's subcutaneous or sub-conjunctival tissues. Microfilaria in day blood taken up by chrysops fly which spreads infection to others near West African rain forest areas.

Complications
Calabar swellings, arising from an allergic reaction to the adult worm, may transiently limit the use of joints and, if near the eye, may cause eye lesions. Infrequently, serious eye lesions result from the presence of the worm in the eye.

Diagnosis
Blood collected during the day and stained by Giemsa or Leishman stains usually shows the characteristic microfilaria. The adult worm may be seen when extracted from the eye. The serum filarial CFT is positive, particularly when there is eosinophilia.

Treatment
Diethylcarbamazine is rapidly effective for treating loiasis.

Prevention
Eradication of the chrysops vector would prevent the disease, but progress with this is slow.

Onchocerca volvulus
Onchocerciasis is a very important cause of blindness, near fast-flowing rivers ('river blindness') where the simulium black fly vector breeds in Africa and Latin America. The patients usually have an eosinophilia.

Geographical distribution

West Africa—Cameroons, Zaire and Nigeria; Latin America—especially Guatemala.

Life cycle

Adult worms in man migrate to skin where dermal nodules, about 1 cm diameter, surround them. Within the nodules, the worms produce microfilaria which do not leave the skin. The microfilaria are taken up by the simulium black fly vector which spreads the infection to other people on biting them.

Complications

1. Ocular. Iridocyclitis, choroiditis, keratitis and cataract, and glaucoma, can result from the worms affecting the eye directly and indirectly by hypersensitivity reactions. Blindness frequently results and most of the older inhabitants of communities in endemic areas may be blind and are led about by children.
2. Skin lesions. Papules, nodules and thickened 'elephantine' wrinkled lesions frequently occur.

Diagnosis

Skin snips (especially of nodules taken from the thigh and near the iliac crests of African patients), immersed in saline, may show microfilaria emerging from them during microscopy. Histology of whole nodules excised under local anaesthetic may show the adult worm. The serum filarial CFT is usually positive.

Treatment

Diethylcarbamazine is effective against microfilaria and helps relieve symptoms; antihistamine and steroid cover may be necessary at the start of treatment, since the killing of microfilariae exacerbates the lesions (positive Mazzotti reaction). Suramin, a toxic drug, is occasionally used against the adult worms but these are usually best removed surgically where possible.

Prevention

Eradication of the simulium vector with DDT has been successful in Kenya where the disease has now disappeared. Unfortunately, it appears more difficult to eliminate the simulium fly in other endemic areas.

TREMATODES (FLUKES)

Schistosoma Species (Bilharzia)

Schistosomiasis affects hundreds of millions of people in the world. Its incidence is increasing due to irrigation developmental schemes which provide further opportunities for the fresh water snail vectors to breed and spread. There are three species—*S. haematobium*, *S. mansoni* and *S. japonicum*. The adult schistosomes live in the pelvic mesenteric and portal venous veins of man and disease is caused mainly by the deposition of ova from the worms in the liver, the walls of the large bowel and the walls of the bladder and ureters. Fibrosis and granulomata occur around deposited ova sometimes also resulting in strictures, polyp formation and possibly pre-malignant change. *S. haematobium* mainly affects the inferior pelvic venous system and the urinary tract whereas *S. mansoni* and *S. japonicum* more frequently affect the liver, the mesenteric venous systems and the colon and rectum. In endemic areas, many children and young people are asymptomatic or have minor symptoms, such as lethargy, only. However, complications, especially in later life, are common and the disease is associated with widespread serious morbidity.

Geographical distribution

S. haematobium is endemic in Egypt and many other parts of the Middle East and Africa. *S. mansoni* also occurs in the Middle East and Africa, but is also found in Latin America and the West Indies. *S. japonicum* occurs in the Far East only, is rarely seen in patients coming to Britain and causes similar complications to *S. mansoni*.

Life cycle

The adult male and female worms lie paired together in the human veins and the female deposits ova which pass through the vein wall to surrounding tissues or embolize to other sites. Many ova penetrate the bladder wall (*S. haematobium*) to be excreted in the urine or through the colonic rectal wall to be excreted in the faeces (*S. mansoni* or *S. japonicum*). When the excreta of man reach fresh water, the ova hatch into miracidium larvae which infect particular species of snails that are intermediate hosts. The larvae continue development inside the snail and emerge from the snails as fork-tailed cercariae that swim in the water and penetrate the skin of man. After penetration, the larvae invade the bloodstream and finally the adult worms develop and migrate down the portal, mesenteric or pelvic veins.

Complications

S. haematobium may cause fibrosis (sandy patches) or calcification in the bladder wall which is apparent on cystoscopy or radiograph and granulomatous polyps or strictures in the bladder or ureters. The distortions in the urinary tract anatomy, including obstructive hydroureter, may lead to secondary bacterial infections and ultimately to serious renal damage. *S. mansoni* may cause pipe stem cirrhosis in the liver, portal hypertension and 'Egyptian splenomegaly' with bleeding oesophageal varices. The colon and rectum may develop strictures or polyps. Rarely adult worms or ova may reach other sites such as the central nervous system and cause serious complications, such as encephalopathy or myelitis.

Diagnosis

During the early and middle stages of the schistosomiasis, when the disease is still active, the characteristic ova of *S. haematobium* (terminal spine) (*Fig. 23.3*)

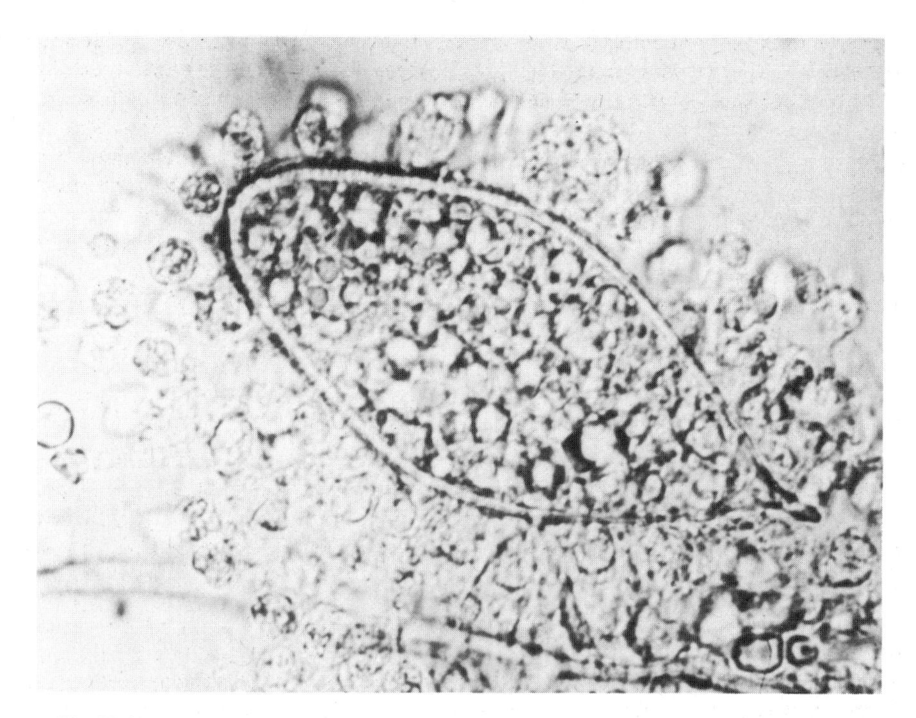

Fig. 23.3. Schistosoma haematobium ovum in urine.

or *S. mansoni* (lateral spine) may be seen during microscopy of urine or faeces, respectively. Patients with *S. haematobium* infestation often have haematuria and the best specimen for looking for ova is a terminal specimen of urine. The ova of *S. mansoni* or *S. japonicum* (lateral knob) may sometimes be seen in microscopic examination of rectal biopsy tissue when the faeces examination gives negative results. Repeated examinations of urine or faeces may be necessary over several months after recent exposure to contaminated fresh water and serology should be tested in exposed visitors returning from endemic areas. The serology is positive before ova become apparent. When eosinophilia is present associated with active schistosomiasis, the serum schistosome enzyme-linked immunosorbent assay (ELISA test), or the CFT, is nearly always positive. Serology is less useful once the patient is known to have had the disease in the past as positive results may persist for a long time after treatment.

Treatment

1. *Niridazole* is effective for treating *S. haematobium* and almost as effective for treating uncomplicated intestinal *S. mansoni* infestation. Side effects are common and toxicity may prevent its use when there is known liver disease or neuro-psychiatric illness.
2. *Metriphonate* is very effective against *S. haematobium* only and can sometimes be used when niridazole is contraindicated.

3. *Praziquantel* is effective against all three *Schistosoma* species and is administered as a single oral dose. This drug appears to be free of serious toxicity. Only the active disease requires treatment with anti-schistosomal drugs.

Surgery is frequently required to treat complications, such as fistulae, preferably after treatment with an anti-*Schistosoma* drug.

Prevention

Control of the disease is becoming more difficult than ever due to the expanding irrigation schemes in many countries. New effective measures to control the snail vector are needed. Public health measures to educate children particularly not to urinate near fresh water and to introduce modern sewage disposal facilities may help to reduce the incidence of the disease. Research on immunity to the schistosomal larvae might lead to a useful vaccine in the future. Visitors to endemic areas should not walk barefoot near to and not bathe in fresh water.

Fasciola hepatica

Fascioliasis is a zoonosis which is encountered sporadically in some patients returning from abroad, but outbreaks have occasionally occurred in Britain following the consumption of contaminated watercress during wet summers.

Geographical distribution

Worldwide including Britain, especially in sheep-rearing areas.

Life cycle

The adult liver fluke usually occurs in the bile duct of sheep or cattle. Other animals can also be affected. The ova from the fluke are passed in the faeces and miracidium larvae develop in the soil and enter snails as the intermediate host. Cercariae emerge from the snail that encyst, as metacercariae, on grass, or watercress. The metacercariae on grass are eaten by the animal and the larvae develops in the alimentary tract into the adult fluke which reaches the bile duct. Man is incidentally infected when metacercariae on watercress is eaten and the fluke develops in the human bile duct.

Complications

Cholangitis, cholecystitis and liver abscess may occur.

Diagnosis

Characteristic ova may sometimes be seen during microscopy of faeces. Serology is the only reliable method of diagnosis when ova are not apparent in the faeces, using a serum immunofluorescent antibody test against the fasciola antigen.

Treatment

Spontaneous cure occasionally occurs. Emetine is effective for curing the majority of patients.

Prevention

Only properly supervised growing of watercress should be allowed where manure is not used and where measures are taken to reduce the likelihood of snail infestation. Wild watercress should never be eaten.

Clonorchis sinensis (Chinese Liver Fluke)

Rarely cases of clonorchiasis are seen in patients returning to Britain from the Far East.

Geographical distribution

Japan, Korea and China are the main areas affected.

Life cycle

Cats and other animals are the usual definitive host where the fluke lives in the bile duct. The ova passed in the faeces develop into miracidium larvae which invade snails. Cercariae from the snails infect fish and the cycle is perpetuated when the fish are eaten by the animals. Man is infected and becomes the definitive host on eating undercooked infected fish.

Complications

Cholangitis, liver abscess and, in chronic cases, gall stones, cirrhosis and primary carcinoma of the liver.

Diagnosis

Characteristic ova are seen usually during the microscopy of faeces. A serum clonorchis CFT may also be positive.

Treatment

Chloroquine, possibly combined with emetine for heavily infested cases. Dithiazamine iodine may be given for light infections.

Prevention

Proper cooking of fish. Preventing dogs and cats having access to offal from fish and good public health measures to prevent pollution of water.

Paragonimus westermani

Rarely a patient from the Far East with pulmonary disease may be seen in Britain suffering from paragonimus infection.

Geographical distribution

Far East, especially Korea, China and Japan. Also parts of Africa.

Life cycle

The adult fluke is in the lung of animals of the cat or canine families and the ova are passed in the sputum or faeces which become miracidia in water. The miracidia invade snails and cercariae emerge which encyst (metacercariae) in crabs and crayfish. Animals and man become infected on eating metacercariae-infested crabs or crayfish. The larvae pass through the abdominal cavity and the diaphragm to reach the lungs.

Complications

Haemoptysis, lung infections, pneumothorax and pulmonary effusion may occur. Abdominal complications are also possible.

Diagnosis

Characteristic ova may be seen during microscopy of sputum, faeces or discharge from sinuses. A serological test, paragonimus CFT, is positive in most cases.

Treatment

Bithionol is effective for curing the disease.

Prevention

Eradication of the snail vector and educating people to eat only adequately cooked crabs and crayfish are important preventive measures.

Further Reading

Gillies H. M. (1976) Disease of the alimentary system: treatment of intestinal worms. *Br. Med. J.* **2**, 1314–1316.

Maegraith B. G. (1980) *Adams and Maegraith: Clinical Tropical Diseases,* 7th ed. Oxford, Blackwell Scientific Publications.

Peters W. and Gillies H. M. (1977) *A Colour Atlas of Tropical Medicine and Parasitology.* London, Wolfe Medical.

Warren K. S. (1979) Schistosomiasis. In: Beeson P. B., McDermott W. and Wyngaarden J. B. (ed.) *Cecil Textbook of Medicine.* Philadelphia, U.S.A., Saunders.

Woodruff A. W. (ed.) (1974) *Medicine in the Tropics.* Edinburgh, Churchill Livingstone.

Chapter 24

Hospital infection

'Hospital infection' includes both (1) infections acquired while in hospital and (2) infections acquired in the community which are then brought into hospital. This chapter is mainly concerned with 'hospital-acquired infection' and the means of controlling it. Recent surveys in Britain indicate that about half of all the infections occurring in hospital in-patients are hospital acquired. These studies also show that between 8 and 16% of hospital patients acquire infections while in hospital. In North America, 'hospital-acquired infections' are referred to as 'nosocomial' infections.

GENERAL CONSIDERATIONS

The majority of hospital-acquired infections are of minor or moderate clinical importance but nevertheless may cause distressing morbidity, lengthen hospital stay and increase costs. Some hospital infections can have catastrophic local consequences, such as infection of a hip joint prosthesis or a prosthetic heart valve, although these do not necessarily result in death. Serious hospital infections due to Gram-negative bacilli have increased greatly in incidence during the last 30 years and the ultimate consequence of these may be fatal Gram-negative septic shock (*see* Gram-negative septicaemia, in Chapter 5). 'New' or previously unrecognized serious problems have occasionally occurred in recent years, such as hospital-acquired Legionnaires' disease. Members of the hospital staff are also sometimes at risk from diseases such as tuberculosis or hepatitis.

There are three main routes of spread of organisms causing hospital-acquired infections: self-infection (autogenous infection), cross-infection and environmental infection (*Fig. 24.1*). Colonization rather than infection occurs with each of these three routes in many instances. This is particularly relevant when considering the epidemiology of outbreaks of hospital infection as the colonized patient or member of staff may cause symptomatic infection in another patient.

Four main factors will determine whether a patient will acquire a hosptial infection (*Fig. 24.2*):

1. *Impaired general host defences of the patient*
   This is due either to extremes of age, the nature of the disease or of the treatment that the patient is receiving (*see* Chapters 5 and 6).
2. *Impaired local host defences of the patient*
   The intact skin or mucosa is normally a barrier to the entry of organisms into the deeper tissues that are, of course sterile in health. This barrier is mainly a mechanical one but other factors, such as local immunoglublin A, or inhibitory substances, such as fatty acids or lysozyme, may also contribute to an effective local barrier against infection. When the skin or mucosal surfaces are breached or are grossly abnormal because of trauma,

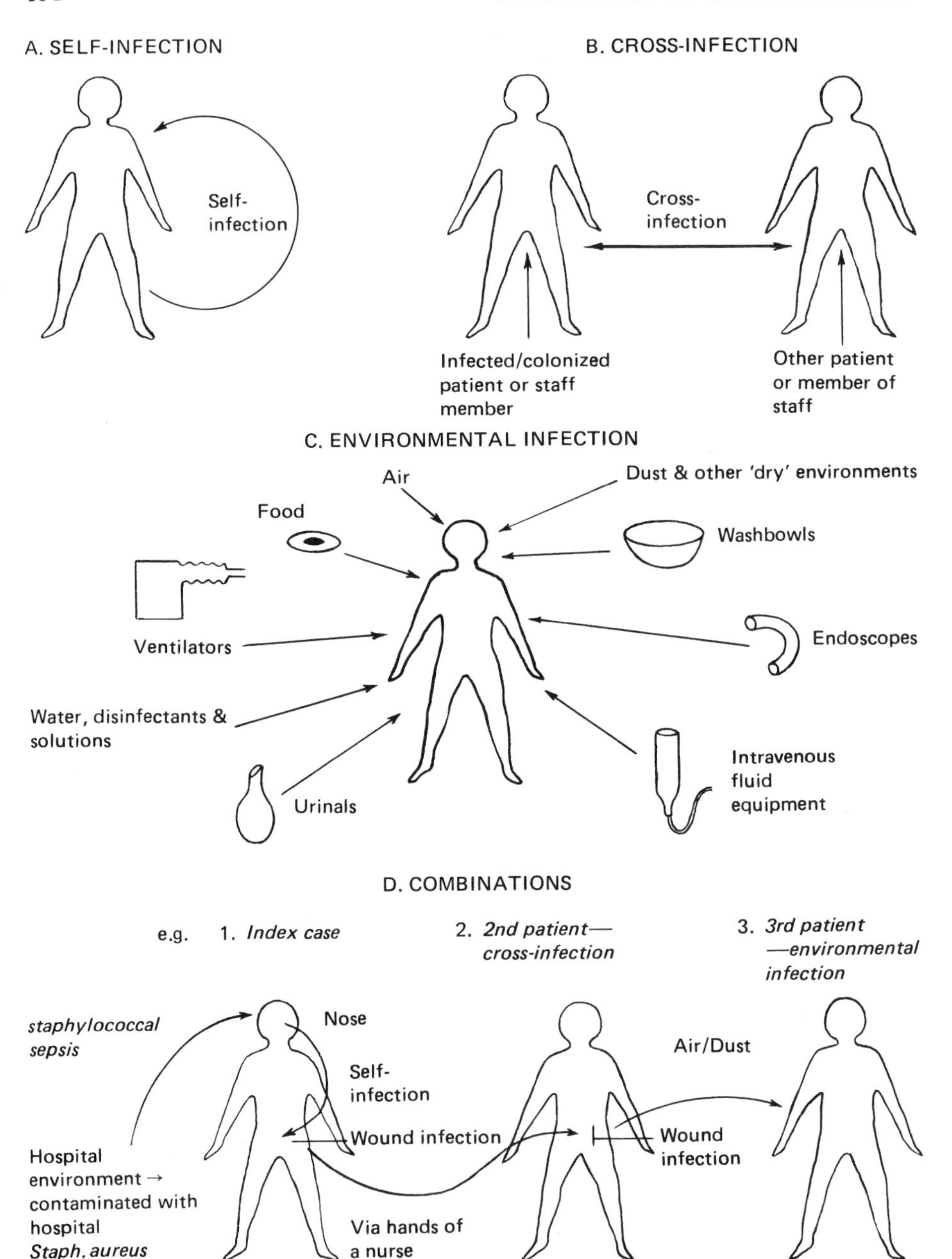

Fig. 24.1. Hospital-acquired infection—major routes of spread.

disease, surgery or instrumentation, infection often results. Examples of conditions where the skin surface is breached include surgical and traumatic wounds, burns, pressure sores and varicose ulcers, intravenous infusion therapy, and insertion of cardiac pacemakers. Examples of conditions

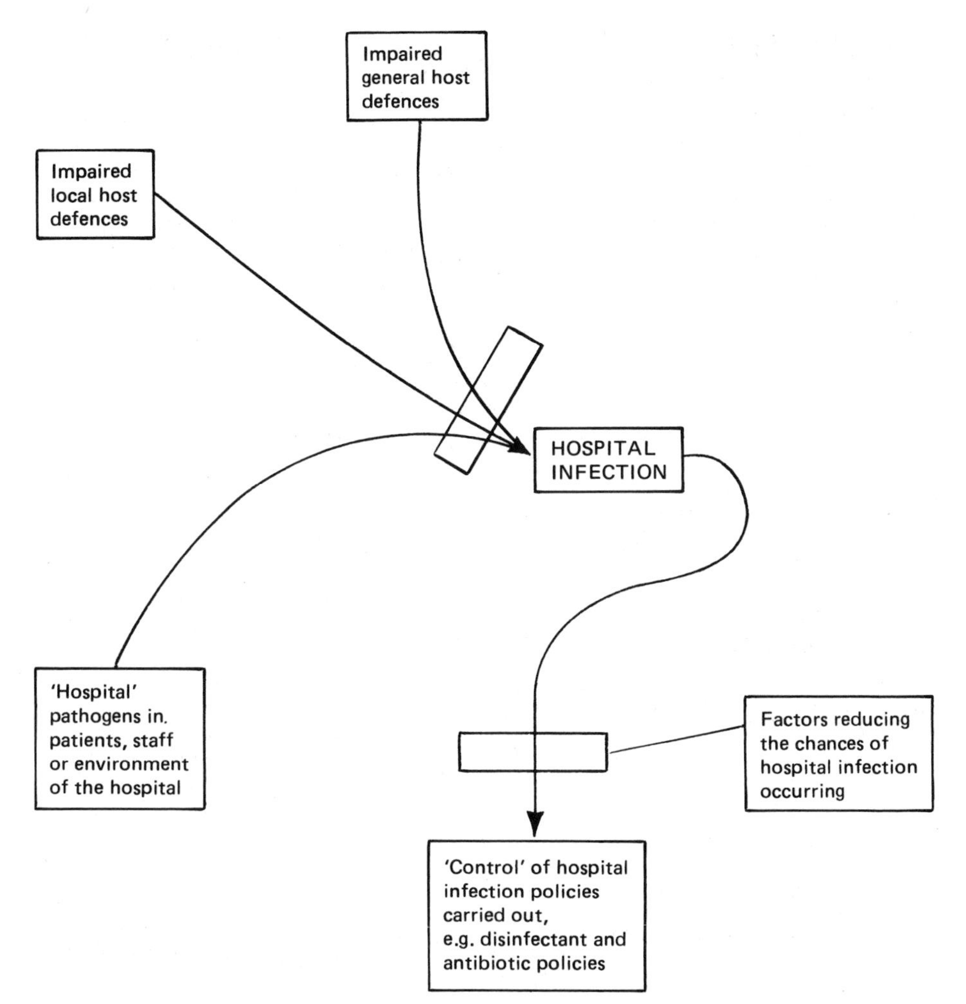

Fig. 24.2. Factors influencing the development of hospital infections.

where the mucosal surface is breached or grossly abnormal include surgery or instrumentation of the gastro-intestinal, genito-urinary or respiratory tract, and diseases such as a perforated appendix or ulcerative malignant disease.

3. *'Hospital' pathogens*

The main types of 'hospital pathogen' encountered are similar in most general hospitals although each hospital may also have its own endemic or epidemic strains of particular types of organism in certain areas at different times. If a hospital has large special units, such as renal transplant, intensive care, liver, neuro-surgical, burns, oncology, plastic surgery, dermatology, and special care baby units, unusual 'opportunist' organisms as well as the common pathogens are likely to cause problems at different times. The various types of hospital pathogen and 'opportunist' organisms are described below (and in Chapter 6).

4. *Control of hospital infection*
Each hospital has many procedures and policies which attempt to reduce the chances of hospital infection occurring but the extent to which these policies are effectively carried out on a day-to-day basis varies greatly between different hospitals or different areas in the hospital. Relevant procedures include those carried out for the sterilization and disinfection of contaminated items and disposal of infected rubbish or linen, aseptic techniques in the operating theatre and in the wards for procedures such as changing of wound dressings, urinary catheterization, setting up an intravenous drip; the 'source' isolation of infected patients or 'protective' isolation of highly susceptible patients; the administration of appropriate antibiotic prophylaxis for certain surgical procedures and the discriminate use of antibiotics for treating patients, preferably according to an agreed policy; the education of staff in hospital hygiene; good staff health facilities; the adequate use of the clinical microbiology department for the precise bacteriological diagnosis.
An essential administrative requirement for the effective control of hospital infection is an active infection control team guided by the Control of Infection Officer who is usually the Consultant Microbiologist. The Consultant Microbiologist needs a trained Infection Control Nurse to help him who is in daily contact with nursing and other hospital staff on the wards. The ideal is to have a Consultant Microbiologist, who is interested in the control of hospital infection, supported by both a trained infection control nurse and junior medical microbiology staff. In many hospitals in Britain, there is also a Control of Infection Committee which helps to design hospital policies and discusses any difficulties encountered during the implementation of these policies.

DIFFERENT TYPES OF HOSPITAL-ACQUIRED INFECTION

The three most frequent types of hospital-acquired infections are, in order, urinary tract infections, wound infections and lower respiratory tract infections. Skin sepsis, affecting especially pressure sores and varicose ulcers, is also common. Alimentary tract infections are only occasionally acquired in hospitals and these occur mainly in psychiatric, geriatric or maternity/paediatric units.

Almost all of the bacterial infections may ultimately lead to fatal septicaemia, especially when the patient's host defences are greatly reduced and there has been surgery or instrumentation (*see also* Chapter 5). Some of the main types of hospital-acquired infections, with their principal sources and means of spread, are included in *Table 24.1*. Further details of the infections are found in other chapters.

ORGANISMS CAUSING HOSPITAL-ACQUIRED INFECTIONS

'Conventional' pathogens, such as *Strep. pyogenes*, can cause clinical infections in previously healthy people. 'Conditional' pathogens, such as *Bacteroides*, may cause clinical infection at an appropriate site where there is an obvious predisposing factor present, for example an abdominal surgical wound. 'Opportunist' pathogens, such as *Pneumocystis carinii*, are usually of low pathogenicity in healthy people, but may cause clinical infection when the patient's general resistance to infection has been greatly compromised. One example of such compromise is prolonged immunosuppression associated with the immunosuppressive agents used in the treatment of leukaemia. This classification based on the 'pathogenicity' of organisms is very approximate and in practice many organisms, such as *Pseudomonas aeruginosa*, can behave as both conditional and opportunist pathogens, while others, such as *Staph. aureus*, can behave as both conventional and conditional pathogens, depending on the circumstances.

Staph. aureus is by far the most frequent cause of hospital infections due to Gram-positive organisms, and is mainly associated with surgical and skin sepsis. *Strep. pneumoniae* is the next most frequent Gram-positive organism and is associated particularly with lower respiratory tract infections, such as post-operative pneumonias (although most of these are self-infections). Gram-negative bacilli cause more hospital infections today than Gram-positive cocci and *E. coli* is in fact the most frequent single bacterial species associated with hospital infection. The majority of *E. coli* infections occur in association with disease, surgery or instrumentation of the urinary or gastro-intestinal tracts. *Bacteroides*, *Klebsiella* and *Proteus* species are next in frequency amongst the Gram-negative causes followed by *Pseudomonas*. Other bacterial species are relatively infrequent causes of hospital infection in Britain. Fungal and viral infections are only occasionally acquired in hospital and protozoal hospital acquired infections are rare.

Many hospital infections are self-infections with the organisms coming originally from the patient's own normal faecal flora, such as *E. coli* and *Bacteroides fragilis*, of from sites such as the skin or upper respiratory tract, where the organism may be transiently carried, such as with *Staph. aureus*. Exogenous infections due to cross or environmental infection also commonly occur. The majority of Gram-negative bacilli, haemolytic streptococci and staphylococci can survive for 20 minutes or longer on the hands of hospital staff and the hands are the most important means of spreading infection from one patient to another in hospital wards or special units. Hands may become contaminated by organisms in the hospital environment as well as directly while handling infected or colonized patients. Gram-positive organisms, such as *Staph. aureus* or *Strep. pyogenes*, often survive well in a dry environment such as the ward dust, air or bed clothes while many of the Gram-negative bacilli, such as *Pseudomonas* or *Klebsiella*, usually only survive well and multiply at room temperature in moist sites such as solutions, wet bed pans or urinals, wash bowls and soap trays, and moist equipment such as suction apparatus, humidifiers or ventilators.

The dose of organisms required to initiate an infection, the invasiveness of the organism and the ability to spread to other patients, are features which vary greatly between different species and also between different strains of the same species. *Strep. pyogenes* can more readily establish itself in subcutaneous tissues than *Staph. aureus* as a lower dose of organisms is required to start infection and there is more rapid spread of infection through the tissues. Gram-negative bacilli are also much less invasive from a skin site of inoculation than haemolytic

Table 24.1. Some hospital-acquired infections

Type	*Main organisms*	*Usual sources*	*Means of spread to other patients include:*
1. *Urinary tract infections* Catheterized patients or those undergoing cystoscopy, prostatic biopsy or urological surgery	Gram-negative bacilli e.g. *E. coli* *Klebsiella* *Proteus* *Pseudomonas* *Serratia*	1. Patient's own faecal flora 2. Contaminated equipment, e.g. urinary catheters or endoscopes	1. Hands of staff contaminated by infected urine, while handling patient, or infected urinary equipment 2. Inadequately decontaminated urinary equipment
2. *Post-operative wound sepsis* 'Clean' surgery	1. *Staph. aureus* 2. *Strep. pyogenes* (much less common than *Staph.*)	1. Patient's own skin or nasal flora 2. *Staph.* or *Strep.* from septic lesions of other patients or hospital staff 3. 'Dry' environment—air, bedclothes, dust, etc.	1. Hands or clothing of staff contaminated by an infected patient 2. Carriage by staff or patients of an epidemic strain 3. Dispersal of *Staph.* or *Strep.* from infected lesion or carriage site into air or dust
Abdominal and gynaecological surgery (also frequently complicated by intra-abdominal or pelvic abscesses due to similar organisms)	1. Gram-negative bacilli e.g. *E. coli* 2. Non-sporing anaerobes e.g. *Bacteroides fragilis* } 3. *Staph. aureus*	1. Patient's own faecal flora	1. Usually not applicable—'self'-infections 2. *Staph.* (*see* 'Clean' surgery *above*)
Orthopaedic surgery	1. *Staph. aureus* 2. Haemolytic streptococci } 3. *Clostridium welchii*	Same as 'Clean' surgery above Patient's faecal flora: spores on skin may germinate unless adequate prophylaxis given, especially for cases of ischaemic arterial disease and lower limb amputations	Usually not applicable—'self'-infection

Orthopaedic surgery	4. *Staph. epidermidis* 5. Gram-negative bacilli and 6. Non-sporing anaerobes	Skin of patient or surgeon when hip joint replacement operation involved Patient's faecal flora when extensive lower limb surgery involved	Usually not applicable—'self'-infection
3. *Respiratory tract infection* Pneumonias in post-operative and debilitated cases	1. *Strep. pneumoniae* 2. *Staph. aureus*	1. Patient's own upper respiratory flora 2. Patient's nasal flora or from hospital 'dry' environment	Usually not applicable Air and dust
Pneumonias in aspiration cases	1. *Strep. pneumoniae* 2. *Staph. aureus* 3. *Haemophilus influenzae* 4. Non-sporing anaerobes 5. Gram-negative bacilli	As above Patient's own upper respiratory flora From hospital 'moist' environment	As above Not applicable Hands of staff and 'moist' environment
Pneumonias in intensive care cases	Similar to aspiration pneumonia	As for aspiration pneumonia (*see* ICU, p. 486)	As for aspiration pneumonia and *see Fig. 24.8*
Immunosuppressed cases	Similar to aspiration pneumonia + cytomegalovirus, *Nocardia*, *Legionella pneumophila*, pneumocystis, fungi, *Mycobacterium tuberculosis*	← *See* Chapters 6, 8 and 12 →	
Tuberculosis	*Mycobacterium tuberculosis*	Respiratory droplets and sputum from open TB cases	Air and dust
Influenza	Influenza viruses	Respiratory droplets from infected patients or staff	Air

Table 24.1. (cont.)

Type	*Main organisms*	*Usual sources*	*Means of spread to other patients include:*
Upper respiratory tract and 'childhood' infections	*Strep. pyogenes* Rhinoviruses Respiratory syncytial virus Measles Varicella-zoster and other 'respiratory' viruses	Respiratory droplets from infected patients or staff	Air
	Herpes simplex	Patient's latent mouth flora	
4. *Alimentary tract infections* Gastro-enteritis	1. *Salmonella* species 2. *Clostridium welchii* 3. *Campylobacter jejuni* 4. *Staph. aureus* 5. Enteropathogenic *E. coli* (infants) 6. Rotaviruses (infants)	*a.* Infected food from hospital kitchen or contaminated infant milk feeds *b.* Infected or asymptomatic carrier patient—faeces	1. Hands of kitchen, nursing or other staff or 2. Direct spread in maternity or paediatric units 3. Contaminated 'moist' sites, e.g. infected bedpans (NB *Clostridium welchii* food poisoning does not spread from patient to patient)
Bacillary dysentery	1. *Shigella sonnei* 2. *Shigella flexneri* 3. Other shigellae	Faeces of infected patients	1. Direct spread in mental, paediatric and geriatric wards 2. Hands of staff and patients 3. Moist sites in toilets, bedpans
Enteric fever	*Salmonella typhi*	Infected or carrier patient—faeces, urine, exudate	1. Contaminated hands of staff 2. Contaminated moist sites—e.g. endoscopes
5. *Hepatitis*	1. Hepatitis B virus	Infected or carrier patient—blood, serum, exudate, tissues, etc.	1. Contamination of hands, mucous membranes or eyes of ward, theatre or laboratory staff 2. Contaminated machines, 'sharps', bed pans and other environmental items
	2. Hepatitis A virus	Faeces of infected patient (before start or less than 1 week of jaundice)	

6. *Maternity/neonatal infections*			
Breast abscess in mother (develops later outside hospital) Neonatal skin/eye/umbilical cord sepsis Ritter's disease	*Staph. aureus* (penicillin resistant)	Skin or nasal flora of hospital staff or infected patient	1. Hands of hospital staff 2. Air and dust in nursery—especially if neonates close to each other
Puerperal sepsis, septic abortion, intra-uterine sepsis	Haemolytic streptococci, Lancefield groups A, B, C or G	1. Vaginal or respiratory flora of patient 2. Upper respiratory flora of hospital staff	1. Hands of hospital staff (although most group B *Strep.* 'self'-infection)
	Non-sporing anaerobes e.g. *Bacteroides* species *Clostridium welchii* *E. coli* and other coliforms	Faecal or lower vaginal flora of patient	2. Not applicable—'self'-infection
	Staph. aureus	(As for *Staph.* above)	
Neonatal septicaemia or meningitis (often following soft tissue or umbilical cord sepsis)	Group B haemolytic streptococcus *E. coli* and other coliforms	Maternal faecal or lower vaginal flora	Usually not applicable—occasionally hands of hospital staff
	Pseudomonas aeruginosa	Maternal flora or contaminated antiseptics, water, baby incubator or resuscitation equipment	
7. *Skin sepsis*			
Infected eczema, burns pressure sores and varicose ulcers	*Staph. aureus* *Strep. pyogenes* and other haemolytic streptococci	Pus and skin scales of infected patients Also *Staph. aureus* self-infection from patient's own carrier sites	1. Hands of hospital staff 2. Air and dust
	'Coliforms', *Pseudomonas* and *Bacteroides*	1. As above 2. Patient's own faecal flora	1. Hands of hospital staff 2. Contaminated moist environment

streptococci or *Staph. aureus*. However, the dose of any organism required to start a clinical infection is much reduced when there is an obvious predisposing factor present at a particular site, such as a wound caused by or containing a foreign body, or when the patient's immunity is compromised. *Strep. pyogenes* is also associated with greater 'spreading' capacity than most strains of *Staph. aureus* or Gram-negative species. The spread of a bacterial strain to cause an outbreak of hospital infection depends on the combination of many of the factors previously outlined as well as on the intrinsic characteristics of the organism. The antibiotic sensitivity characteristics may be of great importance when the spread of a strain is considered. *Strep. pyogenes* is fortunately always very sensitive to penicillin and it is difficult for this species to cause persistent outbreaks of infection once the first cases are treated. However some epidemic strains of *Staph. aureus, Klebsiella aerogenes, Pseudomonas aeruginosa*, and *Serratia marcescens* are resistant to many different antibiotics and this antibiotic resistance may help the organism to spread amongst patients who are already receiving these antibiotics. 'Typing' of strains of a bacterial species may help in the investigation of an outbreak (*see* Appendix, p. 495).

HOSPITAL-ACQUIRED URINARY TRACT INFECTIONS

Urinary tract infections probably account for at least 25% of hospital acquired infections. The organisms responsible usually come from the patient's own faecal flora. However, the Gram-negative bacilli in the faecal flora may have come originally from a moist site in the hospital environment, such as a wash bowl or homogenized food from the diet kitchen. Colonization of the patient's large intestine by 'hospital' antibiotic-resistant strains of Gram-negative bacilli is particularly likely to occur when the patient stays in hospital for more than a few days or when antibiotics are administered. In addition to 'self-infections', there are frequently incidents of 'cross-infection' once the infecting bacterial strain has caused infection of the urinary tract of another patient. *E. coli* strains, often resistant to both sulphonamides and ampicillin, cause over 50% of hospital urinary tract infections. *Klebsiella aerogenes, Proteus mirabilis* and *Pseudomonas aeruginosa* are other important causative agents that may also be associated with outbreaks of urinary tract infections occurring in a ward. In recent years, *Serratia marcescens* and *Staphylococcus epidermidis* have increasingly become recognized as occasional causes of hospital urinary tract infection, especially in catheterized patients. Patients with impaired general host defences may suffer from rarer types of urinary tract infection due to *Candida albicans, Mycobacterium tuberculosis, Nocardia asteroides, Salmonella* species or papovaviruses. Most patients are infected by one organism only but patients with indwelling catheters often suffer from infections due to two, or occasionally more, organisms simultaneously. The reader is referred to Chapter 19 for differences in the organisms causing infection inside, compared with outside, hospital (*Table 19.2*) and for the general features of urinary infection.

Effects of Hospital-acquired Urinary Tract Infection

Some adult patients develop asymptomatic urinary tract infections which do not necessarily require specific antibiotic treatment and which are not followed by any complications. When the predisposing factor, such as an indwelling bladder catheter, is removed the urinary infection often resolves spontaneously.

When urinary tract infections become symptomatic, antibiotic therapy is usually necessary. This may result in the hospital stay being prolonged by several days or more and occasionally problems with drug reactions occur.

More serious local complications may arise from urinary tract infection including pyelonephritis, or secondary haemorrhage post-operatively. In a few patients with a serious abnormality of the urinary tract, the urinary infection may contribute to the development of renal failure and death.

Patients with a urinary tract infection, possibly asymptomatic, who undergo instrumentation such as cystoscopy or surgery, without appropriate antibiotic cover, are at great risk of developing bacteraemia and Gram-negative shock within a few hours of the procedure. This complication is sometimes fatal. In the past, bacteraemia also often occurred following the withdrawal of a catheter ('catheter fever') but this is less common today. Instrumentation or surgery on an apparently sterile urinary tract carries very little risk of bacteraemia except when the instrument passes through a heavily contaminated area, such as during a transrectal prostatic biopsy.

In a high proportion of patients with hospital-acquired urinary tract infections, increased hospital costs result.

Precipitating Factors

A procedure performed in hospital on the urinary tract precedes the development of a hospital-acquired urinary tract infection in at least 40% of cases. Such procedures include bladder catheterization, cystoscopy, suprapubic catheterization, ureteric catheterization, certain local radiological and hydrodynamic invasive investigations, prostatic biopsy and all kinds of urological or gynaecological surgery. However, catheterization of the bladder is by far the most frequent procedure associated with the development of hospital urinary tract infections.

Catheterization of the Bladder

The risk of urinary tract infection following insertion of the catheter in the bladder, with reasonable precautions, is between 1 and 3%, as long as the catheter is removed within a short time of its insertion. However, when the catheter is left in the bladder for some days the likelihood of acquiring a urinary tract infection is enormously increased depending on the duration of catheterization. When an open drainage system was commonly used years ago, the infection rate reached virtually 100% by the fifth day; retrograde spread of the infection up the lumen of the catheter was probably aided by ascending air bubbles. Closed, rather than open, drainage dramatically reduced the incidence of urinary infections but, even with the best techniques, between 15 and 30% of patients still acquire infections by the fifth day. Patients who still require continuous bladder drainage after 2 or 3 weeks usually develop infections. The routes of infection and types of catheter drainage are shown in *Fig. 24.3*.

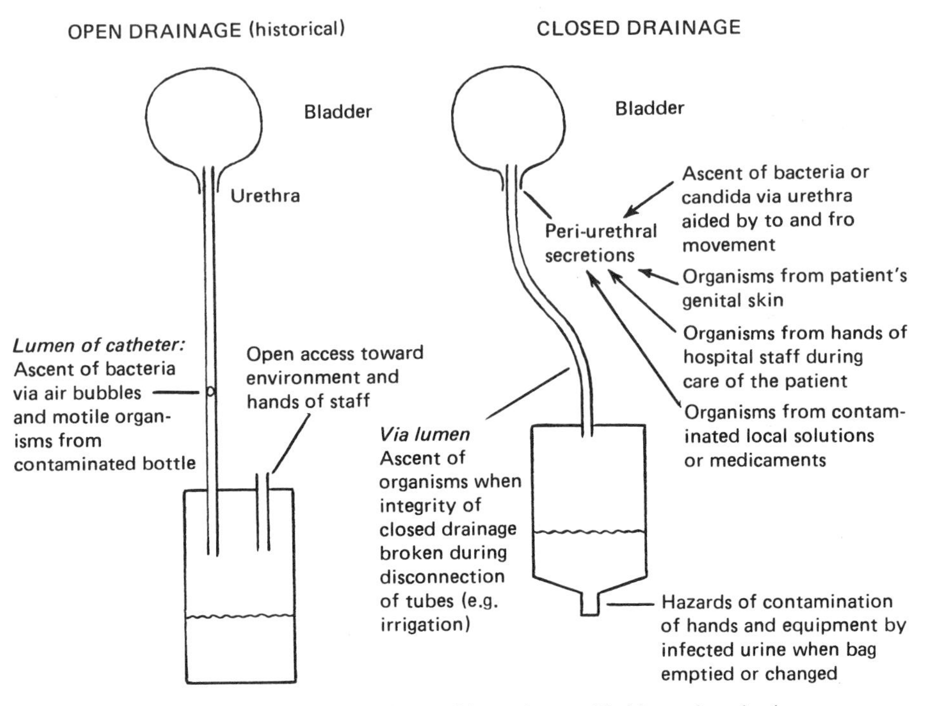

Fig. 24.3. Routes of infection in patients with continuous bladder catheterization.

Prevention of Catheter-associated Urinary Infection

At the time of insertion of a sterile disposable catheter, great care is necessary to avoid the touching of the distal catheter by the hands of the operator, even when gloves are worn, and avoiding the skin of the patient at the perineal or genital sites not immediately adjacent to the urethral orifice. In addition to scrupulous asepsis, good antisepsis is necessary. Before the procedure, the operator must carefully wash the hands, preferably with an antiseptic solution of a chlorhexidine-containing detergent. The genitalia and distal urethra are normally colonized by skin or faecal flora, so both sites need prior adequate antisepsis, chlorhexidine-containing solutions and creams often being suitable. Once the catheter is inserted, some authorities also suggest the immediate instillation of a chlorhexidine solution into the bladder for local prophylaxis. Repeated daily instillations of this antiseptic into the bladder has also been suggested.

The most important measure for patients requiring indwelling bladder catheterization is to ensure that the catheter is not left in any longer than is absolutely necessary. Changing of the catheter every few days should not normally be carried out. Where unnecessary handling of the catheters occur, it is more likely that infections will result. If the catheter becomes blocked or is obviously dirty, then clearly it will have to be changed. It is vital that the integrity of the closed drainage system is maintained at all times. Great care is necessary to avoid contamination of the hands of hospital staff by urine when drainage bags are emptied or changed, and when the bladder is irrigated or samples are taken for investigation. These procedures present great risks of cross-infection via the hands of staff once a patient with a catheter has a urinary infection. If urine does contaminate the hands of a member of staff, immediate washing with an antiseptic and thorough drying of the hands is required. Disposable gloves should always be worn when care of urinary equipment or urethral toilet is carried out on a patient with a known urinary tract infection due to an antibiotic-resistant bacterial strain. Patients with infection due to gentamicin and multiple antibiotic-resistant strains of *Klebsiella, Serratia* or *Pseudomonas* should be isolated and extra precautions observed (*see* Stool/needle/urine isolation in Appendix, p. 497).

Organisms may ascend from the perineal or genital flora by means of the periurethral secretions between the outside of the catheter and the urethral mucosa when the catheter remains in the bladder for more than a few days. This especially applies to the female since the urethra is much shorter than in the male. The restriction of 'to-and-fro' movement of the catheter, using a sponge impregnated with antiseptic around the catheter where it enters the urethra, may help to prevent organisms reaching the bladder by this route. In all patients, regular application of an antiseptic cream around the catheter at the urethral meatus may also be helpful.

The value of adding an antiseptic to the drainage bag itself is uncertain at present and not widely practised.

Before a catheter is withdrawn, instillation of chlorhexidine solution into the bladder is recommended.

Paraplegic Patients

Patients requiring long-term catheterization for many months can sometimes be managed better by repeated self-catheterization, resulting in lower infection rates, than continuous catheterization. With both methods, local antisepsis using chlorhexidine or other appropriate antiseptic solutions has a place. The use of systemic antibiotics is only rarely beneficial in these patients as usually one strain is simply replaced by another bacterial strain resistant to the last antibiotic used.

Outbreaks of Urinary Tract Infection

Most outbreaks of urinary tract infection occur in the wards or special units where there are catheterized patients or patients recovering from instrumentation or surgery on the urinary tract. Rarely operating theatre outbreaks of infection occur because of the use of contaminated antiseptic solutions or contamination of instruments such as endoscopes due to faulty sterilization and disinfection techniques.

Sometimes the index case is admitted from another hospital with the epidemic strain in the faeces, or urine, or both (*Fig. 24.4*). Klebsiella outbreaks have greatly increased in frequency during the last 10 years, probably due in part to widespread overuse of ampicillin in hospital patients. Such strains are virtually always resistant to ampicillin and often become selected out in the faeces of hospitalized patients. The skin of the perineum or genital tract is therefore often contaminated by *Klebsiella* strains and 'self-infection' is frequent. When an epidemic *Klebsiella* strain is introduced into a ward it can sometimes colonize the

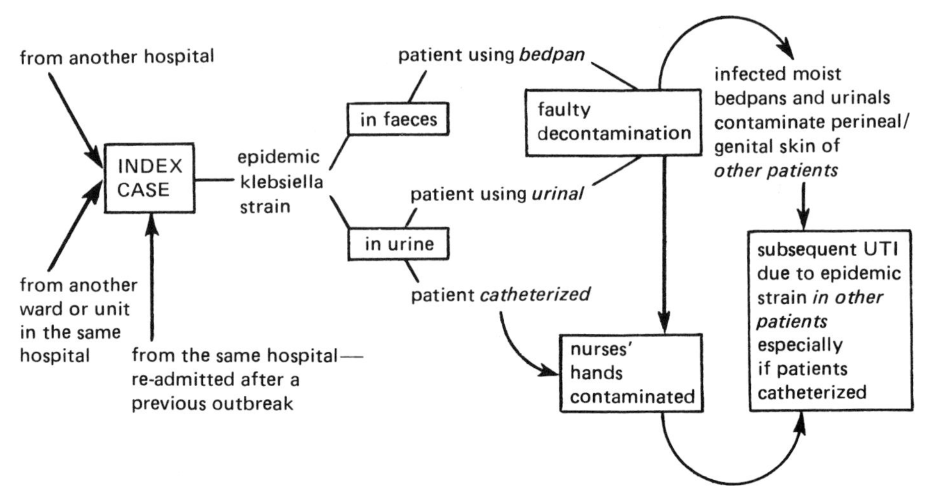

Fig. 24.4. Ward outbreaks of urinary tract infections (UTI) due to multiple antibiotic-resistant epidemic strains of *Klebsiella*.

large bowel or perineal skin of many of the patients in the ward and some of these patients eventually develop urinary tract infections due to this strain. Once the urinary tract of a catheterized patient is infected by the epidemic strain of *Klebsiella*, the organism can rapidly spread to other catheterized patients via contaminated hands of nursing staff. The most important measure to reduce the chains of cross-infection by *Klebsiella* and other organisms in the ward is by scrupulous hand hygiene. Thorough washing of hands, using a chlorhexidine or iodophor detergent preparation, drying of hands, use of gloves and scrupulous aseptic techniques are all important. Recently, the use of alcoholic chlorhexidine on hands has also proved useful in specialized units. Adequate disinfection and dry storage of urinals and bed pans is also necessary.

The investigation of outbreaks in infection due to *Klebsiella, Serratia, Acinetobacter, Pseudomonas* and other Gram-negative bacilli depends on correlating careful epidemiological data about the time and place of each infection or colonization, with information about the bacterial isolate from each patient, member of staff or environmental site. The bacterial isolates are compared for antibiotic sensitivity patterns and further 'typing' information (*see* Appendix I). *Klebsiella* strains are often successfully typed according to their capsular serotype.

Recent outbreaks of infection due to gentamicin-resistant *Klebsiella* strains carrying R factors for many different antibiotics, have mainly affected catheterized men, and have been caused by various serotypes, including K16, K2 and K21. In some serious klebsiella outbreaks in Britain, many patients have had to be isolated and wards temporarily closed before the outbreaks are brought under control. Combined with these measures temporary antibiotic policies to discourage the use of antibiotics to which the epidemic strain was resistant were introduced. In particular, it has often been found useful to ban the use of both ampicillin and cotrimoxazole temporarily in the affected areas of the hospital. (*See* Casewell et al., 1977; Houang et al., 1979; Speller, 1980.)

SURGICAL WOUND INFECTIONS

Types of Wound and Other Factors Affecting Incidence of Wound Sepsis

The type of surgical wound is the most important single factor associated with the development of wound infections. The major types of surgical wound can be classified as follows:

a. 'Clean' operation wounds
Clean surgery that does not involve incisions through the gastro-intestinal, respiratory or genito-urinary tracts is usually associated with very low sepsis rates of less than 2–5%. Examples of such operations include elective repair of an inguinal hernia and excision of a subcutaneous lipoma. The most frequent infecting bacterial species for this type of wound is *Staph. aureus.*

b. 'Contaminated' operation wounds
Surgery that involves a site with known normal flora (apart from the skin) is bound to present additional risks of contamination of the wound, such as operations on the colon, gall bladder, mouth or vagina. Where the contamination is light, such as occurs when removing a non-inflamed appendix, the sepsis rate may be only a little higher than with clean surgery. However in many instances, there is significant spillage from the operation area which results in heavy contamination, as when faecal material enters a wound or peritoneal cavity during some operations on the colon or following a perforated gangrenous appendix. High sepsis rates may then occur, possibly between 10 and 40%. Gram-negative bacilli such as *E. coli* and anaerobes such as *Bacteroides fragilis* predominate in these wound infections.

c. 'Infected' operation wounds
The operation site may occasionally be infected at the time of surgery, as with the incision of an abscess. The sepsis rates in this type of wound will naturally approach 100%.

There are several other important factors that influence the development of wound sepsis (*Table 24.2*). When a prosthesis or foreign body is present, low grade pathogens, such as *Staph. epidermidis*, may also cause clinically significant infections of the wound; this is especially important in patients with a prosthetic hip joint or a prosthetic heart valve. When a drain is inserted, there is an increased risk of wound sepsis but this depends, to some extent, on the site and type of the drain. A suction drainage system usually presents less of a risk than an open separate 'stab' drain. A long operation is more likely to become complicated by infection than a short operation.

The surgical team

The sepsis rates undoubtedly reflect on the skill of an individual surgeon. A careful surgeon who handles the tissues gently, securing good haemostasis and who works moderately quickly with excellent aseptic techniques may have lower sepsis rates than another surgeon who is possibly less skilled. If a member of the surgical team is a heavy skin carrier of *Staph. aureus*, and especially if a skin

Table 24.2. Factors influencing the development of wound sepsis

1. *Type of surgery*
a. Clean, contaminated or infected operation site? *b.* Prosthesis or foreign body (e.g. bullet) present? *c.* Drain inserted? *d.* Duration of surgery *e.* 'Place' in the operation list
2. *Surgical team*
a. Skill of individual surgeon *b.* Good aseptic techniques; adequate protective clothing including gloves *c.* Carriage of *Staph. aureus*?
3. *Age and general condition of the patient*
4. *Persistence of local structural abnormality*
5. *Extra precautions taken against the possibility of infection*
a. Duration of stay pre-operatively *b.* Adequate antisepsis for the hands of surgical team and skin of patient at operation site *c.* Adequate preparation of bowel for patients requiring gastro-intestinal surgery *d.* Appropriate antibiotic prophylaxis when indicated *e.* Adequate ventilation of theatre
6. *Ward factors post-operatively*

lesion is also present on the hands, there may be a much increased risk of staphylococcal wound infection (*see below*).

The patient

Elderly patients and those who are severely debilitated, because of malignant or other disease, have higher wound sepsis rates than younger patients who are reasonably fit at the time of operation. Obese or diabetic patients and those receiving steroid therapy also have above average sepsis rates post-operatively. If local structural abnormalities persist at an operation site post-operatively, such as gall stones or leakage from a damaged gall bladder in a patient who has had bile duct surgery, or break down of a gut anastomosis with subsequent leakage, then clearly wound and deep abdominal sepsis are much more likely to develop than when no such structural abnormalities occur.

Ideally, the patient should have the operation within 24 hours of admission to hospital before his skin has a chance to become significantly colonized by the 'hospital' staphylococci. Patients requiring bowel surgery need to have as much faeces removed as possible pre-operatively, for example by saline irrigation methods.

Antibiotic prophylaxis

Antibiotic prophylaxis can reduce the wound sepsis rates if appropriate agents are suitably administered during and for a short period after the operation;

metronidazole, for example, has already contributed to a fall in sepsis rates from anaerobes, such as *Bacteroides fragilis*, following surgery on the colon. Benzylpenicillin (plus cloxacillin) may be used to cover lower limb amputations and major hip surgery so that the chances of post-operative gas gangrene due to *Clostridium welchii* infection are reduced (*see also* Antibiotic prophylaxis, in Chapter 3).

Post-operative factors

When the patient returns to the ward post-operatively, the wound should not be touched unless absolutely essential or else *Staph. aureus*, haemolytic streptococci or other bacteria that may spread from another patient's infected wound could enter while the dressings are changed. The patient should not stay in hospital any longer than is strictly necessary, and sometimes he or she may be discharged within a few days of surgery. However, careful follow up is necessary at home as well as in hospital for a period of a few weeks. During this time, a hospital-acquired wound infection may become recognized. There are numerous other factors relevant to the development of surgical sepsis (*see* Cruse, 1973).

Recognition of Wound Sepsis

Clinically the most obvious feature of a septic wound is the discharge of pus. The incidence of wound sepsis is best measured prospectively for each surgeon for each of the major types of surgery. In practice, this often involves a lot of surveillance and careful record keeping by a dedicated infection control nurse working in conjunction with the theatre staff, the ward sisters and the consultant microbiologist. The results are sent in confidence to each surgeon regularly. Any sudden increase in a surgeon's sepsis rates needs careful investigation.

Effects of Wound Infections and Other Types of Surgical Sepsis

Major wound sepsis may result in significantly delayed wound healing or dehiscence of the wound. When a skin grafted area is infected, the graft may fail to take, especially when the infection is due to *Strep. pyogenes* or *Pseudomonas aeruginosa*. When the adjacent soft tissues and deeper structures such as bones, joints or peritoneal cavity are also infected the effects of wound sepsis are much more serious. A few patients may develop septicaemia and the wound sepsis might then be a significant contributory cause of death. Some examples of the effects of surgical sepsis and the main associated causative organisms are included in *Table 24.3*.

Staphylococcal Surgical Wound Sepsis

Most of the patients who develop septic wounds due to *Staph. aureus* are not infected by an epidemic hospital strain. The origin of the infecting strain of *Staph. aureus* in sporadic cases is not always clear but in many cases is probably derived from the patient's own skin flora. In the latter situation, the organism may sometimes enter the wound during the operation.

Table 24.3. Some effects of surgical sepsis

Type of surgery	*Main organisms*	*Effects of sepsis include*
'Clean' general surgery	1. *Staph. aureus* predominantly 2. *Strep. pyogenes* and other haemolytic streptococci	Wound sepsis
Abdominal and gynaecological surgery	1. Mixed Gram-negative bacilli predominantly: *E. coli* and other 'coliforms' *Bacteroides fragilis* and other anaerobes 2. *Strep. milleri* 3. *Staph. aureus* and haemolytic streptococci	1. Wound sepsis 2. Intra-abdominal—sub-phrenic, paracolic, liver, pelvic abscesses 3. Peritonitis 4. Septicaemia
Urology	1. Gram-negative bacilli predominantly: *E. coli, Proteus, Klebsiella, Pseudomonas* and various 'coliforms' 2. *Staph. epidermidis* and faecal streptococci 3. *Candida albicans*	1. Urinary tract infections including pyelonephritis 2. Wound sepsis 3. Septicaemia
Orthopaedic surgery	1. *Staph. aureus* predominantly 2. *Staph. epidermidis* and diphtheroids, especially when a prosthesis is present 3. Gram-negative bacilli 4. *Clostridium welchii*	1. Wound sepsis 2. Infected bones and joints 3. Chronic osteomyelitis 4. Post-operative gas gangrene

Staph. aureus is always present in large numbers in hospitals since it is carried in warm moist sites on the skin or in the noses of many patients and hospital staff, (*see Fig. 24.5*) and it survives well in the dry environment. The carriage rate is higher in hospital than in the community. Fortunately, most strains do not cause cross-infection as easily as haemolytic streptococci. Nevertheless, small outbreaks of wound sepsis due to epidemic strains of *Staph. aureus,* often resistant to two or more anti-staphylococcal antibiotics, continue to occur in many hospitals. The microbiologist investigating such outbreaks will arrange for the staphylococcal strains isolated from the patients and, if applicable, from staff and the environment to be phage typed. Epidemiological investigations are necessary before extra swabs are taken and these are first aimed at establishing whether the outbreak of infection has occurred in the operating theatre or in the ward (*Table 24.4*). Ward sources of outbreaks of staphylococcal infection are more common than theatre sources. There are numerous possible routes for *Staph. aureus* cross-infection in each of these areas and some of these are described below (*see also Fig. 24.6* and *24.7*). However, in the majority of incidents, the source of infection in a ward is usually a patient with an established wound infection. In an operating theatre outbreak, the source is usually a member of the surgical team, or theatre staff, who either has an infected or colonized skin lesion or else is a heavy carrier of the epidemic *Staph. aureus* strain. Swabs of the potential

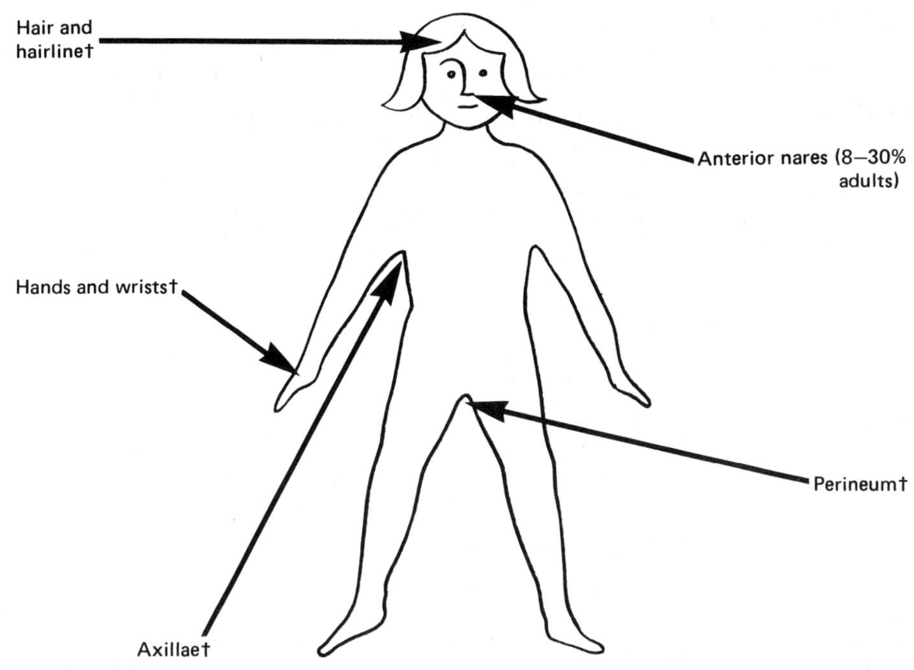

Fig. 24.5. Possible carriage sites for *Staph. aureus*. NB Young to middle-aged adult males are more likely to carry *Staph. aureus* on the perineum or other skin sites than similarly aged females. †Less than 5% carriage rates in adults.

Table 24.4. Factors suggesting a theatre or ward source of outbreak of staphylococcal wound sepsis

Factor	*Theatre source*	*Ward source*
1. Time of first recognition of the septic wound	*a.* Sepsis at the time of removing the first dressing *b.* Sepsis occurring between 1 and 8 days post-operatively	*a.* Sepsis only after the first dressing was removed *b.* Sepsis developing after the third post-operative day
2. Depth of sepsis	Deep or superficial	Superficial
3. Hospital areas affected	Patients in different wards or different hospitals	Patients in the same ward
4. Surgical team and operating theatre details	All the patients: *a.* Operated on by the same person in the surgical team OR *b.* Same operating list OR *c.* Same operating theatre	*a.* Different surgical teams OR *b.* Different operating lists OR *c.* Different operating theatres
5. Further microbiological investigations	*Staph. aureus* strains of similar type isolated from a surgical team member or other theatre source, and from patient's wounds	*Staph. aureus* strains of similar type isolated from patients in the ward and possibly from ward staff

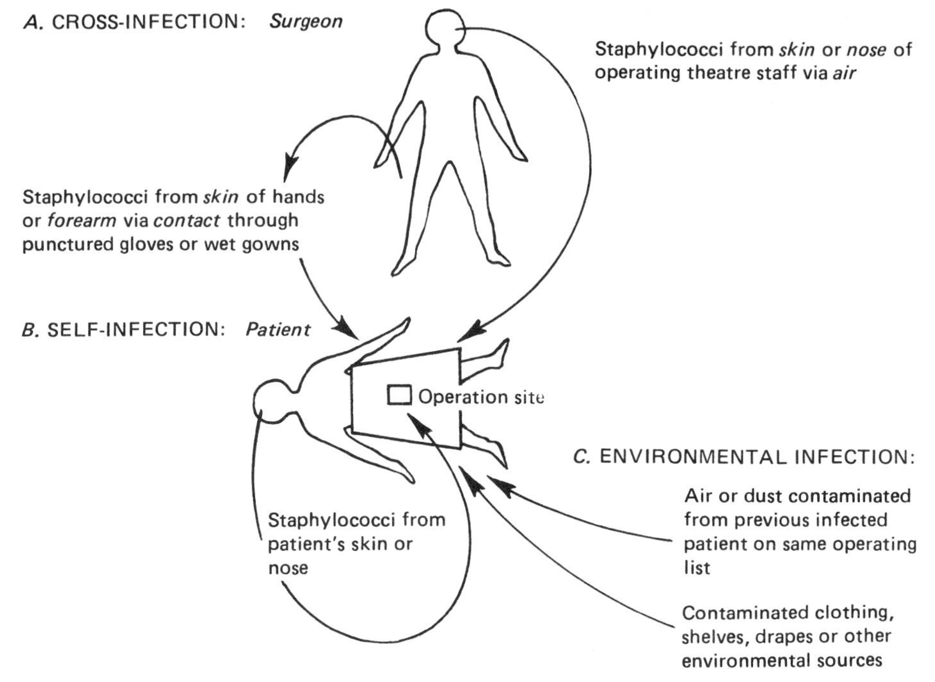

Fig. 24.6. Routes of spread of *Staph. aureus* in the operating theatre.

carriage sites of ward or theatre staff may be collected and swabs of the wounds of all patients in a ward in a suspected ward outbreak.

Operating theatre associated staphylococcal sepsis

1. *The surgical team*

The surgical team is the most frequent source of outbreaks of operating theatre-acquired sepsis (*Fig. 24.6*). Any member of the surgical team who has skin sepsis, or who has skin lesions, including minor eczema which may be colonized by *Staph. aureus*, is particularly likely to be a source of an outbreak. Rarely a person can be a 'broadcaster', i.e. disperses high counts of staphylococci into the air which can spread great distances to infect or colonize other people. Less rare than 'broadcasters' are people who carry a lot of *Staph. aureus* in the perineum and other sites as well as the nose, and perineal carriers particularly can disperse staphylococci into the air which may infect the patient's wound. It has been suggested that sweaty male surgeons, who are most likely to become perineal carriers, should wear sterile disposable well-fitting plastic knickers for each operating list. This would reduce the risk of colonized perineal skin scales being dispersed into the theatre environment.

Gentle handling of the tissues and good haemostasis by surgeons are important factors associated with low sepsis rates in theatre. Other measures which reduce the chance of surgical wound infection involve the use of scrupulous aseptic techniques and also the following:

a. Protective theatre clothing
Caps covering the hair, clean theatre underdress, gowns and masks.

b. Gloves for the hands after adequate cleaning of the hands
Up to 10% of gloves have microscopic punctures so good cleaning of the hands is necessary, preferably involving the use of a hand antiseptic preparation. Chlorhexidine detergent or povidone iodine or alcoholic chlorhexidine solutions are suitable agents for disinfecting surgeons' hands before putting on gloves.

c. Movement of staff in theatre should be reduced to a minimum
This is to decrease the dispersal of skin scales by friction of clothing (and to diminish air turbulence). Only essential staff should be present to keep the total bacterial count around the patient down to the minimum.

d. The theatre environment
Plenum air ventilation is necessary to ensure that an adequate number of air changes per hour are achieved. It is also important that the currents of air flow are in the correct direction, especially near the operating table, to decrease the chances of bacteria-laden particles becoming deposited into the operation site.

The floor should be kept 'socially' clean so that dust does not collect and horizontal surfaces in the main theatre area which are potential dust traps should be reduced to a minimum. Walls and ceilings need not normally be cleaned very often from a bacteriological point of view. Disinfectants as well as thorough cleaning are required if pus or other potentially infected material is spilt on the operating table or floor.

The lights above the operating table should also be kept dust-free, so that potentially bacteria-laden particles do not fall into the wound of the patient.

2. *The patient*

The patient's own skin or nose is sometimes the source of an organism causing the subsequent wound infection. To reduce the chances of organisms from the patient or the ward colonizing the skin of the patient and then causing infection:

a. *Patient's bed linen, clothes, etc.* are not allowed into the theatre area.
b. *Patient's skin at and near the site of the wound* is separated from the rest of the skin surface by drapes.
c. *Patient's skin is disinfected at and near operation site,* for example iodine in spirit, povidone iodine or chlorhexidine in spirit.

Pre-operative baths with anti-staphylococcal agents such as hexachlorophene or chlorhexidine detergents may have a useful role; these are under evaluation at present.

Any known infected case should be kept to the end of the operation list so that a potentially contaminated environment will not affect other patients.

Ward-associated staphylococcal wound infections

Outbreaks of staphylococcal sepsis generally originate in the ward rather than the operating theatre, and the usual source is an infected patient (*Fig. 24.7*). The organism is spread from the infected patient usually by hands of staff, most often

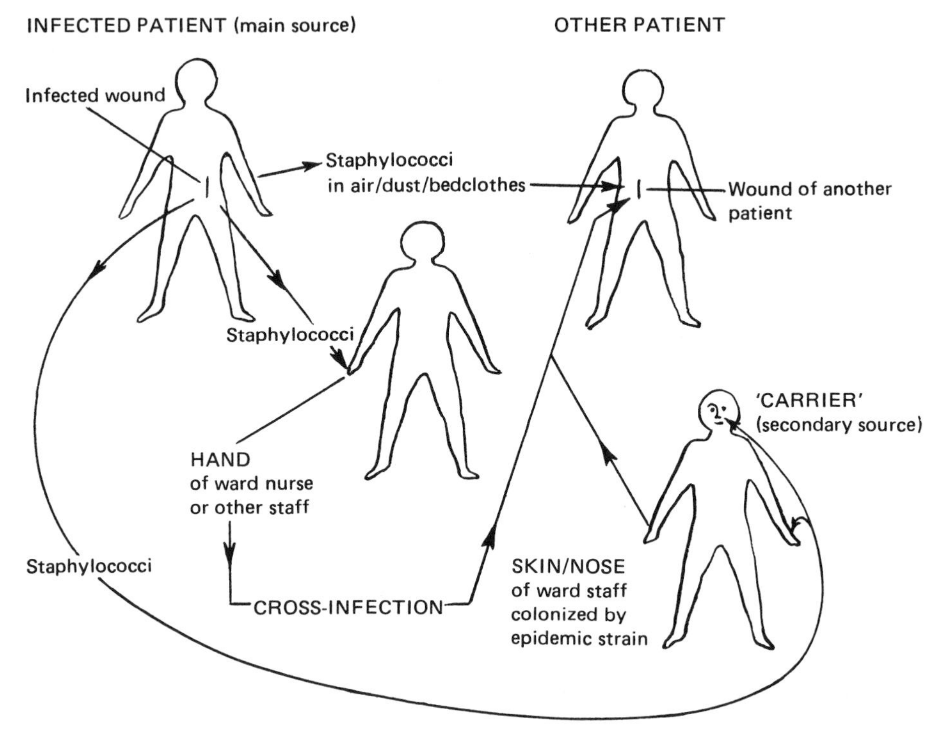

Fig. 24.7. Routes of spread of *Staph. aureus* in the surgical ward.

nursing staff, to one or more of the other patients in the ward. This may occur at the time of changing the dressings. Measures that reduce the chances of ward-acquired *Staph. aureus* wound infection include:

a. Isolation of patients in single rooms and suitable isolation nursing of patients who otherwise would discharge staphylococcal pus from the wound into the surgical ward. This isolation is particularly necessary when there is a lot of pus or the patient has a multiple antibiotic-resistant strain of *Staphylococcus*.

b. No-touch dressing techniques performed carefully—good education of nursing and medical staff is necessary. Medical staff should not touch the skin near the wound when 'peeping' at the wound. Care is also necessary when removing the sutures; adequate washing of hands between patients as well as no-touch techniques should be observed.

c. Suitable bed spacing between patients to decrease air or dust spread (about 8 foot bed centre to bed centre).

d. The patient should be admitted for the shortest time before the operation to decrease the chances of colonization or infection by hospital strains of staphylococci.

e. Antibiotics should be used only when strictly necessary. Virtually all *Staph. aureus* strains in hospital are penicillinase producers but 'hospital' strains may also be resistant to other antibiotics, such as tetracycline, erythromycin, methicillin, fusidic acid or gentamicin as well. Epidemic strains of *Staph. aureus*, which are resistant to many antibiotics, are often encouraged to spread when patients in the ward are receiving antibiotics to which the strain is resistant.

f. Patients with known skin disease are liable to be heavily colonized with *Staph. aureus* and should be excluded from general surgical wards.

g. Members of staff who develop boils, abscesses or other infected skin lesions should not attend surgical patients in the ward or theatre.

Control of staphylococcal outbreaks

When the results of culture of the patient's swabs and swabs of the nose, hands, wrists, perineum and hairline of theatre staff, in theatre-suspected outbreaks, or ward staff, in ward-suspected outbreaks, are known the consultant microbiologist in charge of the investigations can advise appropriate measures to further control an outbreak. He or she will already have arranged for the isolation of patients who have been shown to be infected or significantly colonized by the epidemic strain. The identification of the epidemic strain in practice is easiest when it has a characteristic multiple antibiotic resistance pattern, but in any case results of subsequent phage typing may help to confirm the suspected routes of spread of the epidemic strain. When a carrier of the epidemic strain is identified amongst hospital staff, the staff member may have to temporarily cease work with surgical patients until cleared of the organism. Methods of treating staphylococcal carriers include the repeated use of antiseptics such as hexachlorophane or chlorhexidine on the affected skin sites, hair shampoos and very frequent laundering of bed clothes and underwear. In most cases, the staphylococcal carriage soon disappears unless the person has skin disease or is a rare 'broadcaster' without obvious skin disease. In these latter situations, specialist help from reference centres may be advisable.

In a few recent extensive outbreaks due to *Staph. aureus* strains resistant to methicillin and gentamicin, it has been necessary to temporarily close surgical wards as part of the control measures. Outbreaks due to these multiple, antibiotic-resistant strains, which are resistant to gentamicin, appear to be on the increase in the past few years (*see* Shanson, 1981).

ACUTE LOWER RESPIRATORY TRACT INFECTIONS

Lower respiratory tract infections are the third most common type of hospital-acquired infection, after urinary tract and wound infections. Pneumonia may develop especially in elderly debilitated patients and there is a significant mortality rate. Other patients at risk include comatose patients and those who have been given a general anaesthetic, steroid or immunosuppressive therapy. The majority of these infections occurring amongst adults on general wards are sporadic and in patients with predisposing factors present before admission to hospital. Those with known chest disease or who are heavy cigarette smokers are most likely to become infected. Outbreaks of lower respiratory infections occasionally occur due to influenza A or B, and rare hospital outbreaks of Legionnaires' disease in Britain have been described recently (*see* Fallon, 1981). Epidemics of lower respiratory tract infections are more fequent on paediatric than adult wards and are mainly associated with viruses such as respiratory syncytial virus, para-influenza viruses and measles. The main organisms responsible for acute lower respiratory tract infections are included in *Table 24.1* (*see also* Chapter 12). Certain patients in intensive care units are at risk of developing respiratory infections especially when they receive intermittent positive pressure ventilation. Intensive care units are discussed below.

INTENSIVE CARE UNITS AND HOSPITAL-ACQUIRED INFECTION

Patients in an intensive care unit may suffer from many types of infection including respiratory tract infections, urinary tract infections, wound infections, intravenous infusion-associated infections and peritonitis associated with peritoneal dialysis.

The patients seen in intensive care units have often had major surgery or trauma which may lead to impaired general host defence mechanisms against infection. Other causes of impaired host defences against infection include old age, coma, malignancy, cirrhosis and uraemia, and treatment such as steroid therapy. Local defences against infection are also often greatly impaired in many of the patients in an intensive care unit because of the multiple invasive procedures that are frequently necessary. These procedures breach the intact skin or mucosa; they include intravenous infusion therapy, indwelling urinary catheterization, tracheostomy or intermittent positive pressure ventilation through an endo-tracheal tube, peritoneal dialysis, and suction drainage of lesions in the chest, abdomen or other sites. Patients with many reasons for having a great susceptibility to infection are accommodated in a relatively small area in the intensive care unit where numerous procedures are carried out. A small number of staff frequently work under conditions of great 'pressure' and in these circumstances it is not surprising that there is a high incidence of hospital-acquired infections. Most of the infections that occur are 'self' (autogenous) infections involving organisms from the patient's own faecal, skin or upper respiratory tract flora, although the organisms may have come from the staff or hospital environment originally. Obvious cross-infection incidents, particularly with Gram-negative bacilli, occur at different times in most intensive care units.

Respiratory tract infections due to both Gram-positive organisms (pneumococci and staphylococci) and Gram-negative organisms (coliforms, *Haemophilus*, *Pseudomonas* and *Bacteroides* species) occur in intensive care unit patients. Outbreaks of respiratory infections due to *Pseudomonas aeruginosa*, *Klebsiella aerogenes* and *Serratia marcescens* are also well-known hazards. Widespread use of antibiotics such as ampicillin plus cloxacillin helps to select out *Klebsiella*, *Pseudomonas*, *Serratia* and other Gram-negative bacilli in the saliva, faecal flora and other sites, such as a tracheostomy wound. These Gram-negative bacilli, which may be resistant to several antibiotics because they carry R factors, can reach a new patient from another infected or colonized patient in the unit via the contaminated hands of nursing, or other staff, or by contact with contaminated moist equipment or solutions. In the majority of instances, cross-'colonization', rather than cross-'infection', occurs. Collection of blood cultures, sputum, tracheostomy wound swabs and other relevant specimens is necessary. These are transported promptly to the microbiology department before the start of antibiotic therapy. Careful clinical assessment of the patient's chest and study of a chest radiograph is necessary for the clinical significance of Gram-negative isolates to be reasonably assessed. Moist equipment and solutions that may become easily contaminated and cause Gram-negative respiratory tract infection includes ventilators, humidifiers, suction apparatus, wash bowls, lubricants, water, some disinfectants, and liquid food or milk. Sinks or taps are occasionally contaminated but have rarely been important sources of infection. Some of the many routes of possible respiratory tract cross-infection in intensive care units are included in *Fig. 24.8*.

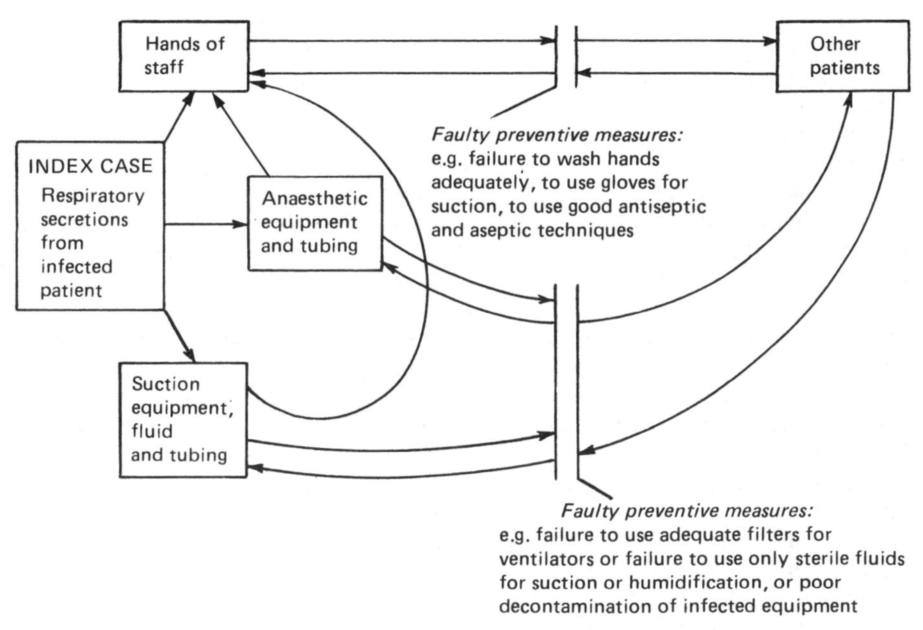

Fig. 24.8. Routes of spread of *Pseudomonas aeruginosa*, or *Klebsiella aerogenes*, in outbreak of respiratory tract infections in intensive care units. ———, Main routes of spread to other patients.

Control of infection in an intensive care unit depends primarily on a well-trained staff there who regularly liaise with the control of infection staff, usually medical microbiologist and infection control nurse, based in the clinical microbiology department. Regular and careful hand washing by the intensive care unit staff and use of appropriate antiseptics on the hands, such as chlorhexidine/alcohol solution, is of paramount importance. For certain procedures, such as tracheostomy suction, gloves are also recommended. Aseptic techniques, and the use of solutions and equipment which are not contaminated, are also essential and constant monitoring of the types of infection seen on the unit is important. Bacteriological surveillance of the equipment in use is also necessary, especially when an increase in infection is apparent. Equipment has to be changed and decontaminated between patients. While the equipment is in use, the prevention of contamination is also necessary. This can be helped by using only sterile fluids which are changed daily, and effective filters, on ventilators. Adequate heating of water in ventilators or humidifiers to a temperature above 50 °C is recommended at least daily. Decontamination of ventilators is easiest where they are of the autoclavable type, otherwise ethylene oxide or formaldehyde gas machines may have to be used. Anaesthetic tubing, bags, some suction apparatus and face masks may be efficiently cleaned and heat disinfected by a purpose-built washing machine or they may be decontaminated in a low temperature steam disinfector. The latter has the advantage in that the items are dry and packed at the end of the cycle. If a washing machine is used, the items need to be placed in a drying cabinet before use. The cleaning and decontamination of apparatus are best carried out in an area separate from the main intensive care unit areas. Chemical methods of disinfection, such as glutaraldehyde, should only be used as a last resort as they are subject to many potential pitfalls, including inadequate immersion of the equipment, and insufficient duration of immersion in an active solution.

When an outbreak of infection occurs in a special unit such as an intensive care unit, or a neurosurgical unit, a restriction of the use of broad spectrum antibiotics may help to bring the outbreak under control more quickly (*see* Price and Sleigh, 1970).

INFECTIVE HAZARDS OF INTRAVENOUS INFUSION THERAPY

Intravenous infusion therapy is frequently complicated by the development of 'minor' degrees of septic thrombophlebitis. However, any degree of sepsis at a drip site is potentially life threatening and between 0·2 and 8% of patients receiving i.v. fluids develop septicaemia. Occasionally patients may also develop potentially fatal endotoxic shock because Gram-negative bacilli that multiply at room temperature in the infusion fluid are introduced with additives into the fluid. Such additions, if necessary, should be added aseptically by trained pharmacy staff wherever possible.

There are numerous possible routes for organisms to enter an intravenous infusion system (*Fig. 24.9*), although in practice entry by way of the drip site is by far the most important of these. The infusion fluid itself may rarely become contaminated by Gram-negative bacilli, aerobic spore bearing or other organisms when there has been a fault in sterilization of the bottles or packs at the manufacturers. During the last decade, outbreaks of septicaemia or endotoxic shock have occurred in the U.S.A. and Britain from this cause (the 'Devonport' outbreak—subject of the Clothier Report). An outbreak of pseudomonas infections occurred in a London teaching hospital due to organisms contaminating the undersurface of the crimpled foil of the bottles. The organisms were introduced by colonized cooling water during the cooling of the bottles in the autoclave. Stringent regulations that include strict physico-chemical monitoring of the sterilization process in approved centres, reduce the chances of further disasters of this type occurring again. Blood or plasma products may contain viable organisms from a blood donor at the time of infusion, such as hepatitis viruses, Epstein-Barr virus, cytomegalovirus, *Treponema pallidum* and malarial parasites. However, screening of blood donors including the use of HBsAg testing considerably reduces this risk.

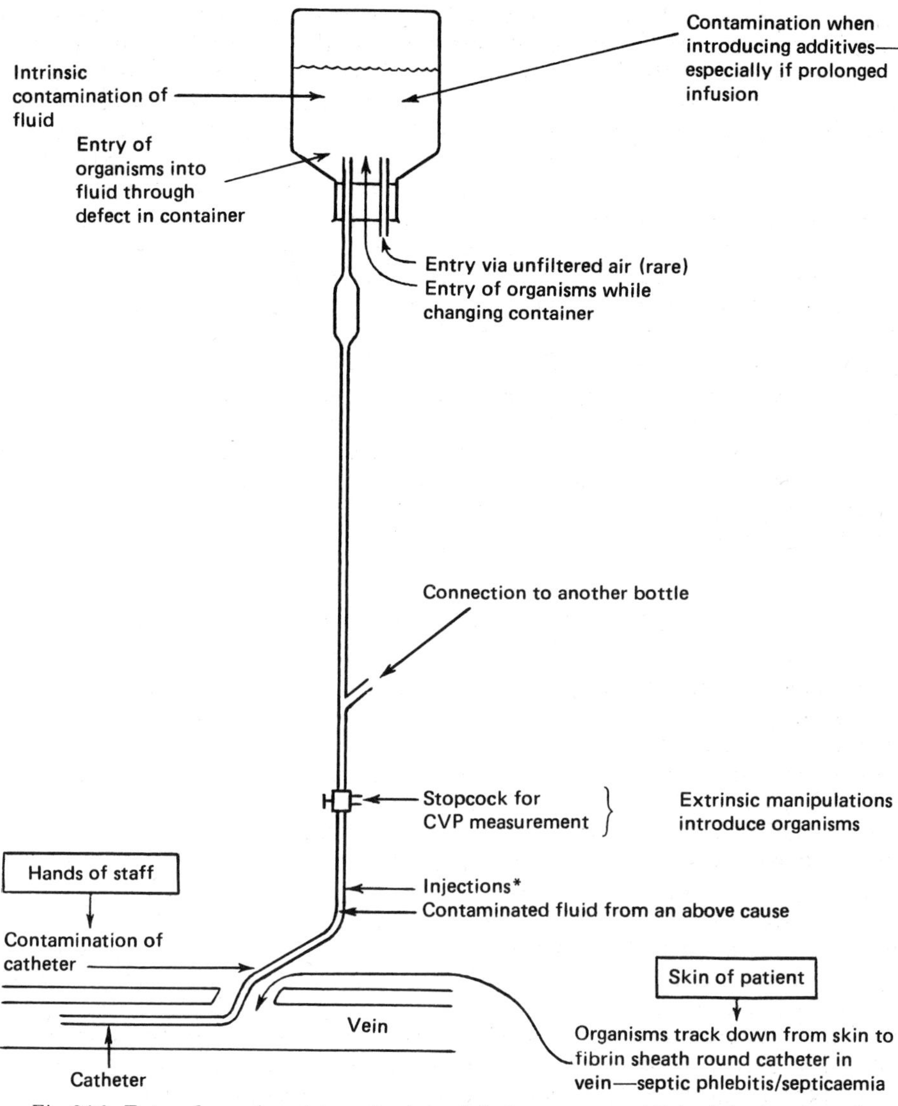

Fig. 24.9. Entry of organisms into patient's i.v. infusion apparatus. *Bolus injection through tubing safer than introducing additive to infusion from infection point of view.

Setting Up and Maintenance of the Intravenous Infusion

Only essential parenteral infusions should be set up. This particularly applies to the insertion of central venous pressure monitoring lines which carry additional infective hazards as they are more invasive, tend to stay inserted longer and have more 'open' moist connection sites that can become contaminated than simple peripheral intravenous drips.

The incidence of septic phlebitis is less with a 'scalp vein' type needle than larger bore plastic cannulae and the former should be used when possible. Aseptic techniques and thorough washing of hands by the operator are always important and the wearing of gloves is preferable. The skin of the patient around the site of the vein should be cleaned and either an alcoholic chlorhexidine solution or an iodine (or iodophor) in spirit mixture applied. Arm veins are less likely to become infected than veins in the legs. If the patient's arm is hairy, a 'dry' shave with a sterile disposable razor blade is preferred before applying the skin antiseptic. After insertion, the needle or cannulae needs to be anchored securely as excessive movement predisposes the site to infection. Topical betadine antiseptic and, where necessary, appropriate antifungal creams applied regularly to the drip site are probably of value in reducing local infection, especially when prolonged intravenous infusion therapy is unavoidable.

Daily inspection of the drip site is necessary and if signs of phlebitis or pus develop or symptoms of pain and tenderness occur, it is important to withdraw all of the infusion equipment and cannula immediately and consider inserting a new drip at a completely different site. Changing of the entire giving set down to the cannula should take place every 24–48 hours, and sooner when blood has been transfused. The cannula itself should also be routinely changed every 48–72 hours. If the patient is receiving broad spectrum antibiotics, such as ampicillin, there is an increased chance of superinfection by antibiotic-resistant organisms, such as *Klebsiella aerogenes* or *Staph. aureus*, at the drip site. It is important to check that the patient still requires such antibiotic treatment during the intravenous infusion.

Diagnosis of Infective Complications of Intravenous Infusion Therapy

The prompt recognition of the local infective complications described above may allow the prevention of the more serious complications of septic shock and septicaemia. However, these serious complications must be suspected if a fever, rigor or sudden fall in blood pressure occurs while the patient is receiving i.v. infusion therapy. In this situation, the drip is withdrawn, blood cultures are collected and the entire infusion set and cannula plus catheter are sent to the microbiology department for immediate investigation.

The microbiologist will examine the bottle or pack for defects (these should, of course, also be looked for by the ward staff before giving the infusion and the container not used if found to be defective), perform microscopy of any fluid left in the bottle and culture remaining fluid at 35 °C, room temperature and 4 °C incubation.

The cannula or catheter tip will also be cultured by putting it in broth, but semi-quantitative cultures, for example by rolling a catheter tip moistened with broth over the surface of a blood agar plate, are also desirable. *Staph. epidermidis* often 'contaminates' the catheter tip as it is withdrawn from the patient's skin site but the same organism may occasionally cause i.v. infusion associated septicaemia, especially in patients who are severely debilitated, or immunosuppressed. Other organisms that may be isolated from the catheter tip which often indicate genuine infection of the i.v. line, include *Staph. aureus, Klebsiella* species, *Serratia marcescens, Pseudomonas* species and *Candida albicans.* The latter yeast is particularly associated with prolonged intravenous total nutrition therapy. Once the infected i.v. infusion is withdrawn, the patient's condition usually improves but shocked patients may require emergency medical measures. A few patients may also require blind specific antibiotic therapy for septicaemia, using a combination such as cloxacillin plus gentamicin, until the results of microbiological investigations are known or until the patient's condition has improved.

Prevention of Intravenous Infusion-associated Infection

The main preventive measures have been discussed above. Skilled setting up and maintenance of drips by specially trained 'IV' teams in hospitals might also reduce the incidence of sepsis associated with i.v. infusion therapy; this practice is increasingly recommended in North America.

TUBERCULOSIS AND VIRAL HEPATITIS

During the last decade, increased attention has been paid in Britain to the health and safety at work of employees in hospitals, and there had been particular interest in reducing the risk to staff from patients with tuberculosis or viral hepatitis. Each hospital needs policies on these matters from the occupational health department which are drawn up in conjunction with the consultant microbiologist.

1. *Tuberculosis*

Staff are Mantoux tested and have a chest X-ray at the start of their hospital employment. Mantoux negative staff may be offered BCG immunization and checked to ensure that they convert to Mantoux positive status. Only Mantoux positive staff should attend patients with known or suspected open tuberculosis or work in laboratories where specimens containing tubercle bacilli are handled. In most hospitals today, it is accepted that the occasional patient with open TB requires single room isolation and special isolation procedures until at least 2–3 weeks of antituberculosis chemotherapy have been given. Staff contacts of patients who expectorate large numbers of tubercle bacilli in the sputum need careful follow up including chest X-ray examinations, supervised by the occupational health department. Patient contacts also may need follow up.

Any sputum expectorated by a patient is regarded with suspicion, even if the patient clinically has no obvious evidence of TB, and sputum containers should not be opened by staff on the wards. Such containers should only be opened and subsequently investigated under an approved 'B1' safety cabinet in the laboratory.

2. *Viral Hepatitis*

The hazards to hospital staff from hepatitis B were dramatically illustrated by several outbreaks occurring in renal dialysis units during the 1960s, which resulted in serious disease and fatalities among staff. All patients and staff should be carefully screened and excluded from renal dialysis units if they are HBsAg positive carriers. Increasing precautions in laboratories during the last 10 years, while working on blood or serum samples in particular, has resulted in a great decline in the number of laboratory staff who develop hepatitis each year. However, hepatitis still occasionally develops in hospital staff who work in the operating theatre, intensive care unit, general wards and non-renal dialysis departments.

In some cases, the infection may occur as a result of contact with a case outside hospital but the increased risks of working in hospital have been recognized and viral hepatitis is now an officially recognized industrial disease which may allow a member of staff who develops it to claim compensation.

Patients who have a clinical diagnosis of suspected viral hepatitis should be isolated (stool/needle/urine isolation techniques). Blood is collected by a member of staff wearing gloves and the specimen is transported to the laboratory in a sealed plastic bag conspicuously marked with a 'hepatitis risk' label. The specimen should be kept upright in a non-leaking screw cap container and be accompanied by a similarly labelled request form in a separate pocket of the plastic bag. Patients may be seen for conditions other than hepatitis, but should be considered as a 'hepatitis risk' if they are drug addicts, patients with previous known hepatitis, known homosexuals, patients with recent or extensive tattoos, or patients from the Middle East, Philippines or other overseas areas known to have a high HBsAg positive carrier rate among the population. It is not necessary to isolate a patient who is an incidental HBsAg positive carrier unless parenteral procedures, such as intravenous infusion therapy or surgery, mean that there are additional hazards present.

Staff who accidentally prick themselves with a needle or 'sharp', that may have been used on a patient with known HBsAg positive blood, need to report immediately to an appropriate senior member of staff so that the incident can be recorded and administration of hyperimmune anti-HBsAg immunoglobulin can be given as soon as possible, and preferably within 24–48 hours of the accident.

About 1 in 800 apparently healthy British people are HBsAg positive and it is clearly impractical to screen every hospital patient. The main advice to staff should be to respect the dangers of contaminating the skin or eye with blood or serum from *any* patient, to avoid such contamination whenever possible, to wash off immediately any blood or serum that contaminates the skin, and to take appropriate action should an accident occur.

Medical and nursing staff who work in the operating theatre and intensive care unit are probably at greater risk than staff on a general ward because of the large number of procedures performed with sharp instruments and the increased chance of contact with blood from patients. There is a very high risk to operating theatre staff when prolonged major surgery is performed on a patient who is incubating hepatitis B, especially when the patient is not known to be a 'hepatitis risk' (*see* Shanson, 1980). Gloves afford some protection, but up to 10% of gloves worn by the principal surgeon and scrub nurse may be microscopically punctured (*see* Church and Sanderson, 1980). During extensive surgery the chances of a needle or instrument causing unnoticed damage to a glove—and a minor inoculation injury—must be quite high. Wearing of two sets of gloves, waterproof apron and goggles together with many other precautions are necessary when surgery is carried out on patients known or suspected of being HBsAg positive (*see* Lowbury et al., 1981). The consequences of acquiring hepatitis B are discussed in Chapter 15.

If a member of staff is found to be a healthy HBsAg positive carrier, he or she can usually continue their normal duties providing they do not work in dialysis units, with transplant patients or possibly oncology units. The risk of hepatitis is almost entirely from patients to staff rather than vice versa.

In the near future, it is hoped that an effective vaccine against hepatitis B will become widely available and then hospital staff could be offered much better specific protection.

Further Reading

Bennett J. V. and Brachman P. S. (ed.) (1979) *Hospital Infections*. Boston, U.S.A., Little, Brown and Company.

Campbell W. B. (1980) Prophylaxis of infection after appendectomy in a survey of current surgical practice. *Br. Med. J.* **281**, 1597–1600.

Casewell M. W., Dalton M. T., Webster M. et al. (1977) Gentamicin-resistant *Klebsiella aerogenes* in a urological ward. *Lancet* **2**, 444–446.

Church J. and Sanderson P. (1980) Surgical glove punctures. *Journal of Hospital Infection* **1**, 84.

Cruse P. J. E. and Foord R. (1973) A five year prospective study of 23 649 surgical wounds. *Arch. Surgery* **107**, 206.

Fallon R. J. (1980) Nosocomial infections with *Legionella pneumophila*. *Journal of Hospital Infection* **1**, 299–305.

Flynn J. T. and Blandy J. P. (1980) Procedures in practice—urethral catheterization. *Br. Med. J.* **281**, 928.

Gillespie W. A. (1976) Hospital infection. In: Williams D. F. and Chisholm G. D. (ed.) *Scientific Foundations of Urology*, Vol. 1, pp. 197–200. London, Heinemann.

Grüneberg R. N. (1980) Antibiotic prescribing policies: a personal view. *Antibiotics and Chemotherapy: Current Topics*. Lancaster, England, MTP Press.

Houang E. T., Evans M. A. and Simpson C. N. (1979) Control of hospital epidemic of gentamicin-resistant *Klebsiella aerogenes*. *Lancet* **2**, 205.

Lowbury E. J. L., Ayliffe G. A. J., Geddes A. M. et al. (1981) *Control of Hospital Infection*, 2nd ed. London, Chapman and Hall.

Meers P. D. (1981) Epidemiology: infection in hospitals. *Br. Med. J.* **282**, 1246.

Parker M. T. (ed.) (1978) *Hospital Acquired Infections: Guidelines to Laboratory Methods*. WHO Regional Publications. Regional Office for Europe, Copenhagen.

Phillips I., Meers P. D. and D'Arcy P. F. (1976) *Microbiological Hazards of Infusion Therapy*. Lancaster, England, MTP Press.

Price D. J. E. and Sleigh J. D. (1970) Control of infection due to *Klebsiella aerogenes* in a neurosurgical unit by withdrawal of all antibiotics. *Lancet* **2**, 1213.

Selwyn S. (1980) Protective isolation: what are our priorities? *Journal of Hospital Infection* **1**, 5.

Shanson D. C. (1980) Hepatitis B outbreak in operating theatre and intensive care unit staff. *Lancet* **2**, 596.

Shanson D. C. (1981) A review: antibiotic-resistant *Staph. aureus*. *Journal of Hospital Infection* **2**, 11–36.

Shanson D. C. and McSwiggan D. A. (1980) Operating theatre acquired infection with a gentamicin-resistant strain of *Staphylococcus aureus:* outbreaks in two hospitals attributable to one surgeon. *Journal of Hospital Infection* **1**, 171–172.

Speller D. C. E. (1980) Hospital infection by multi-antibiotic resistant Gram-negative bacilli. *J. Antimicrob. Chemother.* **6**, 168.

Williams R. E. O., Blowers R., Garrod L. P. et al. (1966) *Hospital Infection, Causes and Prevention*. London, Lloyd-Luke.

Appendix to Chapter 24

1. *Brief notes on 'typing' of organisms*

The main reason for typing organisms is to help clarify the possible routes of cross-infection in an outbreak. There is no point in typing organisms unless relevant accompanying epidemiological information is available.

An ideal typing system would be able to distinguish a large number of different types of a species ('good discrimination'), type all the strains of a species, and also would be highly reproducible. The 'discrimination' is also inversely related to the proportion of strains typable by a given character, e.g. a high proportion of *Sal. typhi* strains (about 30%) have Vi phage type e, and although the Vi phage typing system is highly reproducible, it has low discrimination. In practice, the typing systems available for some organisms are far from ideal, as with *Pseudomonas aeruginosa*, and it is then often necessary to use a combination of two or more different but complementary typing systems for the same species.

Strains of a bacterial species can be typed according to biochemical or cultural differences between strains (biotyping), antigenic differences (serotyping), differences in the susceptibility to lysis by one or more bacteriophages (phage typing), or differences in the susceptibility to inhibitory substances produced by a set of 'indicator' strains of the same species (bacteriocine typing). Other typing systems are also occasionally used. Examples of typing systems available for hospital pathogens are included in *Table 24.5*. The organisms most frequently typed in practice are *Staph. aureus, Strep. pyogenes* (group A haemolytic streptococci), *Pseudomonas aeruginosa* and *Klebsiella aerogenes*.

Table 24.5. Typing systems for hospital pathogens, 1980

	Typing systems				
Pathogen	*Bio*	*Sero*	*Phage*	*Cine*	*Other*
Staph. aureus		+	++		
Coag. neg. *Staph.*	++		+		
Strep. group A		++			
B		++			
D	++	+			
Strep. pneumoniae		++			
Ps. aeruginosa		++	++	++	
Klebsiella	+	++	(+)		
Proteus	+	+			Dienes
E. coli		+	(+)	(+)	
Serratia	++				
Acinetobacter	+				
Salmonella	+	+	++		
Shigella	+	+		++	

++ = Main method.
\+ = Other useful method.
(+) = Developmental.

Phage Typing of Staph. aureus

The great majority of strains of *Staph. aureus* can be reproducibly phage typed using an international set of about 24 phages that are applied to each staphylococcal culture at a standardized dilution (routine test dilution, RTD, and also sometimes RTD × 100). Strains of *Staph. aureus* are usually lysed by a number of phages within a phage 'group'; there are four main phage groups. In the 1950s and early 1960s, many outbreaks of *Staph. aureus* infection were associated with strains of group I phage type, such as 52, 80, 81 type. During the 1970s, many outbreaks of hospital wound infection were caused by *Staph. aureus* strains of group III phage types, such as 83A, 84, 85.

Serological Typing of Strep. pyogenes

Strep. pyogenes strains can usually be successfully compared by identifying T and M protein antigens in the cell wall. Trypsinized suspensions of the organism are used in agglutination tests with known anti-sera against T antigens to obtain the T typing pattern. An acid heat extraction method is used to prepare each strain for M antigen typing with known anti-sera in an immunoprecipitation test.

Typing of Pseudomonas aeruginosa

For many years, *Pseudomonas aeruginosa* strains have been compared according to their pyocine typing patterns. The method is still used but a combination of 'O' serotyping and bacteriophage typing is increasingly used to compare strains that could not previously be distinguished by pyocine typing.

Typing of Klebsiella aerogenes

In recent years, great advances have occurred in the typing of *Klebsiella* strains. The determination of the capsular serotype by a modified 'Quellung' type reaction or an immunoelectrophoresis technique is one of the main methods that have been used. Many gentamicin-resistant klebsiella outbreaks of infection in urology, general surgical and intensive care wards have been successfully investigated using the capsular typing method; K16 and K21 capsular types are two examples that have been implicated in these outbreaks in Britain.

2. *Isolation procedures*

Each hospital needs a policy for the isolation of patients with certain infections that may be transmitted to other patients or staff ('source' isolation) and, if applicable, the isolation of immunocompromised or other patients who are highly susceptible to infection ('protective' isolation). The details of the policy may vary according to local circumstances, but many hospitals adopt three similar categories of isolation that are commonly used—standard isolation, stool–urine–needle and protective isolation. Full details of isolation procedures are included in the book by Lowbury et al. (1981).

Strict Isolation

Infections in this group are rare but highly dangerous and patients require strict isolation procedures in designated high-risk isolation hospitals. These hospitals are often equipped with plastic isolators and staffed by especially trained personnel. Lassa fever and other viral haemorrhagic fevers, anthrax, diphtheria and rabies require strict isolation. Smallpox was included in the past but this disease is now extinct.

Accident and Emergency departments in general hospitals must not admit patients with these diseases. The local Medical Officer for Environmental Health needs to be immediately notified when a patient is suspected of having one of the above diseases and an appropriate 'emergency committee' is also convened.

Standard Isolation

Examples of diseases requiring standard isolation include:

a. Respiratory infections

Respiratory infections and 'childhood' fevers due to organisms which are resistant to antibiotics or are highly transmissible require standard isolation, including staphylococcal pneumonia, open pulmonary tuberculosis, whooping cough, chickenpox, herpes zoster, measles, rubella, influenza and respiratory syncytial virus infections.

b. Skin and wound sepsis

Skin lesions in patients with eczema or psoriasis are often heavily colonized or infected with *Staph. aureus* and these patients should be isolated as they spread large numbers of organisms into the air. Wound or skin sepsis due to *Strep. pyogenes* or to multiple antibiotic-resistant (e.g. gentamicin-resistant) strains of *Staph. aureus, Klebsiella* or other 'coliforms', or *Pseudomonas aeruginosa*, are other indications for standard isolation.

Standard isolation procedures include:

i. Single room isolation accommodation with the door kept closed. Ideally, negative pressure air ventilation also.
ii. Donning of gowns and/or disposable aprons, by all persons after entering the room.
iii. Wearing of gloves when handling patients with skin or wound sepsis.
iv. Washing of hands before leaving the room.

Stool–Urine–Needle Isolation

Examples of diseases requiring stool–urine–needle isolation include:

a. Enteric infections

Salmonella, campylobacter and enteropathogenic *E. coli* gastro-enteritis
Cholera
Enteric fevers—typhoid and paratyphoid fevers
Dysentery
Diarrhoea or vomiting of unknown origin
Threadworm infestation

b. Viral hepatitis

i. Due to hepatitis B, hepatitis A or 'non-A', 'non-B' virus.
ii. Carriers of hepatitis B when high titres are anticipated as in uraemic or immunosuppressed patients, or where there are diseases or procedures associated with spillage of blood or body secretions (e.g. patient with melaena or receiving intravenous infusion therapy).

c. Urinary tract infections

Isolation of the patient is indicated when the infecting organism is a multiple antibiotic-resistant strain of *Klebsiella aerogenes, Serratia marcescens,* other coliforms or *Pseudomonas aeruginosa,* resistant to several antibiotics or to gentamicin—especially when the patient is catheterized.

Stool–urine–needle isolation procedures are designed to limit the spread of infection from excreta and blood of infected patients by including:

i. Single room or side room isolation accommodation if possible.
ii. Wearing plastic apron and a gown over the apron after entering the room when handling the patient, or the bed linen, disposing of excreta.
iii. Washing of hands before and after completing duties in the room.
iv. Wearing disposable gloves before direct contact with patient or handling of equipment for the disposal of the excreta.
v. Addition of a phenolic, such as hycolin, or strong fresh hypochlorite solution, to excreta containing bacterial or viral pathogens respectively, before safe disposal in an adequate bed pan washer.
vi. Disposable crockery used for patients with enteric infections.

Specimens, Linen, Rubbish and 'Sharps'

For all patients requiring either standard or stool–urine–needle isolation a safe policy for the collection and transportation of pathology specimens, decontamination of infected linen by a heat process, disposal of infected rubbish and disposal of sharps is required.

Protective Isolation

Immunosuppressed patients, especially those with prolonged severe neutropenia, and patients with extensive burns require protective isolation.

Precautions necessary include:

i. Single room accommodation, preferably also with positive pressure air ventilation.

ii. Gowns or aprons, and masks, worn by all persons before entering the room.
iii. Hands washed before entering the room.

Patients who are severely immunosuppressed, such as bone marrow transplant cases, may require isolation in special units possibly including Trexler tents (*see* Selwyn, 1980).

Chapter 25

Disinfection and sterilization

Satisfactory removal of pathogenic organisms from the hands of hospital staff and from the environment is often achieved by adopting a high standard of cleanliness using a detergent such as soap and water. Additional methods involving heat or chemicals are only occasionally necessary for certain high-risk areas or procedures or for particular items of equipment.

DEFINITION OF TERMS

Sterilization implies the *complete* removal of *all organisms* including vegetative bacteria, bacterial *spores*, viruses, fungi and protozoa. Spores (e.g. of *Cl. tetani*) are especially resistant to physico-chemical processes. The usual concept of sterilization is an 'absolute' one; an item is either sterile or it is not sterile. However, the concept of sterility really depends on statistical rather than absolute considerations. The usual aim in practice is to render an article 'safe' for the procedure to be undertaken and a sterilizing process that reduces the count of spore-forming organisms by more than 10^6 in a short time is generally satisfactory (*see* Kelsey, 1972).

Disinfection implies the removal of *some types of pathogenic organisms*, usually not including spores, rather than the removal of all types of organisms and is associated with only a partial reduction in the total number of organisms present. It is not as effective a method for the removal of organisms as is sterilization.

DISINFECTION

The main object of disinfection is to reduce the count of pathogenic organisms in a potential source of infection to below that required to cause infection, rather than to eliminate completely the organism from the source. There are three main types of disinfection, cleaning, heating and disinfecting with chemical agents.

Cleaning

Good cleaning is the most widely used and cheapest method of disinfection. Cleaning is also necessary to give a preliminary reduction in numbers of organisms and to remove organic matter, dirt or grease which might otherwise protect the organisms from additional disinfection methods involving either heat or chemical agents. In many instances it is also desirable to make a surface dry following a cleaning procedure to reduce the chances of surviving Gram-negative bacilli multiplying in an otherwise moist situation. Examples of cleaning procedures followed by drying include the washing of hands, the cleaning of anaesthetic tubing and apparatus and then drying in a drying cabinet and the dry storage of mops, after they are cleaned.

Heat Disinfection Methods

Heat methods are subject to a smaller number of variables than chemical methods of disinfection and are generally recommended whenever possible. Most types of microbes, apart from spores, may be removed from inanimate objects with appropriate heat disinfection methods. The following types of heat disinfection methods are available.

1. Pasteurization

Pasteurization was first introduced for removing harmful microbes from milk by raising the temperature to either approximately 63 °C for 30 minutes ('holder type process') or to 72 °C for 20 seconds ('flash process'). Pasteurization methods are often recommended for the decontamination of babies' milk bottles in hospitals and for anaesthetic apparatus, such as face masks and tubing. Such methods are often used for the disinfection of bedpans or urinals by the use of a machine with a cycle which raises the temperature to 80 °C for 1 minute. The reliability of pasteurization methods is increased when the temperature reached is monitored regularly and the machine is designed so that an article cannot be removed before it has completed the minimum adequate time in the machine at a suitably high temperature.

2. Boiling

Heating of items to 100 °C will kill the majority of pathogenic microbes in less than a minute. Some bacterial spores, such as those of *Clostridium tetani*, will resist boiling for long periods, but the majority of *Clostridium welchii* spores are killed by boiling for 20 minutes. In the past, boilers were commonly used in the wards, but they were associated with misuse since contaminated items were not always fully immersed and boiled instruments could be contaminated when new dirty items were introduced into the boiler.

3. Low-temperature steam disinfection

Steam is generated at 75 °C in this method by using sub-atmospheric pressure in a specially designed autoclave. This is probably the best heat disinfectant method for decontaminating many types of articles, such as ventilator tubing, since steam has good penetrating properties, the process is automatic and the items are packed and dry at the end of the cycle. A commonly used cycle which is extremely effective for disinfection involves heating the items to 75 °C for 20–30 minutes. A combined low-temperature steam plus formaldehyde process is useful when sporicidal activity is also desired or when a greater degree of disinfection is needed than can be achieved by low temperature steam without formaldehyde. The low-temperature steam formaldehyde process has been recommended by some authorities for disinfection of some endoscopes. (However, some fibre-optic endoscopes may be damaged by the heat process, irrespective of the presence of formalin, and a chemical disinfectant method is then preferable.)

Chemical Disinfection Methods

Chemical disinfectants are often used to reduce the count of pathogenic microbes on inanimate objects which are heavily contaminated, but their action is greatly limited unless adequate cleaning of the object has first been carried out. 'Antiseptics' are particular types of chemical disinfectants that may be applied to living tissues, such as skin, to remove harmful microbes without causing undue tissue toxicity. Chemical disinfectants and antiseptics are frequently restricted in the types of pathogenic organisms that they may act against; for example, quaternary ammonium compounds (QACs), such as cetrimide or benzalkonium chloride, have good activity against *E. coli* but poor activity against *Pseudomonas aeruginosa*, spores and viruses. A few chemical disinfectants may be active against spores and viruses as well as vegetative bacteria including formaldehyde which is very toxic, glutaraldehyde, also toxic, chlorine, iodine and ethylene oxide gas (toxic).

Factors determining the effectiveness of chemical disinfection methods

The following questions should be asked to determine whether chemical disinfectants or antiseptics will actually work in use on the wards or departments of a hospital:

a. Is the correct type of chemical agent being selected for the purpose required?
A phenolic agent, such as hycolin, would be unsuitable for wiping a floor contaminated by hepatitis B positive blood. 'Flooding' the area with strong hypochlorite solution instead is necessary.

b. Has a suitable concentration of chemical agent been used?
Inadequately supervised, or untrained, members of hospital staff frequently use too low concentrations of disinfectant. 'Topping up' of old dilute disinfectant solutions is occasionally carried out instead of the correct preparation of measured dilutions of fresh disinfectant. Many disinfectants, such as hypochlorite solutions, lose a lot of activity after storage in a dilute form for longer than 24 hours. In most situations dilute 'in-use' solutions should be discarded within 24 hours of opening the container. Where dilute disinfectants are stored for any length of time bacterial contamination may occur with such organisms as *Pseudomonas*. *Pseudomonas* and other organisms may multiply at room temperature in the disinfectant and the contaminated solution may be a source of outbreaks of hospital infections (*see* Chapter 24).

c. Is the time of exposure to disinfectant sufficient, and has adequate prior cleaning been carried out?
Even highly active chemical disinfectants such as 2% glutaraldehyde need to be in contact with an article for more than a few minutes to kill some pathogens, such as *Pseudomonas aeruginosa, Mycobacterium tuberculosis* or hepatitis B virus. These particular organisms may contaminate fibre-optic

endoscopes and will not be adequately removed from a cleaned instrument which is only immersed in the glutaraldehyde for 5 minutes. However, this is the time commonly used in practice by clinicians. The time required for adequate chemical disinfectant will be much longer when there has been heavy contamination since the number of organisms and amount of organic matter which may inactivate the disinfectant is greater than when only light contamination is present. Therefore prior cleaning to reduce the level of contamination is essential. Some parts of complex instruments, such as fibre-optic gastroscopes, are difficult to clean completely even with the brushes that are supplied and a correspondingly longer exposure time to disinfectant is desirable. As a general rule, the endoscope should be immersed for 3 hours in 2% glutaraldehyde, but when only one expensive endoscope is available for a busy endoscopy list this may be totally impractical; at least 10 minutes' immersion has been suggested for the routine disinfection of endoscopes.

d. Has the correct pH been used?
The activity of some disinfectants varies remarkably with pH. One commercial type of glutaraldehyde requires an 'akaline activator' to be added just before use so that an adequate bactericidal effect is achieved.

e. Are inactivating materials present?
Organic matter, i.e. pus, blood, vomit, faeces and other body fluids, is frequently present on the surface of an article requiring first cleaning and then disinfection by a chemical agent. When organic matter remains after cleaning, it may markedly inactivate some chemical disinfectants, such as hypochlorites, and quaternary ammonium compounds, such as cetrimide. Pus also inactivates chlorhexidine. Phenolics, such as sudol or hycolin, are less inactivated by organic matter than hypochlorites or QAC compounds. Organic matter also limits the contact between the pathogenic organisms and the chemical disinfectant used.

Cork inactivates some disinfectants such as chlorhexidine and this is the reason why cork stoppers on disinfectant bottles were replaced by screw-capped tops preferably without cork liners! Many other substances such as cotton mopheads, rubber and certain types of plastics may inactivate various chemical disinfectants. These factors need taking into account when considering the use of specific disinfectants for decontaminating a particular item. Soap is an anionic detergent and may inactivate QACs, which are cationic detergents, and also to some extent chlorhexidine. Even tap water may inactivate some disinfectants such as QACs especially when the water is hard.

f. What is the temperature and volume of the disinfectant in use?
Chemical disinfectants are generally more active against microbes at higher than lower temperatures. Hot rather than cold water is therefore preferable for diluting disinfectants.

Larger volumes are safer than small volumes since the chance of inactivation is less and the contaminating organisms are further diluted following a preliminary cleaning process. An example of this is when there has been spillage of HBsAg positive blood onto the floor. Large volumes of strong hypochlorite solution should be flooded over the contaminated area as soon as possible.

g. *Has 'sterile' antiseptic been applied topically to a patient?*
As mentioned previously dilute antiseptics may become contaminated by Gram-negative bacilli, such as *Pseudomonas* species. This has been described with chlorhexidine, cetrimide or a mixture of these disinfectants which have been used topically and subsequently carried infection. The risks of contamination of a disinfectant is greater when it is stored in non-sterile containers or containers made of certain plastics which may inactivate the antiseptic. Dilute antiseptics ready for use on patients should therefore be heat sterilized and suitable sachets containing sterile antiseptic solutions are available commercially. An alternative is to store the disinfectant in a strong solution and then dilute with sterile distilled water just before topical use. This contamination problem is less with fresh antiseptic containing alcohol, such as 1·5% iodine in spirit or alcoholic chlorhexidine solution.

h. *Are the containers for disinfectant cleaned adequately?*
All used containers and dispensers should be returned to an agreed department, usually the pharmacy, for adequate cleaning and drying before they are considered for re-use.

Testing of chemical disinfectants

Manufacturers have traditionally compared disinfectants with phenol for killing *Salmonella typhi* in a Rideal-Walker test or in later modifications of this test. Phenol coefficients are calculated for each disinfectant; the higher the coefficient the more active is the disinfectant under the conditions of the test. However, these tests have little practical value in an 'in-use' hospital situation where organisms much more resistant than *Salmonella typhi* have to be removed and where organic matter or other inactivating substances are frequently present. More realistic tests include the Kelsey-Sykes test, which is carried out by a reference laboratory, and 'in-use' tests which are carried out by hospital clinical microbiology laboratories.

Kelsey-Sykes test

The Kelsey-Sykes test uses standard test strains of *Pseudomonas aeruginosa* and other Gram-negative bacilli as well as *Staph. aureus*. The activity of different disinfectants can be compared under standard test conditions in the presence of yeasts, which are included as potentially inactivating organic matter.

'In-use' tests

'In-use' tests are realistic as they are intended to test a disinfectant's action in use in the hospital at the time of the tests. An example is hypochlorite disinfectant being used for decontaminating babies' milk feed bottles, or a phenolic disinfectant in a laboratory discard jar containing contaminated pasteur pipettes. The microbiologist visits the ward or department, collects 1 ml of the disinfectant in use and immediately adds it to 9 ml of the nutrient broth. Sometimes it is necessary for a substance such as thiosulphate or Tween 80 to be added to the broth to neutralize specifically the chemical disinfectant added. On returning to the laboratory, the 1 in 10 dilution of disinfectant in nutrient broth is inoculated on to two agar plates using 10 drops of diluted disinfectant per plate. The drops are delivered from a calibrated sterile pasteur pipette which delivers 50 drops for each 1 ml of broth. One plate is incubated at 32–35 °C for 3 days and the other plate is incubated at room temperature. After incubation of the plates, the appearance of a few colonies would not imply failure of the 'in-use' test since disinfection is a partial removal of organisms rather than a complete removal and small amounts of contamination might be acceptable medically. However, if more than five colonies appeared on one plate this would signify at least 250 viable organisms per ml of disinfectant in use and would suggest that the disinfectant process was not working satisfactorily. An investigation to explain the failure of the 'in-use' test may then be mounted and often there is a simple explanation based on one or more of the possibilities discussed under the questions above. Regular 'in-use' tests are valuable for helping supervise the correct use of disinfectants in the hospital.

Main types of disinfectants available

Alcohols

Examples

Iso-propyl alcohol and ethyl alcohol.

Advantages

Kills most vegetative bacteria on clean surfaces in less than 30 seconds.

Iso-propyl alcohol is more antibacterial than ethyl or methyl alcohol.

Disadvantages

Relatively inactive against spores and fungi.

Inflammable.

Must be used with correct amount of water present to allow optimal antibacterial activity by coagulation of protein, i.e. 65–80% alcohol (70% usually used).

Iso-propyl alcohol impregnated swabs—expensive. Industrial methylated spirit is less expensive and suitable for use on inanimate surfaces but not on the skin.

Use

Skin antiseptics before injections or venepuncture: iso-propyl alcohol recommended.

Disinfection of clean inanimate surfaces such as trolley tops.

Aldehydes

Examples

Glutaraldehyde and formaldehyde.

Advantages

Good activity against spores as well as vegetative bacteria, viruses and fungi.

Disadvantages

Glutaraldehyde has only a fair activity against tubercle bacilli.

An exposure of at least 3 hours is desirable to kill all microbes although most vegetative bacteria are killed in less than 10 minutes on a clean surface.

Glutaraldehyde is markedly affected by pH—the solution should be alkaline and fresh for reliable bactericidal activity.

Both aldehydes are toxic and may cause sensitivity reactions affecting skin, eyes or lungs, although glutaraldehyde is safer to use than formaldehyde. Glutaraldehyde must be removed after disinfection of equipment, usually by rinsing with sterile water. Formaldehyde gas or solution must also be removed and neutralization with ammonia is sometimes necessary.

Uses

Glutaraldehyde solutions are widely used at 2% concentration for disinfection of fibre-optic endoscopes and other equipment. It is also a useful alternative to hypochlorites for disinfecting environmental surfaces possibly contaminated by hepatitis B virus.

Formaldehyde solution is used in post-mortem rooms for decontaminating tuberculous material as well as for fixing specimens. Formaldehyde gas is sometimes used in special machines for decontaminating respiratory ventilators and other anaesthetic equipment and babies' incubators. Rarely the formaldehyde gas may be used by Public Health authorities for fumigating areas potentially contaminated by dangerous organisms such as Lassa fever virus.

Diguanides

Example

Chlorhexidine.

Advantages

Good activity against *Staph. aureus.*

Moderate anti-Gram-negative activity including some activity against *Pseudomonas.*

Compatible with alcohol or QACs such as cetrimide.

Relatively non-toxic to skin and mucous membranes.

Disadvantages

Poor activity against tubercle bacilli, spores, fungi and viruses.

Inactivated by pus, soap, some plastics and many other materials—not suitable for disinfecting most equipment or the inanimate environment.

Pseudomonas aeruginosa and other bacteria may multiply in deteriorating chlorhexidine solutions.

Uses

Useful antiseptic for skin and mucous membranes.

Pre-operative skin preparation of a patient, and also before such procedures as lumbar puncture or bone marrow aspiration; 0·5% chlorhexidine in 70% alcohol is preferable to aqueous chlorhexidine solution.

Chlorhexidine–cetrimide mixture (Savlon or Savlodil) is sometimes a useful antiseptic for dirty wounds.

Chlorhexidine, 4%, in detergent ('Hibiscrub') is a useful antiseptic for the hands of staff, especially those staff working on high-risk units, such as in intensive care units. It is also a preoperative 'scrub' for surgeons.

Chlorhexidine–alcohol–glycerine solution ('Hibisol') is an alternative preparation for rapid hand antisepsis in busy intensive care, neurosurgical and other units. The alcohol present results in a rapid antibacterial effect together with drying of the hands.

Chlorhexidine ointments or solutions have been used to provide local antisepsis in the urethra before catheterization and also in the bladder of certain patients with indwelling catheters (*see* Hospital acquired urinary tract infections, in Chapter 24).

Halogens

Examples

a. *Hypochlorites and chlorine*

Advantages

Active against viruses as well as bacteria including spores and fungi. Particularly useful because of its activity against hepatitis B virus.

Disadvantages

Easily inactivated by organic matter including blood, pus and milk. Surfaces must be cleaned thoroughly before applying hypochlorite. Concentration best stated as parts per million (ppm) available chlorine. Freshness and pH are critical factors. Activity deteriorates rapidly when dilute solutions used—discard dilute solutions within 24 hours. Corrosive to metals.

Uses

'Extra strong' hypochlorite solution (10 000 ppm available chlorine) is occasionally necessary for dealing with blood spillage from a HBsAg positive patient. 'Strong' hypochlorite solution (2500 ppm available chlorine) is used for blood spillage in general, laboratory pipette jars, and as an antiseptic for certain dirty or infected wounds, such as infected pressure sores.

Hypochlorite solution (0·1%) (1000 ppm available chlorine) may be used for general environmental disinfection on those few occasions when an additional disinfectant is indicated following cleaning. 'Weak' hypochlorite solution (125 ppm available chlorine) is suitable for disinfecting cleaned infant feeding utensils; a 'stabilized' hypochlorite solution containing added sodium chloride is available commercially ('Milton'). This is diluted just before use to give the chlorine concentration of 125 ppm. Chlorination is also used, together with filtration and other methods, to remove potentially harmful microbes from drinking water supplies. A high concentration of available chlorine has also been recommended for the water of evaporative condensers and cooling towers of air conditioning plants to reduce the risk of multiplication of *Legionella pneumophila* in institutions where outbreaks of Legionnaires' disease have occurred.

b. *Iodophors and iodine*

Advantages

Highly active against vegetative bacteria and some sporicidal activity. Some antiviral and antifungal activity also. Iodophors include a surface active non-ionic detergent and are less likely to sensitize skin. Unlike iodine they need not be removed from the skin after use. Both iodophors and iodine are compatible with alcohol.

Disadvantages

As with other halogens inactivation by blood and other organic matter is important.

Iodine may cause local skin reactions as well as staining of the skin.

The iodophor preparations are moderately expensive.

Uses

Iodine or iodophor containing 1% available iodine mixed with alcohol is excellent for pre-operative skin disinfection.

An aqueous iodophor solution (povidone iodine) may be used as an alternative to chlorhexidine detergent as a surgical 'scrub'.

Povidone iodine powder has been used topically on skin ulcers as an antiseptic.

Phenolics

Examples

a. Phenol (carbolic acid)
b. Chloroxylenol
c. Clear soluble phenolics such as 'sudol' and 'hycolin'
d. Hexachlorophane

a. *Carbolic acid*

Carbolic acid is a phenol of historic interest only as it is too irritant for general use.

b. *Chloroxylenol* has good anti-staphylococcal activity, but only fair activity against Gram-negative bacilli. It also has only poor activity against other microbes and is relatively easily inactivated. These phenolics are not recommended for use in hospital.

c. *Clear soluble phenolics*

Advantages

Good activity against both staphylococci and Gram-negative bacilli including *Pseudomonas aeruginosa*. It is also active against tubercle bacilli. It is relatively resistant to inactivation by organic matter when suitable concentrations are used.

Disadvantages

Relatively inactive against spores and viruses.

Too toxic to be used routinely as an antiseptic.

Repeated contact on the skin may cause irritation.

'Hycolin' may leave a sticky surface on floors and other surfaces if not washed off.

Use

Good antibacterial chemical disinfectants for decontaminating soiled environmental surfaces following a cleaning process.

d. *Hexachlorophane*

Advantage

Good activity against *Staph. aureus* which is cumulative on repeated applications on the skin.

Disadvantages

Poor activity against Gram-negative bacilli and other microbes. Toxic to the central nervous system in high concentration during repeated application of solutions to low-birth-weight infants.

Uses

Hexachlorophane solution (Phisohex) has been used as a valuable preparation for surgeons' hands before operations, but care is necessary to prevent contamination by Gram-negative bacilli.

Hexachlorophane has helped to reduce staphylococcal sepsis in many maternity and neonatal units throughout the world. When a powder rather than a solution is used at restricted sites only (such as the umbilical stump, perineum, groins and axillae), the hexachlorophane can continue to contribute to the control of staphylococcal sepsis in neonatal units without causing toxicity.

Quaternary ammonium compounds (QACs)

Examples

Cetrimide and benzalkonium chloride. These are catonic surface active detergents.

Advantages

Good detergent properties and good activity against staphylococci.

Compatible with chlorhexidine.

Disadvantages

Only moderate activity against Gram-negative bacilli and poor activity against *Pseudomonas aeruginosa*. (A selective medium for the culture of *Pseudomonas aeruginosa* contains cetrimide.) Outbreaks of hospital infection due to *Pseudomonas* have occurred through the use of contaminated cetrimide on the skin of surgical patients.

QACs are relatively easily inactivated by many substances including water, cork and anionic detergents such as soap.

Use

These agents are not routinely recommended for use by hospitals but are valuable when mixed with certain other agents such as chlorhexidine to make 'Savlon' or 'Savlodil'—*see above*.

Filtration Methods of Disinfection

Filters can trap bacteria and other organisms passing through them by direct impaction or electrostatic attraction by the filter material. Both the pore size and the nature of the material determine the efficiency of the filter for removing organisms from fluids or air.

'Seitz' filters have a pore size of between 0·5 and 0·75 µm and consist of asbestos; they were particularly useful in the laboratory for removing bacteria from serum and fluid culture media. In recent years they have become replaced by membrane filters made of cellulose acetate—'Millipore' filters. Membrane filters with different pore sizes are available including those which can even remove some viruses from fluids.

Glass wool, gauze and other filters are useful for removing bacteria and bacteria-laden particles from air in air ventilation systems in special areas of the hospital such as the operating theatres and the isolation unit. If the filters become wet or damaged they clearly become less efficient and the filter needs regular checking. Other examples of air filters include those used to protect respiratory ventilators from contamination by the patient in an intensive care unit (such as the William's siliconized filter), filters in autoclaves to allow bacteria-free cooling air to be delivered, and filters in category B safety cabinets in microbiology laboratories that protect the outside world from tubercle bacilli which are released inside the cabinet during the investigations of specimens. Masks worn in the theatre and wards by hospital staff are not usually very efficient filters especially when they become moist. For high-risk operations surgeons can wear relatively efficient masks although these are often uncomfortable.

Disinfectant policies

A detailed policy for the use of both heat and chemical methods of disinfection is necessary in each hospital. It is not necessary to use more than about half a dozen main chemical agents, e.g. alcohol, chlorhexidine solutions, glutaraldehyde, hypochlorite solutions, a clear soluble phenolic and povidone iodine solutions. The reader is referred to other texts for examples of policies, their design and supervision (Lowbury et al., 1981; Maurer, 1978).

STERILIZATION

'Complete' removal of all types of microbes can be attempted by one of the following methods of sterilization:

1. Heat methods—dry heat or moist heat
2. Ionizing radiation
3. Ethylene oxide gas

Heat Methods

Whichever method is used, a 'sterilization cycle' consists of a 'heating period', a 'sterilization period', a 'safety period' consisting of half the sterilization period, and a 'cooling period'. The term 'holding period' is sometimes referred to and this is the sum of the sterilization and safety periods.

Dry heat

Flaming of bacteriological loops and incineration of infected dressings are simple examples of dry heat methods.

Hot air ovens which have controlled cycles, such as 160 °C for 1 hour, are suitable for killing bacteria on materials which are not penetrable by steam. The dry heat gradually oxidizes the bacterial cytoplasm.

Many materials such as plastics are burnt or damaged by the high temperature of hot air ovens. Examples of items that may be sterilized in a hot air oven include glassware, although glass syringes are less commonly used today, powders such as talc, oils and petroleum jelly. In practice sufficient time is necessary for the heat to penetrate the item to sterilize it safely and to allow it to cool.

The physical process can be checked regularly by Browne's tubes or preferably by thermocouple temperature recorders which can tell whether sufficient heat is evenly distributed in the oven by the fan fitted to it. A biological test piece can also be inserted consisting of sand or soil containing non-toxigenic *Clostridium tetani* spores.

Moist heat

Steam kills bacteria by coagulating the cytoplasm and is an extremely efficient sterilizer when present under increased pressures where the temperature exceeds 100 °C. The simplest form of 'autoclave' is a domestic pressure cooker; steam displaces air upward and then can sterilize items under increased pressure in less than 30 minutes. The main advantages of steam are:

a. At the points of contact with the cooler item to be sterilized there is condensation to form water and the latent heat of evaporation is then delivered locally.

b. At these points, there are local potential 'vacuums' since the gaseous steam has contracted to form water and then more steam rushes in under pressure to replace the condensed steam; hence there is a particularly good penetration of the article by steam at a high temperature.

Air within the pressure chamber of an autoclave can impair the contact between the article and the steam and result in relatively cold pockets where the items may not be safely sterilized; the removal of air from the autoclave is critically important for the efficient sterilization of many articles including dressings. The simplest types of autoclaves with an automatic cycle were downward displacement type autoclaves which were based on a similar principle to the pressure cooker, except that air was displaced downwards instead of upwards. These types of autoclave have largely been replaced in hospital by sophisticated automatic high pre-vacuum autoclaves which are more efficient at removing the air from the autoclave chamber than downward displacement autoclaves. These two main types of autoclaves are now briefly described.

Downward displacement autoclaves

Steam enters the top of the chamber and displaces most of the air out through the air–steam outlet and the steam trap (*see Fig. 25.1*). The steam trap stays open until no more air or condensate passes through it; it may reopen again when condensate reforms and more steam then enters the chamber. A common sterilizing cycle in this type of autoclave involves raising the temperature to 121 °C for 15 minutes at 15 lb/in^2 pressure. The jacket surrounding the chamber is also heated separately by steam and this helps to dry the load.

Careful packing of the autoclave is necessary so that steel bowls are placed on their sides and not the 'right way up', otherwise air cannot effectively be displaced downwards and the items may not reach the desired sterilization temperature. This type of autoclave may be suitable for sterilizing instruments, but in practice today is mainly used in the laboratory. Suitably modified they may also be suitable for sterilizing bottled fluids. Dressings should not be sterilized by this type of autoclave.

High pre-vacuum autoclaves

A high vacuum, less than 20 mmHg (2·5 kPa), is generated within the chamber of the autoclave and almost all of the air is removed before the steam is introduced.

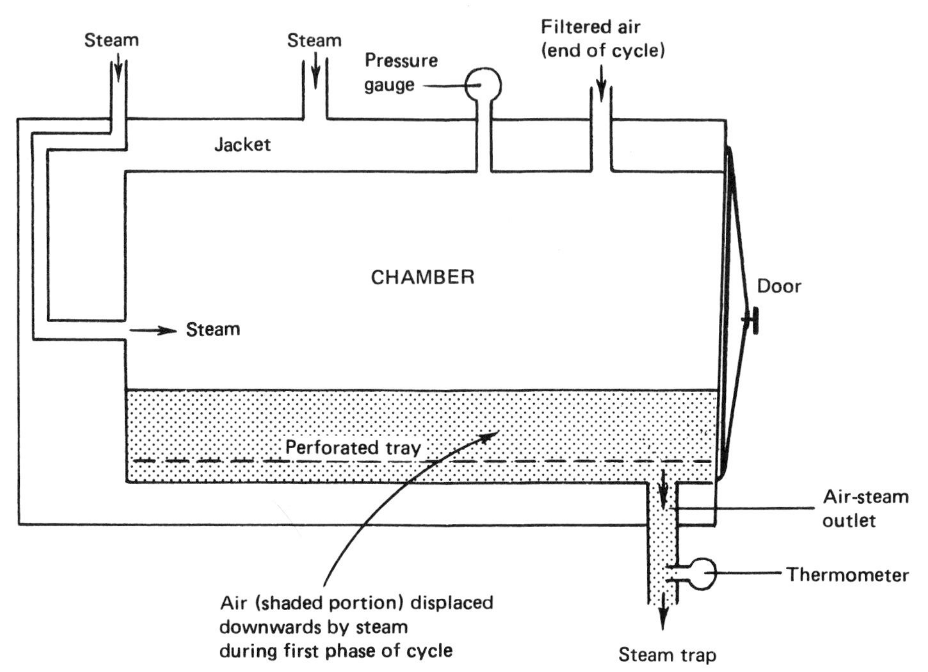

Fig. 25.1. Downward displacement autoclave—diagrammatic representation.

Some modern high vacuum autoclaves also have a series of about half a dozen vacuums and pulsings of steam near the start of the cycle so that the removal of air is extremely efficient. When the steam fills the chamber at a pressure of 30 lb/in^2 a temperature of 133 °C or higher is rapidly achieved and there is excellent steam penetration throughout the load. Items are sterilized within 3–4 minutes at 133 °C. When there has not been a pulsing of the steam a small amount of air, up to 3% of the volume of the chamber, can become concentrated in the centre of the pack; this potential problem is more likely to occur when only a small load is present and most of the chamber is left empty—'the small load effect'.

After the items have been sterilized the steam is automatically withdrawn from the chamber by a post-vacuum cycle and then filtered air fills the chamber. These autoclaves are primarily intended to sterilize porous loads such as dressings and gowns, and wrapped instruments. As with other autoclaves they need regular maintenance and checks.

Tests for heat methods of sterilization

Regular physico-chemical methods to check the sterilizing process are far more important than bacteriological tests on sample test pieces. The frequency and details of the tests required are included in *Hospital Technical Memorandum No. 10* (Department of Health and Social Security, 1980).

a. *Temperature and pressure measurements on record charts*

The temperature reached during each sterilizing cycle of an autoclave or a drying oven are recorded on a chart and should be routinely inspected to check that satisfactory temperatures are in fact reached for a sufficient duration. Thermocouples are more accurate than routine thermometers and must be used regularly to check the performance of the autoclave. The pressure recordings are usually available on the same chart as the temperature recordings and in practice are of less immediate importance than the temperature records.

b. *Browne's tubes*

Each Browne's glass tube contains a red indicator solution that turns green when an adequate temperature has been maintained for a sufficient period. Different types of Browne's tubes are available for use in a drying oven or for autoclaves operated at various temperatures and times. A Browne's tube is included with a load to be sterilized and immediately inspected at the end of the cycle. This type of test is carried out at least daily.

c. *Air leak test (Vacuum leak test)*

This test is suitable for high pre-vacuum autoclaves and should be performed preferably at the start of each day. An initial pre-vacuum is drawn so that the pressure falls below 20 mmHg absolute. The pump is stopped and the pressure observed over a 10-minute period. If there is a loss of vacuum of more than 10 mmHg during this time, the test suggests the presence of an air leak somewhere in the autoclave chamber. An engineer would then be called immediately to attend to the autoclave as it has failed the test.

d. *Bowie-Dick test*

The Bowie-Dick test is also performed daily on porous load high pre-vacuum autoclaves. It is designed to test steam penetration into the centre of a standardized load of towels during a standard sterilizing cycle and tests the degree of air removal in the centre of the pack. The test essentially consists of placing autoclave tape arranged in the shape of a St Andrew's cross into the centre of the pack and examining the tape after the end of the sterilizing cycle which includes a holding time of not greater than 3·5 minutes at 134–137 °C. If the air is satisfactorily removed and there is adequate steam penetration at the centre of the load, the diagonal lines in the tape are all a dark colour and are evenly changed. When air is trapped towards the centre of the St Andrew's cross, the tape does not show a deep colour in the diagonal lines at the centre compared with the tape at the periphery of the cross. There are official regulations that need to be followed concerning the correct performance of a Bowie-Dick test.

Bacteriological tests—spore tests

Spore strips are commercially available that include known numbers of the spores of *Bacillus stearothermophilus*. They are fixed to different parts of the autoclave and also placed in a load. After the sterilization cycle the strips are cultured in a special broth at 55 °C for 5 days. Negative cultures indicate a satisfactory sterilizing cycle during the testing of one load only. They may be used during the commissioning of a new autoclave but have little value during the day-to-day use of the autoclave.

Ionizing Radiation

Gamma-rays are lethal non-charged ultra-short-wavelength rays with great penetrating power from a radioactive isotope such as cobalt 60. They are used by industry to sterilize many disposable items, such as disposable plastic syringes and needles. Disposable suture materials and rubber gloves are other examples of items frequently sterilized by this method.

Sealed packs that would not be suitable for steam sterilizing or heat-sensitive materials are often sterilized by gamma-rays.

The radiation dose usually used is 2·5 Mrad and this kills any microbes present mainly by ionizing their DNA. However, the structure of some plastics or other materials are also altered by gamma-rays and changes in strength or discoloration may result. Checks on the gamma-radiation sterilization process are regularly carried out using a PVC-azo-dye indicator and *Bacillus pumilus* spores. Only a few centres have facilities for gamma-ray irradiation because of the safety precautions required and because of the expense.

Ethylene Oxide

Ethylene oxide is a highly toxic inflammable gas which will kill all types of microbes including bacterial spores, provided it is used with suitable humidity, at the correct temperature and for sufficient time. Carbon dioxide is mixed with the ethylene oxide to reduce the likelihood of an explosion. The gas diffuses well through items such as plastic materials, swabs and paper and is particularly useful for sterilizing any equipment which is heat sensitive. Heart and lung machine components, cardiac catheters and pacers and certain contaminated respiratory ventilators are some of the items that may be sterilized by ethylene oxide. Ventilators are less often sterilized by ethylene oxide today because more ventilators are available with autoclavable components and the machines are better protected from contamination through the use of improved filters. Certain types of complex heat-sensitive endoscopes, such as choleodochoscopes, that are not easily disinfected by glutaraldehyde because of the difficulty of cleaning them effectively, are best sterilized by ethylene oxide. When a fibre-optic endoscope has been used on a patient known to be HBsAg positive, ethylene oxide is preferable to glutaraldehyde for removing hepatitis B virus from the instrument. As with other methods of disinfection or sterilization it is preferable that thorough cleaning of the items is first carried out whenever possible. After sterilization, traces of ethylene oxide must be removed from the item. The process itself is strictly monitored for safety and effectiveness at the few hospitals where ethylene oxide sterilization is carried out on a large scale. Royce's sachet (changes colour from yellow to purple), and *Bacillus globigii* spores on a test piece, are used to test the sterilization process. Small ethylene oxide units are commercially available and may be considered when there is only poor access to a special ethylene oxide unit in another hospital. One small unit in a hospital may be useful in spite of its potential dangers to both the operator and the patient, provided it is supervised carefully and the consultant microbiologist agrees that it is necessary.

CSSD AND TSSU

Central sterile supply departments (CSSDs) often serve a number of hospitals and supply the majority of sterile articles such as dressings. They also receive many used instruments and various items from each hospital that require sterilization. Trained staff and facilities are concentrated on one site where sterilization processes can be more efficiently supervised than when items are sterilized in many different areas. Handling of contaminated items on the wards and departments by staff is also reduced, thereby reducing cross-infection risks.

Theatre sterile supply units (TSSU's) are very desirable in each hospital with busy operating theatres since local needs and instruments vary and there is often a rapid turnover of items required for surgery. Adequate supervision and training of staff is sometimes more difficult in a hospital TSSU than in a CSSD. Engineers play a crucial daily role in maintaining the efficient running of these sterilization units.

Further Reading

Ayliffe G. A. (1980) The effects of antibacterial agents on the flora of the skin. *Journal of Hospital Infection* **1**, 111–124.

Babb J. R., Bradley C. R. and Ayliffe G. A. J. (1980) Sporicidal activity of glutaraldehydes and hypochlorites and other factors influencing their selection for the treatment of medical endoscopes. *Journal of Hospital Infection* **1**, 63–75.

Department of Health and Social Security (1980) *Hospital Technical Memorandum No. 10*. London, H.M.S.O.

Kelsey J. C. (1972) The myth of surgical sterility. *Lancet* **2**, 1301.

Lowbury E. J. L., Ayliffe G. A. J., Geddes A. M. et al. (ed.) (1981) *Control of Hospital Infection*, 2nd ed. London, Chapman and Hall.

*Maurer I. M. (1978) *Hospital Hygiene*, 2nd ed. London, Edward Arnold.

Rubbo J. D. and Gardner J. F. (1965) *A Review of Sterilization and Disinfection*. London, Lloyd-Luke.

Schliessler K. H., Rozendaal B., Taal C. et al. (1980) Outbreak of *Salmonella agona* infection after upper intestinal fibre-optic endoscopy. *Lancet* **2**, 1246.

Selwyn S. (1980) Skin preparation, the surgical 'scrub' and related rituals. In: Karan S. (ed.) *Controversies in Surgical Sepsis*, pp. 23–32. New York, Praeger.

Williams R. E. O., Blowers R., Garrod L. P. et al. (1966) *Hospital Infection, Causes and Prevention*. London, Lloyd-Luke.

* Particularly recommended for further study by undergraduates.

Appendix 1

Basic characteristics of some important Bacterial Pathogens

Notes on some basic characteristics of bacteria that can be Gram-stained are included in this section (*see also Table 24.1*, in Chapter 24; typing methods are also referred to Chapter 24).

A. Gram-positive Bacteria

Staphylococci

Microscopy:	Gram-positive cocci mainly in clusters
Culture:	white, cream or golden yellow 0·5–1·5 mm colonies on blood agar after overnight aerobic incubation

Differential test

COAGULASE TEST

This is the main differential test. Coagulase is an enzyme which converts fibrinogen in plasma to fibrin, thus producing clumping when coagulase-positive staphylococci are mixed with plasma in a slide coagulase test and clot formation in a tube coagulase test.

Coagulase-positive staphylococci	indicates *Staph. aureus*
Coagulase-negative staphylococci	indicates *Staph. albus (Staph. epidermidis)* or *Staph. saprophyticus*

Staphylococcus aureus

Found in the nose of 10–30% of normal people, but only occasionally on healthy skin, it is a common cause of infection in the community and in hospital. Most infections are sporadic but occasional outbreaks occur.

DISEASES INCLUDE:

a. Skin infections including boils, carbuncles, breast abscess, surgical wound infection, neonatal skin sepsis and rare toxic complications such as toxic epidermal necrolysis and vaginal tampon toxic shock syndrome.

b. Deep tissue infections including pneumonia, osteomyelitis, septic arthritis, endocarditis.
c. Septicaemia and complications of septicaemia including disseminated intravascular coagulation, endocarditis and metastatic abscesses.
d. Food poisoning; staphylococcal enterocolitis.

PREDISPOSING HOST FACTORS FOR STAPHYLOCOCCAL INFECTIONS INCLUDE:

Diabetes mellitus, neutropenia, hypogammaglobulinaemia, and rare phagocyte defects as in chronic granulomatous disease.

ANTIBIOTICS

Penicillin, cloxacillin, erythromycin, lincomycin, fusidic acid and vancomycin are examples of narrow spectrum anti-staphylococcal antibiotics.

Greater than 90% hospital strains and 60% community strains are resistant to penicillin because of penicillinase production and these strains would also be resistant to other penicillins, such as ampicillin, but are usually sensitive to cloxacillin (or flucloxacillin).

Multiple antibiotic resistance to two or more different antibiotics may occur, especially in hospital, e.g. *Staph. aureus* resistant to penicillin, tetracycline, erythromycin, lincomycin and fusidic acid. Antibiotic resistance is often plasmid mediated and the spread of plasmids between different strains of *Staph. aureus* is facilitated by transducing phages.

Staphylococcus epidermidis (Staph. albus), and 'Staph. saprophyticus'

Found normally in the nose or skin flora of healthy people.

DISEASES INCLUDE:

Urinary tract infections, endocarditis after heart surgery or in the elderly, shunt infections in infants with hydrocephalus and infections of hip joint prostheses.

ANTIBIOTICS

Antibiotic sensitivity patterns of different strains of *Staph. epidermidis* vary greatly, many strains being resistant to several antibiotics often including cloxacillin.

Streptococci

Microscopy: Gram-positive cocci, either in chains as with β-haemolytic streptococci or viridans streptococci, or as diplococci, as with pneumococci.

Capsules of *Strep. pneumoniae* may occasionally be seen in Gram films and in special stained smears for capsules.

Culture:	Most streptococcal colonies on blood agar are apparent after 24–48 hours incubation aerobically. Some micro-aerophilic or anaerobic streptococci require up to 5 days incubation anaerobically before colonies are seen. Some pneumococcal strains, *Strep. milleri* strains and some viridans streptococci, such as *Strep. mutans*, grow best when 5–10% carbon dioxide is added to the atmosphere for incubation.

Differential tests

CLASSIFICATION ACCORDING TO HAEMOLYSIS ON BLOOD AGAR

Alpha (α) haemolysis	green colour around each colony due to altered haemoglobin, e.g. *Strep. viridans*
Beta (β) haemolysis	complete lysis of red cells around each colony. This is often most obvious on the anaerobic plate, e.g. *Strep. pyogenes*
Gamma (γ) haemolysis	non-haemolytic colonies, e.g. *Strep. faecalis*

a. ALPHA-HAEMOLYTIC STREPTOCOCCI

Strep. pneumoniae and viridans streptococci. However, some viridans streptococci may also appear as non-haemolytic colonies. Pneumococcal colonies often classically have a 'draughtsman' appearance.

Optochin (diethylhydrocuprein) and bile solubility tests

Optochin disc test	pneumococci, but not viridans streptococci, show a zone of inhibition around optochin
Bile solubility test	pneumococci, but not viridans streptococci, are soluble in a bile salt suspension

Biochemical tests for viridans streptococci

Viridans streptococci can be identified further by biochemical tests, such as the production of dextran from sucrose, into species including *Strep. mitior, Strep. sanguis, Strep. mutans, Strep. salivarius* and *Strep. milleri.*

b. BETA-HAEMOLYTIC STREPTOCOCCI

These are differentiated mainly by Lancefield grouping.

Lancefield grouping and the 'bacitracin test'

Polysaccharide antigen is extracted from the streptococcal cell walls for Lancefield grouping and the specific group antigen is identified using known antisera, such as in a precipitin test or in a coagglutination commercially available test.

The Lancefield grouping test may be used to identify some other streptococci which are not necessarily beta-haemolytic. In practice this test is most frequently carried out with beta-haemolytic streptococci. Important examples of different streptococci that can be put into Lancefield groupings include:

i. *Lancefield group A—synonymous with 'Strep. pyogenes'*
Greater than 90% *Strep. pyogenes* strains are sensitive to a bacitracin identification disc. This bacitracin test is often used to presumptively identify beta-haemolytic streptococci on blood agar as *Strep. pyogenes*, especially in cultures of throat swabs. This test is not entirely reliable as other streptococcal species may sometimes by sensitive to bacitracin. Also a few strains of *Strep. pyogenes* may appear with reduced sensitivity to bacitracin.
The group A Lancefield antigen is distinct (polysaccharide) from the other cell wall antigens in *Strep. pyogenes* which are used to type strains in outbreaks such as the M 'virulence' protein and T protein antigens (*see* Typing, p. 496).

ii. *Lancefield group B—'Strep. agalactiae'*
Some group B streptococcal strains are only slightly beta-haemolytic. (There are selective media available to assist the isolation of group B streptococci in specimens from a site with mixed flora such as a vaginal swab.)

iii. *Lancefield group C and Lancefield group G streptococci*
These beta-haemolytic streptococci are frequently isolated from normal (or infected) throat swabs or infected skin sites.

iv. *Lancefield group D*
The main examples include *Strep. faecalis* and *Strep. bovis* although these species usually appear as non-haemolytic colonies on blood agar.

c. NON-HAEMOLYTIC STREPTOCOCCI

These species can be differentiated according to the results obtained with Lancefield grouping, biochemical tests and cultural tests on bile-aesculin agar or MacConkey agar.

Strep. faecalis grows on MacConkey agar (magenta colonies) and on bile-aesculin agar (turning this black).

Examples of streptococcal species that frequently appear as non-haemolytic streptococci include *Strep. faecalis*, *Strep. bovis* and some species of viridans streptococci, such as *Strep. mutans* and *Strep. milleri*.

Normal flora and streptococcal diseases

The main streptococcal pathogens and their associated diseases are included in *Table A1.1*.

Antibiotics

All *Strep. pyogenes* strains are sensitive to penicillin. Nearly all *Strep. pneumoniae* strains are sensitive to penicillin. The majority of '*Strep. viridans*' strains are

Table A1.1. Streptococci and disease

Streptococcus	*Usual haemolysis*	*Normal site*	*Main associated diseases include*
Strep. pneumoniae	α	Throat and nose (up to 70% population)	Otitis media, sinusitis, mastoiditis, pneumonia, meningitis, brain abscess
'*Strep. viridans*' e.g. *Strep. mitior*, *Strep. sanguis*, *Strep. mutans*	α	Mouth	Bacterial endocarditis Dental caries (*Strep. mutans*)
and *Strep. milleri*		Intestine	Collections of pus in abdomen, e.g. liver abscess; or in chest Bacterial endocarditis
Strep. pyogenes (*Lancefield group A*)	β	Throat (up to about 5% population)	Sore throat, scarlet fever, otitis media Later complications—rheumatic fever, acute glomerulonephritis Skin infections including erysipelas, impetigo, infected traumatic or eczematous lesions Wound infections and puerperal sepsis Septicaemia (e.g. complicating cellulitis)
Lancefield group B streptococci	β	Perineal skin lower vagina (5–30% women)	Neonatal septicaemia and meningitis
Lancefield group C or G streptococci	β	Throat	Sore throat (very occasionally), skin infections, septicaemia
Strep. faecalis	Non	Intestine	Urinary tract infection, bacterial endocarditis
Strep. bovis	Non	Intestine	Bacterial endocarditis
Micro-aerophilic or anaerobic streptococci	Non	Skin, throat or lower vagina	Meleney's synergistic gangrene (together with *Staph. aureus*) Cellulitis, such as skin or female genital tract infection Cerebral abscess (often mixed with other organisms)

sensitive to penicillin. *Strep. faecalis* and Lancefield group B streptococci are only moderately sensitive to penicillin.

The great majority of streptococci are sensitive to erythromycin which may be particularly relevant for penicillin-allergic patients.

Bacillus species

These include *Bacillus anthracis, Bacillus cereus* and *Bacillus subtilis*.

Microscopy: *Bacillus anthracis* is typically seen as large square-ended Gram-positive bacilli, sometimes in long chains. (Other aerobic-spore-bearing bacilli including *Bacillus subtilis* may appear as Gram-variable or Gram-negative bacilli.)

Capsules of *B. anthracis* are stained purple in McFadyean's reaction with a polychrome methylene blue stain; other *Bacillus* species do not show capsules.

B. anthracis spores are not apparent in spore stains of clinical specimens from infected patients but may be present in environmental specimens.

Culture: *B. anthracis* colonies are seen after overnight culture on blood or nutrient agar as rough opaque colonies with edges resembling loose curls of hairs. Other *Bacillus* species do not have colonies with this type of edge. (*B. subtilis, B. cereus* and other bacilli are common blood culture contaminants which may sometimes be confused with 'coliforms' when colonies appear on MacConkey's medium.)

B. anthracis gives a characteristic inverted fir tree growth in gelatin.

Differentiation of Bacillus species by animal inoculation tests

B. anthracis, but not the other *Bacillus* species, is pathogenic to mice and guinea-pigs. This test is too dangerous to use in the average hospital animal house. Infected animals may disseminate anthrax spores which could survive for many years in the environment.

Sources and diseases

B. anthracis can infect many different animal species including sheep and the anthrax spores may remain viable in animal products or in the soil for a long period. *B. cereus* and *B. subtilis* are found in the soil, dust and air and *B. cereus* may contaminate food such as boiled rice.

B. anthracis is the cause of anthrax in man and animals (*see* Chapter 16). *B. cereus* is one cause of food poisoning (*see* Chapter 14). *B. subtilis* is nearly always only a contaminant when noticed in cultures. However, it may rarely cause bacteraemia in patients on haemodialysis when the dialysis machines are contaminated or when an intravenous infusion has become contaminated.

Antibiotics

B. anthracis is characteristically sensitive to penicillin.

Corynebacterium species

These include *Corynebacterium diphtheriae*, *Corynebacterium ulcerans*, and 'diph-theroid species' including *Corynebacterium xerosis* and *Corynebacterium hoffmani*.

Microscopy: The Gram-positive bacilli of *C. diphtheriae* are slightly curved and characteristically appear like 'Chinese characters' whereas the diphtheroid bacilli are often seen as palisade rows of bacilli.

Metachromatic granules ('Volutin granules') are sometimes seen in an Albert's stain of diphtheria bacilli. However, these granules do not necessarily indicate that the bacilli are *C. diphtheriae*, nor do they reliably indicate that a diphtheria strain is toxigenic.

Culture: Many 'diphtheroids' can easily be distinguished from *C. diphtheriae* according to the colonial appearances on tellurite media (such as Hoyle's or Downie's medium) and on blood agar. *C. diphtheriae* appears characteristically as grey-black colonies on tellurite. However, a few 'diphtheroid' strains may be difficult to differentiate in this way and any suspicious colonies require further tests.

Loeffler's serum agar slope is also used for the isolation of *C. diphtheriae* and is useful for providing a suitable culture for toxigenicity tests.

Differential tests

Hiss's serum water sugar fermentation tests are inoculated and the pattern of results helps to identify the *Corynebacterium* species. Characteristically *C. diphtheriae* ferments glucose and maltose, rarely sucrose. The *C. diphtheriae* species can be further differentiated into the subspecies *gravis* ('daisy head' classically and ferments starch), *mitis* or *intermedius* but, in practice, this is not important except for epidemiological purposes. *C. ulcerans* can give some biochemical reactions similar to *C. diphtheriae gravis* but the urea slope test reaction is different.

Toxinogenicity tests

These urgent tests on suspicious *C. diphtheriae* cultures are performed by an Elek plate or guinea-pig method (*see* p. 140).

Normal flora and diseases

'Diphtheroids' are commonly isolated skin or throat commensals. Rarely, urinary tract infection or bacterial endocarditis affecting a prosthetic heart valve may be caused by these organisms.

C. diphtheriae is rarely found in the normal throat flora except during convalescent carriage. Toxigenic strains may cause diphtheria in susceptible individuals.

C. ulcerans may cause a severe sore throat and some marked constitutional upset but is rarely associated with the classical toxic complications of diphtheria.

Antibiotics

C. diphtheriae strains are characteristically sensitive to penicillin and erythromycin.

Listeria and Erysipelothrix

Listeria monocytogenes and Erysipelothrix rhusiopathiae

Microscopy: Short Gram-positive bacilli may occasionally be confused with 'diphtheroids'.

Light microscopy of a wet preparation of a peptone water culture of *Listeria monocytogenes*, that has been incubated at room temperature, characteristically shows 'tumbling motility'.

Culture: Small colonies appear on blood agar after overnight incubation at 35 °C. Listeria colonies usually show beta-haemolysis but erysipelothrix colonies are usually alpha- or non-haemolytic. *Listeria*, but not *Erysipelothrix*, grows at 4 °C.

Differential tests

Biochemical tests, as well as cultural characteristics, differentiate *Listeria* from *Erysipelothrix* including tests for aesculin hydrolysis and catalase production.

Diseases

Listeria monocytogenes is a cause of meningitis and/or septicaemia in neonates and in immunocompromised patients. It is a possible but rare cause of still-birth.

Erysipelothrix rhusiopathiae causes erysipeloid (*see* p. 309 and p. 410).

Antibiotics

Listeria and *Erysipelothrix* are both characteristically sensitive to ampicillin (or penicillin).

Nocardia and Actinomycetes

These Gram-positive branching filamentous bacilli cause nocardiosis and actinomycosis, respectively (*see* Chapter 13).

Clostridial species

These include *Clostridium welchii (perfringens), septicum, oedematiens, histolyticum, tetani, botulinum, difficile.*

The main characteristics of Gram-positive spore-forming anaerobic bacilli are described in Chapter 9.

B. Gram-negative Bacteria

Neisseria species

These include *Neisseria gonorrhoeae, meningitidis, catarrhalis, pharyngis* and *lactamis*.

Microscopy: Gram-negative oval diplococci; some are characteristically intracellular when seen in clinical specimens.

Culture: *Neisseria* are fragile and suitable transport of specimens with prompt culture is important (*see* pp. 172, 386).

Small colonies on blood agar after 24–48 hours' incubation in a moist aerobic atmosphere with 5–10% carbon dioxide added. Larger colonies on chocolate agar.

Selective media are used for the isolation of *Neisseria gonorrhoeae* from genital tract or rectal specimens (*see* p. 386). Non-pathogenic *Neisseria* sometimes grow on plain agar.

Differential tests

Neisseria species are oxidase positive. The species are differentiated according to the results obtained with biochemical and immunological tests.

a. Biochemical tests

Serum sugar agar slopes are used usually for carrying out sugar fermentation tests (not horse serum which contains maltose). Hydrocele fluid can be used instead of serum as a growth factor. *G*lucose only is characteristically fermented by *g*onococci. *M*altose and *g*lucose are characteristically fermented by *m*eningococci (although a few strains do not ferment maltose). Sucrose or lactose are sometimes fermented by *Neisseria* species which are neither *Neisseria gonorrhoeae* nor *meningitidis*. The media used for sugar fermentation tests needs to be carefully quality controlled.

b. Immunological tests

An immunological test as well as a biochemical test is desirable for the identification of possible gonococcal strains, especially when the isolate is from a female patient or from an unusual site, such as the throat (because atypical strains of other *Neisseria* species, isolated in these circumstances, may occasionally give similar biochemical reactions to those of gonococci). When an isolate shows strong immunofluorescence with a specific antigonococcal serum, preferably by an indirect immunofluorescent technique, there is good evidence that the isolate is a gonococcus (but the medicolegal differentiation traditionally depends on the results of biochemical tests). Direct immunofluorescent techniques have also been used for the rapid presumptive diagnosis of gonorrhoea by examining smears or early cultures of genital tract specimens.

Immunological tests are also used in reference centres to serogroup meningococci into one of the three main groups, A, B or C. Most strains in Britain are serogroup B.

Normal flora and diseases

Neisseria meningitidis is carried in the naso-pharynx of 5–30% of the general population, and is one of the 'three primary pathogens' causing bacterial meningitis.

Neisseria gonorrhoeae is the cause of gonorrhoea and ophthalmia neonatorum. It is not found in the normal flora.

Antibiotics

All meningococcal strains are sensitive to penicillin. There are increasing reports of gonococcal strains highly resistant to penicillin (penicillinase producers), but sensitive to spectinomycin. However, well over 90% gonococcal strains in Britain are still sensitive to penicillin.

Enterobacteria (Coliforms)

These include scores of different genera and many hundreds of different species. *Escherichia coli, Klebsiella aerogenes, Proteus, Salmonella* and *Shigella* species are examples (*see also Table 1.2,* p. 6).

Microscopy: Gram-negative bacilli—the species are not differentiated by their Gram-stain appearance.

Culture: Good growth on blood agar, MacConkey or Cysteine Lactose Electrolyte Deficient (CLED) medium is characteristic after overnight aerobic incubation.

Selective media such as Desoxycholate Citrate Agar (DCA), which suppress the growth of many *E. coli* strains, are used for the isolation of both salmonellae and shigellae from faeces and require up to 48 hours' incubation.

Enrichment liquid media, such as selenite F, are used to increase the yield of salmonella isolations from the faeces. The organisms are subcultured from these media on to selective media, usually after overnight incubation.

Differential tests

a. Lactose fermentation

Escherichia coli, Klebsiella or other coliforms which are characteristically lactose fermenters appear as pink colonies after overnight culture on MacConkey or CLED media. However, some late lactose fermenting strains of these species may appear as 'non-lactose fermenting' colonies on MacConkey agar. *Salmonella* and *Shigella* species characteristically appear as 'non-lactose fermenters' on MacConkey or DCA media (but *Shigella sonnei* is a late lactose fermenter and may appear slightly pink on MacConkey after 24–48 hours' incubation).

b. Motility and other biochemical tests

A 'hanging drop' of an overnight peptone water culture may be examined by wet microscopy to see if the organism is motile or non-motile. *E. coli* and salmonellae are characteristically motile (they are flagellated coliforms) whereas klebsiellae and shigellae are characteristically non-motile. Semi-solid agar methods are available (e.g. 'Craigie tube') for testing for the motility of a possible salmonella or shigella isolate, which are safer than the hanging drop method.

Biochemical tests, in addition to lactose fermentation, include urea, glucose, mannite, sucrose, indole, citrate, hydrogen sulphide production and decarboxylases for apparent 'non-lactose fermenters' and indole, citrate and inositol for 'lactose fermenters'.

Commercial kits are available to assist this identification process which must be carried out on pure cultures. For the identification of 'difficult' organisms, a computer analysis of the results may be useful at a reference centre.

A few simple characteristic examples of the results of biochemical tests include:

Proteus species	*urease positive*, lactose negative
Salmonella species	*glucose fermented*, *mannite fermented*, lactose negative, *urea negative*, sucrose negative
Shigella species	*glucose fermented* *mannite fermented*—mannitol positive shigellae (e.g. *Sh. sonnei*) *urea negative*, sucrose usually negative *mannite negative*—mannitol negative shigellae
E. coli	indole positive, lactose positive, citrate negative
Serratia marcescens	DNAase positive.

There are also classical 'IMVIC' tests for lactose fermenters isolated from possibly faecally contaminated water supplies—Indole, Methyl Red, Voges–Proskauer, Inositol and Citrate. These biochemical tests may be performed at 44 °C to recognize *E. coli* type I from a possible human faecal source (e.g. from polluted water).

c. *Immunological tests*

Suspensions of suspected pathogenic faecal coliforms can be tested against known specific anti-sera in slide or tube agglutination tests. Specific 'O' (somatic antigen) anti-sera are used for the identification of isolates of salmonellae, shigellae and enteropathogenic strains of *E. coli*. Specific 'H' (flagellar antigen) anti-sera are mainly used to identify *Salmonella* species. A salmonella culture on a nutrient agar is often used for agglutination tests but it may be in a 'non-specific H phase'. To convert the *Salmonella* to a 'specific H phase', a 'phase switch' may be necessary using a Craigie tube method.

Normal flora

E. coli is the most common and most numerous aerobic Gram-negative species in the normal faecal flora. Other coliforms are also often present mixed with the *E. coli*, including *Proteus*, *Klebsiella* or *Citrobacter* species to mention just a few possibilities.

Salmonella and *Shigella* species are not found in the normal flora although they may be found in the faeces of healthy convalescent carriers (or permanently in a biliary tract carrier of *S. typhi*).

Diseases

'Endogenous' infections are most common with lactose fermenting coliforms, such as *E. coli* and certain non-lactose fermenting coliforms, such as *Proteus* species, including urinary tract infections, wound infections, abdominal sepsis and Gram-negative septicaemia.

'Exogenous' infections may also occur with the same organisms as those endogenous infections. Cross-infection or environmental infection in hospital may occur (*see* Chapter 24). Infections of the gastro-intestinal tract are also exogenous, due to salmonellae, shigellae, enteropathogenic *E. coli*, etc. (*see* Chapter 14).

Antibiotics

There is such an enormous variation in the antibiotic susceptibilities of different coliform strains that they can only be predicted to a limited extent.

a. Outside hospital
Many coliforms are sensitive to ampicillin (although *Klebsiella* is an exception), provided no recent antibiotics have been given to the patient. The coliforms are also usually sensitive to cotrimoxazole.

b. In hospital
Coliforms are frequently resistant to ampicillin and are often also resistant to other agents, including sulphonamides, tetracycline and streptomycin. The antibiotic resistance patterns vary between different hospitals and between different places in the same hospital, as well as at different times. The patterns of antibiotic resistance depend greatly on the amounts of particular antibiotics used in a given hospital area, the prevalence of particular R factors which carry genes for multiple antibiotic resistance and the frequency of cross-infection in the hospital. In most hospitals in Britain, the great majority of coliforms are still sensitive to gentamicin and to new cephalosporins such as cefuroxime. However, outbreaks of gentamicin-resistant coliform infections have been increasingly reported during the last few years.

Pseudomonas species

These include *Pseudomonas aeruginosa*, *Pseudomonas cepacia* and other *Pseudomonas* species.

Microscopy: Gram-negative bacilli, indistinguishable from the 'coliforms' above on Gram-stain.

Culture: *Pseudomonas* species are strictly aerobic. Good growth only occurs after overnight incubation in an aerobic atmosphere on a blood or nutrient agar plate in contrast to 'coliform' species which can grow well either aerobically or anaerobically as they are facultative anaerobes.

Pseudomonas aeruginosa also grows well on a selective agar containing the disinfectant 'cetrimide' and in many solutions.

Oxidase test: *Pseudomonas* species are, characteristically, strongly oxidase positive in contrast to 'coliform' species which are oxidase negative.

Differential tests

Pseudomonas aeruginosa (pyocyanea) produces a green 'pyocyanin' pigment on magnesium ion containing media whereas other *Pseudomonas* species do not produce this pigment. It metabolizes glucose by oxidation rather than by fermentation and this can be shown by a 'Hugh and Leifson' test. The other *Pseudomonas* species can be differentiated according to the results of biochemical tests (using ammonium salt sugars).

Normal flora and sources

Pseudomonas aeruginosa occurs infrequently in the faecal flora of patients outside hospital. Hospital patients receiving broad-spectrum antibiotics, such as oral cephalosporins, are frequently colonized by *Pseudomonas aeruginosa* in the lower intestinal tract.

Most *Pseudomonas* species may be isolated from moist environmental sites in the hospital including contaminated suction apparatus, contaminated disinfectants, respiratory ventilators and humidifiers. Bottles containing sterile distilled water or other solutions may become quickly contaminated by Gram-negative bacilli, including *Pseudomonas* species, once the bottles are opened.

Diseases

Endogenous or exogenous *Pseudomonas* infections (cross-infection or environmental infection) include chronic urinary tract infections, wound infections, chronic osteomyelitis, chronic otitis externa, eye infections (rare), and various serious opportunistic infections including pneumonia and septicaemia.

Antibiotics

Pseudomonas aeruginosa is resistant to many antibiotics including ampicillin, sulphonamides, trimethoprim, tetracycline, cephaloridine and the majority of the cephalosporins, streptomycin and kanamycin. Nearly all *Pseudomonas aeruginosa* strains are sensitive to polymyxin but this antibiotic is mainly suitable for treating only superficial infections topically. Most strains are sensitive to the aminoglycosides, gentamicin or tobramycin, which are often valuable for systemic treatment. Many strains are sensitive to carbenicillin, ticarcillin, mezlocillin or azlocillin and these anti-pseudomonas penicillins are usually used systemically together with the above aminoglycosides. There is a lot of variation in the sensitivity of different strains to these penicillins depending on whether the strains produce particular penicillinases.

Vibrios

These include *Vibrio cholerae*, *Vibrio parahaemolyticus* and *Campylobacter* species (previously known as *Vibrio foetus*), such as *Campylobacter jejuni*.

Microscopy: Vibrios characteristically appear as curved Gram-negative bacilli, like 'comma' bacilli, but they may also be indistinguishable from 'coliforms' in a Gram-stain.

Campylobacters are characteristically seen as spiral or small 'S'-shaped Gram-negative bacilli in a Gram-stain.

Vibrios are typically motile when suspensions are examined by 'wet microscopy'.

Culture: Thiosulphate-citrate-bile salt sucrose agar (TCBS) medium is the selective medium used for the isolation of *Vibrio cholerae* and *Vibrio parahaemolyticus* from faeces. *V. cholerae* and *V. parahaemolyticus* usually produce large yellow or green colonies, respectively, on TCBS medium after 24 hours incubation in an aerobic atmosphere.

An alkaline peptone water enrichment culture is used in addition to TCBS selective medium for the isolation of *V. cholerae*.

Campylobacter species grow well after 24–48 hours incubation on a selective blood agar medium containing polymyxin, vancomycin and trimethoprim. The plates have to be incubated in a micro-aerophilic atmosphere with added carbon dioxide, preferably at 40–42 °C. When this medium is used to isolate *Campylobacter* species from the faeces of a patient, a presumptive diagnosis of *Campylobacter* is often possible by seeing 'S'-shaped or slim curved Gram-negative bacilli in a Gram-stain of the characteristic moist-looking, oxidase-positive colonies.

Differential tests for V. cholerae

Suspicious yellow colonies on TCBS medium are further identified by Gram-stain, oxidase test, subculture on to nutrient or blood agar for definitive immunological tests and rapid slide agglutination tests with specific *V. cholerae* anti-serum. A presumptive identification is made by the laboratory which urgently sends the culture to a reference laboratory for confirmatory tests including phage typing (with the Mukerjee phage). The results of phage and polymyxin sensitivity tests, haemolysis and other tests in the reference laboratory can also differentiate between 'El Tor' and the 'Classical' bio-types of *V. cholerae*. Nearly all the patients with cholera seen in Europe, the Middle East and Africa have been infected by the 'El Tor' *V. cholerae*.

Diseases

V. cholerae causes cholera and the strains may be carried during convalesence.

V. parahaemolyticus is an uncommon cause of food poisoning in Britain.

Campylobacter jejuni is a common cause of gastro-enteritis and food poisoning.

Antibiotics

V. cholerae (El Tor) is usually sensitive to tetracycline but the incidence of tetracycline-resistant strains is increasing. Antibiotics are of secondary importance to fluid and electrolyte replacement (*see* p. 288).

Campylobacter species are nearly always sensitive to erythromycin.

Parvobacteria

These include: *Haemophilus influenzae* and other *Haemophilus* species; *Bordetella pertussis* and *parapertussis*; *Pasteurella multocida (septica)*, *Yersinia pseudotuberculosis*, *Yersinia enterocolitica* and other *Yersinia* species; *Brucella abortus* and other *Brucella* species; *Francisella tularensis*; *Pseudomonas mallei*.

Microscopy: The parvobacteria are short Gram-negative bacilli (coccobacilli). Many such as *Haemophilus* species are pleomorphic. Some bacilli, such as *Pasteurella multocida* may show bipolar staining. Occasionally, the capsules of capsulated strains of *Haemophilus influenzae* may be seen, e.g. Pittman type b strain, in stained smears or by immunofluorescent techniques using specific anti-capsular antibody.

Culture: Parvobacteria are relatively fragile and specimens with these organisms need to be promptly cultured and preferably inoculated directly on to media for the best culture results. If delays are inevitable, appropriate transport media may be used for certain species such as *Bordetella* (*see* p. 137).

Most parvobacteria species appear as small colonies on fresh blood agar after 24–48 hours' incubation in an aerobic moist atmosphere with 5–10% added carbon dioxide. A few species will not grow on blood agar, such as *Bordetella pertussis*. Special enriched and selective media such as Bordet-Gengou, Lacey's medium or pertussis charcoal agar are needed for culture of *Bordetella*. Dorset's egg medium is required for culture of *Francisella tularensis*.

Haemophilus species grow better on chocolate agar than on blood agar; moderately large colonies are apparent on chocolate agar after overnight incubation.

Differential tests

a. Haemophilus species

The *Haemophilus* species can be identified according to the results of 'satellitism' tests. *Haemophilus influenzae* will not grow around a disc containing X factor (haemin) or V factor (coenzyme NAD) alone, but will around a combined X plus V disc on plain agar. On blood agar, *Haemophilus influenzae* shows improved satellite growth around *Staph. aureus* colonies due to the release of V factor from the staphylococci. (*Haemophilus parainfluenzae* does not require X factor but does require V factor.)

Haemolysis is another cultural factor that is used for identifying less pathogenic *Haemophilus* species, such as *Haemophilus haemolyticus*, which may be found in the normal throat flora.

Capsulated strains of *Haemophilus influenzae* often grow well with a green sheen on Levinthal's agar. The capsules can be Pittman typed using specific anti-capsular sera (in a Quelling type reaction). The usual capsular type *H. influenzae* infecting infants is Pittman type b. This capsular antigen may sometimes also be detected using an immunoprecipitation test.

b. *Differentiation from coliforms*
Most parvobacteria species will not grow well (if at all) on MacConkey's agar after overnight incubation, in contrast to 'coliforms' and most *Pseudomonas* species. Most of the parvobacteria will not grow in peptone water sugars unlike coliforms, an important exception being *Pasteurella multocida*. Some parvobacteria will not grow anaerobically on blood agar after overnight incubation unlike coliforms.

c. *Yersinia, Pasteurella and Bordetella species*
A range of cultural tests on MacConkey agar, blood agar, enriched and selective media combined with biochemical tests, motility and haemolysis tests help to identify a particular *Yersinia* or *Pasteurella* species. Immunological tests using slide or tube agglutinations of suspensions of the organisms against known anti-sera are also required for *Yersinia* and *Bordetella* species.

Normal flora

Haemophilus species are frequently found in the normal throat flora and occasionally in the nose flora (especially of infants). *Pasteurella multocida* is also occasionally found in the normal upper respiratory tract flora, especially in individuals who may have contact with rodents (because they work in an animal house or have rodent pets).

Diseases

Parvobacteria causing diseases are included in *Table A1.2*. The most common parvobacteria infections in Britain include those due to *Haemophilus influenzae*, *Bordetella pertussis* and *Pasteurella multocida*. Other parvobacteria infections are very uncommon.

Antibiotics

Some parvobacteria species are relatively sensitive to penicillin in contrast to coliforms which are resistant to penicillin, a good example being *Pasteurella multocida*. Many parvobacteria are also sensitive to erythromycin in vitro, such as *Bordetella pertussis*, *Pasteurella multocida*. *Yersinia* and *Brucella* species are characteristically sensitive to tetracyclines.

Haemophilus influenzae strains are usually sensitive to ampicillin but the incidence of ampicillin-resistant β-lactamase-producing strains is increasing and is greater than 10% for Pittman type b capsulated strains in some areas in Britain. Chloramphenicol is nearly always active against *H. influenzae*, including ampicillin-resistant strains and is recommended for treating haemophilus infections such as meningitis or acute epiglottitis. Cotrimoxazole and tetracycline are also useful for treating infective exacerbations of chronic bronchitis due to *Haemophilus influenzae*.

Table A1.2. Some examples of infections due to parvobacteria

Parvobacteria	*Main infections*
Haemophilus influenzae	
i. *Capsulated Pittman type b strains*	*Infections in children mainly, 3 months to 5 years (up to 12 years may occur):* *a.* Respiratory tract infections—pharyngitis, otitis media, sinusitis, acute epiglottitis (rare), pneumonia (very rare) *b.* Septicaemia *c.* Meningitis *d.* Osteomyelitis and septic arthritis *e.* Pericarditis or endocarditis (both rare)
ii. *Other strains*	*Infections mainly in adults:* *a.* Infective exacerbations of chronic bronchitis *b.* Chronic sinusitis *c.* Conjunctivitis
Bordetella pertussis	Whooping cough
Pasteurella multocida (septica)	Wound infections following animal bites: meningitis (rare), septicaemia (rare)
Yersinia pestis	Plague
Yersinia enterocolitica	Gastro-enteritis (possible 'rheumatic fever'-like illness and arthritis possible)
Yersinia pseudo-tuberculosis	Mesenteric adenitis (may clinically mimic acute appendicitis)
Brucella species	Brucellosis
Francisella tularensis	Tularaemia
Pseudomonas mallei	Glanders

Legionella

Legionella pneumophila causes severe pneumonia—Legionnaires' disease.

Microscopy: Gram-negative bacilli in Gram-stains of colonies from culture media; in tissues and clinical specimens the bacilli may stain poorly with an ordinary Gram-stain but better when a prolonged counterstain with carbol fuchsin is used. Gram films made from cultures may show long filamentous forms of the organism. The bacilli are also apparent in silver stains in tissue although they are best seen in tissues by immunofluorescence using specific anti-legionella anti-sera or by electron microscopy using immunoferritin techniques.

Culture: No growth on ordinary media.

Requires 3–5 days' incubation on special legionella media containing blood, added cysteine and iron salts such as ferric pyrophosphate, at pH 6·9.

Guinea-pig inoculation is necessary for the isolation of *Legionella* from environmental samples such as water.

Sources

Environmental: contaminated water in air conditioning plants, shower mixers, etc., causes infection by inhalation of contaminated air.

Disease

Legionnaires' disease ranges from a mild pyrexia of unknown origin (PUO), or mild respiratory symptoms, to severe pneumonia with multisystem complications. It is fatal in about 15% of *Legionella*-infected patients requiring hospital admission for severe pneumonia. Other similar diseases due to ALLO (atypical *Legionella*-like organisms) have been recently reported.

Antibiotics

Legionella is characteristically sensitive to erythromycin and tetracycline but usually resistant to penicillins and aminoglycosides.

Anaerobic Gram-negative Bacilli

Strict non-sporing anaerobic organisms, including Gram-negative bacilli such as *Bacteroides* species, are described in Chapter 9.

Further Reading

See recommended reading list at end of Chapter 1 (p. 15).

Appendix 2

Notes on antimicrobial drugs including some 'new' antibiotics

The purpose of this section is to summarize briefly the principal uses, limitations and main unwanted effects of some major antimicrobial drugs in current use. The antimicrobial spectrum of the drugs and the general principles of antimicrobial chemotherapy are discussed in Chapter 3.

BETA-LACTAM ANTIBIOTICS

These include penicillins, cephalosporins and mecillinam. Patients allergic to penicillin may develop cross-hypersensitivity reactions to all these beta-lactam drugs. Hypersensitivity reactions include skin rashes, drug fevers, 'serum sickness' and rarely fatal anaphylactic shock. Benzylpenicillin, other narrow spectrum penicillins, ampicillin, amoxycillin, carbenicillin and other anti-pseudomonal penicillins are susceptible to staphylococcal penicillinase.

Benzylpenicillin (Penicillin G)

Administration

Intra-muscular (i.m.) or intravenous (i.v.).

Main uses

Valuable for treating severe pneumococcal and streptococcal infections. Effective for treating meningococcal and leptospiral infections. Early treatment essential for serious infections. Useful for the prophylaxis of clostridial gas gangrene.

Antibiotic resistance

Majority of *Staph. aureus* and a small but increasing number of *N. gonorrhoeae* strains are penicillinase producers.

Minority of '*Strep. viridans*' strains and all *Strep. faecalis* strains have reduced sensitivity to penicillin.

Rarely *Strep. penumoniae* strains are penicillin resistant.

Side-effects and toxicity

Penicillin allergy, in up to 5% of patients. When greater than 20 MU per day are given systemically to an adult, neurotoxicity and haemolytic anaemia may occur. It may be toxic when given intrathecally if greater than 10 000 units is administered to an adult (or 2000 units to an infant). Excessive doses intrathecally can result in convulsions and death.

Procaine Penicillin

Administration

Intra-muscular only. Peak levels delayed compared to benzylpenicillin, but serum levels persist for up to 18 hours after each dose. *NB*: Intravenous administration contraindicated.

Main use

Treatment of gonorrhoea and syphilis.

Antibiotic resistance

Gradual increase in MIC to penicillin in many gonococcal strains; large single doses are required (*see* p. 387). Penicillinase-producing gonococci not susceptible to even high concentrations of penicillin.

Side-effects and toxicity

Similar to benzylpenicillin. Rarely hypersensitivity to the procaine component may occur.

Triplopen

This includes a mixture of benzylpenicillin, procaine and benethamine penicillin, BPC.

Administration

Intra-muscular only. *NB*: Intravenous administration contraindicated.

Main use

Prevention of endocarditis in susceptible dental patients.

'Starter' injection for a course of penicillin treatment for severe streptococcal sore throat and other infections.

Side-effects and toxicity

Similar to procaine penicillin.

Penicillin V (Phenoxymethylpenicillin)

Administration

Oral only.

Main uses

Treatment of streptococcal sore throat and other upper respiratory tract infections.

Antibiotic resistance

Same problems as for other penicillins. No *Strep. pyogenes* strains are resistant to penicillin.

Side-effects and toxicity

Penicillin hypersensitivity. Large doses may cause nausea.

'Broad Spectrum' Penicillins Susceptible to Staphylococcal Penicillinase

Ampicillin

Administration

Oral (acid-resistant), intra-muscular or intravenous.

Main uses

Treatment of some lower respiratory tract infections such as infective exacerbations of bronchitis when staphylococcal or mycoplasma infections are not considered likely. Treatment of some urinary tract infections.

Antibiotic resistance

Virtually all *Klebsiella* and *Pseudomonas* strains and greater than a third of hospital *E. coli* and other 'coliform' strains are ampicillin resistant. In general practice, between 10 and 25% *E. coli* strains isolated from urine are ampicillin resistant. Up to 15% Pittman type b capsulated *Haemophilus influenzae* strains are resistant to ampicillin in some areas.

Ampicillin should not be used blindly to treat suspected haemophilus epiglotitis or meningitis (chloramphenicol is preferred).

Side-effects and toxicity

Penicillin allergy. Ampicillin is associated with a higher incidence of drug rashes than penicillin and the incidence is especially high if it is administered to patients with glandular fever. Diarrhoea or nausea is frequent and is most likely if a prolonged course is given.

Superinfection with ampicillin-resistant bacteria, such as *Klebsiella*, or fungi, such as *Candida*, may occur.

Talampicillin

Administration

Oral only. Approximately twice the serum levels of ampicillin occur after a dose compared with an equivalent oral dose of ampicillin.

Main uses, antibiotic resistance, side-effects and toxicity

Similar to ampicillin; possibly slightly lower incidence of diarrhoea with talampicillin.

Amoxycillin

Administration

Oral (or parenteral). After equivalent oral doses of amoxycillin and ampicillin the serum levels of amoxycillin are about twice those of ampicillin. Therapeutic serum amoxycillin levels persist for at least 8 hours after a dose of amoxycillin compared with about 6 hours after an equivalent dose of ampicillin. Absorption is less affected by food than with ampicillin.

Main uses

Similar to ampicillin—the antibacterial spectrum is virtually identical to that of ampicillin. Pharmacodynamically, amoxycillin is a superior drug to ampicillin.

'Special uses' include the oral prophylaxis (high dose) and treatment of streptococcal endocarditis, and the treatment of typhoid fever and carriers.

Antibiotic resistance, side-effects and toxicity

Similar to ampicillin. The incidence of diarrhoea is possibly slightly less with amoxycillin.

Carbenicillin

Administration

Intravenous route usually.

Main uses

For treating serious Gram-negative infections, especially in immunocompromised or neutropenic patients, in combination with an aminoglycoside drug, such as tobramycin or gentamicin, particularly when *Pseudomonas aeruginosa* infection suspected.

Antibiotic resistance

Many strains of *P. aeruginosa* and most *Klebsiella* strains are resistant to carbenicillin due to the production of a beta-lactamase that destroys the drug.

Side-effects and toxicity

Penicillin hypersensitivity reactions, electrolyte imbalance because of sodium overloading when large doses are given to certain patients. Particular care is necessary when renal function is impaired. Rarely haemorrhages, due to platelet dysfunction, may occur.

Carfecillin

Administration

Oral. This ester of carbenicillin is inactive but the active compound is excreted in the urine.

Main use

Occasionally used for treating *Pseudomonas* urinary tract infection in out-patients or general practice (not indicated if renal failure present since insufficient drug is then excreted).

Antibiotic resistance, side-effects and toxicity

Similar problems to carbenicillin. (Sodium ion overloading does not apply.)

Ticarcillin

Administration

Intravenous use mainly.

Main uses

Similar to carbenicillin, in combination with an aminoglycoside.

Antibiotic resistance

Some *Pseudomonas* and other Gram-negative strains are resistant to ticarcillin.

Side-effects and toxicity

Similar to carbenicillin. The main advantage of ticarcillin over carbenicillin is that less sodium ions are infused with ticarcillin.

Mezlocillin

Administration

Intravenous (or intra-muscular).

Main uses

Similar to ticarcillin or carbenicillin for use in combination with an aminoglycoside for treating suspected Gram-negative septicaemias in immunocompromised patients. Mezlocillin is active against many *Klebsiella* strains which are resistant to ticarcillin or carbenicillin, and some *Pseudomonas* strains that are carbenicillin resistant.

Antibiotic resistance

Occasional *Klebsiella, Pseudomonas* and other Gram-negative strains are mezlocillin resistant.

Side-effects and toxicity

Similar to ticarcillin.

Azlocillin

Administration

Intravenous (or intra-muscular).

Main uses

Similar to ticarcillin, for combined use with an aminoglycoside, such as tobramycin, for treating serious pseudomonas infections. Azlocillin is particularly active against *Pseudomonas aeruginosa* strains including some strains which are resistant to mezlocillin, ticarcillin or carbenicillin. However, it is not as active as mezlocillin against some *Klebsiella* strains.

Antibiotic resistance

Azlocillin resistance in *Pseudomonas* strains is rare.

Side-effects and toxicity

Similar to ticarcillin.

Isoxazolyl Penicillins, including Methicillin, Cloxacillin and Flucloxacillin

These penicillins are narrow spectrum anti-staphylococcal drugs which are relatively resistant to staphylococcal penicillinase. The great majority of penicillin-resistant *Staph. aureus* strains are sensitive to these drugs.

Methicillin

Administration

Parenteral only.

Main use

Not used much now, it was the first isoxazolyl drug. It has less anti-staphylococcal activity than cloxacillin (but is less protein bound than cloxacillin).

Antibiotic resistance

Methicillin resistance occurs in less than 1% of strains in Britain at present. Hospital outbreaks due to methicillin-resistant strains of *Staph. aureus* (usually also resistant to other antibiotics) occasionally occur.

Side-effects and toxicity

Penicillin hypersensitivity reactions. Methicillin nephropathy may rarely occur.

Cloxacillin

Administration

Oral, intra-muscular or intravenous.

Main uses

Treatment of suspected and confirmed *Staph. aureus* infections due to penicillinase-producing strains which are sensitive to cloxacillin. Cloxacillin is a valuable narrow spectrum anti-staphylococcal drug which is effective and safe even when used in high dosage. Parenteral administration in high dosage, sometimes combined with another drug such as fusidic acid, or gentamicin, may be indicated for treating some serious infections, e.g. staphylococcal endocarditis, pneumonia or osteomyelitis.

Antibiotic resistance

Cross-resistance with methicillin (*above*).

Side-effects and toxicity

Penicillin hypersensitivity reactions.

Flucloxacillin

Administration

Oral, intra-muscular or intravenous. Oral flucloxacillin is slightly better absorbed than oral cloxacillin and many authorities recommend that flucloxacillin be used as the isoxazolyl penicillin of choice.

Main uses

Similar to cloxacillin.

Antibiotic resistance, side-effects and toxicity

Similar to cloxacillin. Nausea may occur if high doses are given orally.

Clavulanic acid

This novel new drug (available commercially as sodium clavulanate combined with amoxycillin) can protect some beta-lactam antibiotics from inactivation by beta-lactamase-producing bacteria.

Administration

Oral.

Main uses

Clavulanic acid combined with amoxycillin has been effective for treating some urinary tract and other infections due to beta-lactamase-producing strains of *E. coli, Klebsiella* and some other Gram-negative bacilli. (These strains would be ampicillin resistant and therefore amoxycillin resistant.) It is still under evaluation.

Antibiotic resistance

A few strains of *E. coli* and other coliforms have already been reported which are resistant to the combination of sodium clavulanate and amoxycillin. *Pseudomonas* strains are always resistant.

Side-effects and toxicity

Similar to amoxycillin. Sodium clavulanate may infrequently cause nausea or other mild gastro-intestinal side-effects, especially when higher doses are used.

Cephalosporins

General comments

This group of drugs now includes more than 15 different agents and new cephalosporins are becoming available each year. All of these drugs, like isoxazolyl penicillins, are relatively stable to staphylococcal penicillinase (although the degree of stability varies between different cephalosporins). However, a patient who has a known or suspected *Staph. aureus* infection is probably best treated with effective narrow spectrum anti-staphylococcal drugs such as cloxacillin, erythromycin and fusidic acid rather than cephalosporins which are 'broad spectrum' antibiotics. When a patient is seriously infected by a methicillin-resistant strain of *Staph. aureus*, cephalosporins cannot be relied on to treat the infection since there is generally cross-resistance between methicillin and cephalosporins.

Cephalosporins are of particular interest because of their activity against Gram-negative bacilli. Apart from the problem of occasional cross-hypersensitivity with penicillin these drugs are relatively safe. *E. coli, Klebsiella* and other Gram-negative bacteria causing infections are often resistant to ampicillin, carbenicillin or other beta-lactam drugs because of the production of beta-lactamases. Some beta-lactamases can also destroy certain cephalosporins and resistance to the first cephalosporins introduced, such as cephaloridine, is now frequently observed. New cephalosporins have been developed which are relatively stable to Gram-negative beta-lactamases. It is hoped that the need for potentially toxic aminoglycoside drugs, such as gentamicin, to treat serious Gram-negative infections will be greatly reduced when the 'right' cephalosporin is introduced and this might be achieved soon.

Stability to beta-lactamases is important but other factors also affect the antibacterial activities of different cephalosporin drugs including the degree of penetration of the bacterial cell wall and the degree of intrinsic activity against each organism. Pharmacodynamic factors also vary a lot between many different cephalosporin drugs (for some examples, *see Table A2* and p. 45). There are relatively few differences between the agents available in their incidence of side-effects and toxicity. Apart from allergy reactions, the only serious unwanted effect is nephrotoxicity which might occur to some extent with any cephalosporin drug.

In clinical practice, there are few specific indications for the use of *any* cephalosporin. The degree to which these drugs should be used clinically is a controversial question. Instead of summarizing each cephalosporin drug separately some personal comments are given on the main uses and limitations of cephalosporins.

A. Main uses of cephalosporins

1. *Penicillin hypersensitivity*

When a patient with a suspected Gram-negative infection has a possible history of a mild penicillin allergy a cephalosporin could be considered. However, cross-hypersensitivity between penicillins and cephalosporins may occur in up to 10% of patients with penicillin allergy. If there is a definite history of penicillin allergy, especially if a severe reaction has occurred, cephalosporins should not be used.

2. *Culture and antibiotic sensitivity test results indicate the suitability of a cephalosporin*

Isolations of Gram-negative bacilli which are resistant to a number of antibiotics but sensitive to a cephalosporin may clearly indicate the need to use a cephalosporin provided the isolate is clinically significant.

In practice this occasionally occurs with urinary tract infections where, for example, a *Klebsiella* strain may be resistant to ampicillin, trimethoprim, sulphonamides and nalidixic acid but sensitive to a cephalosporin and gentamicin; a cephalosporin, such as cephalexin, may be a suitable choice. Pregnant women with urinary tract infections due to ampicillin-resistant strains of *E. coli* can often be treated safely with a cephalosporin. Another example is the use of a cephalosporin, such as cephazolin, to treat a chronic Gram-negative osteomyelitis infection in an elderly patient in hospital, where the multiple antibiotic-resistant infecting coliform is sensitive to cephazolin and gentamicin. The use of a course of cephazolin injections avoids the need to give potentially ototoxic gentamicin therapy in this situation. Cefuroxime or cefoxitin are often valuable for treating serious infections due to gentamicin-resistant and multiple antibiotic-resistant strains of *Klebsiella*; they should really be kept in reserve for treating these types of difficult infections.

When beta-lactamase-producing strains of *Haemophilus influenzae* are isolated from children with bacteraemia or meningitis, a suitable cephalosporin that is stable to this beta-lactamase can be considered, such as cefuroxime, but most authorities would prefer to use chloramphenicol.

Gonorrhoea, due to strains of *N. gonorrhoeae* that produce penicillinase, can often be effectively treated by a cephalosporin insusceptible to this enzyme, such as cefuroxime. However, at present, most authorities prefer to use spectinomycin to treat the majority of these infections. If, in the future, penicillinase-producing gonococci also develop widespread spectinomycin resistance, cefuroxime or cefotaxime would become particularly valuable.

3. *'Blind' treatment of undiagnosed infections*

'Blind' cephalosporin treatment may be useful for moderately severe infections, where broad spectrum cover is required while awaiting the results of bacteriology tests in hospital patients. Examples of infections suitable for this treatment include:

a. Obstetric or gynaecological infections in patients with post-operative sepsis may be treated by a combination of a cephalosporin plus metronidazole. The cephalosporin would be active against 'coliforms', and *Staph. aureus* and the metronidazole would treat any anaerobic infection present.

b. Neonatal infections of moderate severity are often caused by *E. coli* or other coliforms but *Staph. aureus* is also an occasional cause. A cephalosporin can be used 'blind' in this situation while waiting for culture results. (Of course, severe neonatal infections, such as those due to Lancefield group B streptococci or *Pseudomonas*, would not be effectively treated by a cephalosporin.)

c. A moderately severe infective exacerbation of chronic bronchitis, or pneumonia, in a patient with advanced chest disease may be caused by *Strep. pneumoniae*, a penicillinase-producing *Staph. aureus* and/or an ampicillin-resistant *Haemophilus influenzae* strain. A new cephalosporin active against all of these organisms, such as cefuroxime (or cephamandole), would be a suitable 'blind' choice of drug in this situation.

4. *Use of cephalosporins for 'prophylaxis'*

Cephazolin has been recommended for the peri-operative prophylaxis of biliary tract infections in selected patients undergoing bile duct surgery. Prophylaxis with cephalosporins is, in general, probably 'excessive'; in many situations it is probable that either no prophylaxis is indicated, or only short prophylactic courses for the period at risk, or else a narrow spectrum drug such as cloxacillin is preferable (*see* Prophylaxis, in Chapter 3).

B. Limitations of cephalosporins for treating infections

These include:

a. Pseudomonas aeruginosa serious infections are not effectively treated by any cephalosporin, at present, even though some recently developed drugs, such as cefotaxime, have significant activity against *Pseudomonas* strains in vitro. The incidence of faecal carriage of *Pseudomonas* in hospital patients receiving some cephalosporin drugs, such as cephalexin, is increased. It is possible that when there is widespread use of currently available cephalosporins in a hospital the incidence of pseudomonas infections may become increased. Ceftazidime, not yet released, has promising anti-pseudomonas activity.

b. *Haemophilus influenzae* strains are relatively insusceptible to most cephalosporins. Exceptions include cefuroxime, cephamandole, cefaclor and cefotaxime which have significant activity against *Haemophilus* strains.

c. *Strep. faecalis* is usually resistant to cephalosporins and, therefore, these drugs are not suitable for the prevention or treatment of enterococcal endocarditis.

d. Meningitis due to *Strep. pneumoniae* and *N. meningitidis* is not as effectively treated by cephalosporins as it would be by benzylpenicillin, in spite of sensitivity in vitro of the causative strains to cephalosporins.

e. Some 'coliform' strains, including many *Enterobacter* strains, may be resistant to even the most recently developed cephalosporin drugs.

f. Cephalosporins are not recommended for treating suspected *Bacteroides fragilis* infections. An exception is cefoxitin, a cephamycin drug, which is usually stable to the beta-lactamases produced by *Bacteroides*, and which has been used successfully to treat some patients with serious abdominal sepsis.

g. Nephrotoxicity can occur especially when high doses of cephalosporins are used, or simultaneous aminoglycosides or diuretics are given, or if the patient already has renal damage.

Which cephalosporin?

Most clinicians familiarize themselves with at least a few of the more useful cephalosporins. The hospital consultant microbiologist may be able to help by indicating the up-to-date information that is available on the clinical efficiency of the various drugs, and an antibiotic policy may be adopted by the hospital in order to limit the drugs stocked by pharmacy. Unfortunately, views differ widely on the best choice of agents and the situation is confusing. The main pharmacodynamic and bacteriological differences between major cephalosporins are summarized in *Table A.2*. In addition to the above comments on the uses and limitations of cephalosporins, some further personal comments affecting choice of drug are included in the 'comments' column of *Table A.2*. The more recent cephalosporins, such as cefuroxime, cefoxitin and cefotaxime, are also much more expensive than the earlier cephalosporins, such as cephazolin.

Mecillinam and Pivmecillinam

The amidino-penicillin drug, mecillinam, acts on a different target site in the bacterial cell wall than that of the above beta-lactam antibiotics. Its activity is almost entirely confined against Gram-negative bacilli.

Table A.2. Some cephalosporin or related drugs

Drug	*Route of administration*	*Dose (example) (mg)*	*Peak* serum level (mg/l)*	*Serum half-life (hours)*	*Protein binding, approx. (%)*	*Antibacterial activity against Gram-negative bacteria:* *Klebsiella (typical MIC mg/l)*	*Other coliforms*	*B. fragilis*	*H. influenzae (lactamase strains)*	*N. gonorrhoeae (lactamase strains)*	*Nephrotoxicity†*	*Comment*
Cephaloridine	Parenteral	500	22	1·5	20	3	+	–	–	–	+++	First cephalosporin
Cephalothin	Parenteral	500	10	0·5	70	6	+	–	–	–	++	Painful by intra-muscular route
Cephazolin	Parenteral	500	28	2·0	75	3	+	–	–	–	Not yet reported in humans	*Recommended first line parenteral cephalosporin*
Cephalexin	Oral	500	28	0·7	15	6	+	–	–	–	Not yet reported in humans	Only one of these need be selected as an oral cephalosporin
Cephradine	Oral/Parenteral	500	18	0·7	15	12	+	–	–	–	Not yet reported in humans	Only one of these need be selected as an oral cephalosporin
More recent drugs												
Cefuroxime	Parenteral	500	25	1·2	33	1·6‡	++	–	++	++	Not yet reported in humans	*Valuable 're-serve' cephalosporins* for suspected antibiotic-resistant Gram-negative infections
Cefoxitin	Parenteral	500	11	0·7	75	1·6	++	++	–	–	Not yet reported in humans	*Valuable 're-serve' cephalosporins* for suspected antibiotic-resistant Gram-negative infections
Cephamandole	Parenteral	1000	20	0·6	74	1·6	++	–	+	+	Not yet reported in humans	Uncertain role
Cefaclor	Oral	500	12	0·7	15	6	+	–	+		Not yet reported in humans	? Restrict for treatment of some respiratory infections

* After dose in adjacent column.
† Nephrotoxicity depends on dose used, state of renal function, and is potentiated by simultaneous administration of gentamicin or other aminoglycosides and frusemide.
‡ Cefuroxime has been used successfully to treat some gentamicin-resistant klebsiella infections.

Administration

Pivmecillinam is given orally. This is converted to mecillinam which is ultimately excreted in the urine.

Mecillinam may be also administered parenterally.

Main uses

Treating confirmed urinary tract infections due to *E. coli* or other 'coliform' strains resistant to ampicillin and other antibiotics but sensitive to mecillinam. Oral pivmecillinam is usually given.

Mecillinam may be used to treat systemic infections due to 'food-poisoning' *Salmonella* strains, in synergic combination with another beta-lactam antibiotic, such as ampicillin (according to the results of antibiotic susceptibility tests). Mecillinam has also been used effectively to treat coliform infections of moderate severity in neonates.

Antibiotic resistance

Some beta-lactamase-producing strains of coliforms are resistant to mecillinam. *Pseudomonas* is always resistant.

Side-effects and toxicity

Penicillin hypersensitivity reactions. Occasionally mild gastro-intestinal side-effects.

AMINOGLYCOSIDES

Aminoglycosides are all potentially toxic drugs with a narrow therapeutic margin when administered parenterally to treat systemic infections. They are not absorbed after oral administration. They are all excreted by the kidneys and toxicity is more likely when renal function is impaired. The aminoglycosides should be used with great discrimination to avoid the development of bacterial resistance to these valuable agents as well as to avoid toxic effects. They should not be used topically on the skin, when possible, to reduce the chances of resistant strains developing or spreading. The aminoglycosides mentioned below include streptomycin, neomycin, framycetin, kanamycin, gentamicin, tobramycin and amikacin.

Streptomycin sulphate

Administration

Intra-muscular.

Main uses

Antituberculous chemotherapy in combination with other drugs. Not used as often as previously since the introduction of rifampicin and ethambutol (*see* p. 250). Also used occasionally for the treatment or prevention of streptococcal endocarditis in combination with penicillin.

Antibiotic resistance

Resistance rapidly emerges during treatment if the drug is used alone. Less than 2% *M. tuberculosis* strains are resistant to streptomycin in Britain.

Side-effects and toxicity

Mainly ototoxicity (predominantly vestibular), which is most likely to occur in the elderly, in patients with a previous eighth cranial nerve defect and those with impaired renal function. Streptomycin assays may be indicated to avoid excessive peak levels or accumulation of the drug during treatment.

Neomycin

Administration

Oral and topical only. (Systemic administration is contraindicated due to serious toxicity of the drug.)

Main uses

Treatment of hepatic encephalopathy by oral administration to suppress faecal flora. Topical nasal application in combination with chlorhexidine to treat carriage of an epidemic neomycin-sensitive strain of *Staph. aureus*. Topical neomycin ear preparations are used to treat otitis externa, but are contra-indicated if a perforated ear drum is present.

Antibiotic resistance

Neomycin-resistant *Staph. aureus* strains may cause outbreaks of infection and associated with widespread use of topical neomycin. *Pseudomonas* strains always resistant.

Side-effects and toxicity

Local hypersensitivity reactions. If the drug is exceptionally absorbed from a diseased gut, eighth cranial nerve deafness and nephrotoxicity might result.

Framycetin

Administration

Oral and topical only.

Main uses

Similar anti-bacterial spectrum to neomycin. Included in 'FRACON' non-absorbed oral combined drug prophylaxis of infections in neutropenic leukaemic patients (p. 109). Topical treatment of superficial skin or ear infections; probably preferable to topical neomycin as there may be slightly less risk of antibiotic resistance developing.

Antibiotic resistance, side-effects and toxicity

Similar to neomycin.

Kanamycin

There are many kanamycin-resistant 'coliforms' which are sensitive to gentamicin or tobramycin and these latter drugs have superseded kanamycin. Kanamycin also has no activity against *Pseudomonas*.

Gentamicin

Administration

Intra-muscular or intravenous. Dosage régimes should be adjusted according to the results of serum gentamicin assay (*see* Chapter 3, p. 55). Topical use should rarely be necessary on the eye or ear, and is best avoided completely on the skin.

Main uses

'Blind' treatment of acute life-threatening Gram-negative infections in hospital until the results of cultures and antibiotic sensitivities are known.

Treatment of *Pseudomonas* and confirmed Gram-negative bacillus infections due to strains resistant to several other antibiotics, such as ampicillin, cotrimoxazole and cephazolin, but sensitive to gentamicin.

'Blind' treatment of infective endocarditis in combination with benzylpenicillin, and sometimes cloxacillin to treat suspected streptococcal or staphylococcal causes, pending the results of cultures and antibiotic tests. Gentamicin is often preferable to streptomycin for treating enterococcal endocarditis in combination with penicillin.

Antibiotic resistance

High degrees of gentamicin resistance are usually plasmid mediated and associated with aminoglycoside-destroying enzymes produced by Gram-negative bacilli or *Staph. aureus* strains. Development and spread of gentamicin resistance in staphylococcal strains has occurred following topical use of gentamicin on skin. In Britain, less than 8% of 'coliforms' and *Pseudomonas* and less than 1% of *Staph. aureus* isolates in many hospitals are resistant to gentamicin.

Side-effects and toxicity

Ototoxicity—usually vestibular and reversible after stopping gentamicin. High tone deafness may also occur. The risk is greatest in patients with impaired renal function, elderly patients and those receiving prolonged therapy. Also rapidly acting diuretics, such as ethacrynic acid, may increase the risk of gentamicin ototoxicity developing. Ototoxicity is associated with raised serum trough levels, greater than 2·0 mg/l, and high peak levels such as greater than 15·0 mg/l. Repeated gentamicin assays are often necessary to help avoid accumulation of the drug.

Nephrotoxicity is less frequent than ototoxicity but can occur especially when there is simultaneous use of a cephalosporin, or when there is previous impairment of renal function or hypotension associated with septic shock.

Neuromuscular blockade by muscle relaxants used by the anaesthetist in surgical patients may be potentiated by gentamicin.

Tobramycin

Administration
Intra-muscular or intravenous.

Main uses
Similar to gentamicin for treating some serious Gram-negative infections. Tobramycin was about twice as active as gentamicin against *Pseudomonas* strains and is occasionally active against gentamicin-resistant strains of *Pseudomonas aeruginosa*. Tobramycin may be particularly suitable for treating serious pseudomonas infections in combination with an anti-pseudomonad penicillin such as ticarcillin or azlocillin. However, tobramycin often has less activity than gentamicin against *Klebsiella* strains.

Antibiotic resistance
Tobramycin resistance in coliforms and *Pseudomonas* strains is still relatively rare in Britain.

Side-effects and toxicity
Similar to gentamicin. Repeated serum tobramycin assays are necessary to avoid toxicity as well as to ensure effective treatment is given.

Amikacin

Administration
Intra-muscular or intravenous.

Main uses
Similar to gentamicin and tobramycin for treating serious Gram-negative infections. However, it should be used only as 'reserve' drug for treating infections due to strains of Gram-negative bacilli (including 'coliforms' and *Pseudomonas*) that are resistant to gentamicin and tobramycin, but sensitive to amikacin.

Antibiotic resistance
Very rare at present amongst coliforms and *Pseudomonas*.

Side-effects and toxicity

Similar toxicity to gentamicin except that auditory rather than vestibular eighth cranial nerve damage may occur. Serum amikacin assays are necessary. Toxicity is more likely if high peak levels, greater than 30 mg/l, or accumulation of the drug occurs, suggested by trough levels greater than 4 mg/l.

Spectinomycin

This is an aminocylitol antibiotic, related to the aminoglycosides.

Administration

Intra-muscular (single dose).

Main use

Treatment of uncomplicated gonorrhoea due to penicillinase-producing strains of gonococci.

Antibiotic resistance

Rapidly may emerge in bacteria when repeated doses of the drug are given alone; drug only indicated for single dose treatment of gonorrhoea.

Side-effects and toxicity

No significant unwanted effects when only a single dose is used.

TETRACYCLINES

These broad spectrum bacteriostatic agents are especially useful for treating some infections due to intracellular organisms, such as *Brucella* and chlamydiae, since they penetrate macrophages well. A few examples are mentioned below of drugs for systemic use.

Oxytetracycline

Administration

Oral mainly; intra-muscular or intravenous but caution necessary when using parenteral route (below).

Main uses

Tetracyclines may be useful for treating bacterial infections, including infective exacerbations of bronchitis, pneumonia in some general practice patients, brucellosis, El Tor cholera, severe acne and gonorrhoea in some penicillin-allergic patients. Other conditions that may be susceptible to treatment include Q fever, mycoplasma pneumonia, psittacosis, non-specific urethritis associated with chlamydia infection and lymphogranuloma venereum.

Antibiotic resistance

Tetracycline resistance in *Strep. pneumoniae* and *Strep. pyogenes* strains may occur in a substantial minority of strains in some areas. 'Hospital' multiple antibiotic-resistant strains of *Staph. aureus* are usually tetracycline resistant. Gram-negative bacilli and *Bacteroides* strains are frequently tetracycline resistant. Gonococci with a reduced sensitivity to penicillin also often have a reduced sensitivity to tetracycline.

Side-effects and toxicity

Discoloration of teeth; avoid tetracyclines in children up to 8 years and in pregnant or lactating women. Diarrhoea and nausea, associated with unabsorbed tetracycline after oral administration and the antibiotic disturbance to bowel flora. Overgrowth with *Candida* frequent in mouth or bowel, occasionally leads to 'thrush'. In surgical patients receiving 'prophylactic' tetracycline, staphylococcal enterocolitis may rarely occur post-operatively. Azotaemia is worsened in patients with renal insufficiency—tetracycline should be avoided or else the dose reduced. Hepatotoxicity, occasionally fatal, can occur especially when excessive intravenous doses are given; in patients with impaired hepatic function the dose should be reduced and the intravenous route avoided.

Doxycycline

A 'long acting' tetracycline, with once or twice daily dosage.

Administration

Oral—absorption not affected by milk or food as much as oxytetracycline.

Main uses and antibiotic resistance

Similar to oxytetracycline

Side-effects and toxicity

Similar to oxytetracycline. However, azotaemia not worsened so much as by oxytetracycline in patients with renal insufficiency. Also bowel disturbances possibly less frequent than with oxytetracycline.

Minocycline

Administration

Oral—more reliable absorption than with oxytetracycline and usually twice daily dosage.

Main uses

Similar to oxytetracycline. In practice the main uses suggested have been for treating selected cases of gonorrhoea (e.g. when mixed infection with *Chlamydia*) and nasopharyngeal carriage of sulphonamide-resistant meningococcal strains. However, most authorities prefer to use rifampicin for the latter purpose.

Antibiotic resistance, side-effects and toxicity
Similar to oxytetracycline but, in addition, some ambulant patients may develop vestibular disturbances and complain of vertigo.

OTHER ANTIBACTERIAL DRUGS

Chloramphenicol

Broad spectrum antibiotic with good penetration of tissues, macrophages, sputum and CSF. Potentially fatal bone-marrow toxicity restricts its systemic use to treating life-threatening infections.

Administration
Oral (well absorbed); i.v. (i.m. associated with poor serum levels); topical.

Main uses
The drug of choice for treating enteric fevers and also often effective for treating septicaemias due to 'food-poisoning' salmonellae. Also the drug of choice for treating *Haemophilus influenzae* meningitis and acute epiglottitis. Valuable for treating neonatal meningitis due to coliforms and some other bacteria and meningitis due to meningococci or pneumococci in penicillin-allergic patients. Useful for treating brain abscess in conjunction with surgical drainage of pus and may be used in combination with metronidazole. Treatment of some rickettsiae infections such as 'scrub' typhus in the Far East. Topical use in the eye for treating pyogenic conjunctivitis.

Antibiotic resistance
Main problems include increasing chloramphenicol resistance in strains of *S. typhi, H. influenzae*, some *Salmonella* species and coliforms, in various parts of the world. However, chloramphenicol resistance in *Salmonella* and *Haemophilus* strains in Britain is rare.

Side-effects and toxicity
Idiosyncratic fatal aplastic anaemia is the most important complication. Bone marrow depression can also occur which is related to the dosage and duration of treatment. 'Grey syndrome' is a serious toxic complication affecting neonates; this is related to dose and is less likely when treatment is closely monitored by serum chloramphenicol assays. Simultaneous administration of other drugs metabolized by the liver, such as phenytoin, may result in excessive effects since chloramphenicol may inhibit their metabolism.

Sulphonamides, Trimethoprim and Cotrimoxazole

Sulphonamides

There are many sulphonamides available and only a few examples are mentioned below. The sulphonamides are acetylated in the liver after absorption and excreted by the kidneys. Most modern sulphonamides have little risk of crystallizing in the urine but patients should still be encouraged to drink a lot of fluids.

Sulphonamides absorbed after oral administration, mainly used for treating 'simple' urinary tract infections in general practice

Examples include sulphadimidine, sulphafurazole, sulphamethizole. About one-third of *E. coli* strains in general practice patients and up to two-thirds of *E. coli* strains in hospital patients with urinary tract infections are resistant to sulphonamides.

Side-effects and toxicity of sulphonamides

Serious toxic hypersensitivity reactions are most often seen with long-acting sulphonamides such as sulfametopyrazine but may rarely occur with any sulphonamide. These reactions include exfoliative dermatitis, Stevens-Johnson syndrome and photosensitivity reactions. Many types of blood dyscrasia may occur including haemolytic anaemia (especially if glucose-6-phosphate dehydrogenase deficiency is present), thrombocytopenia and agranulocytosis. Neonatal kernicterus can occur if sulphonamides are given to neonates or mothers in late pregnancy. In practice, the more common problems are hypersensitivity side-effects of mild to moderate severity, such as drug rashes of fever occurring after 1 week's treatment.

Sulphadiazine

Administered orally for the immediate chemoprophylaxis of meningococcal infection in close family or institution contacts of a case of meningococcal meningitis, where the infecting organism is likely to be sensitive to sulphonamides. This sulphonamide is preferable to other drugs as it is particularly potent against meningococci. As the drug also crosses the blood–brain barrier well, it may be given to treat meningococcal meningitis. However, benzylpenicillin is the drug of choice as some meningococcal strains are sulphonamide resistant and if sulphadiazine is used it should be in addition to penicillin.

Antimicrobial resistance in meningococci

Between 10 and 25% of meningococcal strains are sulphonamide resistant in England and Wales, but in some areas, such as London, the incidence of resistance is probably less than 5%.

Trimethoprim (alone)

In Britain trimethoprim is usually given as a component of cotrimoxazole but trimethoprim alone is now also available commercially.

Administration

Oral trimethoprim is well absorbed and twice daily doses are adequate. Intravenous or intra-muscular.

Main uses

Long term chemoprophylaxis of urinary tract infection in selected patients. Treatment of acute urinary tract infections in general practice. Widespread use not yet recommended, especially in hospitals, because of uncertainties about development and spread of trimethoprim resistance in Gram-negative bacilli.

Antibiotic resistance

Less than 10% of *E. coli* strains in Britain are resistant to trimethoprim at present. Plasmid or transposon-mediated trimethoprim resistance in strains of *Klebsiella* or other coliforms has increased in recent years. The development and spread of resistance might be greater when trimethoprim is used alone compared with trimethoprim used in combination with sulphonamides. This is controversial (*see also* Richards and Datta, 1981, in Chapter 3).

Side-effects and toxicity

Nausea and other mild gastro-intestinal side-effects, especially with higher doses. Prolonged courses may infrequently cause megaloblastic marrow changes, reversible by administering folinic acid. Haematological toxic effects are rare.

Cotrimoxazole

Combination of trimethoprim and sulphamethoxazole (a sulphonamide with similar pharmacodynamics to trimethoprim) in optimum proportions for obtaining a significant synergic effect against some bacterial strains (1 : 20, trimethoprim to sulphonamide in the serum). In practice the optimal ratio for synergy is sometimes not achieved in infected tissues or purulent secretions such as sputum. In some sites, such as urine, the concentrations of each component is so great that the 'synergistic' effects may also not be relevant clinically.

Administration

Oral (b.d. usually). Intravenous or intra-muscular. Dosage reduced when renal function is impaired.

Main uses

Common treatment of urinary tract infections and valuable for long term low dose chemoprophylaxis or suppression of chronic urinary tract infection. Treatment of lower respiratory tract infections including infective exacerbations of chronic bronchitis and pneumonia. Parenteral treatment (initially) of enteric fever (*see* p. 266). Treatment of brucellosis and other uncommon infections such as pneumocystis lung infection (high dosage). Prophylaxis of infection in certain leukaemic patients.

Antibiotic resistance

See trimethoprim resistance and sulphonamide resistance above. Cotrimoxazole may be used to treat infections due to *E. coli* resistant to sulphonamides but sensitive to trimethoprim (not vice versa). Patients who have received long-term cotrimoxazole outside hospital have rarely developed resistant strains in the faecal flora. The use of cotrimoxazole in some hospital units, such as urological wards, has occasionally encouraged the spread of multiple antibiotic-resistant strains of *Klebsiella*, resistant to cotrimoxazole and gentamicin, during outbreaks. A few *Haemophilus* strains isolated from chronic bronchitis patients have developed resistance to cotrimoxazole. Trimethoprim-resistant coliforms, *Haemophilus* and *Staph. aureus* strains from patients who have received cotrimoxazole are occasionally 'thymidine dependent' and difficult to isolate unless special culture techniques are used. Less than 2% of *Staph. aureus* strains are trimethoprim resistant; thymidine-dependent staphylococci have mainly been isolated from the sputum of cystic fibrosis patients who have been treated with cotrimoxazole.

Side-effects and toxicity

Hypersensitivity reactions to sulphonamides resulting in rashes and drug fevers are the most frequent side-effects. Serious toxicity is rare and includes severe skin reactions and blood dyscrasias. The incidence of unwanted effects is greater with cotrimoxazole than with trimethoprim alone because the reactions are mainly associated with the sulphonamide component (*see also* Sulphonamides and Trimethoprim *above*).

Impairment of renal function has occasionally followed the administration of cotrimoxazole especially when there is already some renal disease. The dosage needs reduction in accordance with the creatinine clearance results, as suggested by the manufacturer.

Trimethoprim combined with rifampicin

This broad spectrum antibiotic combination may have a valuable place for treating some infections in the future (some strains of coliforms and *Neisseria* are synergistically inhibited by these drugs). It is still under evaluation and is not yet commercially available.

Nalidixic acid

This orally administered antibacterial agent is only suitable for treating 'simple' urinary tract infections due to 'coliforms'. Mutant strains resistant to nalidixic acid may occasionally rapidly emerge during a course of treatment.

Side-effects and toxicity

Mild gastro-intestinal side-effects including nausea. Skin photo-sensitivity reactions may rarely occur. Neurological side-effects including convulsions and psychosis can occur especially when patients have impaired renal function or previous neurological disease. The drug should not be given to patients with severe degrees of impairment of renal function (it also would be less effective for treating urinary infection as less drug would be excreted in the urine).

Nitrofurantoin

Another orally administered antibacterial agent which is mainly used for treating 'simple' urinary tract infections due to coliforms or *Staph. saprophyticus* and occasionally for 'prophylaxis' (*see* Chapter 19). Not usually suitable for treating proteus urinary infections. Resistance probably does not emerge during a course of treatment as frequently as with nalidixic acid.

Side-effects and toxicity

Mild gastro-intestinal side-effects may occur. Peripheral neuropathy is an important toxic effect which may infrequently occur. Rarely serious blood dyscrasias or acute allergic pulmonary infiltration can also occur. The drug is, like nalidixic acid, contraindicated in patients with severely impaired renal function.

Rifampicin

Rifampicin is well absorbed after oral administration and can also be given intravenously. The drug is widely distributed in the body and penetrates macrophages well so that intracellular organisms may be also susceptible to it. It crosses the blood–brain barrier and high concentrations are reached in the bile where it is mainly excreted.

Main uses

Treatment of mycobacterial infections in combination with other antituberculous drugs. Short-course prophylaxis for close contacts of meningococcal meningitis in an area with a significant incidence of sulphonamide-resistant meningococci. Treatment of 'difficult' *Staph. aureus* or other infections in combination with other drugs such as fusidic acid when indicated (close collaboration between clinician and microbiologist essential).

Antibiotic resistance

Primary rifampicin resistance in *M. tuberculosis* strains is rare. Most strains of coliforms, *Salmonella, Neisseria,* staphylococci and streptococci are initially sensitive to rifampicin but rifampicin-resistant mutants may rapidly emerge during treatment if the drug is used alone.

Side-effects and toxicity

There are numerous potential side-effects although in practice the great majority of TB patients receiving the drug do not develop any serious toxicity. Possible unwanted effects include nausea and other mild gastro-intestinal side-effects, brown-red discoloration of urine and other body fluids, and hepatotoxicity. Serious hepatotoxicity is uncommon and is more likely when there is already some impaired hepatic function; the drug may then need to be stopped. Oral contraceptives may be less effective due to hepatic enzyme induction by rifampicin. Drug hypersensitivity reactions can occur infrequently causing many different clinical effects including fever, 'flu-like syndrome', various types of rash and, rarely, thrombocytopenic purpura.

Narrow Spectrum, Non-beta-lactam Antibiotics with Activity mainly against Gram-positive Bacteria

These include erythromycin, lincomycin and clindamycin, fusidic acid and vancomycin.

Erythromycin

After absorption, erythromycin is widely distributed and it may also penetrate macrophages well which may be useful for inhibiting some intracellular organisms, such as *Legionella.*

Administration

Oral, intravenous (or intra-muscular).

Main uses

Treatment of many Gram-positive infections, especially useful in penicillin-allergic patients, including soft tissue infections due to *Staph. aureus* and/or *Strep. pyogenes,* and respiratory tract infections due to *Strep. pyogenes, Strep. pneumoniae* or *Staph. aureus.* Ideally, if erythromycin is used to treat *Staph. aureus* infections in hospital patients, it should be used together with another suitable anti-staphylococcal drug, such as fusidic acid; this is particularly relevant if treatment is continued for longer than 5 days. Useful for prophylaxis of '*Strep. viridans*' endocarditis in some penicillin-allergic susceptible patients undergoing dental procedures.

Valuable also for treating other infections including mycoplasma pneumonia, Legionnaires' disease and more severe attacks of campylobacter gastro-enteritis. Effective for treating chlamydial urethritis and T.R.I.C. conjunctivitis.

Antibiotic resistance

Most *Staph. aureus* strains are now sensitive to erythromycin. In the past, erythromycin resistance was common in hospital staphylococcal strains when erythromycin was widely used alone and when cloxacillin was not yet available. There is still a high incidence of erythromycin resistance in *Staph. aureus* strains in many dermatology wards or burns units due to cross-infection. Resistance only infrequently emerges in a staphylococcal strain during a course of treatment but it is more likely during a prolonged course—in hospital practice there is the danger of cross-infection with an erythromycin-resistant strain of *Staph. aureus* if erythromycin is widely used alone.

Erythromycin resistance only rarely occurs in *Strep. pyogenes* or *Strep. pneumoniae* strains. Less than 8% of *Campylobacter* strains are erythromycin resistant.

Side-effects and toxicity

Mild gastro-intestinal side-effects such as nausea. Drug rashes are rare. The use of erythromycin estolate should be avoided as this may cause jaundice.

Lincomycin and clindamycin

Clindamycin is better absorbed than lincomycin after oral administration and has about 100 times greater activity against *Bacteroides fragilis* strains than lincomycin. After absorption, both drugs are widely distributed in tissues including bone (but the blood–brain barrier is not penetrated well). Clindamycin can be given intravenously also. They should only exceptionally be used because of the risks of pseudo-membranous colitis (*see below*).

Main uses

Lincomycin was often used effectively in the past to treat staphylococcal osteomyelitis, sometimes in combination with fusidic acid. This drug can still have a place for treating difficult staphylococcal infections in selected penicillin-allergic patients. Clindamycin was used to treat some staphylococcal and streptococcal infections but its main promise was for treating serious *B. fragilis* infections; it has now become largely superseded by metronidazole for the treatment of anaerobic infections because of its potential toxicity.

Side-effects and toxicity

Mild diarrhoea is a frequent side-effect. The main but rare toxic effect is the development of pseudo-membranous colitis which can be fatal, and this may follow only a couple of doses. This problem was not widely recognized until after the introduction of clindamycin (*see* pp. 165 and 290).

Fusidic acid

This drug is well absorbed after oral administration and penetrates many tissues well including bone and the depths of an abscess. It can be administered topically and also intravenously.

Main uses

Valuable for the systemic treatment of severe *Staph. aureus* infections including those affecting the lungs, bones or heart; always recommended in combination with another anti-staphylococcal drug such as cloxacillin, erythromycin or rifampicin.

Topical fusidic acid can be useful for treating certain staphylococcal soft tissue infections such as carbuncles on the neck. It should be avoided in hospital in-patients because of the risks of fusidic-acid-resistant strains of *Staph. aureus* developing and spreading.

Antibiotic resistance

The majority of *Staph. aureus* strains are sensitive to fusidic acid but resistance may emerge during a course of treatment and this is particularly possible when the drug is used topically. Cross-infection with fusidic acid-resistant staphylococci may also increase the incidence of resistance in some hospital units. When fusidic acid is used in combination with another antibiotic active against a patient's strain of *Staph. aureus*, resistance developing during a course of treatment is very unlikely.

Side-effects and toxicity

Nausea and other minor gastro-intestinal side-effects after oral administration· which are less likely when the drug is given after food. Jaundice has been reported in some patients who have received an intravenous course of fusidic acid and the drug should be used with caution, if essential, in patients who already have some hepatic damage.

Vancomycin

Vancomycin is a potentially toxic drug when administered intravenously for systemic use. It is also occasionally given orally for topical use as it is not absorbed.

Main uses

Intravenous infusions of vancomycin are valuable for treating selected patients with endocarditis or septicaemia due to antibiotic-resistant strains of *Staph. aureus*, sometimes in combination with another anti-staphylococcal drug. Systemic vancomycin is also useful for the treatment and prevention of '*Strep. viridans*' endocarditis in patients with penicillin allergy. Occasionally it is used in synergic combination with an aminoglycoside, such as gentamicin, to treat or prevent enterococcal endocarditis in penicillin allergic patients.

Oral vancomycin is valuable for treating pseudo-membranous colitis.

Antibiotic resistance

Vancomycin resistance has not yet been reported in *Staph. aureus*.

Side-effects and toxicity

Phlebitis may occur but is less common than in the past with modern vancomycin preparations administered by slow i.v. infusion. Serious eighth cranial nerve damage and nephrotoxicity may occur, especially if the patient has impaired renal function or is also receiving an aminoglycoside drug, such as gentamicin. The treatment should be monitored by serum vancomycin assays.

Polymyxins

These are narrow spectrum polypeptide antibiotics with activity against some coliforms and *Pseudomonas aeruginosa*. They are too toxic to be used systemically, except in a few instances and also are not particularly effective for treating most serious Gram-negative infections. Examples include 'Colistin' and Polymyxin B.

Administration

Oral—the drugs are not absorbed. Intravenous or intra-muscular; topical preparations for use in the ear, eye or on the skin; topical administration by inhalation using a sterile solution of polymyxin B.

Main uses

Systemic treatment of serious infections due to *Pseudomonas aeruginosa* strains resistant to aminoglycosides and anti-pseudomonad penicillins—rarely arises in practice.

Inhalation administration of topical polymyxin might be occasionally useful for treating selected patients with lower respiratory tract infections due to *Pseudomonas* including some patients with cystic fibrosis. Oral colistin is used to suppress normal faecal Gram-negative bacilli in 'FRACON', a non-absorbable mixture of drugs used for prophylaxis of Gram-negative infections in certain neutropenic leukaemic patients.

Topical polymyxin can be used to treat superficial pseudomonas or other Gram-negative infections in selected patients with infected varicose ulcers or pressure sores.

Antibiotic resistance

Proteus strains are intrinsically resistant to polymyxins. *Pseudomonas* and other Gram-negative bacilli only rarely develop resistance to these drugs.

Side-effects and toxicity

Systemic administration can cause nephrotoxicity and neuropathy especially when renal function is already impaired. Casts frequently appear in the urine and azotaemia occurs during a course of treatment. Serum polymyxin assays are essential and the dose needs reducing when there is impaired renal function. Neuromuscular blockade can also occur and may rarely result in respiratory insufficiency.

Metronidazole

This drug is well absorbed after oral or rectal administration and is mainly active against strictly anaerobic bacteria and some protozoa. After absorption the drug is widely distributed and it also penetrates the interior of abscesses well and crosses the blood-brain barrier. It is metabolized in the liver and mainly inactive metabolites are excreted in the urine.

Serious anaerobic infections can be treated with intravenous metronidazole.

Main uses

Valuable drug for the treatment and prophylaxis of surgical sepsis due to non-sporing anaerobes, especially *Bacteroides fragilis* (*see* Chapter 24, Chapter 9 and Prophylaxis, Chapter 8). Other examples of its use to treat anaerobic infections include the management of brain abscess, pyogenic liver abscess and Vincent's infection.

The main protozoal infections which are effectively treated by metronidazole include trichomoniasis, amoebiasis and giardiasis.

Antimicrobial resistance

Metronidazole resistance has been reported on a few occasions in *Bacteroides fragilis* strains isolated from patients receiving prolonged courses of treatment. At present metronidazole resistance in anaerobic Gram-negative bacilli is rare. Occasional strains of anaerobic cocci or clostridia have a reduced sensitivity to metronidazole. Resistance is also only rarely reported in *Trichomonas* strains.

Side-effects and toxicity

Nausea and other mild gastro-intestinal side-effects. In some patients taking alcohol an 'antabuse' effect can occur. Peripheral neuropathy is an important toxic effect which can particularly occur during a prolonged course of therapy. As metronidazole is metabolized by the liver, the dose may need to be reduced when hepatic function is impaired. In the U.S.A., there is concern about a possible carcinogenic effect of metronidazole in experimental animals. In Britain, this is not thought to be relevant to man especially with the relatively small amounts of drug required for the treatment of infections.

ANTI-FUNGAL DRUGS

Amphotericin B

Polyene broad spectrum anti-fungal drug used intravenously in gradually increasing dosage to treat systemic opportunistic infections due to *Aspergillus, Candida* or *Cryptococcus* species. Also used in the American continent to treat serious infections due to *Histoplasma, Blastomyces* and *Coccidioides* species. Resistance does not develop in fungal strains. Topical amphotericin is also available to treat localized *Candida albicans* infections (e.g. candida mouth and urinary tract infections).

Side-effects and toxicity

Nephrotoxic—glomerular filtration is reduced in nearly all patients receiving i.v. amphotericin B. Phlebitis and febrile drug reactions commonly occur. Serum amphotericin B assays may be indicated.

Nystatin

Topical anti-candida polyene drug for treating localized *C. albicans* infections.

5-Fluorocytosine

Narrow spectrum drug mainly used to treat systemic candida or cryptococcal infections mainly after oral administration. Can also be given by the i.v. route. Resistant mutants can rapidly emerge during therapy. Best used in combination with amphotericin B for systemic infections to reduce chances of mutants emerging resistant to 5-fluorocytosine and for a possible synergic effect between the two drugs against yeasts. Before treatment the sensitivity of the isolated fungus to 5-fluorocytosine should be ascertained. Repeat tests should be carried out to check that resistance does not emerge during or after treatment. 5-Fluorocytosine is probably the drug of choice for treating *Candida albicans* urinary tract infections when the strain is sensitive and in this situation the drug may be used alone.

Side-effects and toxicity

Hepatotoxic in some patients and bone marrow depression can also occur resulting in neutropenia. If renal function is impaired, excessive levels can accumulate and increase the risks of toxicity; the dose should be reduced and serum 5-fluorocytosine assays carried out.

Griseofulvin

An orally administered narrow spectrum anti-fungal drug which is useful for treating some dermatophyte infections affecting the nails or scalp. Prolonged treatment for up to 1 year may be necessary. A few patients may have low serum levels because of inadequate absorption of the drug or because of increased inactivation by the liver through enzyme induction by the drugs such as phenobarbitone. Griseofulvin serum assays may rarely be necessary.

Side-effects and toxicity

Mild gastro-intestinal side-effects occasionally. Serious toxicity very rare.

Imidazole Derivatives

These broad spectrum drugs include clotrimazole, econazole, miconazole and ketoconazole. Resistance only very rarely occurs mainly during prolonged therapy.

Clotrimazole

Topical drug used for treating dermatophyte skin infections or *Candida albicans* infection of the skin or vagina.

Econazole

Topical drug effective for treating dermatophyte skin infections and superficial candida infections—including candida vaginitis.

Miconazole

Topical use similar to econazole. Systemic use, after intravenous administration. The drug is metabolized rapidly by the liver and is minimally excreted by the kidneys. Treatment of systemic yeast or yeast-like fungal infections including some non-urinary tract candida infections, cryptococcosis and coccidiomycosis. However, it may sometimes not be as effective as amphotericin B and is often used as a 'reserve' drug if amphotericin B has to be stopped because of serious toxicity. It is still under evaluation.

Side-effects and toxicity
Mild phlebitis occasionally. No serious toxicity.

Ketoconazole (the most recent imidazole drug)

Oral broad spectrum anti-fungal drug which is effective for treating superficial candida, dermatophyte and some other fungal infections. It is also effective for treating histoplasmosis in North America and para-coccidiomycosis in South America. However, it is less effective, so far, for treating disseminated aspergillus opportunistic infections. Still under evaluation.

Side-effects and toxicity
No serious unwanted effects so far reported.

ANTI-VIRAL DRUGS

Idoxuridine

This drug interferes with DNA synthesis and is active against herpesviruses and vaccinia. Administration is topical, usually in dimethyl sulphoxide or, rarely applicable, by the intravenous route for systemic use.

Main uses
The main value of topical idoxuridine is to treat conjunctival or corneal infection due to herpes simplex. Topical idoxuridine may be used to increase the rate of

healing of extensive skin or mucous lesions due to varicella-zoster or herpes simplex, e.g. in immunosuppressed patients. Also useful in strong concentrations for treating 'herpetic whitlow' on the finger of a nurse or doctor.

Systemic use superseded by other agents.

Side-effects and toxicity

Serious toxicity frequently associated with systemic use on central nervous system, skin, liver and other organs. Topical applications contraindicated in pregnancy in case some drug is absorbed and causes teratogenic effects in the foetus.

Cytosine arabinoside (cytarabine)

Similar activity to idoxuridine against herpesviruses. Seriously toxic on liver, kidneys, bone marrow and other organs after intravenous administration. Superseded by other drugs.

Adenine arabinoside (Vidarabine or 'Ara-A')

This drug is less toxic than cytarabine or idoxuridine. It is particularly useful for treating herpes simplex encephalitis, after intravenous administration, provided treatment is started early enough. Also may be useful for treating serious varicella-zoster infections in immunosuppressed patients. Nausea is the most frequent side-effect.

Acycloguanosine (Acyclovir)

Not yet available commercially. This drug is still under evaluation but promises to be a very useful systemic agent for treating serious varicella-zoster infections, including zoster pneumonitis in an immunosuppressed patient, and serious herpes simplex infections. Topically it also could prove helpful for treating extensive superficial herpes infections. It appears to be relatively non-toxic.

Methisazone

Drug given orally.

Active against DNA viruses including vaccinia and variola viruses. It was partially effective for the prophylaxis of smallpox (disease extinct now). Accidental inoculation of vaccinia into the eye may be an indication for immediate methisazone treatment, together with other measures including the administration of vaccinia immunoglobulin. Methisazone may be effective for the treatment of some vaccinial complications including eczema vaccinatum, combined with administration of vaccinia immunoglobulin.

Side-effects and toxicity

Nausea and vomiting frequently occur. Toxic effects on the skin, hair and liver also may occur.

Amantadine

This orally administered expensive drug is active against influenza A viruses. Prophylaxis of influenza A_2 infections can be achieved in about 75% of individuals who are exposed to influenza if it is started early enough. The drug may also be effective to some extent for treating influenza A_1 due to certain strains. It might have a limited place for prophylaxis during influenza A outbreaks in hospital.

Side-effects and toxicity

Numerous psychiatric or neurological toxic effects can occur including hallucinations, loss of vision and ataxia, especially in elderly patients and those with existing neurological disease. Skin rashes, gastro-intestinal and cardiovascular side-effects may also occur. The drug is contraindicated in pregnancy, in patients with central nervous system diseases and in those receiving certain drugs acting on the nervous system.

Further Reading

Garrod L. P., Lambert H. P. and O'Grady F. (1981) *Antibiotic and Chemotherapy*, 5th ed. Edinburgh, Churchill Livingstone.

Kucers A. and Bennett N. M. (1979) *The Use of Antibiotics*, 3rd ed. London, Heinemann.

See also Further reading list of Chapter 3.

Index